To Patrick and our children,
Kimberly, Elizabeth, and Patricia

COPING WITH CHRONIC ILLNESS

OVERCOMING POWERLESSNESS
Edition 3

JUDITH FITZGERALD MILLER, RN, PhD, FAAN

Associate Dean for Academic Affairs
and
Professor
Marquette University College of Nursing
Milwaukee, Wisconsin

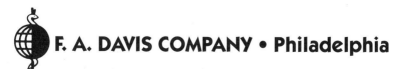

F. A. DAVIS COMPANY • Philadelphia

F. A. Davis Company
1915 Arch Street
Philadelphia, PA 19103

Copyright © 2000 by F. A. Compa..,

Printed in the United States of America

Last digit indicates print number: 10 9 8 7 6 5 4 3 2 1

Acquisitions Editor: Alan Sorkowitz
Managing Publisher, Nursing Department: Lisa A. Biello
Production Editor: Jessica Howie Martin
Cover Designer: Louis J. Forgione

As new scientific information becomes available through basic and clinical research, recommended treatments and drug therapies undergo changes. The author and publisher have done everything possible to make this book accurate, up to date, and in accord with accepted standards at the time of publication. The author, editors, and publisher are not responsible for errors or omissions or for consequences from application of the book, and make no warranty, expressed or implied, in regard to the contents of the book. Any practice described in this book should be applied by the reader in accordance with professional standards of care used in regard to the unique circumstances that may apply in each situation. The reader is advised always to check product information (package inserts) for changes and new information regarding dose and contraindications before administering any drug. Caution is especially urged when using new or infrequently ordered drugs.

Library of Congress Cataloging-in-Publication Data

Miller, Judith Fitzgerald.
    Coping with chronic illness : overcoming powerlessness / Judith Fitzgerald Miller. — Ed. 3.
        p.   cm.
    Includes bibliographical references and index.
    ISBN 0-8036-0298-7 (pbk.)
    1. Chronic diseases—Nursing.   2. Chronic diseases—Psychological aspects.   3. Control (Psychology)—Health aspects.   I. Title.
    [DNLM: 1. Chronic Disease—nursing Case Report.   2. Chronic Disease—rehabilitation Case Report.   3. Models, Psychological Case Report.   4. Nurse-Patient Relations Case Report.   5.   Sick Role Case Report.   WY   152   M648c 2000]
    RT120.C45M55   2000
    610.73'61—dc21
    DNLM/DLC
    for Library of Congress   99-14320
                                                                        CIP

➤ PREFACE

The purpose of this book is to facilitate understanding of the world of the chronically ill and to develop nursing's repertoire of strategies to care for persons with long-term health problems. The ultimate goal of nursing care is to maintain and enhance client and family quality of life. As with all other individuals, quality of life for the chronically ill includes aspirational and spiritual dimensions of self, such as playing roles important to the individual, giving and receiving love, balancing dependence with independence, being satisfied with self, being at peace, having a feeling of self-worth, having energy to enjoy life's special pleasures, coping effectively, and having hope.

Although there are some undeniably negative characteristics associated with chronic illness such as uncertainty, declining physical trajectory, dependence, role transition, and feelings of powerlessness, an expanded perception is needed that takes into account the rich attributes of human life such as the ability to think, create, rationalize, experience joy, learn, and appreciate art and music. Humans have limitless potential for growth, unfolding, and being. During illness a special caring advocate can support adaptation and nurture that unfolding and enable growth through confronting adversity. Persons who are ill are to be viewed as having multiple resources to enable them to be in control of their lives. Despite compromised physical integrity, other resources such as social support, psychological stability, knowledge, self-esteem, energy, and hope can be developed and maintained. Select chapters are devoted to developing client and family power resources.

Client autonomy characterizes the current era of health care; benevolent paternalism of a health-care team or health-care system that determines client and family decisions and directs passive clients and families is no longer tolerated. Nursing care now ensures client and family autonomy, self-determination, and competence in self-management.

This third edition of *Coping with Chronic Illness: Overcoming Powerlessness* contains four new chapters on coping with specific chronic health problems and strategies to alleviate powerlessness. The integrated human system response to stress and coping is included in a review of psychoneuroimmunology. Chronic sorrow in dealing with chronic illness throughout the life span and courage in young adults are analyzed, and nursing strategies presented. Another new chapter in this edition focuses on empowering persons with acquired immunodeficiency syndrome (AIDS). Additional creative strategies are explored, such as the use of imagery, literature, behavior change, and unique coping modalities. All chapters have been expanded and current research reviewed.

Related theories of various authors are explored, including uncertainty (Mishel, 1988); self-regulation (Leventhal & Johnson, 1983), cognitive control (Meichenbaum, 1985); adaptation (LaRocca, Kalb, & Kaplan, 1983) and behavior change, to name a few. Endurance factors such as hardiness and salutogenic factors are reviewed.

Models presented in this edition include care of the client with multiple sclerosis, a model of factors affecting functioning in persons with chronic obstructive pulmonary disease, healing through bibliotherapy, enhancing self-esteem, and inspiring hope.

In addition to the previously selected prototypical chronic health problems discussed in the first edition, client and family responses to AIDS and cancer are explored in relation to coping and control. In-depth analyses of persons with multiple sclerosis and chronic lung disease, including the pathophysiology, factors influencing coping, and adaptation, have been added. Nursing interventions and the related research are the foundations of this book.

Analyses of client and family exemplars provide "real-world" clinical decision making, application of research findings, and generation of nursing strategies, all geared to promote holistic caring. The case study method is a useful research approach to document a sequence of events and responses over time to validate indicators of nursing diagnoses and the immediate and long-term effects of nursing. Diverse methods of client and family coping are also documented in this book.

More precise and in-depth assessments of clinical phenomena are presented, as are reviews of research instruments to measure coping, stressors (of hemodialysis), fatigue, helplessness (of arthritis), quality of life, self-esteem, and hope.

Despite the linking of a diagnostic category such as energy with a specific health problem (arthritis or chronic lung disease), it is hoped that readers will study the chapters and transfer insights regarding nursing diagnoses and treatments to other clients and families and do not restrict the nursing content to a medical diagnosis.

Part I provides a model of persons composed of power resources and a foundation for understanding coping and powerlessness. Part II includes developmental vulnerabilities throughout the life span. Client and family responses to specific prototypical chronic health problems are reviewed in Part III. Caring strategies are presented in Part IV, with an emphasis on maintaining client and family control.

Some sections of this book are entirely new, but despite additions and revisions in each chapter, a work of this nature is never complete. Various theories and perspectives need continued exploration, research, and discovery. More ideas for nursing interventions need to be developed. Expanded perceptions of the chronically ill client and family are needed. It is hoped that this work will provide an impetus for continued work and development. Expansion of nursing's healing power is limited only by the bounds of one's creativity.

JUDITH FITZGERALD MILLER

REFERENCES

Leventhal, H., & Johnson, J. (1983). Laboratory and field experimentation: Development of a theory of self-regulation. In P. Wooldridge, M. Schmitt, J. Skipper, & R. Leonard (Eds.), *Behavioral science and nursing theory* (pp. 189–262), St. Louis: CV Mosby.

LaRocca, N., Kalb, R., & Kaplan, S. R. (1983). Psychological changes. In L. C. Scheinberg (Ed.), *Multiple sclerosis: A guide for patients and their families* (pp. 175–194). New York: Raven Press.

Meichenbaum, D. (1985). *Stress innoculation training.* New York: Pergamon Press.

Mishel, M. H. (1988). Uncertainty in illness. *Image—Journal of nursing scholarship, 20,* 225–232.

➤ Contents

➤ Contributors

JoAnne Bennett, RN, PhD, CS ACRN
Community Health Consultant
New York, New York

Lucille Sanzero Eller, RN, PhD
Assistant Professor and Co-
  Director
Center for Health Promotion
  Research
College of Nursing
Rutgers, the State University of
  New Jersey
Newark, New Jersey

**Deborah L. Finfgeld, RN, PhD,
  AP/MHCNS**
Assistant Professor
Sinclair School of Nursing and
Post-Doctoral Fellow
Family and Community Medicine
  Department
University of Missouri–Columbia
Columbia, Missouri

Debra Hastings, RN, MSN
Milwaukee, Wisconsin

Ruth Hobus, RN, MSN (Deceased)
Instructor
South Dakota University
Brookings, South Dakota

Carolyn L. Lindgren, RN, PhD
Associate Professor and
Interim Assistant Dean of Family,
  Community, and Mental Health
  Nursing
Wayne State University
School of Nursing
Detroit, Michigan

Anne M. McMahon, RN, MSN
Nursing Faculty
Milwaukee Area Technical College
Milwaukee, Wisconsin

**Judith Fitzgerald Miller, RN, PhD,
  FAAN**
Associate Dean for Academic
  Affairs and
Professor
Marquette University College of
  Nursing
Milwaukee, Wisconsin

Christine Bohm Oertel, RN, MSN
Racine, Wisconsin

Polly Ryan, RN, PhD
Assistant Professor
Marquette University College of
  Nursing
Milwaukee, Wisconsin

Patricia S. Schroeder, RN, MSN, MBA
Regional Director
Outcome-Based Care Management
Covenant Health Care Systems
  Inc.
Milwaukee, Wisconsin

Susan Stapleton, RN, MSN, CNM
Certified Nurse Midwife
Reading Birth and Women's
  Center
Reading, Pennsylvania

Rebecca Stephens, RN, PhD
Chair, Division of Nursing
Thomas College
Thomasville, Georgia

PART I ➤

Current Status

➤ A model for understanding nursing care of the chronically ill client that promotes client control through development and support of the individual's power resources is presented in Chapter 1. A common core of client resources is presented in the power resource model; however, it is not possible to enumerate all the human strengths that are to be supported by nurses. The model provides a frame of reference for the book in that some chapters are devoted to developing select resources.

Coping with perceived powerlessness is a major demand throughout chronic illness. All persons have a capacity for coping. Coping is stimulated in individuals with chronic health problems. Unlike acute crises, during which denial of the impact of the threat is the usual means of coping, chronic illness brings about a confrontation with reality, adaptation, and participation in care. The individual and family must respond to the requirements of the external situation (e.g., adhere to the medication regimen, participate in exercises, maintain a weight-reduction program, or complete treatments such as self-dialysis), as well as respond to their own feelings about the situation (powerlessness, depression, or low self-esteem). Other specific coping tasks that have been identified in chronically ill clients are discussed in Chapter 2.

The research base and the resulting theoretical propositions and nursing practice speculations for powerlessness are presented in Chapter 3. Although the research base about concepts of powerlessness, locus of control, helplessness, and reactance theory has been derived from behavioral science literature, its relevance to nursing is noted.

Psychoneuroimmunology is reviewed in depth in Chapter 4. The interrelationships among the neuroendocrine, immune, and psychosocial systems are described. Research on psychoneuroimmunology, chronic illness, stress, and coping is also included.

1

Client Power Resources

> JUDITH FITZGERALD MILLER

There are varied theoretical perspectives on chronic illness that include emphases on client response processes and integration, client and family adjustment and adaptation, and anticipation of illness-related demands and crises aversion (Brown, Rawlinson, & Hilles, 1981; Charmaz, 1983; Craig & Edwards, 1983; Lawrence & Lawrence, 1979; Radley & Green, 1987; Strauss et al., 1984). A model of chronic illness that stems from the commonsense viewpoints of the client and family suffering with the illness has particular relevance to the focus of this book on patient empowerment. Turk, Rudy, and Salovey (1986) proposed a four-dimensional structure of illness interpretation based upon client and family perceptions: seriousness, personal responsibility, controllability, and changeability. These dimensions, derived from Leventhal, Meyer, and Nerenz's (1980) commonsense representation of illness, were validated using the Implicit Model of Illness Questionnaire (Turk, Rudy, & Salovey, 1986). *Seriousness* refers to the individual's knowledge about the degree to which the illness is difficult to manage and the amount of intense medical surveillance that is needed. *Personal responsibility* is the degree to which individuals perceive themselves to cause or cure the illness. *Controllability* is the extent to which the illness is viewed to be controllable by the ill person or other agents. *Changeability* refers to knowledge about the rate and degree to which symptoms vary over time. The expected trajectory of illness events and desired treatment effects may be included in the changeability dimension. The degree of powerlessness perceived by clients is influenced partly by their interpretation of each of these four dimensions.

3

There is a way for individuals with chronic illness to be and feel in control of what is happening to them; power is a resource for living that is present in all individuals. In the most elemental sense, power is the ability to influence what happens to oneself. May (1972) described five types of power: exploitative, manipulative, competitive, nutrient, and integrative. The type of power that is relevant to this book is nutrient power. May defines nutrient power in terms of providing for, caring for, or having concern for the welfare of others. For our purposes, power will be defined as nurturative, that is, providing for and caring for self, directing others regarding self-care, and being the ultimate decision maker regarding care. With power comes the ability to effect change or prevent it; power and control are used as synonymous terms.

Powerlessness is the perception that one lacks the capacity or authority to act to affect an outcome. The greater the individual's expectation to have control and the greater the importance of the desired outcomes to the individual, the greater the perceived powerlessness experienced when the individual does not, in fact, have control (Wortman & Brehm, 1975). Powerlessness in chronically ill clients occurs for a variety of reasons. The client may experience uncertain health with remissions and exacerbations or, in some instances, progressive physical deterioration. There are physical and psychological losses. Overwhelmingly strange, invasive, and threatening experiences may occur as part of ongoing diagnostic and treatment measures. What is routine to the healthcare worker may be anything but routine to the client. The language system of health workers may create the impression that they are sophisticated masters of the situation, while clients feel isolated and unaware of what is happening to them. Exacerbations result in the client's being unable to maintain a front of normalcy and may cause the individual's personal world to stop while the rest of the world does not slow down (Donoghue & Siegel, 1992). As a result, the client may fall behind in work, school, and life in general. Some or all of these factors may influence the chronically ill person's perceived lack of control.

CHRONIC ILLNESS DEFINED:
SELECT FACTORS INFLUENCING RESPONSES

Chronic illness refers to an altered health state that will not be cured by a simple surgical procedure or a short course of medical therapy. Although each chronic illness presents unique demands on the client and family, two generalizations can be made: (1) the person with a chronic illness experiences impaired functioning in more than one—often multiple—body-mind (Turk, Sobel, Follick, & Youkilis, 1980) and spirit systems; and (2) the illness-related demands on the individual are never completely eliminated. Lubkin (1994) critiqued traditional definitions of chronic illness and suggests that chronic illness is "the irreversible presence, accumulation, or latency of disease states or impairments that involve the total human environment for supportive care and self-care, maintenance of function and prevention of further disability" (p. 6).

Many demands are made on the client and family. The client must endure close medical scrutiny regarding symptoms, response to therapy, and compliance, and acquire a knowledge of self and therapy so that self-monitoring is possible. The family also needs to develop and refine skills for daily monitoring and management. Finally, all these efforts must be directed toward keeping the problem controlled and in remission while also controlling anxiety over the threat of full-blown incapacitation during exacerbations.

Reif (1975) identified three general features of chronic illness: (1) the disease symptoms interfere with many normal activities and routines, (2) the medical regimen is limited in its effectiveness, and (3) treatment, although intended to mitigate the symptoms and long-range effects of disease, contributes substantially to the disruption of the usual patterns of living.

Individuals and families have varied responses to the stress of illness; Antonovsky (1985) suggested that this is because of varied resistance resources that are salutary (promote health and prevent illness). The resistance resources include the following variables: physical, biochemical, artifactual-material (money, shelter), cognitive-emotional, valuative-attitudinal, interpersonal-relational, and macrosociocultural (place in the world, familiar rituals). For example, cognitive-emotional characteristics include knowledge and intelligence, ego identity, and a sense of coherence. A sense of coherence is an enduring perception that one's life has worth, meaning, and purpose. A feeling of being in control is part of coherence, as is confidence that "things will work out well." In addition to the variables identified by Antonovsky, another personality variable, hardiness, may promote coping and enable client and family resistance to stress. Kobasa and associates described three components of hardiness: control, commitment, and challenge (Kobasa, 1979a, 1979b, 1982; Kobasa, Maddi Puccetti, & Zola, 1985). Hardy persons tend to believe in their own ability to influence life events rather than being helpless; they are actively involved, not passive or alienated, and they perceive change as an opportunity for growth. Pollock (1985; 1989) extended the construct to include a disposition toward health and resistance to illness. Hardiness in the chronically ill is said to influence the use of social resources for successful coping (Pollock, 1986), psychological health (Nowack, 1989), and psychological well-being (Lambert, Lambert, Klipple, & Mewshaw, 1989; Lambert & Lambert, 1987). Hardiness bolsters endurance throughout unpredictable challenges of chronic illness.

Unpredictable dilemmas that characterize chronic illness and promote powerlessness include symptom exacerbation, failure of therapy, physical deterioration despite adherence to the prescribed regimen, the side effects of drugs, iatrogenic alterations, breakdown in the client's family or significant-other support network, and breakdown in the client's psychological stamina.

Mishel's work on uncertainty has particular relevance for understanding the individual's cognitive and coping response to chronic illness (Mishel, 1981, 1983, 1988; Mishel & Braden, 1987, 1988; Mishel, Hostetter, King, & Graham, 1984; Mishel & Murdaugh, 1987). Mishel's middle-range theory views uncertainty as the inability to arrive at meaning in the illness-related events. Sources of uncertainty stem from inconsistency in symptom patterns, inconsistency between expected and experienced illness-related events, and unfamiliarity and complexity of cues and events. Persons with chronic illness experience remissions and exacerbations, disrupting a predictable pattern of their symptoms. Event congruence in the chronically ill may not take place if the patient expects to be healed yet experiences recurrence of the illness, or when treatment does not produce immediate desired results. The treatment setting remains alien as complexity of surveillance of the chronic condition continues over long periods of time. The client's cognitive capacity is affected by the illness, pain, nutrition, and fear. All these incongruities and decreased cognitive capacity create uncertainty. Select mechanisms referred to as *structure providers* can increase or decrease uncertainty. These include use of education, social support from significant others, and trust in the nurse and health-care providers as "credible authorities." Uncertainty is appraised by clients by use of inference and illusion. Inferences are based upon personality dispositions such as a sense of mastery and general beliefs about oneself and control of the environment. Illusion results in viewing uncertainty as positive. It protects persons when they encounter situations that are difficult to accept such as during the downward trajectory of chronic illness. Coping strategies used by clients will be determined in part by whether uncertainty was appraised as a danger or an opportunity. If viewed as a danger, methods to control negative emotions may be used. If viewed as an opportunity, buffering coping strategies including avoidance, selective ignoring, reordering priorities, and neutralizing are used. The desired end result is adaptation (Mishel, 1988).

Psychodynamics of chronically ill clients have not been well described. Strain (1979) identified the following seven categories of psychological reactions to chronic medical illness:

- Perceived threat to self-esteem and body intactness that challenges individuals' beliefs that they are masters of their own bodies

- Fear of loss of love and approval that evolves from clients' fears that illness and dependence on others will cause significant others to withdraw
- Fear of loss of control of achieved body functions and/or parts with resulting loss of independence
- Anxiety resulting from separation from loved ones and familiar environment that provided support, gratification, and a sense of intactness
- Guilt and fear of retaliation for having incurred the health problem in the first place or for having lost control
- Fear of pain
- Fear of strangers providing intimate care

A prevalent theme throughout all these reactions is a lack of control. The lack of control seems to pervade all aspects of chronic illness—from etiology of the disease itself to events and experiences within the health-care system while the patient seeks treatment for the disease.

Strain (1979) explained the regressive behavior that occurs in children during stress is likely to occur in chronically ill adults. Lack of involvement in their own care promotes regression in chronically ill clients. The regression to unwarranted dependency and passivity can be prevented through nursing care. Nursing measures to prevent negative dependency are discussed throughout this book, and specific measures to empower the chronically ill person are described in Part IV.

Feldman (1974) used the term readaptation in referring to rehabilitation of chronically ill patients. He stated that readaptation "is coming to terms existentially with the reality of chronic illness as a state of being, discarding both false hope and destructive hopelessness, restructuring the environment in which one must now function" (p. 287). Readaptation for chronically ill clients requires reorganization and acceptance of self on a level that transcends the illness. This is a sizable challenge in light of the multiple stresses and unpredictable dilemmas that accompany chronic illnesses.

Factors that are said to influence positive adjustment to chronic illness include knowledge, coping resources, problem-solving attitude, sense of personal mastery, and motivation (Turk, 1979). *Knowledge* of the illness and desired effects of therapy, as well as understanding of client and family roles, facilitates adjustment. Turk (1979) attested that personal meaning is imposed when individuals have the cognitive structure to accurately assign such meaning. *Coping resources* are those that are available to help persons master, tolerate, or reduce a problem or demand. Merely knowing that a coping response is possible helps reduce the threat of a situation. *Problem-solving attitude* is a perspective of active resourcefulness in confronting problems. Persons with this attitude perceive problems accurately, have the ability to pose several alternative responses to problems, and have a history of success in confronting problems. *Personal mastery* means individuals have confidence in their ability and demonstrate a sense of control and self-efficacy to handle situations related to their illness. Although most clients become depressed at times and question the worth of their involvement with illness treatment, these thoughts serve to *motivate* adjusted persons to continue with requisite behaviors compliant with therapy demands, whereas persons who are poorly adjusted tend to manifest a negative, defeated, demoralized attitude.

Perceptions of greater personal control over the care regimen in 92 persons with rheumatoid arthritis were associated with positive mood states and psychosocial adjustment. In contrast, perceptions that health providers had control over clients' daily symptoms were associated with negative mood states in clients (Affleck, Tennen, Pfeiffer, & Fifield, 1987).

Despite the unpredictable dilemmas of living with illness, chronically ill persons have goals similar to those of any well person: to live life fully and to function optimally in all aspects of life, that is, to have quality of life. Quality of life encompasses being able to engage in roles that are important to individuals: to perceive themselves as worthwhile; to achieve a sense of independence; to feel satisfaction with self, accomplishments, and relationships; to have a sense of well-being despite the limitations imposed by illness; to give and receive love; to have energy to enjoy life's special pleasures; to cope effectively; and to have hope. Measurement of quality of life in persons with varied chronic health problems is reviewed by Spilker (1990). The central focus of nursing in empowering the chronically ill is to maintain and enhance the quality of life.

Instruments to assess quality of life in various types of chronically ill persons and in elderly persons have been developed (Ferrans & Powers, 1985; George & Bearon, 1980; Padilla, Peasant, Grant, Metter, Lipsett, & Heide, 1983). A perception of lack of control over most aspects of one's life interfered with achieving quality of life. Living with chronic illness means grieving over an alteration of who one is (Agich, 1995).

Maximizing the client's power resources facilitates the client's ability to cope with chronic illness. An individual's power resources (Fig. 1.1) include physical strength (physical reserve), psychological stamina and social support, positive self-concept, energy, knowledge, motivation, and belief system—hope. Individuals with chronic illnesses may have deficits in several power resources, that is, physical strength and energy; therefore, remaining power components may need to be developed to prevent or overcome powerlessness. The client's unique and varied coping strategies compensate for deficient resources and build up remaining resources such as hope and positive self-concept (specifically

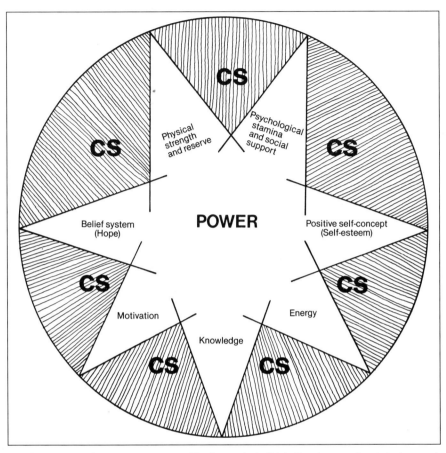

FIGURE 1.1 ➤ Patient power resources. CS refers to the individual's unique coping strategies, used when resources are compromised.

self-esteem). The power resources are discussed in more detail in later chapters and are described only briefly here.

POWER RESOURCES

Physical Strength

Physical strength refers both to the individual's ability for optimal physical functioning and to physical reserve. When any body system is compromised by illness, the individual's power to act is decreased. The present status of an individual's physical strength will influence the client's power—whether the client is on a downward course with more physical symptoms arising (a deteriorating health state) or the client is improving physically. Physical reserve is the ability of the body to maintain physical balance when confronted with threats or extra demands.

For example, individuals with acquired immunodeficiency syndrome (AIDS) or those on long-term therapy with immunosuppressive drugs have less reserve in fighting infection than others. Persons with arthritis may have accompanying muscle atrophy and weakness.

Psychological Stamina: Social Support

Psychological stamina refers to a unique resiliency present in humans. Despite the crisis of illness and day-to-day uncertainty, some clients are able to maintain psychological equilibrium. Somehow, events that could be viewed as threats are interpreted as meaningful. At the other extreme, chronic illness may cause psychological imbalance. Depression and anxiety are two prevalent symptoms in chronically ill individuals (Adams & Lindemann, 1974). The client with a chronic health problem may need help to maintain a positive outlook and to prevent or alleviate paralyzing anxiety, depression, and hopelessness.

Social support refers to relationship qualities of attachment, social integration, opportunity for nurturance, reassurance of worth, sense of reliable alliance, and guidance from a trustworthy, caring person (Weiss, 1974). Additional perspectives describe the types of social support to include tangible support (instrumental support such as help with activities of daily living), emotional support, and informational support (Schaefer, Coyne, & Lazarus, 1981). Social support is said to both buffer the stress of illness and enhance health regardless of the level of stress (Cohen & Syme, 1985). Corbin and Strauss (1984, 1988) noted that couples who worked together were able to prevent and resolve problems and were able to manage the chronic illness demands. Social support has been found to be related to coping effectiveness (McNett, 1987), quality of life (Burckhardt, 1985), and adaptation (Bramwell & Whall, 1986; Dimond, 1979; Maybury & Brewin, 1984; Northouse, 1988; Winert, 1983; Zedlow & Pavlou, 1984) in the chronically ill. Pattison (1974) found that the life spans of patients with chronic obstructive lung disease were not predicted by the amount of remaining respiratory function (extent of pathology), but rather depended on their having someone in their social network who cared about them. Maintaining intact social support systems and supporting the family coping with the burden of caring for and worrying about their chronically ill family member is a challenge for nursing.

Positive Self-Concept

Self-concept is the individual's total thoughts and feelings about self (Rosenberg, 1979). Components of self-concept include physical self (body image), functional self (role performance), personal self (moral self, self-ideal, and self-expectancy) (Driever, 1984), and self-esteem (self-worth). Epstein (1973) stated, "There is a basic need for self-esteem which relates to all aspects of the self systems, . . . in comparison to which, almost all other needs are subordinate" (p. 404). Self-esteem is therefore a crucial component of self-concept and a determinant of functioning. Feeling worthwhile is basic to taking action to achieve improved health.

Chronic illness has an impact on self-concept. The illness may promote a feeling of being "permanently different" or of having less worth—as compared with a defective mechanical device. Cooper (1976) referred to the world of chronic illness as the "fourth world." The fourth world is made up of millions of persons alienated from ideal everyday life and denied interactions because of the effects of disease and its treatment.

Self-concept reconstruction is one phase of adjusting to the illness. The goal in self-concept reconstruction is to integrate an accurate perception of the altered body part into a positive concept of self, while understanding that the ability or potential ability for managing care of the health problem resides within the self. Allowing the illness to be the dominant component in defining self needs to be avoided. Individuals with multiple sclerosis, for example, may need nurses' help to define themselves in terms of continuing roles, strengths, abilities, and goals, rather than simply in terms of the neurological impairment. Chapter 18 discusses enhancement of self-esteem as a method of alleviating powerlessness.

The nature of an individual's personality influences self-concept. One personality characteristic that is directly related to this subject is locus of control. Unlike powerlessness, which is a situationally determined perception that outcomes are beyond the individual's control, an internal locus of control is a stable tendency to perceive events and outcomes to be within the person's own control regardless of the situation. Persons with internal loci of control tend to perceive positive and negative life events as being a result of their own actions—under personal control (Lefcourt, 1966; Rotter, 1966). Persons with external loci of control tend to perceive life events as being unrelated to their own behavior and instead being contingent on chance, fate, or the powers of others. It is important to determine the individual's usual perceptions of life events and how much or how little control and/or involvement in self-care management the ill individual needs. In caring for chronically ill clients, nurses need to be concerned with whether or not the individual with an internal locus of control experiences more intense feelings of powerlessness when dealing with the illness than does an individual with an external locus of control. Locus of control is discussed in more detail in Chapters 9 and 10.

Energy

Energy is the capacity of a system for doing work; energy potential is stored energy. There must be a balance between energy uptake and energy expenditure. Energy sources include nutrients, water, rest, and motivation. Energy is expended to restore or heal physical states, to actively cope with daily living demands, and to cope with unusual stress. Energy is also spent for growth through learning, work, and play (Ryden, 1977). Absence of energy for the most basic levels of energy utilization, referred to as the compensatory level needed for physical balance, contributes to powerlessness of the individual and prevents energy utilization for higher-level expenditure needs, for example, growth and learning. Action is possible if strength and energy are present. Actions of the ill person include measures initiated by the person to protect and/or improve health. Routine daily activities may become difficult for the person who is ill. Healthy persons are described as buoyant and free floating in life; illness, however, weighs one down and is seen as lethargy (Agich, 1995). Coping with uncertainty of energy availability is discussed in Chapter 13.

Knowledge and Insight

Having knowledge and insight about what is happening to them enables clients to feel more in control and helps to alleviate the anxiety of uncertainty. It has been documented many times that clients who were informed and had accurate expectations about an anticipated experience would exhibit less anxiety during the stressful event (Johnson, 1972, 1973; Johnson, Kirchhoff, & Endress, 1975; Johnson, Morrissey, & Leventhal, 1973; Johnson & Rice, 1974).

The care regimens that chronically ill persons are required to implement are difficult in that they require learned skills, take time to execute, usually require changes in habits and routines, and entail physical and psychological stress (Reif, 1975). The regimen's difficulty is not only due to the individual's having to learn psychomotor skills such as an injection technique or having to learn technical information such as actions of drugs, but also to the individual's having to cope with psychological reactions to the health problem. Engaging in the learned therapy is a constant reminder of being different and of having the chronic illness.

Client knowledge allows involvement in decision making and awareness of the alternatives and the anticipated consequences of each alternative course of action. Knowledge is one "structure provider" that decreases uncertainty (Mishel, 1988) and enables development of a cognitive map for ongoing interpretation of events, enabling persons to find meaning in illness-related events (Turk, 1979). Lack of understanding contributes to lassitude and inaction, both of which are characteristic of powerlessness.

Internal awareness (Kinsman, Jones, Matus, & Schum, 1976) is a concept for discussion in relation to the power of knowledge and insight. Internal awareness is the ability to detect and interpret physical and psychological cues so as to take appropriate action to control symptoms and maintain psychological balance (Miller, 1982). This refers to developing a sensitivity to one's own body and means having an accurate perception of alterations in health such as changes in fatigue, pain, appetite, skin color, elimination, mood states, tension, anger, depression, guilt, and other physical and psychological states. For example, a young client with insulin-dependent diabetes may discover that circumoral numbness is the earliest symptom of impending insulin shock. Taking the appropriate action—ingesting glucose, followed by a protein food, for example—could avoid an emergency-room visit. Internal awareness also means knowing the desired effect of the therapy and self-monitoring in light of this effect. The client on diuretics with congestive heart failure who notes a daily weight increase of 2 pounds would be aware of the seriousness of this sign and would contact the physician. The client would not wait a week until the respiratory distress could be severe. Having this sensitivity to one's own signs and symptoms and reactions to therapy empowers the person to take action to control symptoms and avert crises. The outcome of client teaching is self-management, which is an informal process to manage day-to-day demands of illness, to carry out desired life roles, and to enjoy an emotionally satisfying life while confronting illness (Braden, 1993; Lorig, 1996).

Motivation

The theory of motivation based on competence and self-determination was reviewed by Deci (1985). This theory of motivation is congruent with approaches proposed in this book, namely, to develop the client's sense of control over self and environment. Competence theory refers to the individual's ability to deal effectively with the environment by manipulating the environment not only to meet basic needs (e.g., food and comfort) but also to have a feeling of efficacy (Deci, 1985).

Kagan (1972) described the human being as having a motive for mastery. He proposed that the origins of mastery were human beings' desires to achieve standards, predict the future, and define themselves. Reduction of uncertainty is a component of Kagan's concept. In the same sense, deCharms (1968) stated that individuals strive to be their own causal agents (for producing change in the environment, as well as in self and self-behavior). The desire to control one's destiny influences all other human motives. Deci also described competence behaviors as being geared to "dissonance" reduction. That is, the individual strives to reduce the amount of incongruity among beliefs, expectations, and actual actions and outcomes of events. Deci (1985) concluded his review of motivational theories by stating that intrinsically motivated behaviors enable persons to feel competent and self-determining. He summarized intrinsically motivated behaviors as being of two kinds: (1) those seeking stimulation and (2) those reducing incongruity (dissonance).

In chronic illness, motivation is important in maximizing potential, promoting social and work roles, and developing self-confidence through risk taking (e.g., being able to risk rejection when applying for a new job despite the chronic illness). Motivation is also needed to learn new skills and engage in therapies. Humanistic means of motivation especially relevant for nurses are discussed in Chapter 17. Motivation is one aspect of enabling behavior that empowers individuals.

Belief System

The belief system of the individual encompasses belief in God to provide strength and ability to cope with stress and overcome it; belief in therapeutic regimens, with the accompanying autosuggestion that the therapy will be effective; belief in caregivers; and belief in self, that is, confidence in one's own capabilities. Kraines (1943) stated if the client believes strongly in a caregiver, by that very belief the client obtains moral support and can face problems with a new degree of equanimity. Frank (1975) described how clients' expectations for therapy influence outcomes. Clients' self-suggestions about success of therapy may have self-fulfilling prophecy effects. The psychiatric clients' expressed optimism about treatment was a determinant in their symptomatic improvement in a 6-week course of therapy (Uhlenhuth & Duncan, 1968).

Spiritual malaise does not appear to be conducive to healing (Frank, 1975). The chronically ill person needs relief from the isolation of suffering, and having a relationship with God may alleviate the feeling of aloneness. Some individuals may find meaning in the misfortune of chronic illness through religion and faith. The knowledge that chronic illness affects mind, body, and spirit systems directs nurses' attention to developing spiritual well-being in their clients. "Spiritual well-being is the affirmation of life in a relationship with God, self, community, and environment that nurtures and celebrates wholeness" (Moberg, 1979, p. 5). A new hope is derived from renewed spiritual well-being. The presence of faith and hope empowers an individual to have a perceived sense of control and may enhance therapeutic results. Inspiring hope is discussed in Chapter 19.

The more power resources are compromised in an individual, the more nursing strategies will be needed to help the patient overcome a lack of control. These nursing strategies must consider the individual's unique coping style and focus on specific deficient power resources.

SUMMARY

The continuous ups and downs of chronic illness present a threatening sense of uncertainty that may range from an inability to predict whether one will have enough physical energy for an upcoming event, pain or comfort, nausea resulting from chemotherapy, or the internal motivation needed to follow through with an expectation. Not being able to predict how well symptoms will be controlled often prevents the individual from planning and engaging in social activities. Because social activities play a role in the development of a positive self-concept, these types of interactions are especially important for chronically ill persons. However, the uncertainty that accompanies the illness may cause ill individuals to isolate themselves. Eventually, the cure-oriented medical profession may demonstrate its own discouragement to the patient.

The ultimate uncertainty in the question "When will this end in death?" is always with the client. How much more loss the family and patient will suffer before death is a query seldom voiced. Psychological stability and social support help clients balance these fears with recognition of abilities and potential in their lives. The three-staged progression of the chronically ill person's relationship with health workers of *naive trust,* to *disenchantment,* and finally *guarded alliance* (Thorne, 1993; Thorne & Robinson, 1988, 1989) is not the type of full-partnership, participative relationship envisioned to be created by nurses to empower clients. All care is dependent upon a helping, caring nurse-client relationship that becomes the vehicle for client empowerment.

Clients who are chronically ill need to have power to be managers of their own care. They should not forfeit the role of self-management to health-care personnel. Nurses can maximize clients' resources for power by developing the strengths that remain as well as by supporting the clients' select coping strategies while recognizing that individual client and family responses are influenced by salutary resources (Antonovsky, 1980), hardiness, and their developed coping ability.

The power resources model provides the general framework for this book. Chapters are devoted to examining causes, indicators, and measurement of power resource deficits in specific health problems and/or age groups. Strategies to alleviate powerlessness are described for specific chronic health problems. Empowerment strategies specific to components of the power resources model are developed; individual chapters are devoted to enhancing self-esteem, inspiring hope, overcoming energy deficits, and developing enabling strategies (motivation and knowledge), all of which are directed at alleviating powerlessness of chronic illness. The many explicit challenges confronting chronically ill clients are discussed in Chapter 2, in which a typology of coping tasks for chronically ill clients is presented.

REFERENCES

Adams, J., & Lindemann, E. (1974). Coping with long-term disability. In G. Coehlo, D. Hamburg, & J. Adams (Eds.), *Coping and adaptation* (pp. 127–138). New York: Basic Books.

Affleck, G., Tennen, H., Pfeiffer, C., & Fifield, J. (1987). Appraisals of control and predictability in adapting to a chronic disease. *Journal of Personality and Social Psychology, 53,* 273–279.

Agich, G. (1995). Chronic illness and freedom. In S. K. Toombs, D. Barnard, & R. Carson (Eds.), *Chronic illness: From experience to policy* (pp. 129–153). Indianapolis: Indiana University Press.

Antonovsky, A. (1985). *Health, stress and coping.* San Francisco: Jossey-Bass.

Braden, C. (1993). Research program on learned response to chronic illness experience: Self-help model. *Holistic Nursing Practice, 8,* 38–44.

Bramwell, L., & Whall, A. N. (1986). Effect of role clarity and empathy on support role performance and anxiety. *Nursing Research, 35,* 282–287.

Brown, J., Rawlinson, M., & Hilles, N. (1981). Life satisfaction and chronic disease. Exploration of a theoretical model. *Medical Care, 19,* 1136–1146.

Burckhardt, C. S. (1985). The impact of arthritis on quality of life. *Nursing Research, 34,* 11–16.

Charmaz, K. (1983). Loss of self: A fundamental form of suffering in the chronically ill. *Sociology of Health and Illness, 5,* 168–195.

Cohen, S., & Syme, S. L. (1985). Issues in the study and application of social support. In S. Cohen & S. L. Syme (Eds.), *Social support and health* (pp. 3–21). Orlando: Academic Press.

Cooper, I. S. (1976). *Living with chronic neurologic disease.* New York: WW Norton.

Corbin, J., & Strauss, A. (1984). Collaboration: Couples working together to manage chronic illness. *Image—The Journal of Nursing Scholarship, 14,* 109–115.

Corbin, J., & Strauss, A. (1988). *Unending work and care: Managing chronic illness at home.* San Francisco: Jossey-Bass.

Craig, H. M., & Edwards, J. E. (1983). Adaptation in chronic illness: An eclectic model for nurses. *Journal of Advanced Nursing, 8,* 397–404.

deCharms, R. (1968). *Personal causation: The internal affective determinants of behavior.* New York: Academic Press.

Deci, E. (1985). *Intrinsic motivation.* New York: Plenum Press.

Dimond, M. (1979). Social support and adaptation to chronic illness. The case of maintenance hemodialysis. *Research in Nursing and Health, 2,* 101–108.

Donoghue, P. J., & Siegel, M. E. (1992). *Sick and tired of feeling sick and tired.* New York: WW Norton.

Driever, M. (1984). Theory of self-concept. In C. Roy (Ed.), *Introduction to nursing: An adaptation model* (pp. 169–191). Englewood Cliffs, NJ: Prentice-Hall.

Epstein, S. (1973). The self-concept revisited: Or a theory of a theory. *American Psychologist, 28,* 404–416.

Feldman, D. (1974). Chronic disabling illness: A holistic view. *Journal of Chronic Disease, 27,* 287–291.

Ferrans, C., & Powers, M. (1985). Quality of Life Index: Development and psychometric properties. *Advances in Nursing Science, 8,* 15–24.

Frank, J. (1975). *Persuasion and healing.* New York: Schocken Books.

George, L., & Bearon, L. (1980). *Quality of life in older persons.* New York: Human Sciences Press.

Johnson, J. (1972). The effect of structuring patients' expectation on their reactions to threatening events. *Nursing Research, 21,* 499–504.

Johnson, J. (1973). Effects of accurate expectations about sensation on the sensory and distress components of pain. *Journal of Personality and Social Psychology, 27,* 261–275.

Johnson, J., Kirchhoff, K., & Endress, M. (1975). Altering children's distress behavior during orthopedic cast removal. *Nursing Research, 24,* 404–410.

Johnson, J., Morrissey, J., & Leventhal, H. (1973). Psychological preparation for an endoscopic examination. *Gastrointestinal Endoscopy, 19,* 180–182.

Johnson, J., & Rice, V. (1974). Sensory and distress components of pain: Implications for the study of clinical pain. *Nursing Research, 23,* 203–209.

Kagan, J. (1972). Motives and development. *Journal of Personality and Social Psychology, 22,* 51–66.

Kinsman, R., Jones, N., Matus, I., & Schum, R. (1976). Patient variable supporting chronic illness. *The Journal of Nervous and Mental Disease, 163,* 159–165.

Kobasa, S. (1979a). Personality and resistance to illness. *American Journal of Community Psychology, 7,* 413–423.

Kobasa, S. (1979b). Stressful life events, personality, and health: An inquiry into hardiness. *Journal of Personality and Social Psychology, 37,* 1–11.

Kobasa, S. (1982). Commitment and coping in stress-resistance among lawyers. *Journal of Personality and Social Psychology, 42,* 707–711.

Kobasa, S., Maddri, S., Puccetti, M., & Zola, M. (1985). Effectiveness of hardiness, exercise and social support as resources against illness. *Journal of Psychosomatic Research, 29,* 525–533.

Kraines, S. (1943). *The theory of neuroses and psychoses.* Philadelphia: Lea & Febiger.

Lambert, C., & Lambert, V. (1987). Hardiness: Its development and relevance to nursing. *Image: Journal of Nursing Scholarship, 19,* 92–95.

Lambert, V., Lambert, C., Klipple, G., & Mewshaw, E. (1989). Social support, hardiness and psychological well-being in women with arthritis. *Image—Journal of Nursing Scholarship, 21,* 128–131.

Lawrence, S. A., & Lawrence, R. M. (1979). A model of adaptation to the stress of chronic illness. *Nursing Forum, 18,* 33–42.

Lefcourt, H. (1966). Belief in personal control: Research and implications. *Journal of Individual Psychology, 22,* 185–195.

Leventhal, H., Meyer, D., & Nerenz, D. (1980). The commonsense representation of illness danger. In S. Rachman (Ed.), *Contributions to medical psychology* (Vol. 2, pp. 3–26). Oxford: Permagon Press.

Lorig, K. (1996). Chronic disease self-management. *American Behavioral Scientist, 39,* 676–683.

Lubkin, I. (1994). *Chronic illness: Impact and interventions.* Boston: Jones and Bartlett Publishers.

May, R. (1972). *Power and innocence.* New York: WW Norton.

Maybury, C. P., & Brewin, C. R. (1984). Social relationships, knowledge and adjustment to multiple sclerosis: An exploratory study. *Social Science and Medicine, 11,* 245–250.

McNett, S. C. (1987). Social support, threat, and coping effectiveness in the functionally disabled. *Nursing Research, 36,* 98–193.

Miller, J. F. (1982). Categories of self-care needs of ambulatory patients with diabetes. *Journal of Advanced Nursing, 7,* 25–31.

Mishel, M. H. (1981). The measurement of uncertainty in illness. *Nursing Research, 30,* 258–263.

Mishel, M. H. (1983). Parents' perception of uncertainty concerning their hospitalized child. *Nursing Research, 32,* 324–330.

Mishel, M. H. (1988). Uncertainty in illness. *Image: Journal of Nursing Scholarship, 20,* 225–232.

Mishel, M. H., & Braden, C. J. (1987). Uncertainty: A mediator between support and adjustment. *Western Journal of Nursing Research, 9,* 43–57.

Mishel, M. H., & Braden, C. J. (1988). Finding meaning: Antecedents of uncertainty. *Nursing Research, 37,* 98–103.

Mishel, M. H., Hostetter, T., King, B., & Graham, V. (1984). Predictors of psychosocial adjustment in patients newly diagnosed with gynecological cancer. *Cancer Nursing, 7,* 291–299.

Mishel, M. H., & Murdaugh, C. (1987). Family experiences with heart transplantation: Redesigning the dream. *Nursing Research, 36,* 332–338.

Moberg, D. (1979). *Spiritual well-being: Sociological perspectives.* Washington, D.C.: University Press of America.

Northouse, L. L. (1988). Social support in patients' and husbands' adjustment to breast cancer. *Nursing Research, 37,* 91–95.

Nowack, K. (1989). Coping style, cognitive hardiness, and health status. *Journal of Behavioral Medicine, 12,* 145–158.

Padilla, G., Presant, C., Grant, M., Metter, G., Lipsett, J., & Heide, R. (1983). Quality of Life Index for patients with cancer. *Research in Nursing and Health, 6,* 117–126.

Pattison, E. M. (1974). Psychosocial predictors of death prognosis. *Omega, 5,* 145–159.

Pollock, S. E. (1986). Human responses to chronic illness: Physiologic and psychosocial adaptation. *Nursing Research, 35,* 90–95.

Pollock, S. E. (1989). The hardiness characteristic: A motivating factor in adaptation. *Advances in Nursing Science, 11,* 53–62.

Radley, A., & Green, R. (1987). Illness as adjustment: A methodology and conceptual framework. *Sociology of Health and Illness, 9,* 179–207.

Reif, L. (1975). Beyond medical intervention strategies for managing life in face of chronic illness. In M. Davis, M. Kramer, & A. Strauss (Eds.), *Nurses in practice: A perspective on work environments* (pp. 261–273). St. Louis: CV Mosby.

Rosenberg, M. (1979). *Conceiving the self.* New York: Basic Books.

Rotter, J. (1966). Generalized expectancies for internal versus external control of reinforcement. *Psychological Monographs, 80,* 1–28.

Ryden, M. (1977). Energy: A crucial consideration in the nursing process. *Nursing Forum, 16,* 71–82.

Schaefer, C., Coyne, J., & Lazarus, R. (1981). The health-related function of social support. *Journal of Behavioral Medicine, 4,* 381–406.

Spilker, B. (1990). *Quality of Life Assessments in Clinical Trials.* New York: Raven Press.

Strain, J. (1979). Psychological reactions to chronic medical illness. *Psychiatric Quarterly, 51,* 173–183.

Strauss, A., et al. (1984). *Chronic illness and the quality of life.* St. Louis: CV Mosby.

Thorne, S. (1993). *Negotiating health care: The social context of chronic illness.* Newbury Park: Sage.

Thorne, S., & Robinson, C. (1988). Health care relationships: The chronic illness perspective. *Research in Nursing and Health, 11,* 293–300.

Thorne, S., & Robinson, C. (1989). Guarded alliance: Health care relationships in chronic illness. *Image—Journal of Nursing Scholarship, 21,* 153–157.

Turk, D. (1979). Factors influencing the adaptive process with chronic illness. In I. Sarason, & C. Spielberger (Eds), *Stress and anxiety* (Vol. 6, pp. 291–311). New York: John Wiley & Sons.

Turk, D., Rudy, T., & Salovey, P. (1986). Implicit models of illness. *Journal of Behavioral Medicine, 9,* 453–474.

Turk, D., Sobel, H., Follick, M., & Youkilis, H. (1980). A sequential criterion analysis for assessing coping with chronic illness. *Journal of Human Stress, 6,* 35–40.

Uhlenhuth, E. H., & Duncan, D. B. (1968). Subjective change with medical student therapists: Some determinants for change in psychoneurotic outpatients. *Archives of General Psychiatry, 18,* 532–540.

Weiss, R. S. (1974). The provisions of social relationships. In Z. Rubin (Ed.), *Doing unto others* (pp. 17–26). Englewood Cliffs, NJ: Prentice Hall.

Winert, C. (1983). The physiological and psychosocial stress of long term illness and the effects of social support on the "healthy" functioning of the families. *Western Journal of Nursing Research, 5,* 34.

Wortman, C., & Brehm, J. (1975). Responses to uncontrollable outcomes: An integration of reactance theory and learned helplessness. In L. Berkowitz (Ed.), *Advances in experimental social psychology* (Vol. 8, pp. 277–336). New York: Academic Press.

Zedlow, P. W., & Pavlou, M. (1984). Physical disability, life stress, and psychosocial adjustment to multiple sclerosis. *Journal of Nervous and Mental Diseases, 172,* 80–84.

2

Analysis of Coping with Illness

➤ Judith Fitzgerald Miller

The unique manner in which individuals and families deal with the demands of chronic illness influences the degree and nature of lifelong adjustment and well-being. Clients and families must develop skills, not only to manage the physical care demands and lifestyle modifications accompanying illness, but also to cope with a taxonomy of psychosocial tasks accompanying illness. Some stressors of chronic illness are transitory; however, uncertainty is ever present (Auerbach, 1989). It may not be possible to reverse disability, but knowledge about coping strategies can moderate the psychological impact of illness (Johnson, Lauver, & Nail, 1989).

COPING DEFINED

There are varied clinical and research traditions on coping, each having a slightly different emphasis. Psychoanalysis and some psychologists view coping as a stable personality-based emotional and behavioral mode of responding. Some experimental psychologists study coping as learning escape and avoidance of threatening stimuli (Roth & Cohen, 1986). Physiological perspectives consider coping as cortical and subcortical stimulation by the hypothalamus resulting in activation of the pituitary and adrenocortical system. Others such as Lazarus and Folkman (1984) view coping as context-specific behavioral and emotional processes in which an individual appraises, encounters, and recovers from contact with a stressor, whether a minor daily hassle or a major life change. Mechanic's (1974) social-psychological view is that coping deals with social environmental demands. From an education perspective, coping is problem solving; confronting the realities of the problem while maintaining integrity of functioning (Bruner, 1966). Coping is the constantly changing cognitive and behavioral efforts used to manage specific external and/or internal demands that are appraised as taxing and that exceed the resources of the person (Lazarus & Folkman, 1984). Coping is what an individual does about a problem to bring about relief, reward, quiescence, and equilibrium (Weisman, 1979). Focusing specifically on illness, Lipowski (1970) defines coping as all the cognitive and motor activities a sick person uses to preserve bodily and psychic integrity, to recover reversible impaired function, and to compensate to the limit for any irreversible loss. Although Haan (1977) differentiates defense mechanisms (defending) from coping, in this book defense mechanisms are viewed as a part of the individual's coping repertoire. Haan views defense mechanisms as rigid psychological mechanisms regardless of the nature of the problem and defines coping as an open dynamic process that permits new information to be used and behavior modified in light of new insights.

Throughout this chapter, coping refers to dealing with situations that present a threat to the individual to resolve uncomfortable feelings such as anxiety, fear, grief, and guilt. Problems precipitating these uncomfortable affects may be thought of as coping tasks. Coping tasks are external stimuli such as dealing with pain, threat of surgery, and impending death, as well as internal psychic phenomena such as threatened body image, perceived alterations in role function, and unresolved anger. Coping strategies are the specific techniques that a sick person selects to deal with the illness and its consequences. An individual's coping style is one's enduring disposition to deal with challenges and stress by employing a specific group of techniques (Lipowski, 1970). Weisman (1979, p. 27) stated, "Coping combines perception, performance, appraisal, correction, followed by further activity and directed motivated behavior." The aim of coping is mastery, control, or resolution (Weisman & Worden, 1976–1977).

Coping Process

The coping process may include a two-staged cognitive process of primary and secondary appraisals (Lazarus & Folkman, 1984). With the primary appraisal, the individual determines whether the conditions or stimuli are a threat ("Am I O.K.?"), and the secondary appraisal includes a review of choices of action if a threat is perceived ("What can I do?"). Responses include behaviors such as emotional, cognitive, and physical activities.

The coping process may have differing results such as mastery, resilience, or crisis (resolved or unresolved) (Garland & Bush, 1982). If the threat is resolved, the coping behavior will be used in similar situations and a sense of *mastery* will be achieved. In some cases, the threat may not be averted, yet the individual gets through the event without lasting psychic trauma and manifests *resilience* (successful coping). If the threatening situation is not handled effectively (ineffective coping), a *crisis* may result, and if unresolved, psychological and physiological disequilibrium may occur. The crisis may be resolved with or without professional intervention, and the individual returns to previous or higher levels of functioning.

Coping Functions

The function of coping varies with the differing coping theoretical frameworks used (Lazarus & Folkman, 1984) and may include:

- Reduction of tension and maintenance of equilibrium (adaptation)
- Sound decision making
- Maintenance of autonomy and freedom
- Motivation to meet social environmental demands
- Maintenance of stable social, psychological, and physical state
- Control of the meaning of potential stressors before they become a threat, and according to Beutel (1985)
- Avoidance of negative self-evaluation

Pearlin and Schooler (1978) described four types of functions: (1) prevention of stress from events or situations, (2) alteration of the situation or problem, (3) change in the meaning of the situation, and (4) management of the symptoms or reactions to the stress. Lazarus and Folkman (1984) divided coping functions into emotion-focused and problem-focused coping. Emotion-focused coping is said to be prevalent when persons conclude that they cannot control the stressful stimuli; that is, nothing can modify the harmful threatening event. Examples of emotion-focused strategies include avoidance, minimization, distancing, selective attention, mediating, venting feelings, and increasing physical activity as a distractor. Problem-focused coping is the use of a problem-solving process including defining the problem, enumerating alternatives, comparing alternatives in terms of costs and benefits, and finally, selecting an action. Problem-focused strategies are enacted when the threat is appraised as being changeable. Learning new self-care skills to confront the demand is a problem-focused strategy.

Jalowiec (1989) reported three types of coping strategies as a result of confirmatory factor analysis of her Coping Scale based on 1400 respondents. The three factors were confrontive (e.g., discuss problems, seek information, set goals, maintain control), emotive (e.g., worry, expect the worst, blame others), and palliative coping (e.g., sleep, laugh it off, pray, let someone else solve it).

Effective Coping

Coping behavior is effective when the behavior used resolves the uncomfortable feeling associated with threat and/or loss, preserves the integrity of the individual, and preserves the ability of the individual to function effectively in relationships, life roles, and maintenance of a positive self-concept. Visotsky et al. (1961) described coping as being effective when it (1) kept distress within manageable limits, (2) generated encouragement and hope, (3) maintained or restored a sense of personal worth, (4) maintained or restored relationships with significant others, (5) enhanced prospects for physical recovery, and (6) enhanced prospects for favorable situations (interpersonal, social, and economic). Caplan (1963) identified effective coping strategies such as actively exploring reality issues and searching for information; freely expressing both positive and negative feelings, and having tolerance for frustration; actively invoking help from others; breaking problems into manageable bits and working them through one at a time; being aware of fatigue and tendencies toward disorganization, pacing activities, and engaging in problem-solving efforts; mastering feelings when possible and accepting the inevitable when not; trusting in oneself and others, and maintaining optimism about the outcome.

COPING STYLES

Coping changes with situational demands. Flexibility is favored over a rigid style. Some consistency in terms of coping style, yet variability in use of selected strategies depending upon seriousness of the threat, has been noted to be effective. The repeated manner in which the chronically ill individual responds to the presenting coping task is the individual's coping style. Coping style can be identified by noting the individual's range of behaviors over time. Coping styles can be divided into three categories: approach, avoidance, and nonspecific defense (Goldstein et al., 1965; Lazarus, 1966; Lipowski, 1969, 1970; Lomont, 1965). The term *approach* (Lazarus, 1966) is synonymous with the style Goldstein et al. (1965) labeled *sensitizer* and Lipowski (1970) labeled *vigilant focuser*. The term *avoidance* is synonymous with minimization (Lipowski, 1970) and repression (Lomont, 1965). Figure 2.1 illustrates the coping continuum.

To be effective, the coping response should match the nature of the demand (Roth & Cohen, 1986). Mullen and Suls (1982) found that avoidance strategies were effective for short-term outcomes, but approach strategies were more effective for long-term outcomes. Denial

Approach	Nonspecific defenders	Avoidance
(Vigilant focuser)		(Minimizer)
(Sensitizer)		(Repressor)

FIGURE 2.1 ➤ Continuum of coping styles with synonymous terms identified.

might be helpful early in the chronic illness, during an acute traumatic event, or when a threatening situation is uncontrollable (Roth & Cohen, 1986). However, if this method of avoidance continues to such extremes that treatment is not sought or abandoned, then the denial is no longer effective.

Roth and Cohen (1986) summarized the benefits and costs for both extremes of coping. The benefits of approach include: action is taken to alleviate the problem; emotions are accurately perceived and ventilated; and effects of the trauma *may* be integrated, preserving a positive self-concept. The cost or risk of approach may be increased distress and excessive anxiety. Benefits of avoidance include obtaining a reprieve from nonproductive worry and having time to find reasons for hope. Eventually these effects of avoidance may lead to approach methods. The cost or risk of avoidance is that appropriate problem solving and/or treatment may be delayed, true feelings are not perceived and disclosed, and accurate information may intrude and heighten anxiety.

Individuals who practice avoidance use repression, denial, projection, and any other strategy that minimizes the threat. Avoidance includes intellectual strategies that diminish the seriousness of the threat for the individual. Selective inattention and ignoring or rationalizing the facts or consequences of the illness are avoidance strategies (Kiely, 1972).

Approach behaviors on the other end of the coping continuum include tackling, vigilant focusing, and sensitizing. Tackling is energetically fighting the illness and actively engaging in therapy. Vigilant focusing refers to an obsessional alertness and compulsive attention to details of therapy. Vigilant focusers need detailed explanations of procedures and treatment (Kiely, 1972) and have more evident anxiety than do minimizers. Sensitizers are those who readily acknowledge threatening emotions of hate, fear, disgust, and love (Andrew, 1973). They are on the approach end of the coping continuum because of their direct confrontation with emotional states.

Neutrals, or nonspecific defenders, use combinations of approach and avoidance strategies. On the Mainord Coper-Avoider Sentence Completion Test (an instrument to measure coping), the individuals classified as neutrals score in the middle; they are neither avoiders nor sensitizers (Andrew, 1973).

Impact of Client's Coping Style on Care

Does being able to recognize an individual's coping mechanisms serve any real therapeutic purpose? Identifying clients' coping styles and specific coping strategies is imperative for a holistic nursing approach. Nurses need to be made acquainted with how the client is confronting the ups and downs of chronic illness. Nurses may unwittingly stifle helpful client strategies, making judgments about what they themselves would do in similar circumstances instead of objectively evaluating the client's selected strategies and supporting those that are effective.

Judgments cannot be made about the value of approach versus avoidance strategies unless criteria for effective coping are used (see Fig. 2.1). Coping is effective if uncomfortable feelings of anxiety, fear, grief, or guilt are contained; hope is generated; self-esteem is enhanced; relationships with others are maintained; and a state of wellness is maintained or improved. Cohen and Lazarus (1973) studied 61 surgical clients to determine the relationship between the mode of coping and recovery from surgery. Clients were classified as using avoidance, vigilance, or both types of behavior according to results of the Andrew version of the Goldstein Coper-Avoider Sentence Completion Test (1967). The variables studied were number of days in the hospital, number of analgesics used, minor medical complications, and negative psychological reactions. The 10 vigilant clients had slower recoveries that required more days of hospitalization and had more minor complications than did the 14 clients who used avoidance or the 37 clients who manifested both vigilance and avoidance. There were no significant differences in the other variables (Cohen & Lazarus, 1973).

Nurses need to be aware that clients who are vigilant focusers are active seekers of information who master situations in active roles. Persons using this coping style must be kept informed of minute details of care and alternative methods available. The vigilant focuser needs to participate fully in providing care, setting goals, and evaluating progress. Vigilant focusers may test staff by asking several persons the same questions to compare responses and verify information already received. These clients need the same approaches used by nurses for various personal-care activities. Variation in approaches will heighten already-present anxiety. Being forced into powerlessness situations of pain and disability may be more devastating to the vigilant focuser than to an avoider.

It is particularly relevant for nurses to note that instruction programs need to be tailored to the individual's coping style. To give an individual who is an avoider the precise details of an anticipated stress may cause more harm than good. On the other hand, the vigilant focuser needs to feel in control, and the sense of control is rooted in knowledge and competent participation in care. To bombard the avoider with information may diminish ability to cope. To avoid the details of what will occur in dealing with a vigilant focuser heightens anxiety and diminishes coping ability.

Shanan, De Nour, Kaplan, and Schak (1976) studied 59 terminally ill clients with renal failure who were on hemodialysis and a matched sample of 59 subjects to determine if prolonged stress reduced active coping and to determine the effect of the clients' backgrounds on coping. The results of the Shanan Sentence Completion Test indicate that clients on dialysis obtained lower coping scores and had passivity, negative self-perception, and a tendency to withdraw by using denial. The only background variables related to illness and coping were the individual's sex and education. Women were more negative than men. Education helped prepare the client to cope with specific problems.

Miller and Mangan (1983) studied types of surgical preparatory information provided clients with differing coping style preferences. Persons were assigned to one of two conditions: high amount of presurgical information and low amount of information. Persons whose coping style was consistent with the depth of information presented had less distress than those with a discrepancy between style and the intervention. That is, vigilant focusers needed detailed information, whereas avoiders benefited from less detail.

Coping Determinants

The way in which a person copes with illness is influenced by the nature of the power resources of belief system (faith and hope), family–social support, psychological well-being, self-esteem, motivation, type and meaning of the illness, number and seriousness of the illness-related demands, stage of illness progression, developmental and family influences, previous success using varied strategies, accurate appraisal of the threat, self-insight, and self-efficacy. Intrapersonal factors affecting coping may include age, personality, culture, specific self-care skills, values, beliefs, emotional state, and cognitive capacity. Environmental factors may include presence of a support system, access to health services, physical resources for living, and financial resources.

In analyzing the stages of progression of an illness, differences in coping energy utilization can be easily understood. Charmaz (1973) presented a three-stage progression of chronic disease. Stage 1 is labeled interrupted time, when daily activities are temporarily adjusted to obtain a diagnosis. Stage 2 is the time intrusion phase, when daily activities need to be adjusted to control the effect of the disease. The illness consumes time and energy. Stage 3 is time encapsulation, during which the individual is consumed by the illness; the individual is engulfed with care management throughout the day.

The meaning of the illness to the individual affects coping behavior. Differences in coping can be expected if one individual perceives the illness to be a threat to sexual role functioning and another views the illness as insignificant. Illness may be viewed as a loss or gain, or of no significance.

Perceiving illness as a loss refers to loss of pleasures, role fulfillment, functional abilities, self-esteem, self-satisfaction, love, recognition, and normalcy. Illness may be viewed as a threat to life. Grief and anxiety accompany the perception of illness as a loss.

Illness may be perceived by some as a gain if it provides relief from the stress of other life roles. The suffering of illness may be viewed as having spiritual value for the individual and as an opportunity to relieve guilt, repent perceived past offenses, and accept this plight as a punishment. Illness may provide respite from intrapersonal conflict or an opportunity to withdraw and resolve conflict. It may also afford some individuals the opportunity to receive kindness, attention, and signs of affection they might otherwise not get.

If the individual views the illness as insignificant, little importance is assigned to the symptoms (Lipowski, 1969) or possible consequences of the illness and treatment.

The nurse's understanding of the client's perception of the illness will enhance the nurse's ability to identify and support the coping strategy the client selects. Clear differences in coping would exist between individuals perceiving illness as a threat or loss and those perceiving illness as a gain or as insignificant.

COPING TASKS OF CHRONICALLY ILL INDIVIDUALS

Coping tasks are those particular challenges that must be faced and overcome so that the individual preserves integrity, restores or maintains a positive concept of self, and functions effectively in relationships and life roles. Individuals with chronic health problems may be challenged to cope with multiple complex tasks.

Kiely (1972) categorized three types of stresses that initiate coping responses: (1) loss or threat of loss of psychic "objects," that is, personal relationships, body functions and image, and social roles; (2) injury or threat of injury to body involving notions of pain or mutilation; and (3) frustration of biological drive satisfaction—especially nurturant or libidinal drives—as well as frustration over lack of avenues for aggressive discharge.

To identify the coping tasks of chronically ill persons, nursing diagnoses of 118 chronically ill clients were reviewed. These nursing diagnoses were made by 44 graduate nursing students enrolled in a graduate nursing practicum course entitled "Nursing Strategies for Adults: Long-Term Health Problems." Each student studied and cared for a

Table 2.1 ➤ **TYPOLOGY OF COPING TASKS OF CHRONICALLY ILL ADULTS***

Broad Task Category	Subconcepts in the Category
1. Maintaining a sense of normalcy	Hiding, minimizing illness, and/or responding to curious inquiries of others
	Living as normally as possible despite daily therapy and obvious symptoms
2. Modifying daily routine, adjusting lifestyle	Including therapy and symptom control in daily routine
	Providing for safety
3. Obtaining knowledge and skill for continuing self-care	Having internal awareness
	Monitoring effects of therapy
4. Maintaining a positive concept of self	Integrating illness into self-concept
	Maintaining or enhancing self-esteem
5. Adjusting to altered social relationships	Experiencing loneliness and social isolation
	Undergoing patient- or other-initiated disengagement
	Preserving relationships with friends and family who satisfy dependency needs
	Maintaining family solidarity
6. Grieving over losses concomitant with chronic illness	Losing physical abilities, function
	Losing status
	Losing income and social relationships
	Losing roles and dignity
	Dealing with financial losses
7. Dealing with role change	Losing roles—social, work, family
	Gaining roles—dependent help seeker, self-care agent, chronically ill patient
8. Handling physical discomfort	Handling illness-induced discomfort
9. Complying with prescribed regimen	Handling pain caused by therapy
10. Confronting the inevitability of one's own death	
11. Dealing with social stigma of illness or disability	
12. Maintaining a feeling of being in control	Exerting cognitive control
	Exerting behavioral control
	Exerting decisional control
13. Maintaining hope despite uncertain or downward course of health	Experiencing effects of hope
	Finding meaning in physical changes

*Supported by HEW Grant No. 1 D23 NU00038-62.

small case-load of clients (no more than three) for the duration of the academic semester. Coping tasks were also identified in literature review and through Stapleton's (1978) and this author's clinical practice. Table 2.1 lists the coping tasks identified; each will be discussed briefly.

Striving to Feel Normal

Maintaining a sense of normalcy includes keeping signs and symptoms of illness under control or out of view of persons surrounding the individual. It includes a mental review of existing abilities and functions. When the chronically ill individual engages in a personal reaffirmation of being as capable as coworkers or the individuals in the person's social network, the ideal of being and feeling normal (having abilities similar to those of others in the social network) is fostered.

Normalization is a process by which individuals and families cope with chronic illness (Deatrick, 1988; Knafl & Deatrick, 1986; Riding, 1997). That is, individuals view and describe their lives as normal despite severe impairment or disruption within the family routine. Normalization depends upon cognitive reframing of a difficult life challenge into one that is manageable and "normal." Normalization supports hope.

Wiener (1975) described individuals with rheumatoid arthritis using the normalizing strategies of covering up, keeping up, and pacing. Covering up means keeping signs of disability and pain hidden and may include not using an assistive device—a cane or other external sign of handicap such as a wheelchair. Controlling evidence of discomfort and fatigue is an imperative behavior for successful covering up. Chronically ill individuals expend much energy covering up, not only to maintain a sense of normalcy, but to avoid curious questioners and to avoid making those around them feel uncomfortable. Persons interacting with the chronically ill individual may feel uncomfortable about not knowing how much assistance with mobility to provide, how to respond to obvious evidence of pain, and how to minimize their own vigor and vitality so as to lessen the discrepancy between themselves and the chronically ill person's impairment. Covering up is not a form of denial; it is a refusal to allow the disability to interfere with social interactions.

Keeping up refers to the ill individual's successful carrying through with a planned event (Wiener, 1975), while covering up, expending increased energy, and causing overwhelming fatigue and perhaps exacerbation of symptoms. Events, such as hosting a family get-together or preparing a holiday meal, call for frantic keep-up activity.

Pacing refers to balancing the activities of covering up and keeping up with the rest needed to avoid unnecessary periods of immobilization to restore energy wasted in covering up and keeping up. Pacing results from understanding limitations in abilities and appropriately engaging in activities that satisfy ego needs without causing undue exhaustion.

Modifying Routines and Lifestyles

To control symptoms and live as normally as possible, the individual may need to alter habits and routines. Habits of overeating, lack of exercise, lack of relaxation, or smoking may need to be modified. Daily routines may need to be interrupted to obtain needed therapy for the chronic disease, for example, postural drainage and intermittent positive-pressure breathing for individuals with emphysema. Activities that exacerbate symptoms must be learned and avoided. (The elementary school teacher with rheumatoid arthritis may need to avoid playground duty on cool, damp days, for example.)

Obtaining Knowledge and Skill for Continuing Self-Care

Self-care is a key concept for the chronically ill individual's maintenance of optimal health. Achieving desired outcomes depends on the client's self-care practices and not on the power of the health-care team. Being competent in ministering to self means acquiring the necessary skills, knowledge, and motivation. It also means having an awareness of body cues, interpreting physical changes accurately, and taking appropriate action either to alter therapy or to seek help from health-care resources to prevent a crisis.

Maintaining a Positive Concept of Self

When previous abilities are gone, energy and ability to successfully engage in desired activities that satisfy ego needs have disappeared, changes in physical self have occurred, and maintaining a positive concept of self is a major coping task. The individual must avoid allowing the disability or illness to become one's entire identity. Instead, the illness, related changes, and therapies must be integrated into a positive concept of self that helps the individual maintain a sense of competence and normalcy. Activities that enhance self-esteem need to be identified, and the remaining personal strengths need to be emphasized. Helping the client review accomplishments and remaining intact roles enhances self-esteem. Balancing the self-ideal with the altered body image is necessary to maintain a positive self-concept and self-esteem (see Chap. 18).

Adjusting to Altered Social Relationships

Chronic illness may cause social isolation and loneliness. The sick person may withdraw because of a depleted energy reserve or poor self-concept, feeling unworthy of previous social contacts, or simply being physically unable to participate in former social events. As the illness encapsulates more of the person's time, thought processes may be dominated by the illness, controlling symptoms, and obtaining relief. Only the most loyal friends may persist in being supportive during this repetitive pattern of interaction. In other words, isolation may be initiated by significant others' withdrawal to obtain relief from the difficult scene of physical deterioration. Davis (1975, p. 253) quoted a chronically ill woman as saying, "Anyone who is sick for longer than 6 months won't be remembered except for birthdays and holidays."

The ill individual may need to adjust to having fewer interactions with fewer people and to receiving decreased confirmation of being a capable individual. The ill person must also strive to preserve relationships with those friends and family members who satisfy physical and emotional dependency needs.

Grieving over the Losses of Chronic Illness

Chronically ill individuals grieve over multiple losses. Loss of physical abilities includes losses of mobility, organ functioning, energy availability, physical stamina, sexual attractiveness, and sexual function. Other losses may include loss of self-esteem, role performance, and social relationships. Grief work takes place to deal with these losses and to preserve a sense of personal integrity and dignity. The cumulative effect of significant losses may create doubts in ill persons' minds about their own ability to maintain quality of life. Reformulating goals and examining aspirations require coping skills.

Dealing with Role Change

Role changes of chronically ill persons may be analyzed in terms of loss and gain. The role losses may include loss of social roles (church participant, member of bowling team, officer in a community group) and employment role, and diminishing of the role of family decision maker and disciplinarian. The individual has to take on the roles of being chronically ill, dependent help seeker, self-care agent, and client of a complex health-care system.

Role change encompasses giving up roles, accompanied by grief work, and taking on new roles, accompanied by role insufficiency. "Role insufficiency is any difficulty in the cognizance and/or performance of a role or of the sentiments and goals associated with the role behavior as perceived by self or by significant others" (Melies, 1975, p. 264). In adoption of the role of self-care agent, rehearsal of role enactment may be an important prelude to actual role taking. Kassebaum and Baumann (1965) pointed out that Parsons' sick-role theory (Parsons, 1951) is inadequate for the chronically ill person because of Parsons' emphasis on the temporary surrendering of roles and the person's desire to get well. Kassebaum and Baumann identified four dimensions of the sick role in chronically ill persons. The dimensions include dependence, reciprocity (mutual expectations for exemption from some role obligations), role-performance alteration, and denial of sick role. The incapacity for role performance is not a total, temporary incapacity as described by Parsons, but rather may be a partial, permanent alteration in roles and performance of roles (Kassebaum & Baumann, 1965).

Learning the role of dependent help seeker, maintaining a positive dependence, is another component of this coping task. Positive dependency "requires honest acceptance of one's differentness and the special needs and conditions it imposes" (Feldman 1974, p. 290). Seeking help for physical and emotional needs without feeling weak and inadequate is necessary. The client is challenged to resolve feelings of conflict over wanting to be totally independent yet needing to be dependent at a time in adult life when independence is expected. Manipulating a complex health-care system to have needs met is also a challenge to the individual. Accepting the role of being chronically ill and having a less-than-ideal state of health is included in coping with role changes.

Handling Physical Discomfort

Virtually all chronic illnesses are accompanied by some discomfort, either from the disorder itself (e.g., joint pain of arthritis) or from the prescribed therapy (e.g., insulin injections or hemodialysis treatment). The individual needs to discover personally satisfying and adequate means of dealing with pain. Modalities adjunctive to medications that have been effective include relaxation, autosuggestion, distraction (as with music), and biofeedback.

As pain becomes chronic, the sufferer devotes time and energy describing the discomfort so as to reinforce with others the idea that the pain is legitimate. The pain of a specific chronic illness such as arthritis is not as overt as pain of a fracture or surgical incisions. When the pain experience is prolonged and the chronically ill client's pain experience is not congruent with health-care workers' perception of the usual course of pain, the client may need constantly to reaffirm that the pain is real.

Complying with the Prescribed Regimen

It is one thing to make temporary adjustments in habits and daily patterns and quite another to alter habits for the rest of a lifetime. Acquiring new behaviors, taking medications, and so forth are less difficult compliance problems than altering personal habits and routine behaviors of smoking, drinking, and eating (Haynes, 1976). Helping sick individuals realize that their actions will result in desired outcomes is a challenge to health professionals, especially when the actions demand discipline and result in uncomfortable side effects.

Confronting the Inevitability of One's Own Death

Having a chronic illness causes reflection on life's accomplishments and a direct realization of the temporary nature of earthly existence. There may be thoughts of having "little time left," especially in comparison with the life expectancies of healthy friends. The goal is to confront this task, interpreting it as a challenge to make the most of life instead of giving in to paralyzing depression and anticipating one's own demise.

Dealing with Social Stigma

How does the chronically ill individual handle the second looks, the stares from children, and the embarrassment of being unable to enter buildings or use toilet facilities unassisted? Wright (1983) described three types of responses of individuals to stigmatizing behavior: (1) ignore it, bury one's head in the sand; (2) overreact with rage, retaliation, and overt hostility; and (3) use humor, which may cause further self-deprecation. Nurses can help chronically ill persons develop mature acceptance of self and undaunted self-confidence despite the disability.

Maintaining a Feeling of Being in Control

Chronically ill persons may find it difficult to maintain control because of intrusions into privacy by health-care teams and the sharing of intimate information on medical records for all interested onlookers to review. One client with brittle diabetes stated, "It's as though you're a butterfly with a pin stuck through you. The MDs come around to view you as a specimen on exhibit." The ability to control environmental intrusion while maintaining a sense of privacy preserves personal dignity.

Controlling a deteriorating physiological state may not always be possible, even in the best of compliance situations. Enhancing the client's knowledge of what is happening—physiological changes and improvements, and effects of therapy—increases a sense of control. Having the client make decisions about routine timing of therapy and altering habits gives the client psychological control. Nurses can plan for increasing client control according to Averill's (1973) categories: (1) behavior control—the individual's direct action on the environment; (2) cognitive control—the way in which an event is interpreted or appraised by the individual; and (3) decisional control—the opportunity to choose among various courses of action.

Maintaining Hope Despite Uncertainties or Downward Course of Illness

As the chronic health problem progresses, and as physiological deterioration and loss of function continue, hope is a sustaining force that helps the individual avoid despair and actually "prolongs life against all odds" (Korner, 1970). The course of events is unpredictable in chronic illness, in which remissions and exacerbations occur. There may be uncertainty in day-to-day functioning; for example, clients with rheumatoid arthritis may find planning ahead impossible because of unexpected pain and stiffness. To augment and confirm an individual's values and purposes in life and to help the individual establish realistic goals are challenges to the nurse and the individual's significant others. Pattison (1974) studied three types of predictors of death prognoses in 12 men with pulmonary emphysema over an 18-month period. He found that neither the physiological measures (blood gases and pulmonary studies) nor the psychological measure (Inpatient Multidimensional Psychiatric Scale) was correlated with death or clinical improvement. The only measure that correlated with death was the sociological tool that determined the nature of family and friend relationships. Clinical improvement correlated with intact and positive family relationships; death correlated with disruption and negative family relationships. Hope for life and the will to live are related to having something and someone to live for (Pattison, 1974).

COPING WITH CHRONIC ILLNESS: A DESCRIPTIVE STUDY

A study of 56 chronically ill adults was completed to determine the specific coping strategies used to deal with the tasks of being ill. The study sample consisted of the caseloads of 19 graduate students enrolled in a seminar-practicum course entitled "Nursing Strategies for Adults: Long-Term Health Problems" during two academic semesters. The graduate students, with the author's guidance, cared for and studied the clients for 3 months. The students used field notes to record the impact of chronic illness on the client's life; daily activities of leisure and work, family interaction, role disturbances, self-esteem, patterns of self-care, and grief work. Coping behaviors were documented and summarized from a review of field notes that were recorded throughout the semester. The coping strategies were recorded on a data collection tool "Impact of Chronic Illness." The aim of this tool was to enhance the students' understanding of the world of chronically ill persons as well as to collect data about coping.

Adults with chronic health problems hospitalized during exacerbations in a 700-bed metropolitan hospital were included in the sample. Clients in the sample ranged from ages 20 to 79, with the largest number being in the 40- to 69-year-old age group; 25 subjects were men and 31 were women (Table 2.2).

The medical diagnoses reported in Table 2.3 are the clients' major presenting diagnoses, which caused problems and/or incapacitation at the time of the study. Many clients had multiple diagnoses; for example, clients with coronary artery disease also had underlying diabetes. Only one diagnosis was tabulated for each client. The most frequent diag-

Table 2.2 ➤ **SAMPLE AGE AND SEX CHARACTERISTICS**

Age	Number of Men	Number of Women
20–29	2	5
30–39	2	3
40–49	5	7
50–59	7	6
60–69	6	8
70–79	3	2
Total	25	31

noses were cancer, 12 clients; diabetes, 9 clients; coronary artery disease, 9 clients; and ostomies, 5 clients. (See Table 2.3 for complete tabulation.)

Data on coping using the Impact of Chronic Illness Tool were analyzed to determine the various coping strategies used by 56 clients. The intent was not to categorize the clients as minimizers, focusers, or neutrals, but rather to discover as many effective coping strategies as possible. Coping strategies were considered effective if they met any one of the criteria listed in Figure 2.2 as modified from Visotsky, Hamburg, Goss, and Levobits (1961). More than one strategy was identified for each client. The coping behaviors were categorized as approach or avoidance strategies. Approach strategies are behaviors that indicate a willingness to confront the realities of the threat, an awareness of personal reactions and feelings, and an attempt to deal with these feelings. Avoidance strategies are behaviors that protect the individual from con-

Table 2.3 ➤ **NUMBER OF PREVALENT CHRONIC DISEASES**

Chronic Disease*	Number
Cancer	12
Coronary artery disease	9
Diabetes	9
Ostomies	5
Congestive heart failure	4
Arthritis	3
Chronic renal failure	3
Multiple sclerosis	3
Amputation	2
Paraplegia	2
Cerebral vascular accident	1
Hypertension	1
Peripheral vascular disease	1
Systemic lupus erythematosus	1
Total	56

*Many clients in the sample had multiple diagnoses. Only the major presenting diagnosis of each client that is causing problems at this time is listed.

Uncomfortable feelings
(anxiety, fear, grief, or guilt) contained

Hope generated

Self-esteem enhanced

Relationships with others maintained

State of wellness (self-actualized well-being)
maintained or improved

FIGURE 2.2 ➤ Criteria for effective coping.

scious confrontation with the threat. Table 2.4 summarizes the approach and avoidance behaviors.

Approach Strategies

The approach strategy most frequently used to deal with the tasks of chronic illness had to do with seeking information. Being attentive to the details of care and symptom control, participating in managing requirements of the illness, and raising questions without hesitation are examples of this approach strategy.

Enhancing one's spiritual life was the second most frequently used approach strategy. Specifically, individuals renewed their faith in God, prayed for strength to endure the threats, and received a sense of peace and hope as a result of "asking God for help." Clients related that they felt God's love and had strong convictions about His goodness to all earthly creatures. They felt that God would challenge them only with tasks He knew they could handle. When individuals interpreted handling the challenge as an expectation of God, they established a self-expectation to be successful.

Methods of self-distraction—diverting attention from illness to other facets of living—included submerging oneself in work and performing mental exercises such as solving problems and meditating. More passive self-distraction activities were watching television and doing needlework. Self-distraction was classified as an approach strategy when the client consciously selected these activities as a means of dealing with otherwise continuous thoughts about the illness. Another

Table 2.4 ▶ APPROACH AND AVOIDANCE COPING STRATEGIES OF 56 CHRONICALLY ILL ADULTS

Approach Coping Strategies	Number Using Strategy
1. Seeks information	14
—Focuses vigilantly on details of care	
—Eagerly learns illness-related modifications in habits, diet	
—Questions rationale for therapy	
—Compares staff responses to same questions	
2. Gains strength from spirituality	13
—Prayer	
—Faith	
3. Diverts attention	10
—Recognizes when becoming anxious; engages in extreme physical exertion or compulsive activity	
—Meditation	
—Pain distraction	
—Television	
—Needlework	
4. Expresses feelings and emotions	8
—Cries	
—Expresses hostility, anger	
—Describes powerlessness	
5. Uses relaxation exercises	6
6. Maintains control	5
—Of environment	
—Of daily activity schedules in hospital	
—Of ostomy care	
—Of advice-giving to spouse and nurse	
7. Verbalizes concerns	4
8. Maintains a positive healthy dependence on others	4
—For physical needs (shopping, housework)	
—For emotional needs (love, support)	

Avoidance Coping Strategies	Number Using Strategy
1. Uses denial, suppression, repression	11
2. Minimizes problems, signs, and symptoms of illness	9
3. Social isolation	6
—Disengages from previous activities and social relationships	
—Becomes preoccupied with self	
—Withdraws	
4. Avoids talking about self, feelings or thinking about health problem	6
5. Passive acceptance	5
—Belief in spiritual predestination	
—It's God's will; nothing can be done	
—Shows little or no emotional concern over existing problems	
6. Sleeps	3
7. Delays decision making on personal health matters	2
8. Considers alternative modes of therapy	2
—Unconventional diets	
9. Blames others	2
—Physician	
10. Refuses to participate in treatment	1
11. Excessive dependence on significant other	1
12. Manipulates others	1
—Significant other performs care tasks the patient could do	
13. Sets unrealistic goals	1
14. Unrealistic hope for future	1
—Functional abilities to return	
—Remission	

9. Uses positive thinking techniques — 4
   — Tries to see good in every situation
   — Autosuggestion for pain relief
10. Seeks help — 4
   — From diabetes nurse-specialist when patient determines it is needed
11. Maintains realistic independence — 4
   — Completes self-care activities within the limitations of illness
   — Relates past health experiences to future actions in caring for self (responding to insulin reactions)
   — Manipulates prescribed therapy, tranquilizers
   — Has realistic expectations for outcome of therapy
12. Maintains social activities — 3
   — Retirement activities
   — Church activities
13. Sets goals, strives to achieve them — 3
   — Attacks problems, "digs in" to get things done
14. Reminisces over past accomplishments — 3
   — Life review
15. Conserves energy — 3
   — Analyzes daily activity; saves energy for most desirable activity
   — Daily rest periods
16. Uses humor — 3
17. Intellectualization — 3
   — Mental mechanisms used to devise rational, personally meaningful explanations for occurrences (physical deterioration)
18. Engages in activities covering up disability, discomfort — 2
19. Role rehearsal — 2
   — Visualizes what it will be like as illness progresses
   — Rehearses a variety of personal outcomes as a result of therapy
20. Uses problem-solving approach — 2
21. Finds comfort in realizing there are other persons who are in the same boat — 1

15. Does not actively seek help — 1
16. Uses cigarettes, drugs, alcohol — 1

39

approach strategy was to be keenly aware of emotions and reactions to personal dilemmas and sharing these feelings with a helper. Some patients coped with stress by using a specific routine of physical relaxation exercises. Other specific strategies are listed in Table 2.4.

Avoidance Strategies

The mental mechanisms of denial, repression, and suppression are included in the most frequently used avoidance strategies. These influence all the avoidance strategies; that is, if the individual denies the fact that diabetes is serious, participation in treatment may be haphazard, or no help will be sought when assistance is needed. Both of the latter are other avoidance strategies. One client who was blind because of retinopathy of diabetes believed that her eyesight would return. Clients avoid the serious nature of their illness by minimizing symptoms and therapy, playing down consequences of their illness. This is noted in the way the clients describe the illness and refer to their being little affected by it. The third most common avoidance strategy was withdrawing from others, either to avoid disclosure about the impact of the illness or to continue preoccupation with self. In not talking about themselves and their health problems with health-care workers, clients use avoidance; other specific avoidance strategies are listed in Table 2.4.

Although the isolated strategies have been categorized as either approach or avoidance, it should be noted that many clients are in the center of the approach-avoidance continuum, using combinations of approach and avoidance strategies. Figure 2.3 illustrates a model for coping with chronic illness that identifies the tasks and depicts clients' use of coping strategies in which they characterize themselves as approachers, avoiders, or nonspecific defenders (combined approach and avoidance). Criteria for effective coping are included in the model.

Weisman and Worden (1976–1977) studied 120 clients coping with newly diagnosed cancer. A tool based on the coping scale of Sidle, Adams, and Cady (1969) was developed to categorize coping strategies of the clients with cancer. This tool included 15 coping behaviors such as seeking more information (rational inquiry), sharing concerns (mutuality), making light of the situation (affected reversal), doing something else (distraction), taking action regarding the problem (confronting), seeking direction (cooperative compliance), and blaming self (masochism). The coping behaviors used by each client were compared with their scores on three other indices: (1) the client's total mood disturbance was measured by the Profile of Mood States, (2) the client completed a self-rating revealing how adequately the problem was resolved, and (3) the client's vulnerability index was determined by a psychological interview. Weisman and Worden concluded that good copers used confrontation, redefinition of the problem (accepting the problem

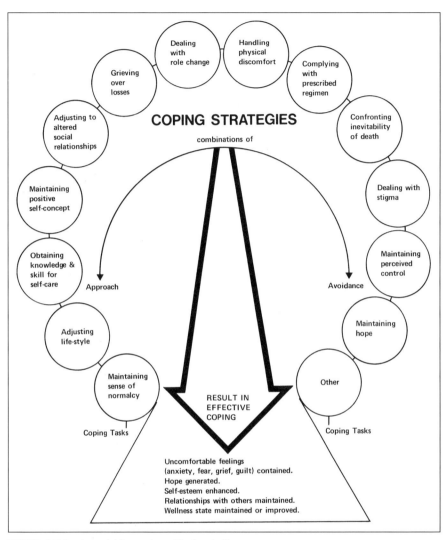

FIGURE 2.3 ➤ A model for coping with chronic illness.

and looking for positive aspects), and compliance with authority. Good copers had high resolution, low vulnerability, and low total mood disturbance. Poor copers used suppression, passivity, submission, and tension-reducing measures (such as drinking and drugs), and had low resolution, high vulnerability, and high total mood disturbance.

Weisman (1979) described good copers in more detail. Good copers are resourceful and are not rigid; they are characterized by the fact that they avoid denial and take action based on confronting reality, redefine problems into solvable forms—consider alternatives, maintain open communications, seek help and accept support, maintain high morale, and maintain hope.

ASSESSMENT AND STRATEGIES TO ENHANCE COPING

Nurses should avoid prescribing a favored coping technique without assessing the client's perceptions, feelings, suggested ways of dealing with the problem, and usual modes of coping. The nurse needs complete awareness of the nature of the threat. Information about coping can be obtained by selected interview questions. Paper-and-pencil coping instruments can be used for a quantitative evaluation.

Examples of coping interview questions to uncover primary and secondary appraisal information may include the following:

- Can you identify what makes you stressful or anxious? If so, what?
- How are you feeling about (mention the specific threat such as impending diagnostic test, treatment protocol, or living with the specific health problem)?
- What helps you deal with these feelings?
- How have you handled these kinds of situations in the past?
- Has this (e.g., arthritis) changed your life? If so, in what way(s)?
- What helps you handle these changes and/or stresses? How do you deal with the ups and downs?
- What has helped you through difficulty in the past? Have you tried these methods now?
- Do you generally like all the detailed information you can get about a difficult event or threatening situation, or do you prefer not facing it head-on?

Specific ideas may be stimulated in the assessment by reviewing a list of strategies and inquiring whether they are meaningful for the client.

- Are religion and prayer important to you?
- Do you use specific distractions?
- Do you know any relaxation exercises?
- Have you tried mental imagery?
- Do you share your perceptions, reactions, and fears with someone else who is close to you?
- Are you able to find and concentrate on positive aspects of most situations?
- Do you readily seek help from others?
- Do you try to put difficulties out of your mind?

- Do you rely on your problem-solving ability?
- Has daydreaming or fantasizing helped you?

Instruments to evaluate coping to be used in a research context or to validate clinical impressions and nursing diagnoses have been developed. Those most appropriate for nursing include the Jalowiec Coping Scale (Jalowiec, 1989); Coping Strategies Inventory (Quayhagen & Quayhagen, 1982); Ways of Coping Checklist (Lazarus & Folkman, 1984); Coping Responses Scale (Moos, Cronkite, Billings, & Finney, 1984); Coping Strategies Scale (Weisman & Worden, 1976–1977); Coping Scale (Sidle, Adams, & Cady, 1969); Pain Management Strategies (Brown, Nicassio, & Wallston, 1989); Daily Coping Checklist (Stone & Neale, 1984); Chronicity Impact and Coping Instrument, for parents with ill children (Hymovich, 1984); and Family Crisis Oriented Personal Evaluation Scale: F-COPES (McCubbin, Olson, & Larsen, 1987).

Expanding Coping Repertoires

Strategies to develop or expand coping repertoires include use of a self-regulation approach, cognitive control strategies such as stress inoculation, and other miscellaneous approaches.

Self-Regulation

Self-regulation theory is based on developing a cognitive scheme (mental map) to guide incoming information, retrieve stored information, focus attention, and guide behavior (Johnson, 1984; Leventhal & Johnson, 1983). Preparatory information and past experience influence the composition of the scheme clients develop regarding impending health-care events, threatening intrusive procedures, or deterioration in health. Clients are helped to focus attention on the objective characteristics of the experience rather than on the subjective emotions provoked and negative evaluative reactions. Information is given in a clear and unambiguous manner, describing as exactly as possible the event to be experienced. Physical sensations to be experienced are reviewed, including what will be felt, seen, heard, smelled, and tasted. These physical sensations are those experienced by most persons going through this event. The environment in which the event will take place needs to be described as well as the duration and sequence of happenings during the anxiety-provoking event. When possible, self-care activities to promote comfort are also shared (Johnson & Lauver, 1989; Johnson, Lauver, & Nail, 1989). In summary, the self-regulation approach to coping enhancement includes providing concrete objective information about physical sensations to be experienced, environmental features, and temporal characteristics. The goal in implementing this coping strategy is to enhance understanding of the experience, reduce its abstract nature, and increase confidence in dealing with the situation by focusing attention on the objective, not on the unpleasant, uncomfortable nature of the experience.

The effects of using self-regulation were evaluated in 84 men having radiation therapy for prostatic cancer who were randomly assigned to an experimental or control group (Johnson, Lauver, & Nail, 1989). The self-regulation procedure used a series of four tape recordings administered: (1) before treatments began, informing patients of the treatment plan; (2) just before the first treatment, describing the size and location of the treatment room, sound of the treatment machine, length of treatment; (3) at the fifth treatment, providing information about the nature, timing, and pattern of side effects of therapy; (4) at the last week of treatment, describing changes in side effects following completion of the therapy. Self-care activities to prevent or minimize side effects were included in the third and fourth tapes. The same researcher spent the same amount of time with men in the control group discussing the clients' well-being and using social conversation. Measurements of function and mood were taken during the first, third, and last week of treatment and at 1 and 3 months posttreatment (Johnson, Lauver, & Nail, 1989). Persons receiving the experimental procedure experienced less disruption in function as measured by the recreation and pastime subscale of the Sickness Impact Profile (Bergner, Bobbitt, Carter, & Gilson, 1981). No differences were found on negative mood scores measured by the Profile of Mood States (McNair, Lorr, & Doppelman, 1971).

The primary purpose of the self-regulation strategies is to create cognitive schemata that enable the person to cope with threatening events. The goal is to decrease any discrepancy between what clients expect and what actually happens to them. Key types of information are (1) physical sensations to be experienced, (2) characteristics of the environment, and (3) temporal information. Baker and Stern (1993) described a process of mobilizing self-care in chronic illness by: (1) assenting to the chronic illness and (2) reframing the implications of illness into a positive optimistic mindset, thus controlling one's thoughts and eliminating a negative outlook.

Cognitive Control Strategies

Stress inoculation training (SIT) is a technique aimed at desensitizing individuals to events they perceive as threatening. It combines teaching, discussion, cognitive restructuring, problem solving, relaxation, behavioral rehearsal, self-monitoring, self-instruction, and self-reinforcement (Meichenbaum, 1985). Persons develop a sense of *learned resourcefulness* and become immune to coping failure when confronting stress. Meichenbaum (1985) highlights the specific purposes of SIT:

- Teach clients that stress and coping are transactional
- Develop clients' skills to monitor maladaptive thoughts and behavior
- Develop clients' problem-solving skills
- Develop emotion regulation and self-control coping skills
- Sensitize clients to recognize and use maladaptative responses as cues to implement substitutive coping behaviors

Overall SIT should help patients become knowledgeable, enabling them to use self-understanding and coping skills to handle the stress of illness. The phases of teaching this coping strategy include conceptualization, skill acquisition and rehearsal, and application and follow-through.

During the conceptualization phase, a helping relationship is established between the client and nurse. The stress-related problems and the client's responses and feelings are clarified. Nonthreatening probes may be used by the nurse such as, "Is this what I hear you saying? I get the feeling that repeated doctor visits create anxiety about discovering cancer recurrence; is this the way you see it? Tell me more about that." Clients may be asked to re-create an image of the stress-provoking event and share reactions to it. Clients are taught that thoughts and emotions play a role in creating and maintaining a stressful state. After clients are helped to identify their reactions, they are taught to monitor their thoughts, feelings, and behaviors related to stressors of interest.

During the skill acquisition and rehearsal phase, relaxation training, elimination of negative self-talk and substitution of positive self-statements (Table 2.5), role playing, and mental rehearsals take place. The newly learned behaviors are then used in stress-provoking situations and their effects are evaluated. Modifications of SIT have been effective with clients with cancer (Moore & Altmaier, 1981; Weisman & Sobel, 1979) and with clients in rehabilitation (Corburn & Manderino, 1986).

Table 2.5 ➤ **EXAMPLES OF NEGATIVE AND POSITIVE SELF-TALK**

Negative Self-Talk	Positive Self-Talk
I can't handle this.	I need to take one day at a time.
	I'm doing the best I can.
This is the worst thing that could have happened to me.	I am strong and will not be defeated.
How can this happen to me?	Life on earth means confronting difficulties.
This place is terrible.	I am lucky to be where the latest technology and know-how exist.

Other Strategies

Emotion-focused strategies are attempts to eliminate or control emotional responses to aversive events by using relaxation, deep breathing, focusing on calmness, practicing calming self-talk ("It will be over soon. I'll be fine. I'm fortunate to be in such good hands."), redirecting attention by using pleasant mental images. *Problem-focused* strategies are those using information providing accurate expectations about sensory and procedural properties of an impending stimulus. Martelli, Auerbach, Alexander, and Mercuri (1987) found that combinations of problem-focused and emotion-focused interventions were most helpful in 46 clients' responses to oral surgery. Emotion-focused interventions, when used alone, resulted in the lowest adjustment levels measured by the Krantz Health Opinion Survey Information (Krantz, Baum, & Wideman, 1980). Preoperative anxiety was directly related to postoperative pain and inversely related to postoperative adjustment.

COPING WITH SPECIFIC HEALTH PROBLEMS

Cancer

Persons may experience differing stressors (coping tasks) depending on the type of chronic health problem they have. Cancer may provoke emotional distress including depression, anxiety, and anger; physical symptoms; disruption in daily life patterns and relationships including marital and sexual activities; and fears regarding disease progression and death (Meyerowitz, Heinrich, & Schag, 1983). Hinton (1973) identified six major stressors of 100 clients with cancer to be pain, disfigurement, concern over the future (dying), loss of work role, dependency, and alienation. Woods, Lewis, and Ellison's (1989) review of living with cancer confirmed sexuality, communication, intimacy, and role changes as family concerns. Living with a chronic illness such as cancer requires behavioral skills such as relaxation, assertiveness, and problem solving (Heinrich & Schag, 1984; Miller & Nygren, 1978). Gotay (1984) discovered that women with breast cancer and their spouses used different coping strategies at the beginning and advanced stages of the illness. During the early stages, women sought information, used self-talk, tried to put it out of their minds, found something favorable in their situation, and took firm action. Spouses sought direction, sought information from an authority, took firm action, and accepted the inevitable. During the advanced stage, women used self-talk and prayer, had faith and hope, found something favorable about the situation, and talked with others. Their mates took firm action, used prayer and self-talk, and shared with others. Taking firm action was prevalent for both spouses in both stages of the illness and refers to taking care of one's business in the early stages, and in the advanced stage involved actions that enabled others to plan for life after death of the woman. Hope was a prevalent coping strategy during the advanced stage for both spouses (Gotay, 1984). Herth (1989) found a significant relationship between hope and successful coping in 120 adults with cancer undergoing chemotherapy.

Forty spouses of men with cancer, identified as having difficulty coping, disclosed in interviews that their major difficulties were emotional, social, family, and financial needs (Kalayjian, 1989). Uncertainty was a problem for 50 percent of the wives. The following nursing behaviors were identified as helpful to their coping: listening, talking, caring, availability, sensitivity, empathy, and honesty. Nursing interventions that family judged helpful to their coping were discovered from 62 family members responding to vignettes of persons with cancer in an initial, adaptational (transitional), and terminal phase of illness (Lewandowski & Jones, 1988). The most helpful interventions during the initial phase were giving a clear explanation of what is being done for the ill member and keeping the ill member comfortable. Being kept informed was the most helpful intervention during the adaptation phase, and providing time alone for the client and family member was the most important for the terminal phase.

Cardiac

Perception of adequate social support has been related to effective coping by wives of men with coronary artery disease and myocardial infarctions (MIs) (Riegel, 1989; Riffle, 1988). As a result of studying 40 wives of clients who had an MI, Nyamathi (1987) made the following nursing care recommendations to enhance the spouses' coping:

- Involve the couple in the plan of care, particularly planning for postdischarge.
- Provide explicit, pertinent information to the couple.
- Consistently provide reassurance, concern, and a positive attitude as a communication style.
- Prepare for discharge including specifics about diet, exercise, sexual activity, preparation for cardiac emergency, follow-up, and cardiac rehabilitation program as appropriate.
- Review existing coping resources such as social support.

Of the 60 adults who underwent cardiac surgery studied by Anderson (1987), those who were in the experimental groups (receiving preoperative information or the group receiving preoperative information plus coping preparation) had significantly less preoperative anxiety and fear and postoperatively had more positive affect and less incidence of sudden hypertension than the control group.

Preparation of 60 adults for cardiac catheterization using one of five methods was studied to determine the impact of those coping methods on client anxiety. The experimental group consisted of variations of self-regulation (Johnson & Lauver, 1989) using videotapes presenting (1) sensory procedural information; (2) modeling—a client describing the experience; (3) cognitive behavioral coping (procedural information plus relaxation, reframing with self-reinforcing statements and distraction); (4) modeling plus coping; (5) attention to placebo group receiving information about the structure and function of the heart. Persons in all four of the treatment groups had less anxiety than those in the placebo group (Anderson & Masur, 1989).

Other Health Alterations

Langer, Janis, and Wolfer (1975) studied the effectiveness of a coping strategy on reducing stress in surgical clients. The coping device was based on use of distraction and perception control. Clients were taught to direct attention toward favorable aspects of the anticipated stressful situation. The client was made to feel in control by using the strategy of cognitive reappraisal of the anxiety provoking events and calming self-talk. Clients were taught that it is rarely the events themselves that cause stress, but rather the views people take of events and attention given to these views. Clients were taught to rehearse the positive aspects of hospitalization (improving health, receiving care and attention, having a rare opportunity to relax, and enjoying temporary relief from the pressures of the world).

Sixty clients were divided into four groups of preparation. Group 1 received the coping device described. Group 2 received preparatory information only, that is, preoperative skin preparation instructions and information about medications, anesthesia, and how the client would feel after surgery, with incisional pain, nausea, and constipation described as possible discomforts. Group 3 received a combination of preparation information and the coping device. Group 4 served as a control and received only information about hospital routines. Nurses blindly rated the subjects' anxiety and ability to cope with discomfort before and after the researcher intervention. There was a rapid decrease in anxiety and increase in ability to cope in the group given the coping strategy. Postoperatively, the group given the coping device required fewer pain medications and fewer sedatives than the groups not given the device. There was no significant difference among the groups in the number of days of hospital stay (Langer, Janis, & Wolfer, 1975).

The strategy described by Langer is appropriate for nurses to use to help clients cope not only with stresses that are short term in nature, such as facing surgery, but also with stresses lasting a lifetime, as in the case of chronic disease.

Dimond (1980) studied the effects of two coping strategies used by 36 clients on hemodialysis to adapt to chronic hemodialysis. The two coping strategies were client-perceived progress in managing dialysis (cognitive control) and client use of short-term planning (behavioral control). Adaptation was determined by subjects' morale scores (Behavior-Morale Scale), changes in social function (Sickness Impact Profile), number of medical problems, and stability of physical status. Those subjects who used the two coping strategies had significantly higher scores at the 0.05 level on the four measures of adaptation. Dimond emphasized that short-term planning was one way that clients on dialysis could control their daily lives. She suggested that, in addition to teaching clients with renal failure about the disease and its treatment, teaching specific skills in short-term planning is important to enhance the client's perception of personal competence and control.

Does the coping capacity of chronically ill individuals decrease as the illness continues over long periods? Although there is no conclusive answer based on research, it seems logical that nurses should generate specific strategies clients can try out as the illness progresses. Determining the combinations of strategies that are appropriate to the client's coping style and control orientation is the challenge. Much nursing research on the topic of coping is needed.

Specific tasks confronting chronically ill persons can be labeled coping tasks. Individuals have unique means of responding to the tasks (using coping strategies) in order to master, control, or resolve the tasks. Collectively, the coping tasks of chronic illness precipitate powerlessness. Coping facilitates powerfulness.

REFERENCES

Anderson, E. (1987). Preoperative preparation for cardiac surgery facilitates recovery, reduces psychological distress and reduces the incidence of acute postoperative hypertension. *Journal of Consulting and Clinical Psychology, 55,* 513–520.

Anderson, K., & Masur, F. (1989). Psychologic preparation for cardiac catheterization. *Heart and Lung, 18,* 154–163.

Andrew, J. (1973). Coping style and declining verbal abilities. *Journal of Gerontology, 28,* 179–183.

Auerbach, S. (1989). Stress management and coping research in the health care setting: An overview and methodological commentary. *Journal of Consulting and Clinical Psychology, 57,* 388–395.

Averill, J. (1973). Personal control over aversion stimuli and its relationship to stress. *Psychological Bulletin, 88,* 286–303.

Baker, C., & Stern, P. (1993). Finding meaning in chronic illness as the key to self-care. *Canadian Journal of Nursing Research, 25,* 23–36.

Bergner, M., Bobbitt, R. A., Carter, W. B., & Gilson, B. S. (1981). The Sickness Impact Profile: Development and final revision of a health status measure. *Medical Care, 19,* 787–805.

Beutel, M. (1985). Approaches to taxonomy and measurement of adaptation in chronic disease. *Psychotherapy and Psychosomatics, 43,* 177–185.

Brown, G., Nicassio, P., & Wallston, K. (1989). Pain coping strategies and depression in rheumatoid arthritis. *Journal of Consulting and Clinical Psychology, 57,* 652–657.

Bruner, J. (1966). *Toward a theory of instruction.* Cambridge, MA: Belknap University Press of Harvard University.

Caplan, G. (1963). Emotional crises. In A. Deutsch (Ed.), *The encyclopedia of mental health* (Vol. 2). New York: Franklin Watts.

Charmaz, K. (1973). *Time and identity: The shaping of selves of the chronically ill.* Unpublished doctoral dissertation, San Francisco: University of California.

Coburn, J., & Manderino, M. (1986). Stress inoculation: An illustration of coping skills training. *Rehabilitation Nursing, 11,* 14–17.

Cohen, F., & Lazarus, R. (1973). Active coping processes, coping dispositions and recovery from surgery. *Psychosomatic Medicine, 35,* 375–389.

Davis, M. (1975). Social isolation as a process in chronic illness. In M. Davis, M. Kramer, & A. Strauss (Eds.), *Nurses in practice: A perspective on work environments* (pp. 253–259). St. Louis: CV Mosby.

Deatrick, J. (1988). The process of parenting a child with a disability: Normalization through accommodations. *Journal of Advanced Nursing, 13,* 15–21.

Dimond, M. (1980). Patient strategies for managing maintenance hemodialysis. *Western Journal of Nursing Research, 2,* 555–568.

Feldman, D. (1974). Chronic disabling illness: A holistic view. *Journal of Chronic Disease, 27,* 287–291.

Garland, L., & Bush, C. (1982). *Coping behaviors and nursing.* Reston, VA: Reston Publishing.

Goldstein, M. F., Jones, R. B., Clemens, T. L., Flagg, G. W., & Alexander, F. G. (1965). Coping style as a factor in psychophysiological response to tension-arousing film. *Journal of Personality and Social Psychology, 1,* 200–302.

Gotay, C. (1984). The experience of cancer during early and advanced stages: The views of patients and their mates. *Social Science and Medicine, 18,* 605–613.

Haan, N. (1977). *Coping and defending: Processes of self-environmental organization.* New York: Academic Press.

Haynes, R. B. (1976). A critical review of the determinants of patient compliance with therapeutic regimens. In D. Sackett & R. B. Haynes (Eds.), *Compliance with therapeutic regimens.* Baltimore: Johns Hopkins University Press.

Heinrich, R., & Schag, C. (1984). A behavioral medicine approach to coping with cancer: A case report. *Cancer Nursing, 7,* 243–247.

Herth, K. (1989). The relationship between level of hope and level of coping responses and other variables in patients with cancer. *Oncology Nursing Forum, 16,* 67–72.

Hinton, J. (1973). Bearing cancer. *British Journal of Medical Psychology, 46,* 105–113.

Hymovich, D. (1984). Development of the Chronicity Impact and Coping Instrument: Parent Questionnaire (CICI:PQ). *Nursing Research, 33,* 218–222.

Jalowiec, A. (1989). Confirmatory factor analysis of the Jalowiec Coping Scale. In C. Waltz & O. Stricland (Eds.), *Measurement of nursing outcomes: Vol. 1. Measuring client outcomes* (pp. 287–308). New York: Springer.

Johnson, J. (1984). Psychological interventions and coping with surgery. In A. Baum, S. E. Taylor, & J. E. Singer (Eds.), *Handbook of psychology and health: Vol. 4. Social psychological aspects of health* (pp. 167–176). Hillsdale, NJ: L. Erlbaum Associates.

Johnson, J., & Lauver, D. (1989). Alternative explanations of coping with stressful experiences associated with physical illness. *Advances in Nursing Science, 11,* 39–52.

Johnson, J., Lauver, D., & Nail, L. (1989). Process of coping with radiation therapy. *Journal of Consulting and Clinical Psychology, 5,* 358–364.

Kalayjian, A. (1989). Coping with cancer: The spouse's perspective. *Archives of Psychiatric Nursing, 3,* 166–172.

Kassebaum, G., & Bauman, B. (1965). Dimensions of the sick role in chronic illness. *Journal of Health and Human Development, 6,* 16–27.

Kiely, W. F. (1972). Coping with severe illness. *Advanced Psychosomatic Medicine, 8,* 105–118.

Knafl, K., & Deatrick, J. (1986). How families manage chronic conditions: An analysis of the concept of normalization. *Research in Nursing and Health, 9,* 215–222.

Korner, I. (1970). Hope as a method of coping. *Journal of Consulting Psychology, 34,* 134–139.

Krantz, D. S., Baum, A., & Wideman, M. (1980). Assessment of preferences for self-treatment and information in health care. *Journal of Personality and Social Psychology, 39,* 977–990.

Langer, E., Janis, I., & Wolfer, J. (1975). Reduction of psychological stress in surgical patients. *Journal of Experimental Social Psychology, 11,* 155–165.

Lazarus, R. (1966). *Psychological stress and the coping process.* New York: McGraw-Hill.

Lazarus, R., & Folkman, S. (1984). *Stress, appraisal and coping.* New York: Springer.

Leventhal, H., & Johnson, J. (1983). Laboratory and field experimentation: Development of a theory of self-regulation. In P. Wooldridge, M. Schmitt, J. Skipper, & R. Leonard (Eds.), *Behavioral science and nursing theory* (pp. 189–262). St. Louis: CV Mosby.

Lewandowski, W., & Jones, S. (1988). The family with cancer. *Cancer Nursing, 11,* 313–321.

Lipowski, Z. (1969). Psychosocial aspects of disease. *Annals of Internal Medicine, 71,* 1197–1206.

Lipowski, Z. (1970). Physical illness, the individual and the coping process. *Psychiatry in Medicine, 1,* 91–102.

Lomont, J. (1965). The repression-sensitization dimension in relation to anxiety responses. *Journal of Consulting Psychiatry, 29,* 84–86.

Martelli, M. F., Auerbach, S. M., Alexander, J., & Mercuri, L. G. (1987). Stress management in the health care setting: Matching interventions with patient coping styles. *Journal of Consulting and Clinical Psychology, 55,* 201–207.

McCubbin, H., Olson, D., & Larson, A. (1987). F-COPES: Family Crisis Oriented Personal Evaluation Scales. In H. McCubbin & A. Thompson (Eds.), *Family assessment inventories for research and practice* (pp. 194–207). Madison: University of Wisconsin Press.

McNair, D. M., Lorr, M., & Doppelman, L. F. (1971). *Manual for the profile of mood states.* San Diego: Educational and Industrial Testing Service.

Mechanic, D. (1974). Social structure and personal adaptation: Some neglected dimensions. In G. V. Coelho, D. H. Hamburg, & J. E. Adams (Eds.), *Coping and adaptation.* New York: Basic Books.

Meichenbaum, D. (1985). *Stress inoculation training.* New York: Pergamon Press.

Melies, A. (1975). Role insufficiency and role supplementation: A conceptual framework. *Nursing Research, 24,* 264–271.

Meyerowitz, B., Heinrich, R., & Schag, C. (1983). A competency-based approach to coping with cancer. In T. Burish & L. Bradley (Eds.), *Coping with chronic disease: Research and applications* (pp. 137–158). New York: Academic Press.

Miller, M., & Nygren, C. (1978). Living with cancer: Coping behaviors. *Cancer Nursing, 1,* 297–302.

Miller, S., & Mangan, C.E. (1983). Interacting effects of information and coping style in adapting to gynecological stress: When should the doctor tell all? *Journal of Personality and Social Psychology, 45,* 223–236.

Moore, K., & Altmaier, E. M. (1981). Stress inoculation training with cancer patients. *Cancer Nursing, 4,* 389–393.

Moos, R., Cronkite, R., Billings, A., & Finney, J. (1984). *Health and daily living form manual.* Palo Alto, CA: Social Ecology Laboratory, Department of Psychiatry, Stanford University Veterans Administration Hospital.

Mullen, B., & Suls, J. (1982). The effectiveness of attention and rejection as coping styles. *Journal of Psychosomatic Research, 26,* 43–49.

Nyamathi, A. (1987). The coping responses of female spouses of patients with myocardial infarction. *Heart and Lung, 16,* 86–91.

Parsons, T. (1951). *The social system.* New York: The Free Press.

Pattison, M. (1974). Psychosocial predictors of death prognosis. *Omega, 5,* 145–159.

Peralin, L. I., & Schooler, C. (1978). The structure of coping. *Journal of Health and Social Behavior, 19,* 2–21.

Quayhagen, M., & Quayhagen, M. (1982). Coping with conflict: Measurement of age-related patterns. *Research on Aging, 4,* 364–377.

Riding, T. M. (1997). Normalization: Analysis and application within a special hospital. *Journal of Psychiatric and Mental Health Nursing, 4,* 23–28.

Riegel, B. (1989). Social support and psychological adjustment to chronic coronary heart disease: Operationalization of Johnson's Behavioral System Model. *Advances in Nursing Science, 11,* 74–84.

Riffle, K. (1988). The relationship between perception of supportive behaviors of others and wives' ability to cope with initial myocardial infarctions in their husbands. *Rehabilitation Nursing, 13,* 310–314.

Roth, S., & Cohen, L. (1986). Approach, avoidance, and coping with stress. *American Psychologist, 41,* 813–819.

Seligman, M. (1995). *Helplessness: On depression, development, and death.* San Francisco: WH Freeman and Co.

Shanan, J., De Nour, A., Kaplan, A., & Schak, G. (1976). Effects of prolonged stress on coping style in terminal renal failure patients. *Journal
of Human Stress, 2,* 19–27.

Sidle, A., Adams, J., & Cady, P. (1969). Development of a coping scale.
Archives of General Psychiatry, 20, 226–232.

Stapleton, S. (1978). *Coping with chronic illness.* Unpublished paper. Milwaukee, WI: Marquette University College of Nursing.

Stone, A., & Neale, J. (1984). New measure of daily coping: Development
and preliminary results. *Journal of Personality and Social Psychology,
46,* 892–906.

Visotsky, H., Hamurg, D., Goss, M., & Levobits, B. (1961). Coping behavior
under extreme stress. *Archives of General Psychiatry, 5,* 27–52.

Weisman, A. (1979). *Coping with cancer.* New York: McGraw-Hill.

Weisman, A., & Sobel, H. (1979). Coping with cancer through self-instruction: A hypothesis. *Journal of Human Stress, 5,* 3–8.

Weisman, A., & Worden, W. (1976–1977). The existential plight in cancer:
Significance of the first 100 days. *International Journal of Psychiatry
and Medicine, 7,* 1–15.

Wiener, C. (1975). The burden of rheumatoid arthritis: Tolerating uncertainty. *Social Science Medicine, 9,* 97–104.

Woods, N., Lewis, F., & Ellison, E. (1989). Living with cancer: Family experiences. *Cancer Nursing, 12,* 28–33.

Wright, B. (1983). *Physical disability: A psychosocial approach.* New York:
Harper & Row.

Development of the Concept of Powerlessness:

A Nursing Diagnosis

➤ Judith Fitzgerald Miller

Development of the concept of powerlessness is the focus of this chapter. The process of concept development involves distinct phases such as developing a commitment to study the concept as a result of experienced challenges and/or piqued curiosity, defining the concept in a working-definition format, reviewing the literature to substantiate current concept development, making observations in the field, drawing conclusions from one's own and others' descriptive research, and designing predictive and prescriptive studies. The phases of concept development emphasized in this chapter include reviewing the literature (deriving theoretical propositions and proposing nursing practice speculations), and reporting field observations. Powerlessness manifested in the specific health problems of acquired immunodeficiency syndrome (AIDS) and cancer are included as prototypes.

Methods of concept analysis and development have been proposed by Chinn and Jacobs (1994), Norris (1982), Rodgers, (1989a, 1989b), Rodgers and Knafl (1993), and Walker and Avant (1988). Wilson's (1970) technique of concept analysis has influenced nursing's methods in explicating the nature of phenomena of concern for this discipline. See Forsyth's (1980) concept analysis of empathy for an example. This research on concept clarification, analysis, and development has provided for development of nursing's body of knowledge.

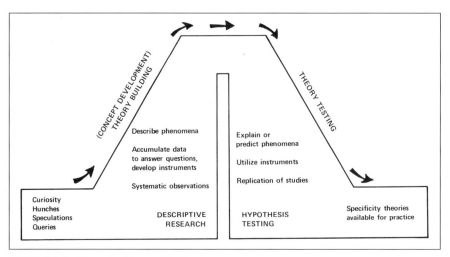

FIGURE 3.1 ➤ Theory building and testing.

Developing and validating new nursing diagnostic categories requires concept analysis and systematic investigation. A descriptive research approach in developing the concept of powerlessness is used throughout this book. Dubin (1978) distinguished between descriptive and hypothesis-testing research. He stated that descriptive research is the questioning, or theory-building, side of research. For purposes of this book, development of the concept of powerlessness takes place on this side of the model. Hypothesis testing is the answer-seeking, theory-testing side (Fig. 3.1).

Before hypotheses can be formulated and tested, systematic observations of phenomena must take place. Observations of clients in states of powerlessness have been made and are reported in this book. Interest and curiosity have been piqued by these observations of individuals whose physical conditions plunged downward despite strict adherence to prescribed regimens.

Nurses are challenged to help clients achieve a sense of control and avoid or alleviate powerlessness. Nurses need to be able to recognize the nursing diagnosis, determine which clients are vulnerable to diagnoses related to powerlessness, design nursing strategies to alleviate the diagnosis, and evaluate outcomes.

RELATED THEORIES AND POWERLESSNESS DEFINED

Constructs such as helplessness, learned helplessness, external locus of control, and powerlessness connote that individuals believe that outcomes of events are not contingent upon their own behaviors. Each construct has some uniqueness and specificity. Learned helplessness and locus of control are presented in the literature as theories.

A person who experiences repeated uncontrollable events may eventually manifest learned helplessness. That is, persons come to expect noncontingency between their actions and the resulting outcomes. This expectancy may be transferred to many life experiences. Three deficits result: (1) motivation deficits—hesitancy to take action; (2) cognitive deficits—the inaccurate expectation of uncontrollability is transferred to other life situations; and (3) affect deficits—apathy, withdrawal, depression, and decreased self-esteem (Seligman, 1995). Because persons assigned reasons for their uncontrollability, the concept or attribution was added to the revised theory of helplessness (Abramson, Seligman, & Teasdale, 1978). Persons attribute their helplessness to stable or unstable, global or specific, and personal or external factors. When persons attribute their helplessness to a broad range of situations and helplessness is present in varied situations, the attributions are said to be global and stable. Persons who attribute their lack of control to personal, stable, and global factors will be more vulnerable to depression and have lower self-esteem than persons who attribute powerlessness to universal, unstable, and specific factors (Abramson, Garber, & Seligman, 1980; Maiden, 1987; Murphy, 1982). Cumulative losses, disabilities, and impairments of elderly people and chronically ill render them vulnerable to perceived helplessness (Slimmer, Lopez, LeSage, & Ellor, 1987).

Locus-of-control theory is founded on social learning theory and posits that potential for a behavior to occur in any situation is a function of the expectancy that the behavior will lead to a valued reinforcement (Rotter, 1975). The generalized expectancy that one's reinforcements are directly the result of one's own behavior is labeled internal locus-of-control orientation. The expectancy that outcomes (reinforcements) are determined by powerful others, fate, luck, or chance is termed an external locus-of-control orientation. Thousands of papers have been published on differences in locus of control, and, generally, people with an internal locus of control (internals) are described as more potent, competent, effective, and able to take action to modify aversive situations (Wallston & Wallston, 1989). Internals seem to be desirable in this age of taking responsibility for one's own health. Wallston and Wallston (1981, 1989) expanded the conceptualization to a multidimensional health locus-of-control concept by developing the scale to measure Internal Health Locus of Control (IHLC) and two external scales: Powerful Other Health Locus of Control (PHLC) referring to doctors, nurses, family, or friends, and Chance Health Locus of Control (CHLC) measuring health and illness as a matter of fate, luck, or chance. Helplessness and locus of control are based on a reinforcement paradigm, whereas powerlessness is an existential construct (Lewis,

1982). An existential focus refers to the "here and now," the current circumstance or situation rather than to an enduring personality trait such as locus of control.

Powerlessness is the perception that one lacks the capacity or authority to act to affect an outcome of a current situation or immediate happening. When one or more of the power resources of physical strength, psychological stamina, self-concept, energy, knowledge, motivation, and belief system are compromised, powerlessness is a potential problem (see Fig. 1.1.) In contrast to locus of control, powerlessness is situationally determined. Locus of control is directly related to powerlessness and is a rather stable personality trait. Locus of control seems to be a long-term tendency or a stable view of why events take place.

The studies on powerlessness were analyzed in the following categories: powerlessness and learning, individuals' beliefs or illusions and control, effects of no control on animals, effects of no control on humans' physiologic response and problem solving, control in selected health-illness situations, and powerlessness as a precipitant of death.

For each section of literature reviewed, theoretical propositions (Newman, 1979) are deduced. Theoretical propositions are translations and conclusions drawn from research findings. Some interpretation for nursing practice are included in each section. These interpretations are labeled practice speculations. They are derived from theoretical propositions, and although they have logical practice relevance, they need to be tested.

LITERATURE REVIEW

Powerlessness and Learning

Seeman (1962) concluded that powerlessness leads to poor learning of control-relevant information. Clients hospitalized with tuberculosis who were high in powerlessness knew fewer facts about the disease and maintaining health than did a matched sample who were low in powerlessness. The clients low in powerlessness were less satisfied with information given by staff and were rated by the staff as being more knowledgeable about their illness. In Seeman's study of prisoners (1963), there was no difference between high-powerlessness and low-powerlessness prisoners' knowledge of life in the correctional institution; however, prisoners who were low in powerlessness had more knowledge about parole matters, that is, how to get out on parole and conditions while on parole. The premise for Seeman's (1967) studies is that "An individual's generalized expectancy for control of his outcomes governs attention to and acquisition of information available in the environment" (p. 105). Seeman also correlated high powerlessness with low political awareness (1972) and low nuclear survival knowledge (1967).

Phares, Ritchie, and Davis (1968) studied acquisition and utilization of information in subjects with internal or external locus of control. Both groups were taught information until they had perfect recall. The subjects then had to use the information in a computer simulation task. They found that, although the internals and externals did not differ in the acquisition of material, internals provided significantly more reasons for decisions made during the simulation task than did the externals, and differential retention of the information did not explain the internals' superior utilization of the information.

Nineteen externals and 21 internals were given personality tests and informed of reports containing negative and positive information about their personalities. The externals had greater recall of the negative information given to them about themselves than did internals. The internals were more willing to try remedial behaviors to improve than were the externals (Phares et al., 1968).

Giving learners a choice, such as determining the series in which to take a test (Stotland & Blumenthal, 1964), resulted in lower anxiety as indicated by palmar sweating than did not giving individuals a choice. Perlmutter and Monty (1973) demonstrated that the group given the choice of lists for word memorization did better than the group given no choice. The theoretical propositions (translation and conclusion statements) and practice speculations are presented in Figure 3.2.

Theoretical Propositions	Practice Speculations
1. Perceived powerlessness leads to poor learning of control-relevant information.	Before beginning client teaching, determine the client's feelings of powerlessness.
2. Involving learners in decision making regarding content to be learned enhances learning.	Clients with an internal locus of control need emphasis on information that gives them a sense of control.
3. The personality trait locus of control influences ability to utilize control-relevant information.	High-powerless clients may need structured approaches, teaching of self-care in small increments so clients can feel a sense of control without being overwhelmed with care demands.
	Involve clients by having them determine what aspects of care they are ready to learn and when they want to learn them.

FIGURE 3.2 ➤ Powerlessness and learning.

DISCUSSION OF PRACTICE SPECULATION

The phrase "start teaching where the client is" has new meaning when we look beyond motivation, psychological readiness, and ability to grasp concepts to determine the client's feelings of powerlessness. Clients with low powerlessness may need multiple avenues of content presentation. They should be encouraged to compare methods of self-care and be given freedom to question and pursue alternate modes of meeting needs for care. Those clients who tend to have an internal locus of control may need added emphasis on information that would give them a sense of control. This may even involve explicit verbalization by the nurse, such as, "Knowing this will give you added ability to be in control of the situation." High-powerless clients, however, may need structured approaches. This could mean teaching self-care in small increments so that clients feel a sense of accomplishment when they are successful with these scaled-down, yet realistic, goals.

A feeling of being controlled by fate, destiny, or others is not conducive to learning new skills such as self-care (Zahn, 1969). Clients with this orientation may believe that learning a self-care skill—such as learning a low-salt and calorie-restricted diet, as well as monitoring the effects of the rest of the antihypertensive regimen—will do no good because what was meant to happen will happen despite client involvement. Despite their locus-of-control tendency, perhaps all clients must perceive some sense of situation control before they can learn health-control information.

Illusions of Control

In situations in which personal competence can affect outcomes, individuals tend to perform more actively and competently than in situations that appear beyond their control. What effect does the individual's belief in having control have on arousal, anxiety, and so forth? The reviewed studies on perceived control report that subjects who believed they had control of an aversive stimulus such as an electric shock or noise manifested less anxiety and tolerated noxious stimuli better than subjects who believed they had no control.

Geer, Davison, and Gatchel (1970) studied autonomic responses of 20 men who perceived they had control over electric shock and 20 men who perceived no control. The subjects in the perceived-control group were led to believe that they could decrease the duration of the shock from 6 to 3 seconds if they pushed a reaction switch with each electric shock. The no-perceived-control group was not given this information. Both groups were told that the researcher was interested in reaction time between receiving the shock and pushing the switch. Even though the perceived-control group did not affect the duration of the shock, their perception of being in control influenced the results. The perceived-control subjects rated the shocks as less painful than did the no-perceived-control subjects; the perceived-control subjects had less galvanic skin response, suggesting that they were less aroused by the shocks than were the no-perceived control subjects. This study was replicated by Glass et al. (1973) on 48 college students. Subjects in the perceived-control group rated their pain as less and performed better on the Stroop Color Word Test than did those in the no-perceived-control group. Contrary to the findings of Geer, Davison, and Gatchel (1970), there was no significant difference in autonomic response, as measured by the galvanic skin response, between the two groups.

Glass and Singer (1972) studied the response to belief of control over aversive stimuli. The subjects received 18 electric shocks while trying to solve graphic puzzles. Half of the group was given solvable puzzles, whereas the other half was given unsolvable puzzles. All subjects received the same number of shocks but were told that solving the puzzles would prevent the next scheduled shock. The subjects who perceived control performed better on postshock tasks, making fewer errors on a proofreading test, and having shorter reading times than the subjects who perceived no control.

Procedures that give subjects the choice of avoiding or not avoiding aversive stimuli are equivalent to giving them perceived control over the potential stress of threat (Corah & Boffa, 1970). Forty subjects were divided into two groups: an escape group, which had the choice instructions, and a no-escape group, which had no choice instructions. The escape group was instructed to press a button to escape white noise if the noise became uncomfortable. The choice was up to them. The no-escape subjects were told not to push the button unless the noise "became so uncomfortable you must." The galvanic skin response was used as an indicator of physiological arousal. The escape group had less arousal than did the no-escape group. The escape group also rated the discomfort as less than did the no-escape group (Corah & Boffa, 1970). A sense of control influences the way in which threats are appraised. This study suggests that choice is a variable that can reduce the aversive quality of the stimulus.

Houston (1972) studied the effects of an illusion of control on anxiety and physiological arousal as measured by the Zuckerman Affect Adjective Check List and heart rate, respectively. He also used no-control situations to compare the physiological arousal of individuals with internal locus of control with the arousal in individuals with external locus of control. The 20 subjects in the avoidable-shock group were led to believe that they could avoid an electric shock by not making mistakes on a memory task. The 20 subjects in the unavoidable-shock group were told there was no way to avoid the shock. Despite the fact that both groups received the same number and intensity of shocks, subjects in

Theoretical Propositions	Practice Speculations
1. An illusion of control causes less physiological arousal during stress events than perception of no control.	Providing client with alternatives to make choices provides an illusion of control.
2. An illusion of control causes threats to be evaluated as less harmful than perception of no control.	Containing anxiety and aversive physiologic arousal is desirable in all phases of health-illness. Helping clients feel a sense of control achieves this end.
3. When individuals are provided with freedom to make choices, an illusion of control is created.	Helping the client feel control over aspects of the immediate environment, personal effects, plants, and so forth.

FIGURE 3.3 ➤ Illusions of control.

the latter group reported more anxiety but demonstrated less physiological arousal. Contrary to Houston's expectations, the group with external locus of control manifested less physiological arousal than did the group with internal locus of control. This could be attributed to the effects of placing individuals with an internal-locus personality trait in no-control situations. More anxiety, as measured by physiological arousal, may be caused in subjects with an internal locus of control because they are not resigned to events being contingent on external forces (Fig. 3.3).

DISCUSSION OF PRACTICE SPECULATION

The illusion of client control has benefits for clients in terms of creating less anxiety and physiological arousal and greater ability to learn than does the perception of no control. Helping clients know when specific events will take place provides an illusion of control. The events may be diagnostic tests or treatments such as a dressing change. Clients can achieve some sense of control by knowing about alternatives for self-care and feeling free to make decisions about the alternatives. Nurses need to help clients become aware of alternatives and enable them to make decisions. An example is having the new client with diabetes realize that a diet restriction of 1200 calories per day involves freedom and variety in meal planning. Good selections will now enhance the client's nutritional state because food of no nutritional value is not included in the selection of six food-exchange lists.

Helping the clients and families be as informed as health-care personnel about their health states is fundamental. Although the perceived absence of control is debilitating, the illusion of control may improve well-being (Langer, 1983).

Effects of No Control on Animals

"The mere knowledge that one can exert control serves to mitigate the debilitating effects of aversive stimuli" (Lefcourt, 1973, p. 419). The reported aversive quality of a stimulus decreases when subjects exercise control over that stimulus.

The original study of control by Mowrer and Viek (1948) demonstrated that rats exhibited less fear of an aversive stimulus (electric shock) if they could exercise control (leap into the air when shocked to terminate the shock). A significant difference in eating inhibition was noted in the group that had no control over the shock. (The animals were presented with food; if they did not eat within 10 seconds, the behaviors were labeled an inhibition.) Mowrer and Viek observed the 20 animals for 15 consecutive days. They described the no-control animals as being helpless, having lost their will, and not actively providing for their self-interest, for example, satisfying hunger.

The effects of subjecting animals to no-control situations have been documented in a series by Seligman, Maier, and Solomon (1971); Overmier and Seligman (1967); Overmier (1968); and Seligman and Maier (1967). In these studies, dogs were restrained in a cloth hammock and given electric shocks by electrodes attached to their feet. The intensity and duration of the shocks varied in the experiments. Another series of shocks was given to the same dogs while they were in an escapable shuttle box. The animals were shocked by a wire grid on the bottom of the box. If the animal crossed the shoulder-high barrier in the center of the box, the shocks would be stopped. Overmier and Seligman (1967) compared responses of dogs that received inescapable shocks and those that received no aversive pretreatment but were placed in the escapable shuttle box. Those animals that had been restrained and shocked when placed in the escape box displayed helpless behavior; at first, they ran around frantically for approximately 30 seconds, and then they lay down and quietly whined. After a few seconds, the dogs seemed to give up and passively accept the shock.

The helplessness induced by the inescapable shock was eliminated if the animal had some experience in controlling the shock (Seligman & Maier, 1967; Seligman, Maier, & Geer, 1968). Seligman (1968) tried to overcome the helplessness in dogs previously in no-escape conditions by calling the animal over a lowered barrier in the box to the no-shock side. One in four dogs crossed the barrier. The other three were then leashed and forced to the escape side. The animals were pulled across the barrier 20 times. It then took 20, 35, and 50 trials for the dogs to escape the shock on their own. The animals' behavior was explained as resulting from learned helplessness. Their having learned a lack of control over reinforcement was difficult to reverse.

Not all animal studies reported that the control subjects have the advantage. Brady, Porter, Conrad, and Mason (1958) reported that the

Theoretical Propositions	Practice Speculations
1. Repeated exposure to threat and/or harm induces a state of helplessness in animals.	
2. Reversal of learned helplessness is difficult but can take place with forceful success experiences provided by someone controlling the situation.	
3. Predictability of aversive stimuli decreases the threat of the stimuli.	

FIGURE 3.4 ➤ The effects on animals of helplessness or lack of control.

four monkeys who pressed levers to escape electric shocks developed ulcers. The paired monkeys who had no control did not develop gastrointestinal lesions. The control monkeys were labeled by Brady's group as "executive" monkeys. The findings were refuted by Weiss' study (1971) of 180 rats, in which ulcers were more common and more extensive among the animals with no control.

Seligman and Meyer (1970) studied the effects of unpredictable shock on rats' bar-pressing behavior for food. A variable number of unpredictable shocks were given to 20 rats. Suppression of bar pressing occurred. After being given a fixed number of otherwise unpredictable shocks in each session, rats resumed bar pressing after the last shock, using its occurrence as a safety signal. Bar pressing resumed more quickly in rats that received milder predictable shocks than in rats that received the mild unpredictable shocks. Fear, measured by the suppression of bar pressing, correlated with the amount of gastric ulceration found in the unpredictable-shock animals (Fig. 3.4).

The implications of this research and these propositions are discussed at the end of the next session.

Effects of No Control on Humans

When subjects administered shocks to themselves and selected the level of intensity of shock, they reported less discomfort at higher levels of shock and endured stronger shock intensity than did matched subjects who were given shocks by the investigator (Staub, Tursky, & Schwartz, 1971). The predictability of self-administered shocks diminished the threat of aversive stimuli (Ball & Vogler, 1971; Pervin, 1963). On a second series of shocks, both control and no-control groups now had shocks administered to them; the groups that previously had control declined in tolerance for shocks and rated shocks as more painful than when they had control. The ability to predict events may reduce the subjective experience of helplessness, even when control is not possible, and may thereby reduce tension or anxiety. When ability to terminate aversive stimuli is lacking, predictability may reduce the impact of the stimuli; and when the ability to predict is lacking, perceived ability to terminate aversive stimuli may have a similar effect (Staub, Tursky, & Schwartz, 1971).

To determine the effect of control over environmental stressors on frustration tolerance and task performance, two groups of subjects were exposed to random noise played on a tape recorder at 110 decibels (Glass, Singer, & Friedman, 1969). One group had control over the noise through use of a button; the other group had no control. The response to the noise stressor was measured by use of the galvanic skin response readings, number of errors made on cognitive tasks, tolerance for frustration by the number of trials made at insoluble puzzles, and a postexperimental questionnaire requesting ratings from the subjects on how distracting, irritating, and unpleasant they felt the noise to be. The group that had control demonstrated much greater tolerance for frustration based on a larger number of trials at solving unsolvable puzzles. The percentage of proofreading errors was less for the group with control. The group with control also rated the noise as less aversive than did the group with no control.

Kanfer and Seidner (1973) studied the effectiveness of self-controlling response in 45 female undergraduate students. The subjects were divided into three groups, and all subjects had one hand immersed in ice water. Subjects in group 1 viewed travel slides that they advanced at their own desired rate. Group 2 had the slides advanced by the experimenter. No slides were used for group 3. The duration of ice-water tolerance was greater for subjects who advanced the slides at their own rate (significant at the 0.01 level). The researchers did not attribute the tolerance for ice water to self-distraction techniques that may have been used by the group controlling the slides. The conclusion was that the self-controlling responses increased tolerance for the aversive stimuli.

Thornton and Jacobs (1971) were able to replicate learned helplessness in humans, as had been done in previous animal studies. After pretreatment in which the subjects had no control, humans transferred helplessness to a second task in which they had control, just as the animals had done. Eighty subjects were divided into four groups. One group could avoid the electric shock by pushing a button in a 30-second reaction time; the second and third groups could not avoid the shock. The fourth group was given no shock pretreatment. The variable-shock group that had less predictability experienced more stress. Groups 1, 2, and 3 transferred their helplessness to a task in which they had control.

In this second phase, pushing a button could eliminate the shock. Fewest attempts to control the shock were made by the variable-shock pretreatment group.

The learned helplessness is due to learning that reinforcement and responding are independent of one another. Miller and Seligman (1973, 1975), in comparing depression and laboratory-induced learned helplessness, determined that learning that reinforcement and responding are independent is central to the symptoms and etiology of both learned helplessness and depression. Seligman (1995, p. 90) drew a parallel between the behaviors of depression and those of learned helplessness, stating that in both there is

1. A lowered initiation of voluntary responses—animals and humans who have experienced uncontrollability show reduced initiation of voluntary responses.
2. A negative cognitive set—helpless animals and humans have difficulty learning that responses produce outcomes.
3. A time course—helplessness dissipates in time when induced by a single session of uncontrollable shock; after multiple sessions, helplessness persists.
4. Lowered aggression—helpless animals and humans initiate fewer aggressive and competitive responses, and their dominance status may diminish.
5. Loss of appetite—helpless animals eat less, lose weight, and are sexually and socially deficient.
6. Physiological changes—helpless rats show norepinephrine depletion, and helpless cats may be cholinergically overactive.

Hiroto and Seligman (1975) and Gatchel, McKinney, and Koebernick (1977) found that depressed subjects and nondepressed subjects exposed to inescapable noise exhibit similar deficits in attempting to solve anagram puzzles.

Johnson and Kilmann (1975) studied the relationship between locus of control and perceived problem-solving ability in 20 internal men, 20 internal women, 20 external men, and 20 external women. Men who were internal rated themselves as more confident in problem-solving ability than did men who were external. No significant difference was found between internal and external women.

Anderson (1977) studied 90 owner-managers of small businesses that were damaged by a hurricane to determine the relationship among locus of control, perceived stress, coping behaviors, and performance. Externals perceived higher stress than did internals. The externals responded with more defensiveness and less task-oriented coping behavior than did internals. The task-oriented coping behaviors of the internals were more successful in solving the problems created by the stressful event, because the performance of the internals' organizations

Theoretical Propositions	Practice Speculations
1. Repeated no-control experiences precipitate a state of helplessness.	Be sensitive to how helplessness is induced in clients: strange language system, strange environment, uncertainty of health-illness and treatment situations, unpredictability of therapy outcomes.
2. Observed behaviors of helpless animals parallel behaviors of depressed human beings.	Eliminate unpredictability of events by informing clients of scheduled tests and procedures.
3. Coping behaviors may vary depending on the personality trait locus of control.	Helping clients be aware of the sensory events that may accompany a threatening procedure will decrease the perception of threat. Recognize that individuals' coping styles will vary.
4. When aversive stimuli are predictable, the stimuli are interpreted by the subject as less threatening than when the stimuli are unpredictable.	Recognize that no control or helplessness in one aspect of the clients life may be transferred to all aspects, creating generalized helplessness. Help the client be aware of those aspects that are client controlled. Prevent generalized helplessness, which is difficult to reverse.

FIGURE 3.5 ➤ The effects on humans of helplessness or lack of control.

was better. (Coping was determined by evaluating the economic position of the company. If the company returned to preflood status, coping was considered effective.) Kahn, Wolfe, Quinn, Snoek, and Rosenthal's (1981) categorization of coping behaviors was employed to categorize coping. Class I coping responses are aimed at dealing with the objective task situation. In class I, coping behavior included problem-solving efforts such as obtaining resources to counter the initial loss. Class II coping behaviors deal with emotional or anxiety reactions to the stimulus. Examples include withdrawal, group affiliation, hostility, and aggression (Fig. 3.5).

DISCUSSION OF PRACTICE SPECULATIONS

Helplessness is a syndrome of behaviors that mimics depression (Seligman, 1995). It is a challenge to the nurse to be aware of how helplessness can be induced in clients in order to take measures to prevent it. This involves the nurse being sensitive to the client's response to a strange language system, strange environment, uncertainty of health-illness and treatment situations, and unpredictability of therapy outcomes. Planning for client control by enabling client decision making and participation is crucial. Determining clients' preferred coping strategies and not suggesting strategies that could be in conflict with their related locus-of-control tendency must also be kept in mind.

Eliminating unpredictability of events is possible for most clients. This may involve keeping clients informed of scheduled tests, anticipated sensations during an examination or test, and the expected outcomes. It may involve, for example, helping the client and family plan for discharge from a health setting to home. The certainty of knowing the date of discharge gives the client a sense of control. Knowledge about anticipated events allows the client to direct activities within the family to prepare for the events.

Control in Health-Illness Situations

MacDonald and Hall (1971) studied the relationship of locus of control and perception of disability. The Rotter Locus of Control Scale and a disability scale were completed by 479 subjects. Externally controlled subjects rated physical disabilities as more debilitating than did the internally controlled subjects. Internals rated emotional disorders as being more debilitating than physical disabilities. The emotional disabilities included having irrational fears, being extremely depressed, and being withdrawn. Physical disabilities included internal disorders such as heart problems and diabetes, sensory disorders such as speech loss and deafness, and cosmetic disorders such as obesity and amputations.

Several studies have been done on the relationship of locus of control to anxiety (Donovan, Smyth, Paige, & O'Leary, 1975; Lowery, Jacobsen, & Keane, 1975; Watson, 1967). Findings of all these studies are the same; that is, external subjects have higher anxiety than internal subjects. In these studies, anxiety was measured by the Taylor Manifest Anxiety Scale and the Zuckerman Affect Adjective Check List. The Lowery, Jacobsen, and Keane study (1975) measured state anxiety in preoperative clients. Both trait and state anxiety are higher in external subjects when self-report is used. Donovan, Smyth, Paige, and O'Leary (1975) also used an unobtrusive measure of anxiety, the Activity Preference Questionnaire. The results of this anxiety measure revealed no difference in anxiety between internals and externals. These authors raise the issue that the Taylor Manifest Anxiety Scale may measure a dimension of neuroticism and/or negative self-concept rather than anxiety. Yet another consideration is that the subject with internal locus of control may be unwilling to disclose anxiety on tools that overtly measure it.

A scale measuring health locus of control was designed by Wallston, Wallston, Kaplan, and Maides (1976) and by Wallston, Wallston, and De-Vellis (1978). These instruments are area-specific for health and have been used to study health behavior and predict the most helpful approaches for clients desiring weight reduction. Wallston et al., (1976) studied 88 subjects and found that internals who valued health sought more information on hypertension as a health risk, by choosing a significantly larger number of pamphlets made available, than did the high- and low-health-value external subjects and the low-health-value internal subjects. The Rokeach (1973) value survey served as a model for developing the health-value scale.

In the study of subjects participating in a weight-reduction program, 34 women completed the Health Locus of Control Scale and were randomly assigned to two different types of weight-reduction treatments. The basic difference in the type of treatment program was that one was self-directed and the other was group-oriented. The 8-week program was completed by 22 women. The externals in the group program lost more weight than did the externals in the self-directed program. The internals in the self-directed program lost more weight than did the internals in the group program (Wallston, Wallston, Kaplan, & Maides, 1976). The results of this study provide some support for the need to tailor diet and behavior modification programs to match the individual's locus-of-control tendency.

In comparing locus of control to pain tolerance, Craig and Best (1977) found that internals had greater pain tolerance to increasing intensities of researcher-administered electric shocks than did the externals (Fig. 3.6).

Theoretical Propositions	Practice Speculations
1. Control is stress reducing.	Ways of ameliorating fear during pain and strategies to enhance control should be used.
2. Individuals with an external locus of control more readily report anxiety than do those with internal locus of control.	Validation of mood states is necessary in that anxiety may not be disclosed by clients with internal locus of control and therefore may not be treated by the nurse.
3. Effectiveness of treatment programs may depend on tailoring the program to an individual's locus-of-control tendency.	Provide support and behavior therapy to clients considering their locus of control. Externals benefit from a group approach, and internals benefit from a one-to-one approach.

FIGURE 3.6 ➤ Control in health-illness situations.

DISCUSSION OF PRACTICE SPECULATIONS

Consideration of the unique client situation and personal meaning of control is necessary for accurate nursing prescriptions. Nurses must recognize that fear of not being in control during painful experiences or of being unable to terminate the pain is a major threat. These fears can be ameliorated somewhat by the nurses' sharing information, demonstrating pain-relief strategies, and teaching the clients relaxation, use of autosuggestion, and many self-control techniques.

One of several variables that influence self-disclosure of anxiety is the locus-of-control tendency. Interpretation of mood states must be validated with the client and not conclusively interpreted and recorded on care plans. Individuals with internal locus of control do not readily self-report anxiety, yet these clients may have more anxiety than clients with external locus of control.

The Health Locus of Control Scale (Wallston et al., 1976) should be considered for nursing research involving locus-of-control tendencies in clients. This tool is area-specific for health and does not have the global political items that are contained in the Rotter Internal-External Locus of Control Scale (Rotter, 1966). Behavioral indicators of locus of control need to be studied in more detail. An initial study is described in Chapter 10.

As programs on nursing care are prescribed, tailoring the program to client's control tendency is essential.

PRECIPITANTS OF DEATH

Richter (1959) concluded that death in rats resulted from a combination of responses to various stresses occurring in rapid succession, which generates a sense of hopelessness in the animals. In wild (non-laboratory-bred) rats, handling, whisker snipping, and confinement to glass jars to swim without knowing that they would be saved caused the animals to die. The death was not attributed to an adrenal response. When hopelessness was eliminated by removing the rats from the water and then immersing them again, the rats did not die. Removal of the rats caused them to become aggressive in trying to free themselves, showing no signs of giving up. Such rats perceived the situation not to be hopeless and swam for 40 to 60 hours, instead of dying within minutes.

Accounts of deaths in humans caused by hopelessness are reported by Seligman (1995), Engel (1968, 1971), Kastenbaum and Kastenbaum (1971), and Lefcourt (1973). A dramatic example of a healthy individual succumbing to hopelessness is reported by Lefcourt (1973):

> A female patient who had remained in a mute state for nearly 10 years was shifted to a different floor of her building along with her floor

mates, while her unit was being redecorated. The third floor of this psychiatric unit where the patient in question had been living was known among the patients as the chronic, hopeless floor. In contrast, the first floor was most commonly occupied by patients who held privileges, including the freedom to come and go on the hospital grounds and to the surrounding streets. In short, the first floor was an exit ward from which patients could anticipate discharge fairly rapidly. All patients who were temporarily moved from the third floor were given medical examinations prior to the move, and the patient in question was judged to be in excellent medical health though still mute and withdrawn. Shortly after moving to the first floor, this chronic psychiatric patient surprised the ward staff by becoming socially responsive such that within a 2-week period she ceased being mute and was actually becoming gregarious. As fate would have it, the redecoration of the third floor unit was soon completed and all previous residents were returned to it. Within a week after she had been returned to the "hopeless" unit, this patient, who like the legendary Snow White had been aroused from a living torpor, collapsed and died. The subsequent autopsy revealed no pathology of note, and it was whimsically suggested at the time that the patient had died of despair.

Ferrari (1962) studied freedom of choice in 75 elderly clients admitted to a nursing home. Of the 17 who said they had no alternative except to move into the nursing home, 8 died after 4 weeks in the home and 16 were dead by the end of 10 weeks. Of the 38 who saw alternatives to being admitted to the nursing home but chose to reside there, only 1 subject died in the 10 weeks. All the deaths were termed unexpected by the nursing home staff. It could be argued that the sicker clients had fewer alternatives and more family pressure to move into a nursing home, yet all the deaths were termed unexpected.

Although skepticism may be expressed by researchers who do not recognize a qualitative approach, it is impossible to validate the happenings with the subjects themselves. To permit these findings to fall on deaf ears would cause needless physiological deterioration and death in situations in which nurses could intervene by instilling a sense of hope. Is it possible to document the passive surrender of some chronically ill individuals? A case is presented in Chapter 8.

Hopelessness is a feeling of giving up. The individual is filled with despair, a sense of "there is nothing left." A feeling that one is completely responsible for the situation contributes to the feeling that nothing can be done to overcome or change the situation. The individual does not feel worthy of help (Engel, 1962). Hopelessness is loss of autonomy, with a feeling of despair coming from the individual's awareness of an inability to provide gratification to self (Schmale, 1964). If powerlessness is not contained, a cycle of lowered self-esteem and depression occurs, followed by hopelessness. The client is immobilized in terms of solving problems, setting goals, and taking action. If this state is permitted to continue, isolation, loneliness, and death may ensue.

Theoretical Propositions	Practice Speculations
1. Hopelessness is a temporary failure of mental coping mechanisms.	Helping clients achieve a sense of control, averting a hopeless state, may be vital to their recovery.
2. When helplessness builds over time and results from various situations, a generalized feeling of hopelessness results.	Inspiring hope affects survival.
3. When a cycle of powerlessness, depression, immobility, and hopelessness is not broken, a deteriorated physical health state may result.	Helping clients realize there is someone and/or something to live for prolongs life.

FIGURE 3.7 ➤ Precipitants of death.

Engel (1968) has identified five characteristics of a hopelessness complex he labels "giving-in-given-up." This complex includes:

- A feeling of giving up, experienced as helplessness or hopelessness
- A depreciated image of self
- A sense of loss of gratification for relationships or role in life
- A feeling of disruption of the sense of continuity between past, present, and future
- A reactivation of memories of earlier periods of giving up

Theoretical propositions on powerlessness and death are listed in Figure 3.7.

Discussion of Practice Speculations

Having someone or something to live for inspires continued life (Pattison, 1974). Building patient endurance and inspiring survival by instilling hope are familiar to nurses. Strategies for inspiring hope are discussed in Chapter 19.

Averill (1973) specified three types of control: behavioral, cognitive, and decisional. Behavioral control is the availability of a response that may directly influence or modify the objective characteristics of a threatening event. Providing the client control over aspects of the environment is an example of behavioral control. Allowing the client to carry out a procedure such as a colostomy irrigation, in a self-determined, therapeutically effective way, is another example. Cognitive control is the way in which an event is interpreted, evaluated, or used in a cognitive plan. Clients can be helped to interpret events as being controlled by them. Decisional control is the opportunity to choose among various alternatives. Clients need to be aware of alternatives and consequences of alternatives. This categorization of control types may be helpful in guiding nurses to provide for client control so as to avert hopelessness. Helping clients perceive a sense of control may be vital to their recovery.

The review of literature reveals that powerlessness has devastating effects on the person's physical and emotional states. This is a diagnosis that is not only amenable to nursing but also unique to nursing—dependent upon nursing as the professional group to take action to alleviate powerlessness. The speculations derived from a research base provide ideas for testing in practice. Whether the interventions proposed alter the powerlessness state needs to be studied.

FIELD OBSERVATIONS AS ANOTHER PHASE OF CONCEPT DEVELOPMENT

Making observations in the field verifies or refutes the need for developing the concept of powerlessness. Questions about whether the concept has real-world relevance are answered by initial field observations. These observations were made to identify factors in the health-care environment and actions of health-care providers that could increase or decrease patient control. Averill's (1973) categories defined in this chapter were used to categorize observations of chronically ill clients in one urban hospital. Observations were made 2 to 3 hours a week for a period of 6 weeks. Examples of factors decreasing and increasing control according to Averill's categories are presented in Tables 3.1 and 3.2. These field observations help us conclude that further development and validation of the nursing diagnostic label of powerlessness is warranted.

INDICATORS OF POWERLESSNESS

The indicators or defining characteristics of powerlessness are those signs and symptoms that lead to the conclusion that powerlessness exists. Indicators of the nursing diagnosis of powerlessness were determined by 27 graduate students enrolled in a clinical nursing course on chronic illness. The students had studied powerlessness as part of the course content and made powerlessness diagnoses in 81 chronically ill clients in their caseloads. The graduate students recorded other indicators that led them to believe their chronically ill clients were experiencing powerlessness. Similar specific signs and symptoms were clustered into 17 categories (broad statements or indicators). The indicators were then rated by a panel of 24 experts (graduate nursing

Table 3.1 ▶ FACTORS DECREASING BEHAVIORAL, COGNITIVE, AND DECISIONAL CONTROL IN HOSPITALIZED CHRONICALLY ILL CLIENTS

Behavioral Control	Cognitive Control	Decisional Control
Blind client was left in a wheelchair in the center of the waiting room and was not told where she was or how long she must wait.	Client was reprimanded for leaving waiting room to go to restroom after waiting 2 hours. "If you aren't here when we call you, you will miss your turn."	Appointment scheduled in ambulatory care department without asking client if date and time are convenient.
Client was left alone in x-ray room on hard table, in cold room, only partially covered.	Client was not informed of his daily lab values, although he had requested that this be done.	Client in x-ray department told to "try to hold it" when he asked location of bathroom.
	Health-care personnel more knowledgeable about client's illness and treatment than he is.	Diagnostic and treatment procedures scheduled without asking client or explaining why they were being done.
	Health-care personnel walked into client's room without knocking.	Patient has little or no choice about who will share room.
	Health-care personnel talk "over" client about their personal activities.	Little choice over scheduling activities— eating, sleeping, bathing, and treatments.
	Health-care personnel are not wearing name tags.	

Table 3.2 ► FACTORS INCREASING BEHAVIORAL, COGNITIVE, AND DECISIONAL CONTROL IN HOSPITALIZED CHRONICALLY ILL CLIENTS		
Behavioral Control	**Cognitive Control**	**Decisional Control**
Nursing care plan: "Allow client to sleep until breakfast trays arrive; do not awaken for TPR." Client moved to another room at her request because of roommate noise. Client in x-ray was told, "We can see you through the window. Hold up your hand if you need something." After clients were taught specific procedures, expectation given for them to take full responsibility for catheter care, urine testing, dressing change, shunt care.	Client informed of weight, blood pressure, lab values. Client taught about medications. Nursing care plan: Detailed description of how to do client's dressing change had been worked out with the client. Client given feedback about lab values, taught how to record results on a flow sheet.	Client given access to refrigerator to get own soft drinks. Client given list of all U.S. dialysis centers and given full responsibility for making own vacation arrangements. Medications left at bedside for clients to take when ready.

faculty and advanced-standing graduate students), to determine which indicators may be characteristic of severe, moderate, low, or no powerlessness (Table 3.3).

The indicators rated as "severe" could be termed "critical indicators" of the nursing diagnosis of powerlessness. That is, when any of these indicators are present, nurses could conclude that the client has a nursing diagnosis of powerlessness. Although the signs and symptoms categorized as "moderate" and "low" are important cues, they may not lead the nurse to conclusively make the diagnosis of powerlessness. Validity and reliability of this tool have not been established.

POWERLESSNESS AND SPECIFIC HEALTH PROBLEMS
Acquired Immunodeficiency Syndrome

Since AIDS was first diagnosed in the United States in 1981 (Grady, 1988), the illness has been synonymous with uncertainty. The few knowns about this illness to date include methods of transmission, methods of diagnosis, the nature of the debilitating clinical course of the illness resulting in death, effects of specific drugs such as azidothymidine (AZT), and types of opportunistic infections that occur.

Methods of transmission known to date include contact with infected blood or semen. Specifically, the human immunodeficiency virus (HIV) is transmitted by sexual contact (vaginal, anal, and oral), blood transfusions, intravenous drug use, and perinatally from infected mother to infant. McMahon (1988) reviewed the literature on body fluids and cells containing HIV and reported it isolated in blood, semen, cervical and vaginal secretions, breast milk, saliva, serum, tears, urine, alveolar fluid, brain tissue, cerebrospinal fluid, and epithelial cells.

It must be noted that data on AIDS change weekly, particularly epidemiological information on deaths and incidence according to the Centers for Disease Control and Prevention Classification. Groups include acutely infected (group I); asymptomatic infected (group II); generalized lymphadenopathy (group III); and HIV with other related diseases such as secondary cancers, infections, neurological involvement (group IV). Readers are referred to the Centers for Disease Control and Prevention AIDS weekly Surveillance Report to obtain the latest statistics. Opportunistic infections include *bacterial infections* such as salmonella in the blood, lungs, gastrointestinal (GI) tract, and gallbladder; *viral infections* (cytomegalovirus, herpes simplex and zoster) in the skin, mucosa, peripheral nerves, retina, lungs, GI tract, and brain; *protozoal infections* of the brain, lymph nodes, muscle, lungs, and GI tract; *fungal infections* of the brain, lungs, bone marrow, skin, GI tract, mucosa, and reticuloendothelial system (Wolfe, 1989).

Table 3.3 ▶ DEFINING CHARACTERISTICS OF POWERLESSNESS		
Severe	**Moderate**	**Low**
Verbal expressions of having no control or influence over situations	Nonparticipation in care or decision making when opportunities are provided	Expressions of uncertainty about fluctuating energy levels
Verbal expressions of having no control or influence over outcomes	Expressions of dissatisfaction and frustration over inability to perform previous tasks and/or activities	
Verbal expressions of having no control or influence over self-care	Expressions of uncertainty about treatment outcomes	
Depression over physical deterioration that occurs despite patient compliance with regimens	Dependence on others that may result in irritability, resentment, anger, and guilt	
Passivity	Inability to seek information regarding self-care	
	Inability to monitor progress	
	Does not defend self-care practices when challenged	
	Hesitant to plan for future, set goals	
	Expressions of doubt regarding role performance	
	Reluctance to express true feelings, fearing alienation of self from caregivers	

The physical and psychosocial complexity of the person with AIDS results in multiple nursing diagnoses and difficult challenges for nurses. It is a multisystem disease having no known cure. Because this health problem has the potential to overload the health-care system as it currently exists and create an economic crisis, AIDS is a concern of all persons. It is a national problem (Lynch, 1989). Three phases of the illness may be considered: (1) diagnosis—HIV antibodies are detected in the blood; (2) AIDS-related complex of symptoms may be experienced such as night sweats, lymph node enlargement; and (3) frank immunologic suppression with rampant opportunistic infections (Lynch, 1989).

NURSING DIAGNOSES

Nursing diagnoses of persons with AIDS have been described (McLaughlin et al., 1987; Rosenthal & Haneiwich, 1988; Ungvarski, 1989) and include alteration in breathing pattern, alteration in nutrition (less than body requirements), alteration in elimination (diarrhea), impaired skin integrity, alteration in thought processes, alteration in comfort, potential for additional infection, and potential for physical injury. Other nursing diagnoses to consider include activity intolerance and fatigue, ineffective family and individual coping, self-care deficits, spiritual distress, social isolation, sensory deprivation, role deprivation, knowledge deficit, self-esteem disturbance, body image disturbance, hopelessness, depression or suicide ideation, anxiety and uncertainty, anticipatory grieving, bereavement overload, and powerlessness. The body wasting, skin lesions from Kaposi's sarcoma, inability to ambulate without assistive devices, and uncontrolled diarrhea (due to protozoal and other opportunistic infections) may result in body image disturbance. Bereavement overload and powerlessness may be due to the large number of irreversible losses such as loss of body function, social support network, livelihood, role performance, financial security, independence, and anticipation of a future.

INTERVENTIONS

Consistent symptoms management is central to enabling the person with AIDS to maintain a sense of control (Bennett, 1988). Control begins with prevention of opportunistic infections if possible, being informed of T4 lymphocyte levels. (Normal levels range from 600 to 1200 per millimeter. Persons with AIDS may have a T4 cell range from 0 to 500 per millimeter.) When the T4 cell level drops to around 400 per millimeter, the person is more vulnerable to opportunistic infections such as the prevalent *Pneumocystis carinii* pneumonia (Grady, 1988). Regardless of symptoms and complications, maintaining adequate nutrition is essential for restoring energy reserves and muscle strength. Providing comfort, preventing falls and injury, anticipating a future, and preserving positive self-worth are categories of nursing interventions. Referrals may be needed to community support agencies specific for AIDS patients and others such as Meals on Wheels, Cancer Care (Bennett, 1988), and Home Hospice Care. Having the person maintain a sense of purpose and meaning in life and feeling in control of the direction of one's own life may be facilitated by reminiscence and goal setting, reflecting on favorable aspects of the past while anticipating a future. Empowerment does not preclude asking for help (Ribble, 1989); clients may need assistance in identifying helpful persons in their social network and soliciting their care.

Information contributes to emotional mastery of uncontrollable events (Furstenberg & Olson, 1984) and is indispensable in enabling coping (Frierson, Lippmann, & Johnson, 1987). Misinformation has contributed to panic, stigmatization, and premature closure of clients' and families' anticipating life's pleasures. Information about the disease transmission and effects, sexual activities that are safe, available community support, treatment choices, compliance with treatments, nutrition, skin care, mouth care, and monitoring for signs of opportunistic infections are examples of information to be provided by the nurse. Providing a climate for ventilation of feelings helps alleviate anger and enables grief work. Grief work also encompasses examining unrealistic guilt, confronting self-protective denial, using peer counseling (Frierson and Lippman, 1987), and avoiding perceptions of illness as punishment. Nurses can help clients plan for a future, helping them realize that AIDS can be a chronic illness and not an immediate death sentence. Listening holistically, providing a caring milieu, and being present nonjudgmentally are meaningful nursing behaviors (Warner-Robbins & Christiana, 1989).

In addition to information, symptom management, stress management, planning for the future, and spirituality can be sources of empowerment. Nurses should establish helping relationships with persons with AIDS and display unconditional positive regard and respect. Issues sensitive to the client's well-being can emerge when the qualities of a helping and therapeutic relationship exist. Spirituality may be a sensitive issue yet a valued coping resource. Spirituality is noted to become more valuable to some persons when the diagnosis of AIDS is confirmed (Belcher, Dettmore, & Holzemer, 1989; Warner-Robbins & Christiana, 1989). Some express that "even when no one else can accept me, God will." Spirituality involves a relatedness (connectedness) with something greater than self, a sense of closeness to a higher being and others (Reed, 1986). Reed found that older terminally ill persons had higher well-being than younger persons (1986) and that terminally ill hospitalized adults had a greater spiritual perspective than nonterminally ill hospitalized adults (1987). Similar findings of greater spiritual well-being and higher religious well-being among chronically ill adults compared to healthy adults were noted by Miller (1985). Reed (1986) attributed spirituality to enabling self-transcendence during suffering of a terminal illness. The love and spiritual strength provided by personal religious practices, faith, prayer, and beliefs need to be recognized and encouraged by nurses if this dimension is valued by clients. The spiritual needs of persons with cancer can be applied as well to the person with AIDS. These include having hope, giving and receiving love, and feeling significant to those around them (Epperly, 1983).

RESEARCH

Feelings of helplessness or lack of control have been a common research finding in studies on psychological responses to AIDS (Archer, 1989; Frierson & Lippmann, 1987; Frierson, Lippmann, & Johnson, 1987; Furstenburg & Olson, 1984; Viney, Henry, Walker, & Crooks, 1989). Viney, Henry, Walker, and Crooks' (1989) review of literature on emotional reactions of persons to physical illness revealed that anxiety, depression, anger, and helplessness are present. Specific psychological issues of 11 persons with AIDS included social isolation, change in body image, helplessness, sexual concerns, and anger and grief (Frierson & Lippman, 1987). Similar responses were found in 50 family members of AIDS patients. Families manifested psychological stress related to fear of contagion—anxiety about contracting AIDS; having to reveal private information about self and family to the public; feeling stigmatized; feeling helpless; and being filled with grief mixed with anger, guilt, and denial (Frierson, Lippmann, & Johnson, 1987). Frierson, Lippmann, and Johnson (1987) described the response of a wife of 15 years who found out her husband had become bisexually active over the past 5 years and contracted AIDS. "At first I felt like killing him, then I realized he was already dying" (p. 64).

Viney et al. (1989) studied 105 men to compare emotional states of 35 HIV-positive men with 35 chronically ill and 35 healthy adult men. Content analysis scales were developed to analyze transcripts of tape-recorded interviews. The two ill groups were more anxious, depressed, and helpless than the well group. The HIV-positive men had more anger yet higher competence than the other clients. Enjoyment was a more prevalent theme (more frequently expressed) in the interviews with the HIV group than the others. These researchers concluded that expressions of enjoyment should be encouraged by health personnel. Expressions of enjoyment result from effective coping.

A poignant finding of a study of spirituality and well-being of 35 persons with AIDS (Belcher, Dettmore, & Holzemer, 1989) is summarized in a client's quote, "AIDS is not all that I am" (p. 24). In general, respondents in this study saw the diagnosis as positively enhancing their spirituality, not destroying it. Select activities of importance to them were meditation, reading spiritual literature, praying, and visualization.

Empowerment is a process by which persons are supported and valued as they learn about themselves, make decisions, mobilize resources, accept control of themselves, and plan for direction in their lives (Ribble, 1989). Nurses themselves may feel powerless striving to change public policy, counteracting stigmatizing behavior of others, and working on prevention of this public health problem. They witness a difficult illness progression including AIDS dementia and, despite today's technology, know the illness will result in death. These nurses experience repetitive grief (Flaskerud, 1994). Dealing with value discrepancies, fears of contagion, and maintaining confidentialities are other nurse stresses (Bolle, 1988) that provoke powerlessness in the practitioner. The ANA Guide for Nursing's response to the person with AIDS (Miramontes, Boland, Corless, & McLoughlin, 1988) is a reminder of nursing's history in providing exemplary care to persons suffering from epidemics and difficult conditions from the Crimean to poliomyelitis. AIDS is another opportunity for nursing health-care leadership. Physical and psychological problems of the clients and families may have a cumulative effect and the affirmation of the goodness of life and continued living may no longer be possible unless skillful nursing intervention takes place.

Cancer

Helplessness in cancer clients may be evident during varied stages of the illness. During the diagnosis phase, clients may experience unfamiliar intrusive procedures. They may feel victimized, having an illness beyond their control. They may view themselves as vulnerable and interpret the diagnosis as synonymous with death. Stoner (1985) provided clinical examples throughout the phases of illness progression. During the diagnostic phase, Stoner described a 65-year-old man who had cared for his wife throughout her long course with cancer, bringing her for chemotherapy three times a week and so forth. Despite all concerted effort, he witnessed her physical decline and death. When he developed lung cancer himself, his initial reaction of helplessness was manifested in his refusal to have treatment and comment, "What good will it do anyway, it did nothing for my wife." Perceptions of uncontrollability are extended beyond receiving the diagnosis to experiencing the effects of treatment.

Bombarding clients with chemotherapy, radiation, or bone marrow transplantation, for example, heightens symptoms and may be a threat to life. Clients and families need to be involved in making informed decisions about treatment choices and know the potential risks involved. If metastasis occurs despite adherence to regimens, feelings of helplessness increase. Cooperating with further treatments may be very difficult for the client. During the terminal stage, cancer is not controllable (Stoner, 1985). Until self-actualized acceptance and peace are achieved, powerlessness may reach its peak at this time for clients and families.

Some research on helplessness and control in persons with cancer has been completed. Men with genitourinary cancer who were anxious at the time of periodic cystoscopic follow-up examinations also tended to feel *helpless,* hopeless, overwhelmed, and depressed (Scott, Oberst, & Bookbinder, 1984). Lewis (1982) studied 57 persons with late-stage (terminal) cancer and found a positive correlation between experienced personal control and quality of life measured by self-esteem and purpose in life. Similar to Scott and associates' findings, a negative correlation was found between control and anxiety (Lewis, 1982). Lewis concluded that well-being in clients with late-stage cancer is not a function of the control they maintain over their health but is a function of a more global sense of control over their lives in general. Relinquishing personal control over health during varied phases of illness may not be negative. Relinquishing control during critical or terminal phases may be a necessary adaptive maneuver. On the other hand, having ability and performing self-care skills is not synonymous with the perception of control (Anderson, 1990). Efficacy training may be used to increase perceptions of control and to reduce anxiety.

Taylor (1983) found that adaptation to chronic illness (cancer) was influenced by cognitive coping processes that enhanced self-esteem and included (1) making social comparisons with less fortunate others, (2) selectively focusing on attributes that make the client feel advantaged, (3) creating hypothetical worse worlds, (4) construing benefits from the event, and (5) manufacturing normative standards of adjustment that make one's own adjustment seem exceptional. Westbrook (1987) found similar coping processes were associated with persons with scleroderma who perceived they had some control over their disease.

Others

The nursing diagnosis of powerlessness is frequently observed in clients with spinal cord injuries (Mahon-Darby, Ketchik-Renshar, Richmond, & Gates, 1988; Richmond & Metcalf, 1986) and other neurological deficits (Boeing & Mongera, 1989; Miller & Hastings, unpublished paper).

SUMMARY

This chapter contains initial work on analysis of the concept of powerlessness. Harmful effects of powerlessness were noted in the early literature. That research was comprised largely of studies by psychologists carried out in laboratory settings. Nurses' clinical observations of factors increasing and decreasing control as well as indicators of powerlessness noted in selected chronic health problems such as in persons with AIDS or cancer provide convincing data that nurses can facilitate coping with chronic illness and alleviate powerlessness. These data also challenge continued study of powerlessness as a maladaptive response to chronic illness. Opposing forces, such as self-efficacy as a strategy to combat powerlessness, are discussed later in this book. The theoretical propositions and practice speculations suggested in this chapter provide direction for nursing. Drawing conclusions that are less speculative but are based on descriptive research is the focus of other chapters as a continued exercise in theory development.

REFERENCES

Abramson, L., Garber, J., & Seligman, M. (1980). Learned helplessness in humans: An attributional analysis. In J. Garber & M. Seligman (Eds.), *Human helplessness: Theory and applications* (pp. 3–34). New York: Academic Press.

Abramson, L., Seligman, M., & Teasdale, J. (1978). Learned helplessness in humans: Critique and reformulation. *Journal of Abnormal Psychology, 87,* 49–74.

AIDS Program Centers for Disease Control (1988). *AIDS weekly surveillance report.* Washington, DC.

Anderson, C. (1977). Locus of control, coping behaviors and performance in a stress setting: A longitudinal study. *Journal of Applied Psychology, 62,* 446–451.

Anderson, J. (1990). Home care management in chronic illness and the self-care movement: An analysis of ideologies and economic processes influencing policy decisions. *Advances in Nursing Science, 12,* 71–83.

Archer, V. (1989). Psychological defenses and control of AIDS. *American Journal of Public Health, 79,* 876–878.

Averill, J. (1973). Personal control over aversive stimuli and its relationships to stress. *Psychological Bulletin, 80,* 286–303.

Ball, T., & Vogler, R. (1971). Uncertain pain and the pain of uncertainty. *Perceptual and Motor Skills, 50,* 1195–1203.

Belcher, A., Dettmore, D., & Holzemer, S. (1989). Spirituality and sense of well-being in persons with AIDS. *Holistic Nursing Practice, 3,* 22–26.

Bennett, J. (1988). Helping people with AIDS live well at home. *Nursing Clinics of North America, 23,* 731–748.

Boeing, M., & Mongera, C. (1989). Powerlessness in critical care patients. *Dimensions of Critical Care Nursing, 8,* 274–279.

Bolle, J. (1988). Supporting the deliverers of care: Strategies to support nurses and prevent burnout. *Nursing Clinics of North America, 23,* 843–850.

Brady, J., Porter, R., Conrad, D., & Mason, J. (1958). Avoidance behavior and the development of gastroduodenal ulcers. *Journals of Experimental Analysis of Behavior, 1,* 69–72.

Chinn, P., & Jacobs, M. (1994). *Theory and nursing: A systematic approach.* St. Louis: CV Mosby.

Corah, N., & Boffa, J. (1970). Perceived control, self observation and response to aversive stimulation. *Journal of Personality and Social Psychology, 16,* 1–4.

Craig, K., & Best, A. (1977). Perceived control over pain: Individual differences and situational determinants. *Pain, 3,* 127–135.

Donovan, D., Smyth, L., Paige, A., & O'Leary, M. (1975). Relationships among locus of control, self-concept and anxiety. *Journal of Clinical Psychology, 31,* 682–684.

Dubin, R. (1978). *Theory building.* New York: Free Press.

Engel, G. (1962). *Psychological development in health and disease.* Philadelphia: WB Saunders.

Engel, G. (1968). A life setting conducive to illness: The giving up-given up complex. *Annals of Internal Medicine, 69,* 293–300.

Engel, G. (1971). Sudden and rapid death during psychological stress, folklore or folkwisdom? *Annals of Internal Medicine, 74,* 771–782.

Epperly, J. (1983). The cell and the celestial: Spiritual needs of cancer patients. *Journal of the Medical Association of Georgia, 72,* 374–376.

Ferrari, N. (1962). *Institutionalization and attitude change in an aged population: A field study on dissidence theory.* Unpublished doctoral dissertation. Cleveland: Case Western Reserve University.

Flaskerud, J. (1994). *AIDS / HIV infections: A reference guide for nursing professionals.* Philadelphia: WB Saunders.

Forsyth, G. (1980). Analysis of the concept of empathy: Illustration of one approach. *Advances in Nursing Science, 2,* 23–42.

Frierson, R., & Lippman, S. (1987). Psychologic implications of AIDS. *American Family Practitioner, 35,* 109–115.

Frierson, R., Lippmann, S., & Johnson, J. (1987). Psychological stresses on the family. *Psychosomatics, 28,* 65–68.

Furstenberg, A., & Olson, M. (1984). Social work and AIDS. *Social Work in Health Care, 9,* 45–62.

Gatchel, R., McKinney, M., & Koebernick, L. (1977). Learned helplessness, depression and psychological responding. *Psychophysiology, 14,* 25–31.

Geer, J., Davison, G., & Gatchel, R. (1970). Reduction of stress in humans through nonveridical perceived control of aversive stimulation. *Journal of Personality and Social Psychology, 16,* 731–738.

Glass, D., & Singer, J. (1972). *Urban stress: Experiments in noise and social stressors.* New York: Academic Press.

Glass, D., Singer, J., & Friedman, L. (1969). Psychic cost of adaptation to environmental stressor. *Journal of Personality and Social Psychology, 12,* 200–210.

Glass, D., Singer, J., Skipton, L., Krantz, D., Cohen, S., & Cummings, H. (1973). Perceived control of aversive stimulation and the reduction of stress responses. *Journal of Personality, 41,* 577–595.

Grady, C. (1988). HIV: Epidemiology, immunopathogenesis, and clinical consequences. *Nursing Clinics of North America, 23,* 683–696.

Hiroto, D., & Seligman, M. (1975). Generality of learned helplessness in man. *Journal of Personality and Social Psychology, 31,* 311–327.

Houston, B. (1972). Control over stress, locus of control and response to stress. *Journal of Personality and Social Psychology, 21,* 249–255.

Johnson, B., & Kilmann, P. (1975). Locus of control and perceived confidence in problem-solving abilities. *Journal of Clinical Psychology, 31,* 54–55.

Kahn, R., Wolfe, D., Quinn, R., Snoek, C., & Rosenthal, R. (1981). *Organizational stress: Studies in role conflict and ambiguity.* New York: John Wiley & Sons.

Kanfer, F., & Seidner, M. (1973). Self-control: Factors enhancing tolerance of noxious stimulation. *Journal of Personality of Social Psychology, 25,* 381–389.

Kastenbaum, R., & Kastenbaum, B. (1971). Hope, survival and the caring environment. In E. Palmor & F. Jerrers (Eds.), *Prediction of life span* (pp. 249–271). Lexington, MA: Health Lexington Books.

Langer, E. (1983). *The psychology of control.* Beverly Hills: Sage.

Lefcourt, H. (1973). The function of the illusions of control and freedom. *American Psychologist, 28,* 417–425.

Lewis, R. (1982). Experienced personal control and quality of life in late-stage cancer patients. *Nursing Research, 31,* 113–119.

Lowery, B., Jacobsen, B., & Keane, A. (1975). Relationship of locus of control to preoperative anxiety. *Psychological Reports, 37,* 1115–1121.

Lynch, R. (1989). Psychological impact of AIDS on individual, family, community, nation, and world in a historical perspective. *Family and Community Health, 12,* 60–64.

MacDonald, A., & Hall, J. (1971). Internal-external locus of control and perceptions of disability. *Journal of Consulting Clinical Psychology, 36,* 338–343.

Mahon-Darby, J., Ketchik-Renshar, Richmond, R., & Gates, E. (1988). Powerlessness in cervical spinal cord injury patients. *Dimensions of Critical Care Nursing, 7,* 346–355.

Maiden, R. (1987). Learned helplessness and depression: A test of the reformulated model. *Journal of Gerontology, 42,* 60–64.

McLaughlin, F., Grant, A., MacIntyre, R., Miramontes, H., Jorrison, C., & O'Brien, M. (1987). *AIDS resource manual.* San Francisco: California Nurses' Association.

McMahon, K. (1988). The integration of HIV testing and counseling into nursing practice. *Nursing Clinics of North America, 23,* 803–822.

Miller, J. (1985). Assessment of loneliness and spiritual well-being in chronically ill and healthy adults. *Journal of Professional Nursing, 1,* 79–85.

Miller, J., & Hastings, D. Unpublished paper. Family and patient response to chronic illness.

Miller, W., & Seligman, M. (1973). Depression and the perception of reinforcement. *Journal of Abnormal Psychology, 82,* 62–73.

Miller, W., & Seligman, M. (1975). Depression and learned helplessness in man. *Journal of Abnormal Psychology, 84,* 228–238.

Miramontes, H., Boland, M., Corless, I., & McLoughlin, S. (1988). *Nursing and the human immunodeficiency virus: A guide for nursing's response to AIDS.* Kansas City, MO: American Nurses' Association.

Mowrer, O., & Viek, P. (1948). An experimental analogue of fear from a sense of helplessness. *Journal of Abnormal and Social Psychology, 43,* 193–200.

Murphy, S. (1982). *Concept clarification in nursing.* Rockville, MD: Aspen.

Newman, M. (1979). *Theory development in nursing.* Philadelphia: FA Davis.

Norris, C. (1982). *Concept clarification in nursing.* Rockville, MD: Aspen.

Overmier, J. (1968). Interference with avoidance behavior: Failure to avoid traumatic shock. *Journal of Experimental Psychology, 78,* 340–343.

Overmier, J., & Seligman, M. (1967). Effects of inescapable shock upon subsequent escape and avoidance responding. *Journal of Comparative and Physiological Psychology, 63,* 23–33.

Pattison, E. (1974). Psychological predictors of death prognosis. *Omega, 5,* 145–160.

Perlmuter, L., & Monty, R. (1973). Effect of choice of stimulus on paired associate learning. *Journal of Experimental Psychology, 99,* 120–123.

Pervin, L. (1963). The need to predict and control under conditions of threat. *Journal of Personality, 31,* 570–587.

Phares, E. J., Ritchie, D. E., & Davis, W. (1968). Internal-external control and reaction to threat. *Journal of Personality and Social Psychology, 165,* 402–405.

Reed, P. (1986). Religiousness among terminally ill and healthy adults. *Research in Nursing and Health, 9,* 35–41.

Reed, P. (1987). Spirituality and well-being in terminally ill hospitalized adults. *Research in Nursing and Health, 10,* 335–344.

Ribble, D. (1989). Psychosocial support groups for people with HIV infection and AIDS. *Holistic Nursing Practice, 3,* 52–62.

Richmond, T., & Metcalf, J. (1986). Psychosocial responses to spinal cord injury. *Journal of Neuroscience Nursing, 18,* 183–187.

Richter, C. (1959). The phenomenon of unexplained sudden death in animals and man. In H. Feifel (Ed.), *The meaning of death.* New York: McGraw-Hill.

Rodgers, B. (1989a). Concepts, analysis and the development of nursing knowledge: The evolutionary cycle. *Journal of Advanced Nursing, 14,* 330–335.

Rodgers, B. (1989b). Exploring health policy as a concept. *Western Journal of Nursing Research, 11,* 694–702.

Rodgers, B., & Knafl, K. (1993). *Concept development in nursing: Foundations, techniques, and applications.* Philadelphia: WB Saunders.

Rokeach, M. (1973). *The nature of human values.* New York: Free Press.

Rosenthal, Y., & Haneiwich, S. (1988). Nursing management adults in the hospital. *Nursing Clinics of North America, 23,* 707–718.

Rotter, J. (1966). Generalized expectancies for internal versus external control of reinforcement. *Psychological Monographs, 80,* 1–28.

Rotter, J. (1975). Some problems and misconceptions related to the construct of internal versus external control of reinforcement. *Journal of Consulting and Clinical Psychology, 43,* 56–67.

Schmale, A. (1964). A genetic view of affects. *Psychoanalytic Study of the Child, 19,* 287–310.

Scott, D., Oberst, M., & Bookbinder, M. (1984). Stress-coping response to genito-urinary carcinoma. *Nursing Research, 33,* 325–329.

Seeman, M. (1962). Alienation and learning in a hospital setting. *American Sociological Review, 27,* 772–798.

Seeman, M. (1963). Alienation and social learning in a reformatory. *American Journal of Sociology, 69,* 270–284.

Seeman, M. (1967). Powerlessness and knowledge: A comparative study of alienation and learning. *Sociometry, 30,* 105–109.

Seeman, M. (1972). Alienation and knowledge-seeking: A note on attitude and action. *Social Problems, 20,* 3–7.

Seligman, M. (1968). Chronic fear produced by unpredictable shock. *Journal of Comparative and Physiological Psychology, 66,* 402–411.

Seligman, M. (1995). *Helplessness: On depression, development and death.* San Francisco: Freeman.

Seligman, M., & Maier, S. (1967). Failure to escape traumatic shock. *Journal of Experimental Psychology, 74,* 1–9.

Seligman, M., Maier, S., & Geer, J. (1968). The alleviation of learned helplessness in the dog. *Journal of Abnormal and Social Psychology, 73,* 256–262.

Seligman, M., Maier, S., & Solomon, R. (1971). Unpredictable and uncontrollable aversive events. In F. R. Bruch (Ed.), *Aversive conditioning and learning.* New York: Academic Press.

Seligman, M., & Meyer, B. (1970). Chronic fear and ulcers as a function of the unpredictability of safety. *Journal of Comparative and Physiological Psychology, 73,* 202–207.

Slimmer, L., Lopez, M., LeSage, J., & Ellor, J. (1987). Perceptions of learned helplessness. *Journal of Gerontological Nursing, 13,* 33–37.

Staub, E., Tursky, B., & Schwartz, G. (1971). Self-control and predictability: Their effects on reactions to aversive stimulation. *Journal of Personality and Social Psychology, 18,* 157–162.

Stoner, C. (1985). Learned helplessness: Analysis and application. *Oncology Nursing Forum, 12,* 31–35.

Stotland, E., & Blumenthal, A. (1964). The reduction of anxiety as a result of the expectation of making a choice. *Canadian Journal of Psychology, 18,* 139–145.

Taylor, S. (1983). Adjustment to threatening events: A theory of cognitive adaptation. *American Psychology, 38,* 1161–1173.

Thornton, J., & Jacobs, P. (1971). Learned helplessness in human subjects. *Journal of Experimental Psychology, 87,* 369–371.

Ungvarski, P. (1989). Nursing management of the adult client. In J. Flaskerud (Ed.), *AIDS/HIV infection: A reference guide for nursing professionals* (pp. 74–110). Philadelphia: WB Saunders.

Viney, L., Henry, R., Walker, B., & Crooks, L. (1989). The emotional reactions of HIV antibody positive men. *British Journal of Medical Psychology, 62,* 153–161.

Walker, L., & Avant, K. (1988). *Strategies for theory construction in nursing.* Norwalk, CT: Appleton & Lange.

Wallston, K., & Wallston, B. (1981). Health locus of control scales. In H. Lefcourt (Ed.), *Research with locus of control construct.* (Vol. 1). New York: Academic Press.

Wallston, K., & Wallston, B. (1989). Who is responsible for your health? The construct of health locus of control. In G. Sandes & J. Suls (Eds.), *Social psychology of health and illness* (pp. 65–95). Hillsdale, NJ: L. Erlbaum Associates.

Wallston, K., Wallston, B., & DeVellis, R. (1978). Development of the Multidimensional Health Locus of Control (MHLC) Scales. *Health Education Monographs, 6,* 161–170.

Wallston, K., Wallston, B., Kaplan, G., & Maides, S. (1976). Development and validation of the Health Locus of Control (HLC) Scale. *Journal of Consulting and Clinical Psychology, 44,* 580–585.

Warner-Robbins, C., & Christiana, N. (1989). The spiritual needs of persons with AIDS. *Family and Community Health, 12,* 43–51.

Watson, C. (1967). Relationship between locus of control, self-concept and anxiety. *Journal of Clinical Psychology, 31,* 682–685.

Weiss, J. (1971). Effects of coping behavior in different warning signal conditions on stress psychology in rats. *Journal of Comparative Physiologic Psychology, 73,* 202–205.

Westbrook, M. (1987). Belief in ability to control chronic illness: Associated evaluations and medical experiences. *Australian Psychologist, 22,* 203–218.

Wilson, J. (1970). *Thinking with concepts.* London: Cambridge University Press.

Wolfe, P. (1989). Clinical manifestations and treatment. In J. Flaskerud (Ed.), *AIDS / HIV infection: A reference guide for nursing professionals* (pp. 58–73). Philadelphia: WB Saunders.

Zahn, J. (1969). Some adult attitudes affecting learning: Powerlessness, conflicting needs and role transition. *Adult Education Journal, 19,* 91–95.

PART II

Vulnerabilities Across the Life Span

➤ Individuals are vulnerable to powerlessness at different times throughout the life cycle. Behavioral manifestations of powerlessness, coping behaviors, and some nursing approaches are discussed in this part.

Chronic sorrow is a response to losses concomitant with chronic illness. Developmental challenges in dealing with loss and specific clinical examples and nursing interventions to manage chronic sorrow are presented in Chapter 5.

The research base for courage in chronically ill young adults is presented in Chapter 6. A model of becoming and being courageous is developed.

A prevalent health problem among some middlescent women is obesity. The relationship of obesity to powerlessness is discussed in Chapter 7. Empowerment strategies for women coping with the stressors of middle years who are also struggling with weight control are presented.

The relationship of long-standing, uncontrolled powerlessness and hopelessness is revealed in the detailed case-study analysis of an elderly client (Chapter 8). Nursing care of elderly clients who are experiencing powerlessness is included. The serious consequence of a feeling of futility is that the ill elderly person may actually invite death.

▶ 4

Stress and Coping: Psychoneuroimmunology

▶ Lucille Sanzero Eller

Psychoneuroimmunology (PNI) is the study of interrelationships between the neuroendocrine and immune systems. It seeks to elucidate the influence of psychosocial factors on health as mediated by bi-directional neuroendocrine-immune system interactions (Blalock, 1989). PNI offers a holistic perspective in which the body and mind are viewed as a single integrated system where communication occurs at the cellular level. In this model, psychosocial phenomena such as stress, depression, social support, and coping style can influence the neuroen-docrine and immune systems. PNI provides a theoretical framework for understanding relationships between psychological factors and health outcomes. The ultimate goals of PNI are to provide: (1) an understand-ing of the complex biopsychosocial factors that may alter the integrity of the immune system, (2) explanation of the mechanisms of bidirectional neuroendocrine-immune interactions, (3) explication of causal relation-ships between biopsychosocial factors and health, and (4) development of psychosocial interventions that can affect health outcomes.

IMMUNE MEASURES IN PSYCHONEUROIMMUNOLOGY

The immune system is described as having two separate branches, humoral immunity and cellular immunity. Humoral immunity is medi-ated by plasma molecules called antibodies (Abs), which are produced by B lymphocytes. Their function is to recognize and neutralize anti-gens, which are foreign substances in the body. This branch of the im-mune system is the primary defense against extracellular microbes and their toxins.

Cellular immunity is mediated by T lymphocytes and natural killer (NK) cells and is the body's primary defense against intracellular pathogens such as viruses. One function of T lymphocytes is the production of proteins called cytokines. Cytokines are responsible for communication among immune cells, and they mediate and regulate the responses of these cells. Cytokine production is an important measure in the assessment of immune function. The cytokines of interest in PNI include the interleukins and interferons.

Other immune cells of interest in PNI research include monocytes, macrophages and granulocytes (usually neutrophils). Monocytes or macrophages perform phagocytic functions, engulfing and destroying particulate antigens in the body. They also produce cytokines and serve as accessory cells, assisting T cells in their function. Neutrophils are the primary cells activated in acute inflammatory responses. They also perform phagocytic functions.

Immune tests used in PNI research include both enumerative and functional assays. Enumerative tests count either the number or percentage of a specific immune cell in peripheral blood. Enumerative tests measure circulating cells and indicate changes in trafficking such as movement of immune cells from compartments such as the spleen and lymph nodes into and out of peripheral circulation. The presence of adequate numbers and types of immune cells is one criterion necessary for effective immune responses. For example, enumerative assays in PNI may measure number and/or percentage of total lymphocytes, helper T (CD4+) or suppressor T (CD8+) lymphocytes, or NK (CD16+56+) cells.

Functional tests of immunity include measures of cellular and humoral (B-cell-mediated) immune responses. These tests may measure in-vitro lymphocyte activity or the individual's in-vivo response to antigen challenge. For example, in-vitro proliferation assays measure the activity of lymphocytes incubated with mitogens, plant substances that initiate an immune response. Three mitogens used are phytohemagglutinin (PHA), concanavalin A (conA), and pokeweed mitogen (PWM).

Natural killer cell cytotoxicity (NKCC) assays measure the ability of these lymphocytes to lyse target cells in vitro. The standard target used to measure NK activity is the K562, a leukemic cell line. NK cells are responsible for immunosurveillance and can spontaneously lyse virally infected cells and tumor cells. Reduced NK cell numbers or activity are associated with cancer development or progression, viral infection, autoimmune disease, and immunodeficiency states (Whiteside & Herberman, 1994).

Three types of in-vivo tests are also often used to measure cellular or humoral immunity in PNI research. Herpes simplex virus (HSV) or Epstein-Barr virus (EBV) may be measured to assess cellular immune function. HSV and EBV are common viruses to which most people have been exposed. The amount of latent virus present in the blood is the result of the immune system's ability to keep the virus in check. Suppression of cellular immunity results in viral replication. In response to viral replication, there is increased production of virus-specific antibodies. Therefore, higher levels of antibody to HSV or EBV provide evidence of suppressed cellular immune function.

Cellular immunity may also be tested using delayed-type hypersensitivity (DTH) responses. Small amounts of antigens to which most people have been exposed (e.g., tetanus toxoid) are injected intradermally. A DTH response is determined by the degree of induration and erythema present at the site within 24 to 48 hours. The reaction is an indication of the competence of the cellular immune system to recall and respond to the specific antigen.

An in-vivo test used to determine the competence of the humoral immune system is the quantification of antigen-specific Ab produced in response to ingestion or inoculation with a novel antigen. The Ab can be quantified from peripheral blood or, in the case of secretory immunoglobulin A (IgA), in saliva. Greater quantities of Ab production indicate a more competent humoral immune response.

BIOLOGICAL BASIS FOR PNI

Neuro-Immune Interactions: Structure and Function

The mind-body link is supported by well-described neural and hormonal common pathways. Evidence of several structural and functional relationships among the central nervous, endocrine, and immune systems provides conceptual support for PNI.

Alpha-adrenergic and β-adrenergic receptors are present on the surface of lymphocytes in different distributions on B cells and CD4+ and CD8+ T cells (Landmann, Burgisser, West, and Buhler, 1985). Lymphocytes also express receptors for endogenous opioids and other neuropeptides. Receptors exist to receive hormonal signals, so the possibility of immune-endocrine communication via signal molecules is structurally supported. Additional structural evidence is provided by findings that noradrenergic fibers of the sympathetic nervous system (SNS) innervate primary and secondary lymphoid tissue, including the thymus, spleen, and lymph nodes (Felten, Ackerman, Wiegand, & Felton, 1987; Felton et al., 1987). It appears, therefore, that the central nervous system (CNS) and immune system are "hard-wired" together. The presence of these fibers implies some relationship between the CNS and immune system.

Functional evidence comes from studies showing that nerve fibers synthesize and release signal molecules in lymphatic organs. The assumption is that if a chemical is released in the region of a cell that has a receptor for it, the cell will respond to the signal molecule. The presence of lymphocyte adrenoreceptors supports the possibility that norepinephrine, epinephrine, and dopamine, which are secreted in response to SNS activation, are capable of binding to lymphocyte receptors and regulating immune responses. It is therefore feasible that stress-induced activation of the SNS and release of catecholamines in lymphatic compartments could alter trafficking of lymphocytes into peripheral circulation. Neurohormones may also affect the function of these cells in defending the body against disease. A recent finding is that the early-immediate gene product c-*fos* is expressed in catecholaminergic brainstem neurons in response to both actual and conditioned stressors. The projection of these fibers into lymphoid organs helps explain how stress can trigger immune modulation (Pezzone, Lee, Hoffman, & Rabin, 1992; Pezzone, Lee, Hoffman, Pezzone, & Rabin, 1993).

Bidirectionality of neuroendocrine-immune system communication is suggested by evidence that lymphocytes synthesize neuropeptides, including β-endorphin, norepinephrine, epinephrine, and corticotropin (ACTH) (Camara and Danao, 1989; Smith, Morrill, Meyer, & Blalock, 1986). The stress response activates a feedback loop of signal molecules between the neuroendocrine and immune systems (Ader, Cohen, & Felten, 1995). Further support for the CNS-immune link came from studies showing that CNS anterior hypothalamic lesions in rats resulted in either reduced or enhanced cellular and humoral immune responses, depending on the location of the lesions (Jankovic, 1989; Keller, Stein, Camerino, Schleifer, and Sherman, 1980; Macris, Schiavi, Camerino, and Stein, 1970). Hypothalamic-pituitary-adrenal (HPA) activation may be one mediator of this effect. Stress-related release of corticotropin-releasing factor (CRF) by the hypothalamus was found to induce autonomic activation and suppression of NK cell activity in rats (Irwin, Hauger, Brown, & Britton, 1988).

In summary, structural support for neuro-immune interactions include direct innervation of the immune system and the presence of shared neuropeptide receptors by neurons and immune cells. Functionally, lymphocytes produce neuropeptides, and both immune and neural cells produce and respond to the same hormones and cytokines.

Neuroendocrine Mechanisms

The HPA axis and sympathetic-adrenomedullary (SAM) system are two pathways that are activated via hypothalamic stimulation in response to stress. First, stressful events initiate hypothalamic stimulation of the SNS and the adrenal medulla. This initiates the release of the catecholamines epinephrine and norepinephrine.

After exposure to a stressor, stimulation of the HPA is also initiated. First, CRF is released from the hypothalamus to the anterior pituitary. CRF stimulates pituitary secretion of pro-opiomelanocortin, which is cleaved into ACTH and β-endorphin, an endogenous opioid. ACTH stimulates the production of corticosteroids by the adrenal cortex.

Effects of endocrine factors on immunity have been studied in several ways. In-vivo studies have explored the effects of endogenous stress-induced hormones or of direct injection with hormones. In-vitro studies have exposed cells of the immune system to endocrine factors and examined changes in their function. There are four potential mechanisms of neuroendocrine effects on immunity that have some support in the literature.

HYPOTHALAMIC-PITUITARY-ADRENAL AXIS

Stress activates the HPA axis, resulting in increased glucocorticoid production. Glucocorticosteroids have been shown to suppress the number of white blood cells, particularly T cells and monocytes (Hillhouse, Glaser, & Glazer, 1990). They also suppress lymphokine production (interleukin-2 [IL-2] and interferon gamma), which affects all immune functions, including lymphocyte numbers and function and NK cytotoxic activity (Gatti et al., 1987; Munck and Guyre, 1991).

In a study of 416 air traffic controllers (a high-stress occupation) at work, plasma cortisol was higher than normal, and further elevated on days of high workload and more "subjective difficulties" (Rose, Jenkins, & Hurst, 1982a, 1982b).

SYMPATHETIC-ADRENOMEDULLARY SYSTEM

Stress also stimulates the SAM system, resulting in the secretion of catecholamines including epinephrine and norepinephrine. The SAM is stimulated mostly in response to acute stressors. In a study of short-term laboratory stress, changes observed in circulating lymphocyte numbers were associated with catecholamine levels (Landmann et al., 1984; Manuck, Cohen, Rabin, Muldoon, & Bachen, 1991; Naliboff et al., 1991).

Monocytes, B cells, and NK cells increased with higher levels of plasma adrenaline, and CD4+ and CD8+ T-cell ratio was reduced. Similarly, in studies in which epinephrine was injected into subjects, changes in proportions of blood lymphocyte populations, and reductions in the function of these lymphocytes in response to plant mitogens were reported (Crary, Borysenko, Sutherland, et al., 1983; Crary, Hauser, et al., 1983).

Hellstrand and Hermodsson (1989) reported that adrenaline added to NK cells in vitro suppressed their cytotoxic activity. This effect was mimicked by a B_2-receptor agonist and inhibited by a B_2-receptor antagonist, confirming the effect via β-adrenergic receptors.

ENDOGENOUS OPIOIDS

A third and less well-characterized PNI mechanism are the effects of the endogenous opioids. These neuropeptides include endorphins, enkephalins, and dynorphins. Endogenous opioids are peptide molecules secreted by the pituitary and adrenal glands in response to pain and stress. In addition, endogenous opioids can be synthesized by CRF-stimulated lymphocytes (Smith, Morrill, Meyer, & Blalock, 1986). They act on cells that have surface opioid receptors. In addition to nerve cells, opioid peptide receptors have been described on lymphocytes, NK cells, macrophages, polymorphonuclear leukocytes, and mast cells.

Stress can result in the release of these morphine-like compounds, which induce stress-induced analgesia (SIA) (Bandura, Ciofi, Taylor, & Brouillard, 1988; Mogil, Sternberg, & Liebeskind, 1993). In animals, inescapability of the stressor (shock) seems to play a role in whether or not SIA is immune suppressive.

Beta-endorphins are produced by the pituitary gland in response to stress, are elevated in response to relaxation techniques, and can also be produced by lymphocytes. In a review of several hundred studies, Fischer (1988) concluded that β-endorphin enhances immunity. This includes enhanced lymphocyte proliferation (Heijnen, Croiset, Zulstra, & Ballieux, 1987) and NK cell activity (Carr & Klimpel, 1986).

In studies of the effects of stress on opioid production, exercise stress enhanced NK cell activity. This enhancement was blocked by naloxone, an opioid antagonist. Although levels of endogenous opioids were not measured, these findings support the possibility of an opioid mechanism for NK enhancement (Morley, Benton, & Solomon, 1991). Relaxation techniques have been shown to increase β-endorphin. Biofeedback therapy increased levels of β-endorphin in clients with chronic pain (Peniston & Kao, 1984), and progressive muscle relaxation had the same effect in healthy male subjects. Neither of these studies examined immune changes; however, it is reasonable to explore the possibility that these interventions may modulate immunity via their effects on expression of endogenous opioids.

In studies in which met-enkephalin was given over several weeks to healthy subjects and those with acquired immunodeficiency syndrome (AIDS), increases in lymphocyte proliferation, NK cell and T-cell activity were observed (Plotnikoff et al., 1986; Wybran & Plotnikoff, 1991).

Taken together, there is good support from multiple studies for the immune-enhancing effects of endogenous opioids. Considering reports of endogenous opioid-mediated analgesia in animals subjected to acute physical stress, and evidence of their immune-enhancing effects, it may be that endogenous opioids are a preparatory mechanism for physiological response to an acute physical threat.

CONDITIONING OF IMMUNITY

A fourth and final PNI mechanism has been mainly explored in animal studies and is possibly the most fascinating. This is a cognitive mechanism, based on learning theory, and is the operant conditioning of immunity, or "learned" immune modulation.

The earliest studies based on this paradigm were conducted with animals. In one study, Ader & Cohen (1975) paired a neutral conditioned stimulus (saccharin solution) with an immunosuppressive drug, cyclophosphamide. Re-exposure to the conditioned stimulus alone, plain saccharine solution without the drug, resulted in suppression of antibody responses.

In a later experiment, behaviorally conditioned immunosuppression was effective in reducing symptoms and increasing survival time in animals prone to autoimmune disease (Ader & Cohen, 1982).

In human studies with a clinical population, Bovbjerg et al. (1990) reported anticipatory immunosuppression in women being treated with chemotherapy for ovarian cancer. Subjects' blood samples taken in the hospital just before their scheduled chemotherapy infusion were compared with samples taken at their homes 3 to 8 days earlier. Lymphocyte proliferation to the mitogens conA and PHA was suppressed in the prechemotherapy samples, even when controlling for anxiety and anticipatory nausea at the time of the hospital blood draw. There was no difference in NK cell activity or in numbers of lymphocyte subsets.

In healthy subjects in the laboratory, a conditioning procedure paired sweetened sherbet with epinephrine injections. The epinephrine suppressed NK cell activity. On later re-exposure to the sweetened sherbet paired with innocuous saline injections, the suppressed NK cell response was again observed (Buske-Kirschbaum, Kirschbaum, Stierle, Lehnert, & Hellhammer, 1992).

The potential for the conditioning of immune responses can have positive and negative health implications. Additional research is needed to clarify the mechanisms and explore whether psychosocial stressors paired with other events can lead to "learning" of immune responses.

PSYCHOLOGICAL FACTORS; NEUROENDOCRINE AND IMMUNE RESPONSES

Much of the preliminary evidence for PNI comes from animal stress studies. These studies provided the basis for exploration of the effects of psychological factors on neuroendocrine and immune responses in humans. The following section focuses on human studies. Four lines of PNI research are explored: laboratory studies, field studies of naturally occurring stressors, studies of psychological states, and finally, intervention studies.

Laboratory Studies

This line of research explores the effects of brief psychological stress on healthy subjects under laboratory conditions. This study model provides well-controlled conditions in which to examine neuroendocrine and immune outcomes. Stressors used included the Stroop test (Bachen et al., 1992; Caudell & Gallucci, 1995; Manuck et al., 1991), mental arithmetic (Cacioppo, 1994; Naliboff et al., 1991), unsolvable puzzles (Brosschot et al., 1992), loud noise (Cacioppo, 1994; Sieber et al., 1992; Wiesse et al., 1990), shock (Weisse et al., 1990), emotional recall (Knapp et al., 1992), and a gruesome film (Zakowski, McAllister, Deal, & Baum, 1991). Exposure to the stressor ranged from 5 to 20 minutes, and measures were taken from immediate poststress to up to 3 days poststress.

Multiple and sometimes inconsistent immune and neuroendocrine changes were observed. These included:

1. Increase, decrease, or no change in natural killer cell activity (Cacioppo, 1994; Caudell & Gallucci, 1995; Naliboff et al., 1991).
2. Suppression or no effect on lymphocyte proliferation in response to PHA (Bachen et al., 1992; Knapp et al., 1992; Manuck et al., 1991), conA (Cacioppo, 1994; Knapp et al., 1992; Zakowski et al., 1992), and PWM (Linn, Linn, & Klimas, 1988).
3. Alterations in numbers of lymphocyte subsets, including CD4+, CD8+, and CD16+CD56+ (NK) lymphocytes (Bachen et al., 1992; Manuck et al., 1991; Naliboff et al., 1991); and B-cell immunity. These increased or decreased, depending on how long after the stressor the measure was taken.
4. Increases in catecholamine levels (Manuck et al., 1991; Naliboff et al., 1991) or decreases in catecholamines and cortisol at some poststress time points (Caudell & Gallucci, 1995).

These studies revealed that changes in immune and neuroendocrine outcomes varied across time, indicating potential differences in responses to acute versus chronic stress. Immediate poststress increases in measures such as NK cell and CD8+ T-cell numbers were followed by decreases over time. Similarly, decreases in CD4+ T-cell numbers were followed by increases later in time (Brosschot et al., 1992). However, it is clear that there were inconsistencies in findings across studies of immunologic changes due to stress. These inconsistencies may be the result of several factors. First, researchers did not use the same stress model. Different stressors may activate different neuroendocrine pathways resulting in varying immune responses. Second, length of exposure to the stressor also varied. In addition, the length of time between the termination of the stressor and measurement of immune response was not consistent across studies, and appeared to play a role in observed differences in findings. Most studies compared baseline measures with only one poststress measure. Others took measurements at varying time points up to 3 days poststress. Third, assay methods and issues of accuracy and precision of immune measures were not addressed in many studies, reducing comparability across studies. And finally, indicators of SNS activation were not consistently measured or controlled across studies.

It may be that the critical difference in responses to acute stress is SNS response. Researchers who divided subjects into "high" and "low" sympathetic reactors, based on changes in heart rate, blood pressure, and catecholamine production, noted immune differences. Those with high sympathetic reactivity had the most pronounced immune responses (Manuck et al., 1991; Zakowski et al., 1992). This was confirmed by studies in which administration of adrenergic blockers prevented the immune responses previously seen in response to stress (Bachen et al., 1995).

It is clear that even in laboratory studies, in which many confounding factors can be controlled, there is a need for consistency and replicability of experimental conditions and measures. In addition, multiple dependent variables must be measured across time to accurately characterize biphasic or multiphasic immune responses.

Stressful Life Events: Field Studies

A second line of PNI research consists of field studies examining the effects of naturally occurring stressors on immune outcomes. Research supports a relationship between exposure to stressful life events and immune changes in healthy persons. These include caregiving, academic stress, natural disasters, chronic illness, divorce or marital separation, bereavement, and interpersonal relationships.

CAREGIVING

Early studies indicated that caregivers of persons with Alzheimer's disease (AD) were at high risk for depression (Crook & Miller, 1985) and demonstrated impaired health and well-being over time (Brocklehurst, Morris, Andrews, Richards, & Laycock, 1981; Sainsbury & Grad de Alarcon, 1970). These observations led to explorations of potential immunologic changes in this population. Researchers compared 34 family caregivers of clients with AD with matched control subjects. They found higher distress and lower immune function, including higher EBV antibody titers and lower T-lymphocyte percent and helper T lymphocytes in the caregiver group (Kiecolt-Glaser, Fisher, Ogrocki, et al., 1987). Spousal caregivers also demonstrated decreases in lymphocyte response to mitogen and reported more days of infectious illness than matched controls (Kiecolt-Glaser, Dura, Speicher, Trask, & Glasser, 1991).

Family caregiving is on the rise with the current changes in the U.S. health-care system and the increase in community-based care. The changing demographics of the country, with an increased elderly cohort, also predict an even greater rise in the number of family caregivers. Evidence of the effects of stress on caregivers to clients with AD may have relevance for this future population of caregivers. Specifically, it speaks to the need for identifying the specific stressors and for testing stress-reducing interventions in this population.

Aᴄᴀᴅᴇᴍɪᴄ Sᴛʀᴇꜱꜱ

A series of studies of the impact of stressful life events on healthy subjects examined the impact of academic stress on immunity (Kiecolt-Glaser & Glaser, 1992). Comparing medical students' baseline post-vacation measures (low stress) with those during examinations, researchers found decreases in NKCC (Glaser, Rice, Speicher, Stout, & Kiecolt-Glaser, 1986; Kiecolt-Glaser, Garner, et al., 1984), lymphocyte response to mitogens (Glaser et al., 1985, 1987, 1993), and interferon gamma production (Glaser et al., 1986, 1987) and increased antibody titers to HSV and EBV (Glaser et al., 1985a, 1987, 1991). An early study, and one of the few prospective studies linking stress, immunity, and health outcomes examined the effects of academic stress. Researchers followed up 1400 West Point cadets for a period of 4 years. Those susceptible to mononucleosis were identified by the presence of EBV antibodies. Cadets who had higher stress, as defined by high motivation to succeed combined with poor academic performance, were more likely to seroconvert and to develop clinical mononucleosis (Kasl, Evans, & Niederman, 1979).

Nᴀᴛᴜʀᴀʟ Dɪꜱᴀꜱᴛᴇʀꜱ

Natural disasters are arguably the least predictable and controllable of stressful life events. Prospective studies after natural disasters have provided information about the effects of stress on health.

In 1979, a damaged nuclear power plant at Three Mile Island (TMI) presented a major threat to residents of the area. During a 6-year study, these residents were compared with control subjects who lived 80 miles away from the power plant. Researchers found consistent indications of autonomic arousal, including higher catecholamine levels, blood pressure, and heart rates in TMI residents, and also reported sporadically elevated cortisol levels (Baum, Gatchel, & Schaeffer, 1983; Davidson & Baum, 1986; McKinnon, Weisse, Reynolds, Bowles, & Baum, 1989). Immunologic changes in this population included reductions in B lymphocytes, NK cells, and CD8+ lymphocytes, and higher antibody titers to HSV compared with control subjects (McKinnon et al., 1989). Another study reported a relationship between psychological distress and an increased incidence of cancer in those living closest to the power plant during the year after the power plant accident (Hatch, Wallenstein, Beyea, Nieves, & Susser, 1991).

Taken together, the TMI studies may indicate a role for chronic stress in mediating neuroendocrine changes, which may lead to immunosuppression and, ultimately, the incidence of disease. The duration or chronicity of stressful events is also a factor in their eventual health effects. However, further work is necessary to describe the effects of chronic stress on immune and health outcomes and to explore the related neuroendocrine mechanisms.

A study of stress in Israeli civilians compared the effects of exposure to Scud missile attacks during and after the Persian Gulf War, a total period of a few weeks. In this study, researchers reported higher NK cell activity, lymphocyte proliferation, and ACTH levels during the war. Findings also included a high level of problem-focused coping during the war (Weiss et al., 1996). The authors suggested that the short-term nature of exposure may explain enhanced immunity as a preparatory response to acute stress. It may also be that active coping modified the stress response, as will be discussed later in this chapter.

CHRONIC ILLNESS

The occurrence of a life-threatening illness can be viewed as a stressful life event. Several researchers have explored the effects of stress and psychological factors on disease progression and clinical outcomes in persons with cancer and HIV. The effects of psychological factors are discussed later in this chapter. Differing findings were reported regarding the effects of the number of life stressors in persons with HIV. Kessler et al. (1991) reported no effect on disease progression. However, Blaney et al. (1992) reported an association between number of life stressors and increase in symptoms 6 months later. Blaney's group controlled for coping style and other variables known to affect clinical progression. Evans et al. (1995) also reported significant association between severity of stress and CD8+ lymphocyte and NK cell numbers in a sample of 99 HIV-positive men.

Funch and Marshall (1983) conducted a 20-year longitudinal study of women with breast cancer. They found that stressful life events were associated with shorter survival in older women, whereas subjective stressors were associated with shorter survival in younger subjects.

Derogatis, Feldstein, and Morrow (1979) found that higher distress and poorer adjustment to illness predicted longer survival in women with breast cancer. This was interpreted by these researchers as a greater ability to express feelings during a stressful event in the high-distress/low-adjustment group.

Divorce and Marital Separation

Interpersonal losses caused by divorce or marital separation, like losses caused by death, can result in immunosuppression. Thirty-two separated or divorced women were reported to have lower lymphocyte responses to mitogen, fewer NK cells, and higher EBV antibody titers compared with a matched sample of married women (Kiecolt-Glaser, Fisher, Ogrocki, et al., 1987).

Similarly, a sample of 32 separated or divorced men were compared with a matched sample of married men. The separated or divorced sample had higher antibody titers to EBV and HSV. This group also had higher depression, distress, and loneliness compared with the control group. There was no difference between the groups in CD4+ or CD8+ lymphocyte percentage (Kiecolt-Glaser, Kennedy, Malkoff, Fisher, Speicher, & Glaser, 1988).

Bereavement

Early PNI studies linked bereavement with immunosuppression. Bartrop, Luckhurst, Lazarus, Kiloh, and Penny (1977) reported reduced lymphocyte proliferation in response to conA and PHA in newly bereaved spouses compared with matched controls at 6 weeks postbereavement. Similar findings were reported by Schleifer, Keller, Camerino, Thornton, & Stein (1983). They compared lymphocyte proliferation responses up to 14 months postbereavement in men whose wives had died of breast cancer. Immune function was suppressed compared with prebereavement levels. A later study compared NK cell function in three groups of women whose husbands were healthy, were being treated for lung cancer, or had died of lung cancer (Irwin, Daniels, Smith, Bloom, & Weiner, 1987). Wives of men in the last group had the lowest NK function. However, Monjan (1984) did not find any changes in immune parameters in bereaved men compared with control subjects. Lymphocyte proliferation to PHA and conA was unchanged at 1 and 3 months after the death of the spouse.

Several studies explored the effects of bereavement on HIV-positive men. Bereavement was associated with reduced lymphocyte responses to PHA and increased levels of serum neopterin, a predictor of risk for progression to AIDS (Kemeny et al., 1995). Bereavement was also related to a more rapid decline in CD4+-cell count over 4 years in this population (Kemeny & Dean, 1995). It may be that depression is the mediating psychological state in bereavement-associated immunosuppression. In studies in which depression was measured, bereaved subjects who scored higher on depression had suppressed immune responses to DTH tests and lower IgG and IgM Ab levels (Linn & Linn, 1984; Linn, Linn, & Jensen, 1982). Irwin, Daniels, Smith, Bloom, & Weiner (1987) also reported that increases in depression scores in women from prebereavement to postbereavement were strongly associated with concomitant reductions in NKCC. In the same study, 1 to 4 months postbereavement, depression scores were higher and NK function lower in bereaved women when compared with a control group. Goodkin et al. (1996) reported decreased NKCC and PHA responses 6 months after the loss in bereaved HIV-positive men. These decrements were associated with increased catecholamine and cortisol levels. However, in another study with HIV-positive men, Kemeny et al. (1994) reported that depressed mood was associated with immunosuppression only in nonbereaved HIV-positive men. These authors suggested that a high depression score in the bereaved group may, in fact, indicate a different psychological process (i.e., grief rather than depression) compared with that of the nonbereaved group.

There are many potential confounding variables that may account for inconsistent findings across these studies. The type and quality of the relationship with the deceased, coping style, differing immunologic methods, and methods of analysis may have a role in the inconsistencies in results.

INTERPERSONAL RELATIONSHIPS STUDIES

There is strong support for the association between interpersonal relationships and immune function. In women with breast cancer, perceived support from a significant other and the physician and actively seeking social support were related to higher NK cell activity (Levy et al., 1990). In spouses of clients with cancer, those who reported greater social support had higher NK cell activity and lymphocyte response to PHA. Depression and negative life events did not influence immune outcomes (Baron, Cutrona, Russell, Hicklin, & Lubardoff, 1990). It may be that the positive effects of interpersonal relationships are related to the ability to disclose and discuss stressful life events.

Loneliness in medical students was associated with higher EBV antibody titers and lower NK cell activity (Glaser, Glaser, Williger, et al., 1985; Kiecolt-Glaser, Garner, Speicher, et al., 1984). In another study, psychiatric patients who scored higher on loneliness had lower levels of NK cell activity and lymphocyte responses to PHA, and higher urinary cortisol than those who were less lonely (Kiecolt-Glaser, Ricker, George, et al., 1984).

Studies of Psychological States and Traits

There are multiple factors that influence the degree to which an event is assessed as stressful. Unpredictability, as noted earlier regarding natural disasters, adds to perceived stressfulness of an event. Inability to prepare mentally and/or physically for an event adds to its stressful nature.

Uncertainty about an event, and particularly about its anticipated outcome, adds to perceived stress. This is relevant in the case of chronic illness.

The timing and duration of an event also influence the degree to which it is appraised as stressful. Timing relates to the proximity in time of a negatively perceived event to other stressful events. Timing also influences the degree to which an event is stressful in terms of the individual's age and developmental stage.

Depression

The psychological state most studied in relation to PNI is depression. A number of studies have examined the relationship between depression and immunity, and depression and neuroendocrine function.

Studies examining depression and immune outcomes differed in their findings. Researchers reported decreases in NK, total lymphocyte, and B-lymphocyte numbers (Schleifer et al., 1984) or no change (Darko et al., 1988; Evans, Pedersen, & Folds, 1988; Schleifer, Keller, Bond, Cohen, & Stein, 1989; Schleifer, Keller, Siris, Davis, & Stein, 1985; Sengar, Waters, Dunne, & Bovar, 1982). Similarly, lymphocyte proliferative responses to PHA, conA, and PWM either decreased (Calabrese et al., 1986; Kronfol et al., 1983; Kronfol, House, Silva, Greden, & Carroll, 1986; Kronfol, Nasrallah, Chapman, & House, 1985; Schleifer et al., 1984) or did not change (Albrecht, Helderman, Schlesser, & Rush, 1985; Darko et al., 1989; Schleifer et al., 1985, 1989; Sengar, Waters, Dunne, & Bover, 1982). Factors such as age and severity of depression were found to be confounding variables. When categorized by age and severity of depression, older subjects had significantly lower proliferative responses. This was also true in more severely depressed subjects in whom lower numbers of helper T cells were observed (Schleifer, Keller, Bond, et al., 1989).

Elevation of corticosteroids is the neuroendocrine mechanism most commonly implicated in depression-related immunosuppression. Increased cortisol (Linowski et al., 1985), ACTH (Pfohl, Sherman, Schlechte, & Stone, 1985) and CRF (Owen, Michael, & Nemeroff, 1988) have been reported in some studies of clients with depressive disorders. However, others reported no difference in these HPA axis hormones (Linowski et al., 1987). Differing findings may be related to reports of two subtypes of depression that differ in neuroendocrine activation. In melanocholic depression, there is hyperarousal, whereas in atypical depression there is hypoarousal (Gold, Goodwin, & Chrousos, 1988). Providing additional support is the finding of differences in dexamethasone suppression of cortisol in the two types of depression. Andrianopoulos and Flaherty (1991) suggested that these differences in hypercortisolism may explain inconsistencies in reports relating depression and immunosuppression. In addition, catecholamine levels may also be elevated in some persons with depression (Roy, Pickar, Linnoila, & Potter, 1985). It may be that there are subgroups of persons with depression in whom immune suppression may be present. It is critical to assess sympathetic and HPA axis activity as well as other potential confounding variables, such as age and severity of depression, along with immune measures. The only thing that is clear about the association between depression and immunity is the complexity of relationships that must be considered in exploring mood states, neuroendocrine mediators, and immunity.

CONTROLLABILITY AND HELPLESSNESS

A large body of work in animal experiments supports the effects of controllability of the stressor and helplessness on neuroendocrine and immune responses. Laudenslager, Ryan, Drugan, Hyson, & Maier (1983) found that uncontrollable, but not controllable, shocks resulted in suppression of lymphocyte proliferative responses. In a later series of experiments, unpredictability and lack of control over electric shocks resulted in lower lymphocyte responses to PHA, conA, and PWM, and higher levels of corticosteroids (Mormede, Dantzer, Michaud, Kelley, & Le Moal, 1988).

Helplessness is defined as "the psychological state that frequently results when events are uncontrollable" (Seligman, 1975, p. 9). Helplessness and hopelessness are usually linked in human studies. Human experiments appear to confirm findings in animal studies. In one experiment, 10 healthy subjects were each exposed to controllable and uncontrollable noise stress on separate days. An aversive noise exposure was followed by a mental task. Helplessness and control were measured and ACTH and cortisol levels were assessed. Uncontrollable noise resulted in higher reported helplessness and lack of control, and elevated ACTH and cortisol levels (Breier et al., 1987, 1991). In a similar study, conducted with depressed patients, subjects had even greater increases in cortisol when exposed to uncontrollable stress (Breier et al., 1991). Sieber et al (1992) reported reductions in NK cell activity immediately poststress and up to 72 hours later in subjects exposed to uncontrollable noise.

In a study of clients with stages I and II breast cancer, Greer, Pettingale, Morris, & Haybittle (1985) reported greater disease recurrence and shorter survival in those who demonstrated a helpless attitude.

Coping Style

Another potential variable in determining how stress affects health is the individual's coping style. Ultimately, it may be the ability to cope with the stressor that determines its effects on neuroendocrine responses, immunity, and health.

Coping is defined as "constantly changing cognitive and behavioral efforts to manage specific external and/or internal demands that are appraised as taxing or exceeding the resources of the person" (Lazarus & Folkman, 1984). Based on Lazarus' transactional model (1986), coping consists of three basic steps: the event, the appraisal process, and efforts to manage the event and its emotional consequences. It is hypothesized that the processes used to cope with stress, not the stress itself, influence health and psychological well-being.

Stone et al. (1994) examined the effects of appraisal of daily events on humoral immunity. Healthy subjects kept diaries reporting positive and negative daily events and mood. They also ingested a capsule containing a novel protein (antigen) daily over an 8- or 12-week period. Daily saliva samples were tested for levels of salivary antibody (sIgA) to the protein. Higher levels of sIgA, indicating a brisk humoral immune response, were produced in response to events perceived as positive. Lower sIgA levels were associated with negatively perceived events. In another study, higher perceived stress resulted in lower antibody production to hepatitis B vaccination among those who seroconverted (Jabaaij, Grosheide, & Heijtink, 1993). However, Moss, Moss, & Peterson (1989) reported no effects of daily stressful events, mood states, and NK cell activity over a 4-week period. It is noteworthy that these studies examined two different types of immune response. It may be that mood in response to minor daily events has an effect on the humoral but not the cellular immune system. Replicated studies are needed that measure both arms of the immune system to more accurately characterize these responses. Pertinent psychological factors should also be measured in these studies. In an early study with healthy subjects, Locke et al. (1984) found that stressful life changes did not influence NK cell activity. However, when the high-stress group was divided into groups of "good copers" and "poor copers" based on psychological symptoms, the poor copers had lower NK cell function.

Two coping processes used are emotion-focused coping and problem-focused coping. Emotion-focused coping is directed at reducing the negative emotional impact of stressors, whereas problem-focused coping is aimed at resolving the problem itself. Research has shown that depression and anxiety were positively associated with emotion-focused coping and negatively associated with problem-focused coping (Folkman & Lazarus, 1986; Vitiliano, Russo, Carr, Maiuro, & Becker, 1985; Vitiliano et al., 1987). Emotion-focused coping also was associated with duration and pain of recurrent genital herpes simplex virus (HSV) infection (Silver, Auerbach, Vishniavsky, & Kaplowitz, 1986). Kemeny (1991) reported that subjects who used emotion-focused coping in stressful situations demonstrated twice as many recurrences of genital HSV compared with those who used problem-focused coping over 6 months. However, there was no difference in CD4+ or CD8+ levels across groups.

Active coping style was positively associated with NKCC and PHA responses in bereaved HIV-positive men (Goodkin et al., 1996). Goodkin, Fuchs, Feaster, Leeka, & Rishel (1992) and Goodkin, Blaney, et al. (1992) also found that, in HIV-positive subjects, active coping was related to increased CD4+ lymphocyte counts and increased NKCC. Active confrontational coping was also significantly associated with less clinical disease progression in HIV-positive men; however, it was not related to CD4+ counts (Mulder, Antoni, Dutvenvooden, Kauffman, & Goodkin, 1995). Therefore, there may be differences depending on the types of active coping used. In supporting the effects of active, or problem-focused, coping versus emotion-focused coping, Ironson et al. (1994) reported that denial, an emotion-focused coping strategy, and distress were both correlated with immune status and predicted 2-year disease progression in HIV-positive men.

Multiple stressful life events and psychological states and traits have been studied and, in some cases, associated with immune changes in healthy and clinical populations. The clinical significance of stress-associated changes in cellular and humoral immunity warrants further study. There are methodological difficulties in retrospective studies, including inability to control other stressful events and confounding variables that influence findings. Lack of comparability across studies also limits the strength of positive results. Future research should consider the use of standardized, reliable, and reproducible models to build a sound body of PNI knowledge in this area.

Intervention Studies in Selected Clinical Populations

Stress management interventions can be aimed at changing a person's perception of events, enhancing his or her coping skills, or altering the pattern of psychophysiological responses to stress. Based on a PNI model, intervening at any of these points can potentially enhance immune function through neuroendocrine-immune system modulation.

Interventions with the potential for reducing stress and augmenting immune function can include education, cognitive restructuring, self-disclosure, support groups, relaxation training, and combination cognitive-behavioral approaches.

Perception of events can be altered through education and cognitive restructuring. Educational interventions for stress reduction can include providing information about the physiological effects of stress, learning to recognize stress symptoms, and learning to analyze stressful life events. In addition, they may provide specific information regarding uncertain events and potential outcomes. For example, this could include information about what to expect regarding an impending medical procedure. Educational interventions enhance feelings of personal control and self-efficacy and reduce uncertainty.

Psychotherapeutic approaches that include cognitive restructuring can change the perception of stress. Cognitive restructuring involves the reappraisal of perceived threats. It provides a method for recognizing negative automatic thoughts and irrational beliefs and assumptions and replacing them with realistic appraisals. Cognitive restructuring can include the identification of common cognitive distortions. One example is "should" or "must" statements. Thoughts or statements prefaced with "I should" or "She should" lead to feelings of pressure or resentment. Cognitive restructuring provides the skills and self-monitoring techniques to identify negative thought patterns and to challenge automatic and irrational thinking.

Coping skills training that helps the individual use active coping strategies can reduce psychological distress. Self-disclosure provides an opportunity to disclose and discuss stressful events. It can be practiced in any supportive interpersonal relationship, including support groups, or in private through journal writing. In a study of the effects of self-disclosure, Pennebaker, Kiecolt-Glaser, and Glaser (1988) compared healthy subjects who wrote about traumatic experiences for 20 minutes on 4 consecutive days with control subjects who wrote about trivial experiences. The group writing about upsetting experiences had decreased distress, higher lymphocyte responses to PHA, and fewer health center visits. Immune responses were most pronounced in subjects who had not previously disclosed their experiences with others.

Fawzy et al. (1990, 1993) showed that a coping-enhancing intervention in clients with malignant melanoma improved immunity at 6 months and survival at 6 years in the intervention group. The intervention included education, relaxation techniques, problem-solving skills, and psychological support. At 6 months, the intervention group demonstrated reductions in psychological distress and increases in NK cell activity and percentage of NK cells. At 6 years, those in the intervention group had lower cancer recurrence and mortality rates than control subjects. Similarly, Spiegel, Bloom, & Kraemer (1989) reported an average increased survival of 18 months in women with breast cancer who were part of a support group intervention that included self-hypnosis for pain management. Unfortunately, Spiegel's study did not include immune or neuroendocrine measures.

However, another support intervention reported in the literature was not successful in influencing immune function. In this study, college students visited residents of a nursing home three times a week for 4 weeks. No effect was seen on immunity in the elderly subjects (Kiecolt-Glaser et al., 1985). It may be that the age difference precluded meaningful disclosure by subjects to the students. It may also be that age-related suppression in immunity is less amenable to intervention.

In addition to reducing psychological distress and improving coping skills, cognitive-behavioral interventions can potentially enhance immune function through neuroendocrine-immune system modulation. Newer approaches to stress management include behavioral techniques aimed at reducing stress reactivity. Relaxation strategies can reduce the sympathetic response and increase β-endorphins, which may enhance immunity. Relaxation strategies include focused breathing, guided imagery and visualization, progressive muscle relaxation, meditation, and biofeedback.

In one study, Jasnoski & Kugler (1987) found elevated sIgA levels and lowered norepinephrine levels in clients practicing relaxation and imagery. Kiecolt-Glaser et al. (1986) reported that frequency of practice of relaxation techniques was associated with higher CD4+ T-lymphocyte percentages in medical students during examinations. The same group also reported significant increases in NK cell activity and lower HSV antibody titers in older adults in response to a 1-month relaxation intervention (Kiecolt-Glaser et al., 1985).

Two studies examined the effects of a relaxation with guided imagery intervention on subjects with a variety of metastatic tumors or stage I breast cancer (Gruber, Hall, Hersch, & Dubois, 1988; Gruber et al., 1993). In both studies, the intervention group demonstrated increases in NK cell activity, lymphocyte response, immunoglobulin levels, and IL-2 production. Eller (1995) compared relaxation and guided imagery interventions to standard treatment in persons with HIV. Depression was decreased in both treatment groups, whereas CD4+ increased only in the relaxation group compared with controls.

The relaxing effects of a back rub may be responsible for findings of Groer, Mozingo, & Droppleman (1993). Postintervention levels of sIga were higher in experimental subjects receiving the back rub compared with control subjects.

Cognitive-behavioral stress management training typically occurs over several weeks and includes education, cognitive restructuring, and some form of relaxation training. Because training usually takes place in a group format, there are also elements of a support group structure that may be present.

Seligman (1991) reported increased NK cell activity in a group of subjects with cancer enrolled in a 12-week program compared with control subjects. The program included relaxation training and cognitive therapy.

In several studies with persons with HIV, subjects in a cognitive-behavioral stress management program had increased CD4+ and NK cell counts, decreased depression and anxiety, decreased antibody titers to HSV, and decreased use of maladaptive coping strategies (Antoni et al., 1991; Ironson, Antoni, & Lutgendorf, 1995). Conversely, Coates, McKusick, Kuno, & Stites (1989) reported no difference in HIV-positive subjects in an 8-week stress management intervention compared with controls. However, this intervention used a confrontational coping strategy, which, the authors suggested, may have induced rather than reduced stress.

Inconsistent results in PNI intervention studies can make interpretation of results difficult at best. Differences in findings may be attributed to several factors:

1. Differences in treatment protocols, especially in combination interventions, make comparability across studies difficult. Techniques were combined differently in each study and therefore may moderate immune and endocrine variables differently.
2. The dose and duration of treatment varied across studies.
3. Immune measures, endocrine mediators, and psychological moderators were not consistently measured across studies.
4. Most studies did not address control of confounding variables.

Despite inconsistencies in research findings, taken together, the studies provide preliminary support for the effects of self-regulatory techniques on multiple immune parameters. The clinical relevance of immune changes in response to self-regulatory strategies is still unclear. A statistically significant increase or decrease in a single or even in several immune parameters may or may not have health implications. However, the clinician should be aware of the possibility that immune modulation may occur and may be either beneficial or harmful to clients. In particular, these effects should be considered in clients with autoimmune diseases and in immunosuppressed populations, such as clients with HIV and those undergoing immunosuppressive pharmacotherapies. Therefore, the clinician using these interventions for symptom management must remain cognizant of the potential for unexpected immune responses.

METHODOLOGICAL ISSUES TO CONSIDER IN PSYCHONEUROIMMUNOLOGY RESEARCH

There are multiple methodological considerations in the design and conducting of PNI research (Kiecolt-Glaser & Glaser, 1988; Zeller, McCain, McCann, Swanson, & Colletti, 1996). Physical activity, alcohol and drug use, nutritional status, medications, smoking, and caffeine intake can have immunosuppressive effects. Exposure to stressful life events can lead to behaviors that can impair immunity. These may also present confounding variables in determining the relationship between stress, neuroendocrine factors and immunity (Cohen and Herbert, 1996). Behavioral changes associated with coping responses to stress or negative emotional states that may influence immunity may include smoking, alcohol or drug use, poor diet, and sleep deprivation. It is impossible to control all potential moderating factors. However, for those elements that cannot be controlled by subject selection, data should be collected to maximize statistical control.

Findings of a study by Girgis, Shea, and Husband (1988) are relevant to the undertaking of any PNI study that includes phlebotomy. These authors reported that the acute stress of the first venipuncture in a study with repeated venipunctures resulted in decreases in total T lymphocytes, CD4+ lymphocytes, and NK cell activity. After a third blood drawing, subjects demonstrated decreased anxiety and increased immune responses. The authors suggested that at least one blood sample be drawn before baseline samples to reduce the effects of venipuncture stress. Alternative methods include the use of a topical anesthetic or the placement of an angiocatheter, allowing sufficient time to elapse before drawing the baseline blood sample.

Issues in laboratory analyses of immune and neuroendocrine variables must also be considered. Variations in immune parameters and neuroendocrine factors due to circadian rhythms can be controlled by collecting samples at the same time of day within and between subjects.

Assay accuracy and precision is another methodological issue. Systematic bias can be minimized by conducting assays on control and experimental subjects at the same time. The use of the same lots of laboratory reagents and supplies can also reduce error in the conducting of assays. Other issues to consider are the use of normal control subjects, standardization of instruments, and routine quality-control measures.

➤➤➤ CASE STUDY

Ann Smith is a 60-year-old housewife and sole caregiver to her 62-year-old husband, who has just been released from the hospital to the home post-CVA. As Mr. Smith's home-care nurse, you realize that Mrs. Smith needs your support. There are several interventions that you can provide to help her to cope and care more effectively for her husband.

SOCIAL SUPPORT

Social support is provided by many religious institutions that have "friendly visitor" or "friendly caller" programs in which members could visit or call Mrs. Smith on a regular basis. You could also contact the local Office on Aging to locate a respite care program to provide care for her husband while Mrs. Smith resumes some of her previous social activities or joins a spouses' support group at the local hospital.

SELF-DISCLOSURE

Encourage Mrs. Smith to begin keeping a journal, writing just 15 or 20 minutes a day, perhaps at bedtime. Explain that the expression of stressful thoughts and feelings on paper can help to lessen their negative impact. Many people have concerns about the confidentiality of such journals, so you can address this and help her to think about a "safe" place where her journal won't be seen. If this is still a concern, another alternative is to tear up the sheets after writing, and view this as eliminating the negative thoughts and feelings of the day.

RELAXATION

Relaxation techniques are useful for beginning the day on a positive note and for reducing stress throughout the day. There are several techniques for relaxation, and individual preferences vary. Some techniques are focused breathing, imagery, progressive muscle relaxation, and meditation. Relaxation should be taught by someone trained in these techniques, and acquisition of relaxation skills requires regular practice. However, one simple technique that you can teach Mrs. Smith is a sort of "time-out" using focused breathing. However, be aware that some people experience anxiety about breathing or may have respiratory problems that preclude this type of exercise.

In teaching focused breathing, you would tell Mrs. Smith, "Find a place where you can sit comfortably for a few moments. Now, take a few deep breaths and begin to turn your attention inward. You can close your eyes if you like. Now, just allow your breath to follow its natural rhythm. Notice the in breath and the out breath. As you exhale, imagine the tension leaving your body with the out breath, and as you inhale, breathe in peace and calm."

SUMMARY

Since the early 1980s, there has been a progression of research that supports the effects of psychological factors on immunity and the potential for interventions to influence immune outcomes. Thus far, there are three broad areas in which some support is provided. First, there is biological evidence to support the potential for communication among the central nervous, endocrine, and immune systems. Second, the mechanisms for self-regulation of immunity include glucocorticoids, sympathetic tone and endogenous opioid secretion, and conditioning. And third, stress studies and studies of self-regulation show that both can affect immune markers, but the results are not consistent, probably because of study design and because the interaction of multiple variables is more complex than we know at this point.

Statistically significant correlations between immune measures and psychological or neuroendocrine measures do not prove causality, nor do they prove the clinical relevance of the relationships. There is a need for more investigation of the role that stress and psychological factors play in human health and disease.

In animals, several laboratory stressors were used to assess the influence of stress on the development of infectious diseases. Generally, stressed animals had higher mortality rates from viral and bacterial infections than nonstressed animals. This was most apparent when the challenge with the infectious agent was conducted at the same time as the stressor (Cohen & Williamson, 1991; Peterson et al., 1991).

Prospective human studies are needed to provide support for causal relationships among psychosocial stressors, immune decrements, and health effects. These longitudinal studies would provide the best, albeit the most costly, methods to explore the relationships between stress and health. The few prospective studies conducted provide preliminary causal evidence for the health effects of stress.

In a prospective study of genital HSV recurrence over 36 months, researchers found that increased stressful life events and changes in CD4+ and CD8+ cells were not related to HSV recurrences over a 6-month period. However, depressed mood was significantly correlated with recurrence, and negatively related to CD8+ levels. CD8+ levels and recurrence rate were also negatively associated (Kemeny, 1991).

Several studies indicated an increased risk of morbidity and mortality for bereaved persons (Helsing & Szklo, 1981; Kaprio, Koskenvui, & Rita, 1987; Stroebe & Stroebe, 1993). The highest relative risk of mortality occurred between 7 to 12 months postbereavement (Schaefer, Quesenberry, & Wi, 1995). Because a large proportion of deaths were caused by infectious illness or cancer, it is reasonable to consider the possibility that these deaths were related to postbereavement immunosuppression.

REFERENCES

Ader, R., & Cohen, N. (1975). Behaviorally conditioned immunosuppression. *Psychosomatic Medicine, 37,* 333–340.

Ader, R., & Cohen, N. (1982). Behaviorally conditioned immunosuppression and murine systemic lupus erythematosus. *Science, 214,* 1534–1536.

Ader, R., Cohen, N., & Felten, D. (1995). Psychoneuroimmunology: Interactions between the nervous system and the immune system. *Lancet, 345,* 99–103.

Albrecht, J., Helderman, J., Schlesser, M., & Rush, A. (1985). A controlled study of cellular immune function in affective disorders before and during somatic therapy. *Psychiatry Research, 15,* 185–193.

Andrianopoulos, G. D., & Flaherty, J. A. (1991). Bereavement: Effects on immunity and risk of disease. In N. Plotnikoff, A. Murgo, R. Faith, & J. Wybran (Eds.), *Stress and immunity* (pp. 129–153). Boca Raton, FL: CRC Press.

Antoni, M. H., Baggett, L., August, S., Klimas, N., Schneiderman, N., & Fletcher, M. A. (1991). Cognitive-behavioral stress management intervention buffers distress responses and immunologic changes following notification of HIV-1 seropositivity. *Journal of Clinical and Consulting Psychology, 59*(6), 906–915.

Bachen, E. A., Manuck, S. B., Marsland, A. L., Cohen, S., Malkoff, S., Muldoon, M. F., & Rabin, B. S. (1992). *Psychosomatic Medicine, 54,* 673–679.

Bandura, A., Cioffi, D., Taylor, C. B., & Brouillard, M. E. (1988). Perceived self-efficacy in coping with cognitive stressors and opioid activation. *Journal of Personality and Social Psychology, 55,* 479–488.

Baron, R. S., Cutrona, C. E., Russell, D. W., Hicklin, D., & Lubardoff, D. M. (1990). Social support and immune function among spouses of cancer patients. *Journal of Personality and Social Psychology, 59*(2), 344–352.

Bartrop, R., Luckhurst, E., Lazarus, L., Kiloh, L., & Penny, R. (1977). Depressed lymphocyte function after bereavement. *Lancet, 1,* 834–836.

Baum, A., Gatchel, R. J., & Schaeffer, M. A. (1983). Emotional, behavioral and physiological effects of chronic stress at Three Mile Island. *Journal of Consulting and Clinical Psychology, 51,* 565–572.

Blalock, J. E. (1989). A molecular basis for bidirectional communication between the immune and neuroendocrine systems. *Physiological Review, 69,* 1–32.

Blaney, N. T., Goodkin, K., Morgan, R. O., Feaster, D., Millon, C., Szapocznik, J., & Eisdorfer, C. (1992). Life events and coping style predict health status in early HIV-1 infection (Abstract). *Proceedings of the VIII International Conference on AIDS, 8,* 84.

Bovbjerg, D. H., Redd, W. H., Maier, L. A., Hollanc, J. C., Lesko, L. M., Niedzwiecki, D., Rubin, S. C., & Hakes, T. B. (1990). Anticipatory immune suppression and nausea in women receiving cyclic chemotherapy for ovarian cancer. *Journal of Consulting and Clinical Psychology, 58*(2), 153–157.

Brier, A., Albus, M., Pickar, D., Zahn, T. P., Wolkowitz, O. M., & Paul, S. M. (1987). Controllable and uncontrollable stress in humans: Alterations in mood, neuroendocrine and psychophysiologic function. *American Journal of Psychiatry, 144,* 1419–1425.

Brier, A., Albus, M., Wolkowitz, O. M., Zahn, T. P., Paul, S. M., & Pickar, D. (1991). The effects of psychological and physical stress in humans. In N. Plotnikoff, A. Murgo, R. Faith, & J. Wybran (Eds.), *Stress and immunity* (pp. 47–60). Boca Raton, FL: CRC Press.

Brocklehurst, J. C., Morris, P., Andrews, K., Richards, B., & Laycock, P. (1981). Social effects of stroke. *Social Science and Medicine, 15A,* 35–39.

Brosschot, J. F., Benschop, R. J., Godaert, G. L. R., De Smet, M. B. M., Olff, M., Heijnen, C. J., & Ballieux, R. E. (1992). Effects of experimental psychological stress on distribution and function of peripheral blood cells. *Psychosomatic Medicine, 54,* 394–406.

Buske-Kirschbaum, A., Kirschbaum, C., Stierle, H., Lehnert, H., & Hellhammer, D. (1992). Conditioned increase of natural killer cell activity (NKCA) in humans. *Psychosomatic Medicine, 54,* 123–132.

Cacioppo, J. T. (1994). Social neuroscience: Autonomic, neuroendocrine and immune responses to stress. *Psychophysiology, 31,* 113–128.

Calabrese, J. R., Skwerer, R. G., Barna, B., Gulledge, A. D., Valenzuela, R., Butkus, A., Subichin, S., & Krupp, N. E. (1986). Depression, immunocompetence and prostaglandins of the E series. *Psychiatry Research, 17,* 41–47.

Camara, E. G., & Danao, T. C. (1989). The pain and immune system: A psychosomatic network. *Psychosomatics, 30,* 140–146.

Carr, D. J., & Klimpel, G. R. (1986). Enhancement of the generation of cytotoxic T-cells by endogenous opiates. *Journal of Neuroimmunology, 12,* 75–87.

Caudell, K. A., & Gallucci, B. B. (1995). Neuroendocrine and immunological responses of women to stress. *Western Journal of Nursing Research, 17*(6), 672–692.

Coates, T. J., McKusick, L., Kuno, R., & Stites, D. O. P. (1989). Stress reduction training changed number of sexual partners but not immune function in men with HIV. *American Journal of Public Health, 79,* 885–887.

Cohen, S., & Herbert, T. B. (1996). Health psychology: Psychological factors and physical disease from the perspective of human psychoneuroimmunology. *Annual Review of Psychology, 47,* 113–142.

Cohen, S., & Williamson, G. M. (1991). Stress and infectious disease in humans. *Psychological Bulletin, 109,* 5–24.

Crary, B., Borysenko, M., Sutherland, D. C., Kutz, L., Borysenko, J. Z., & Benson, H. (1983a). Decrease in mitogen responsiveness of mononuclear cells from peripheral blood after epinephrine administration in humans. *Journal of Immunology, 130,* 694–697.

Crary, B., Hauser, S. L., Borysenko, M., Kutz, I., Hoban, C., Ault, K. A., Weiner, H. L., & Benson, H. (1983b). Epinephrine-induced changes in the distribution of lymphocyte subsets in the peripheral blood of humans. *Journal of Immunology, 131,* 1178–1181.

Crook, T. H., & Miller, N. E. (1985). The challenge of Alzheimer's disease. *American Psychology, 40,* 1245–1250.

Darko, D. F., Gillin, J. C., Risch, S. C., Bulloch, K., Goldshan, S., Tasevska, Z., & Hamburger, R. N. (1989). Mitogen-stimulated lymphocyte proliferation and pituitary hormones in major depression. *Biological Psychiatry, 26,* 145–155.

Darko, D. F., Lucas, A. H., Gillin, J. C., Risch, S. C., Goldshan, S., Hamburger, R. N., Silverman, M. B., & Janowsky, D. S. (1988). Age, cellular immunity and HP axis in major depression. *Progress in Neuro-Psychopharmacology and Biological Psychiatry, 12,* 713–720.

Davidson, L. M., & Baum, A. (1986). Chronic stress and posttraumatic stress disorders. *Journal of Consulting and Clinical Psychology, 54,* 303–308.

Derogatis, L. R., Feldstein, M., & Morrow, G. (1979). A survey of psychotropic drug prescriptions in an oncology population. *Cancer, 44,* 1919–1929.

Eller, L. S. (1995). Effects of two cognitive-behavioral interventions on immunity and symptoms in persons with HIV. *Annals of Behavioral Medicine, 17*(4), 339–348.

Evans, D. L., Leserman, J., Perkins, D. O., Stern, R. A., Murphy, C., Tamul, K., Liao, D., van der Horst, C. M., Hall, C. D., Folds, J. D., Golden, R. N., & Petitto, J. M. (1995). Stress-associated reductions of cytotoxic T lymphocytes and natural killer cells in asymptomatic HIV infection. *American Journal of Psychiatry, 152,* 543–550.

Evans, D. L., Pedersen, C. A., & Folds, J. D. (1988). Major depression and immunity: Preliminary evidence of decreased natural killer cell populations. *Progress in Neuro-Psychopharmacology and Biological Psychiatry, 12,* 739–748.

Fawzy, F. I., Fawzy, N. W., Hyun, C. W., Elashoff, R., Guthrie, D., Fahey, J. L., & Morton, D. L. (1993). Malignant melanoma: Effects of an early structured psychiatric intervention, coping and affective state on recurrence and survival six years later. *Archives of General Psychiatry, 50,* 681–689.

Fawzy, F. I., Kemeny, M. E., Fawzy, N. W., Elashoff, R., Morton, D., Cousins, N., & Fahey, J. L. (1990). A structured psychiatric intervention for cancer patients: Changes over time in immunological measures. *Archives of General Psychiatry, 47,* 729–735.

Felten, D. L., Ackerman, K. D., Wiegand, S. J., & Felten, S. Y. (1987). Noradrenergic sympathetic innervation of the spleen. I. Nerve fibers associated with lymphocytes and macrophages in specific compartments of the splenic white pulp. *Journal of Neuroscience Research, 18,* 28–36.

Felten, D. L., Felten, S. Y., Bellinger, D. L., Carlson, S. L., Ackerman, K. D., Madden, K. S., Olschowaka, J. A., & Livnat, S. (1987). Noradrenergic sympathetic neural interactions with the immune system: Structure and function. *Immunology Review, 100,* 225–260.

Fischer, E. G. (1988). Opioid peptides modulate immune function: A review. *Immunopharmacology, 10,* 265–326.

Folkman, R., & Lazarus, R. S. (1986). Stress processes and depressive symptomatology. *Journal of Abnormal Psychology, 95,* 107–113.

Funch, D. P., & Marshall, J. (1983). The role of stress, social support and age in survival from breast cancer. *Journal of Psychosomatic Research, 27,* 77–83.

Gatti, G., Cavallo, R., Sartori, M. L., del Ponte, D., Masera, R., Salvadori, A., Carignola, R., & Angeli, A. (1987). Inhibition by cortisol of human natural killer (NK) cell activity. *Journal of Steroid Biochemistry, 26,* 49–58.

Girgis, A., Shea, J., & Husband, A. (1988). Immune and psychological responses to acute venipuncture stress. *Medical Science Review, 16,* 351–352.

Glaser, R., Kiecolt-Glaser, J. K., Speicher, C. E., & Holliday, J. E. (1985). Stress, loneliness and changes in herpesvirus latency. *Journal of Behavioral Medicine, 8,* 249–260.

Glaser, R., Kiecolt-Glaser, J. K., Stout, J. C., Tarr, K. L., Speicher, C. E., & Holliday, J. E. (1985). Stress-related impairments in cellular immunity. *Psychiatric Research, 16,* 233–239.

Glaser, R., Pearson, G. R., Bonneau, R. H., Esterling, B. A., Atkinson, C., & Kiecolt-Glaser, J. K. (1993). Stress and the memory T-cell response to the Epstein-Barr virus. *Brain, Behavior and Immunology, 12,* 435–442.

Glaser, R., Pearson, G. R., Jones, J. F., Hillhouse, J., Kennedy, S., & Kiecolt-Glaser, J. K. (1991). Stress-related activation of Epstein-Barr virus. *Brain, Behavior and Immunity, 5,* 219–232.

Glaser, R., Rice, J., Sheridan, J., Fertel, R., Stout, J. C., Speicher, C., Pinsky, D., Kotur, M., Post, A., & Beck, M. (1987). Stress-related immune suppression: Health implications. *Brain, Behavior and Immunity, 1,* 7–20.

Glaser, R., Rice, J., Speicher, C. E., Stout, J. C., & Kiecolt-Glaser, J. K. (1986). Stress depressed interferon production by leukocytes concomitant with a decrease in natural killer cell activity. *Behavioral Neuroscience, 100,* 675–678.

Goodkin, K., Blaney, N. T., Feaster, D., Fletcher, M. A., Baum, M. K., Mantero-Attienza, E., Klimas, N. G., Millon, C., Szapocznik, J., & Eisendorfer, C. (1992). Active coping style is associated with natural killer cell cytotoxicity in asymptomatic HIV-1 seropositive homosexual men. *Journal of Psychosomatic Research, 36,* 635–650.

Goodkin, K., Feaster, D. J., Tuttle, R., Blaney, N. T., Kumar, M., Baum, M. K., Shapshak, P., & Fletcher, M. A. (1996). Bereavement is associated with time-dependent decrements in cellular immune function in asymptomatic HIV-1 seropositive homosexual men. *Clinical and Diagnostic Laboratory Immunology, 3,* 109–118.

Goodkin, K., Fuchs, I., Feaster, D., Leeka, J., & Rishel, D. D. (1992). Life stressors and coping style are associated with immune measures in HIV-1 infection: A preliminary report. *International Journal of Psychiatry in Medicine, 22,* 155–172.

Gold, P. W., Goodwin, F. K., & Chrousos, G. P. (1988). Clinical and biochemical manifestations of depression: Relationship to neurobiology of stress. *New England Journal of Medicine, 319,* 348–353.

Greer, S., Pettingale, K., Morris, T., & Haybittle, J. (1985). Mental attitudes to cancer: An additional prognostic factor. *Lancet, 30,* 750.

Groer, M., Mozingo, J., Droppleman, P. (1993). Measures of salivary immunoglobulin A and state anxiety after a nursing back rub. *Applied Nursing Research, 7,* 2–6.

Gruber, B. L., Hall, N. R., Hersch, S. P., & Dubois, P. (1988). Immune system and psychologic changes in metastatic cancer patients while using ritualized relaxation and guided imagery: A pilot study. *Scandinavian Journal of Behavioral Medicine, 17,* 15–46.

Gruber, B. L., Hersh, S. P., Hall, N. R. S., Waletzky, L. R., Kunz, J. F., Carpenter, J. K., Kverno, K. S., & Weiss, S. M. (1993). Immunological responses of breast cancer patients to behavioral interventions. *Biofeedback and Self-Regulation, 18*(1), 1–22.

Heijnen, C. J., Croiset, G., Zulstra, J., & Ballieux, R. E. (1987). Modulation of lymphocyte function by endorphins. *Annals of the New York Academy of Science, 496,* 162–167.

Hellstrand, K., & Hermodsson, S. (1989). An immunopharmacological analysis of adrenaline-induced suppression of natural killer cell cytotoxicity. *International Archives of Allergy and Applied Immunology, 89,* 334–341.

Helsing, K. J., & Szklo, M. (1981). Mortality after bereavement. *American Journal of Epidemiology, 114,* 41–52.

Hatch, M. C., Wallenstein, S., Beyea, J., Nieves, J. W., & Susser, M. (1991). Cancer rates after the Three Mile Island nuclear accident and proximity of residence to the plant. *American Journal of Public Health, 81,* 719–724.

Hillhouse, J. E., Glaser, J. K., & Glaser, R. (1991). Stress-associated modulation of the immune response in humans. In N. Plotnikoff, A. Murgo,

R. Faith, & J. Wybran (Eds.), *Stress and immunity* (pp. 3–27). Boca Raton, FL: CRC Press.

Ironson, G., Antoni, M., & Lutgendorf, S. (1995). Can psychological interventions affect immunity and survival? Findings and suggested targets with a focus on cancer and human immunodeficiency virus. *Mind/Body Medicine, 1*(2), 85–110.

Ironson, G., Friedman, A., Klimas, N., Antoni, M., Fletcher, M. A., LaPierre, A., Simoneau, J., & Schneiderman, N. (1994). Distress, denial and low adherence to behavioral interventions predict faster disease progression in gay men infected with human immunodeficiency virus. *International Journal of Behavioral Medicine, 1*(1), 90–105.

Irwin, M., Daniels, M., Smith, T. L., Bloom, E., & Weiner, H. (1987). Impaired natural killer cell activity during bereavement. *Brain, Behavior and Immunity, 1,* 98–104.

Irwin, M., Hauger, R. L., Brown, M., & Britton, K. T. (1988). CRF activates autonomic nervous system and reduces natural killer cytotoxicity. *American Journal of Physiology, 255*(5, Pt. 2), R744–747.

Jabaaij, P. M., Grosheide, R. A., & Heijtink, R. A. (1993). The influence of perceived psychological stress and distress of antibody response to low dose rDNA hepatitis B vaccine. *Journal of Psychosomatic Research, 37,* 361–369.

Jankovic, B. D. (1989). Neuroimmunomodulation: Facts and dilemmas. *Immunology Letters, 21,* 101–118.

Jasnoski, M. L., & Kugler, J. (1987). Relaxation, imagery and neuroimmunomodulation. *Annals of the New York Academy of Sciences, 496,* 722–730.

Kaprio, J., Koskenvui, M., & Rita, H. (1987). Mortality after bereavement: A prospective study of 95,647 widowed persons. *American Journal of Public Health, 77,* 283–287.

Kasl, S. V., Evans, A. S., & Niederman, J. G. (1979). Psychosocial risk factors in the development of infectious mononucleosis. *Psychosomatic Medicine, 41,* 445–466.

Keller, S. E., Stein, M., Camerino, M. S., Schleifer, S. J., & Sherman, J. (1980). Suppression of lymphocyte stimulation by anterior hypothalamic lesions in the guinea pig. *Cellular Immunology, 52,* 334–340.

Kemeny, M. E. (1991). Psychological factors, immune processes and the course of herpes simplex and human immunodeficiency virus infection. In N. Plotnikoff, A. Murgo, R. Faith, & J. Wybran (Eds.), *Stress and immunity* (pp. 199–210). Boca Raton, FL: CRC Press.

Kemeny, M. E., & Dean, L. (1995). Effects of AIDs-related bereavement on HIV progression among New York City gay men. *AIDS Education and Prevention, 7*(s), 36–47.

Kemeny, M. E., Weiner, H., Duran, R., Taylor, S. E., Visscher, B., & Fahey, J. L. (1995). Immune system changes after the death of a partner in HIV-positive gay men. *Psychosomatic Medicine, 57,* 547–554.

Kemeny, M. E., Weiner, H., Taylor, S. E., Schneider, S., Visscher, B., & Fahey, J. L. (1994). Repeated bereavement, depressed mood, and immune parameters in HIV seropositive and seronegative men. *Health Psychology 13,* 14–24.

Kessler, R., Foster, C., Joseph, J., Ostrow, D., Wortman, C., Phair, J., & Chmeil, J. (1991). Stressful life events and symptom onset in HIV infection. *American Journal of Psychiatry, 148,* 733–738.

Kiecolt-Glaser, J. K., Dura, J. R., Speicher, C. E., Trask, O. J., & Glaser, R. (1991). Spousal caregivers of dementia victims: Longitudinal changes in immunity and health. *Psychosomatic Medicine, 53,* 345–362.

Kiecolt-Glaser, J. K., Fisher, L. D., Ogrocki, P., Stout, J. C., Speicher, C. E., & Glaser, R. (1987). Marital quality, marital disruption and immune function. *Psychosomatic Medicine, 49,* 13–34.

Kiecolt-Glaser, J. K., Garner, W., Speicher, C. E., Penn, G. M., Holliday, J., & Glaser, R. (1984). Psychosocial modifiers of immunocompetence in medical students. *Psychosomatic Medicine, 46,* 7–14.

Kiecolt-Glaser, J. K., & Glaser, R. (1988). Methodological issues in behavioral immunology research with humans. *Brain, Behavior and Immunity, 2,* 67–78.

Kiecolt-Glaser, J. K., & Glaser, R. (1992). Psychoneuroimmunology: Can psychological interventions modulate immunity? *Journal of Consulting and Clinical Psychology, 60*(4), 569–575.

Kiecolt-Glaser, J. K., Glaser, R., Dyer, C., Shuttleworth, E., Ogrocki, P., & Speicher, C. E. (1987). Chronic stress and immunity in family caregivers of Alzheimer's disease victims. *Psychosomatic Medicine, 49,* 523–535.

Kiecolt-Glaser, J. K., Glaser, R., Strain, E. C., Stout, J. C., Tarr, K. L., Holliday, J. E., & Speicher, C. E. (1986). Modulation of cellular immunity in medical students. *Journal of Behavioral Medicine, 9*(1), 5–21.

Kiecolt-Glaser, J. K., Kennedy, S., Malkoff, S., Fisher, L., Speicher, C. E., & Glaser, R. (1988). Marital discord and immunity in males. *Psychosomatic Medicine, 50,* 213–229.

Kiecolt-Glaser, J. K., Ricker D., George, J., Messick, G., Speicher, C. E., & Glaser, R. (1984). Urinary cortisol levels, cellular immunocompetency and loneliness in psychiatric inpatients. *Psychosomatic Medicine, 46,* 15–24.

Knapp, P. H., Levy, E. M., Giorgi, R. G., Black, P. H., Fox, B. H., & Heeren, T. C. (1992). Short-term immunological effects of induced emotion. *Psychosomatic Medicine, 54,* 133–148.

Kronfol, Z., House, J. D., Silva, J., Greden, J., & Carroll, B. J. (1986). Depression, urinary free cortisol secretion and lymphocyte function. *British Journal of Psychiatry, 148,* 70–73.

Kronfol, Z., Nasrallah, H. A., Chapman, S., & House, J. D. (1985). Depression, cortisol metabolism and lymphocytopenia. *Journal of Affective Disorders, 9,* 169–173.

Kronfol, Z., Silva, J., Gardner, R., Dembinski, S., Gardner, R., & Carroll, B. J. (1983). Lymphocyte function in melancholia. *Life Sciences, 33,* 241–247.

Landmann, R., Burgisser, E., West, M., & Buhler, F. R. (1985). Beta-adrenergic receptors are different in subpopulations of human circulating lymphocytes. *Journal of Receptor Research, 4,* 37–50.

Landmann, R. M. A., Muller, F. B., Perini, C., Wesp, M., Erne, P., & Buhler, F. R. (1984). Changes of immunoregulatory cells induced by psychological and physical stress: Relationship to plasma catecholamines. *Clinical Experimental Immunology, 58,* 127–135.

LaPierre, A. R., Antoni, M. H., Schneiderman, N., Ironson, G., Klimas, N., Caralis, P., & Fletcher, M. A. (1990). Exercise intervention attenuates emotional distress and natural killer decrements following notification of positive serologic status for HIV-1. *Biofeedback and Self-regulation, 15,* 229–242.

Laudenslager, M. L., Ryan, S. M., Drugan, R. C., Hyson, R. I., & Maier, S. F. (1983). Coping and immunosuppression: Inescapable but not escapable shock suppresses lymphocyte proliferation. *Science, 221,* 568–570.

Lazarus, R. S. (1986). *Psychological stress and the coping process.* New York: McGraw-Hill.

Lazarus, R. S., & Folkman, S. (1984). Stress, appraisal and coping. New York: Springer.

Levy, S., Herberman, R., Whiteside, T., Sanzo, K., Lee, J., & Kirkwood, J. (1990). Perceived social support and tumor estrogen/progesterone receptor status as predictors of natural killer cell activity in breast cancer patients. *Psychological Medicine, 52,* 73–85.

Linn, B. S., & Linn, M. W. (1984). Stressful events, dysphoric mood and immunologic systems. *Psychological Reports, 54,* 219–222.

Linn, B. S., Linn, M. W., & Jensen, J. (1982). Degree of depression and immune responsiveness. *Psychosomatic Medicine, 44,* 128–129.

Linn, B. S., Linn, M. W., & Klimas, N. G. (1988). Effects of psychophysical stress on surgical outcome. *Psychosomatic Medicine, 50,* 230–244.

Linowski, P., Mendelwicz, J., Kerkhofs, M., Leclercq, R., Goldstein, J., Brasseur, M., Copinschi, G., & Van Cauter, E. (1987). 24-Hour profiles of adrenocorticotropin, cortisol and growth hormone in major depressive illness: Effect of antidepressant treatment. *Journal of Clinical and Endocrinological Metabolism, 65,* 141–152.

Linowski, P., Mendelwicz, J., Leclercq, R., Brasseur, M., Haubain, P., Goldstein, J., Copinschi, G., & Van Cauter, E. (1985). 24-Hour profiles of adrenocorticotropin and cortisol major depressive illness. *Journal of Clinical and Endocrinological Metabolism, 61,* 429–438.

Locke, S. E., Kraus, L., Leserman, J., Hurst, M. W., Heisel, J. S., & Williams, R. M. (1984). Life change stress, psychiatric symptoms and natural killer cell activity. *Psychosomatic Medicine, 46,* 441–453.

Macris, N. T., Schiavi, R. C., Camerino, M. S., & Stein, M. (1970). Effect of hypothalamic lesions on immune processes in the guinea pig. *American Journal of Physiology, 219,* 1205–1209.

Manuck, S. B., Cohen, S., Rabin, B. S., Muldoon, M. F., & Bachen, E. A. (1991). Individual differences in cellular immune response to stress. *Physiological Science, 2*(2), 111–115.

McKinnon, W., Weise, C. S., Reynolds, C. P., Bowles, C. A., & Baum, A. (1989). Chronic stress, leukocyte subpopulations, and humoral response to latent viruses. *Health Psychology, 8,* 389–402.

Mogil, J. S., Sternberg, W. F., & Liebeskind, J. C. (1993). Studies of pain, stress and immunity. In C. R. Chapman & K. M. Foley (Eds.), *Current and emerging issues in cancer pain: Research and practice* (pp. 31–47). New York: Raven Press.

Monjan, A. A. (1984). Effects of acute and chronic stress upon lymphocyte blastogenesis in mice and humans. In E. L. Cooper (Ed.), *Stress, immunity and aging* (pp. 81–108). New York: Marcel Dekker.

Morley, J. E., Benton, D., & Solomon, G. F. (1991). The role of stress and opioids as regulators of the immune response. In J. A. McCubbin, P. G. Kaufmann, & C. B. Nemeroff (Eds.), *Stress, Neuropeptides and Systemic Disease* (pp. 221–232). New York: Academic Press.

Mormede, P., Dantzer, R., Michaud, B., Kelley, K. W., & Le Moal, M. (1988). Influence of stressor predictability and behavioral control on lymphocyte reactivity, antibody responses and neuroendocrine activation in rats. *Physiology and Behavior, 43,* 577–583.

Moss, R. B., Moss, H. B., & Peterson, R. (1989). Microstress, mood and natural killer cell activity. *Psychosomatics, 30,* 279–283.

Mulder, C. L., Antoni, M. H., Dutvenvooden, H. J., Kauffman, R. H., & Goodkin, K. (1995). Active coping predicts decreased clinical progression over a one-year period in HIV-infected homosexual men. *Journal of Psychosomatic Research, 39,* 957–965.

Munck, A., & Guyre, P. M. (1991). Glucocorticoids and immune function. In R. Ader, D. L. Felton, & N. Cohen (Eds.), *Psychoneuroimmunology* (2nd ed., pp. 447–474). New York: Academic Press.

Naliboff, B. D., Benton, D., Solomon, G. F., Morley, J. E., Fahey, J. L., Bloom, E. T., Makinodan, T., & Gilmore, S. L. (1991). Immunological changes in young and old adults during brief laboratory stress. *Psychosomatic Medicine, 53,* 121–132.

Oleson, D. R., & Johnson, D. R. (1988). Regulation of human natural killer cytotoxicity by enkephalins and selective opiate agonists. *Brain, Behavior and Immunity, 2,* 171–186.

Olness, K., Culbert, T., Uden, D. (1989). Self-regulation of salivary immunoglobulin A by children. *Pediatrics, 83*(1), 66–71.

Owen, S., Michael, J., & Nemeroff, C. B. (1988). The neurobiology of corticotropin releasing factor: Implications for affective disorders. In A. F. Schatzberg & C. B. Nemeroff (Eds.), *The hypothalamic-pituitary-adrenal axis: Physiology pathophysiology and psychiatric implications* (pp. 1–35). New York: Raven Press.

Peniston, E. G., & Kao, P. (1984). The EMG biofeedback relaxation training effectiveness in the production on beta-endorphins and the suppression of chronic pain. *Biofeedback in perspective: Fifteen years of development, proceedings.* Albuquerque, NM: Biofeedback Society of America.

Pennebaker, J. W., Kiecolt-Glaser, J. K., & Glaser, R. (1988). Disclosure of traumas and immune function: Health implications for psychotherapy. *Journal of Consulting and Clinical Psychology, 56,* 239–245.

Peterson, P. D., Chao, C. C., Molitor, T., Muntaugh, M., Straar, F., & Sharp, B. M. (1991). Stress and pathogenesis of infectious disease. *Review of Infectious Disease, 13,* 710–720.

Pezzone, M. A., Lee, W. S., Hoffman, G. E., Pezzone, K. M., & Rabin, B. R. (1993). Activation of brainstem catecholaminergic neurons by conditioned and unconditioned aversive stimuli as revealed by c-Fos immunoreactivity. *Brain Research, 608,* 310–318.

Pezzone, M. A., Lee, W. S., Hoffman, K. M., & Rabin, B. R. (1992). Induction of c-Fos immunoreactivity in the rat forebrain by conditioned and unconditioned aversive stimuli. *Brain Research, 597,* 41–50.

Pfohl, B., Sherman, B., Schlechte, J., & Stone, R. (1985). Difference in plasma ACTH and cortisol between depressed patients and normal controls. *Biological Psychiatry, 20,* 1055–1072.

Plotnikoff, N. P., Miller, G. C., Solomon, S., Faith, R. E., Edwards, L., & Murgo, A. J. (1986). Methionine enkephalin: enhancement of T-cells in patients with Kaposi's sarcoma (AIDS). *Psychopharmacological Bulletin, 22,* 695.

Rose, R. M., Jenkins, D. C., & Hurst, M. (1982a). Endocrine activity in air traffic controllers at work. I. Characterization of cortisol and growth hormone levels during the day. *Psychoneuroendocrinology, 7,* 101–111.

Rose, R. M., Jenkins, D. C., & Hurst, M. (1982b). Endocrine activity in air traffic controllers at work. II. Biological, psychological and work correlates. *Psychoneuroendocrinology, 7,* 113–123.

Roy, A., Pickar, D., Linnoila, M., & Potter, W. Z. (1985). Plasma norepinephrine level in affective disorders. *Archives of General Psychiatry, 42,* 1181–1185.

Sainsbury, P., & Grad de Alarcon, J. (1970). The psychiatrist and the geriatric patient: The effects of community care on the family of the geriatric patient. *Journal of Geriatric Psychiatry, 4,* 23–41.

Schaefer, C., Quesenberry, C. P., & Wi, S. (1995). Mortality following conjugal bereavement and the effects of a shared environment. *American Journal of Epidemiology, 141,* 1142–1152.

Schleifer, S. J., Keller, S. E., Bond, R. N., Cohen, J., & Stein, M. (1989). Major depressive disorder and immunity: The role of age, sex, severity and hospitalization. *Archives of General Psychiatry, 46,* 81–87.

Schleifer, S. J., Keller, S. E., Camerino, M., Thornton, J. C., & Stein, M. (1983). Suppression of lymphocyte stimulation following bereavement. *JAMA, 250,* 374–377.

Schleifer, S. J., Keller, S. E., Meyerson, A. T., Raskin, M. J., Davis, K. L., & Stein, M. (1984). Lymphocyte function in major depressive disorder. *Archives of General Psychiatry, 41,* 484–486.

Schleifer, S. J., Keller, S. E., Siris, S. G., Davis, K. L., & Stein, M. (1985). Depression and immunity: lymphocyte stimulation in ambulatory depressed patients, hospitalized schizophrenics, and patients hospitalized for herniorrhaphy. *Archives of General Psychiatry, 42,* 129–133.

Seligman, M. (1975). *Helplessness: On depression, development and death.* San Francisco: WH Freeman.

Seligman, M. E. P. (1991). *Learned optimism.* New York: Knopf.

Sengar, D. P. S., Waters, B. G. H., Dunne, J. V., & Bover, I. M. (1982). Lymphocyte subpopulations and mitogenic responses of lymphocytes in major depressive disorders. *Biological Psychiatry, 17,* 1017–1022.

Sieber, W. J., Rodin, J., Larson, L., Ortega, S., Cummings, N., Levy, S., Whiteside, T., & Heberman, R. (1992). Modulation of natural killer cell activity by exposure to uncontrollable stress. *Brain, Behavior and Immunity, 6,* 141–156.

Silver, P. S., Auerbach, S. M., Vishniavsky, N., & Kaplowitz, L. G. (1986). Psychological factors in recurrent genital herpes infection: Stress, coping style, social support, emotional dysfunction, and system recurrence. *Journal of Psychosomatic Research, 30,* 153–171.

Smith, E. M., Morrill, A. C., Meyer, W. J., & Blalock, J. E. (1986). Corticotropin releasing factor induction of leukocyte-derived immunoreactive ACTH and endorphins. *Nature, 3211,* 881–884.

Smith, G. R., McKenzie, J. M., Marmer, D. J., & Steele, R. W. (1985). Psychologic modulation of the human immune response to varicella zoster. *Archives of Internal Medicine, 145,* 2110–2112.

Spiegel, D., Bloom, J. R., & Kraemer, H. C. (1989). Effect of psychosocial treatment on survival of patients with metastatic breast cancer. *Lancet, 1,* 888–901.

Stone, A. A., Neale, J. M., Cox, D. S., Napoli, A., Valdimarsdottir, H., Janmsdorf, L., & Kennedy-Moore, E. (1994). Daily events are associated with secretory immune response to an oral antigen in men. *Health Psychology, 13,* 440–446.

Strobe, M. S., & Stroebe, W. (1993). The mortality of bereavement: A review. In M. S. Stroebe, W. Stroebe, & R. O. Hansson (Eds.), *Handbook of bereavement.* New York: Cambridge University Press.

Vitiliano, P., Katon, W., Russo, J., Maiuro, R. D., Anderson, K., & Jones, M. (1987). Coping as an index of illness behavior panic disorder. *The Journal of Nervous and Mental Disease, 175,* 78–84.

Vitiliano, P., Russo, J., Carr, J. E., Maiuro, R. D., & Becker, J. (1985). The Ways of Coping Checklist: Revision and psychometric properties. *Multivariate Behavioral Research, 20,* 3–26.

Weiss, D. W., Hirt, R., Tarcic, N., Berzon, Y., Ben-Hur, H., Breznitz, S., Glaser, B., Grover, N. B., Baras, M., & O'Dorisio, T. M. (1996). Studies in psychoneuroimmunology: Psychological, immunological and neuroendocrinological parameters in Israeli civilians during and after a period of Scud missile attacks. *Behavioral Medicine, 22,* 5–14.

Weisse, C. S., Pato, C. N., McAllister, C. G., Littman, R., Breier, A., Paul, S. M., & Baum, A. (1990). Differential effects of controllable and uncontrollable acute stress on lymphocyte proliferation and leukocyte percentages in humans. *Brain, Behavior and Immunity, 4,* 39–51.

Whiteside, T. L., & Herberman, R. B. (1994). Role of human natural killer cells in health and disease. *Clinical and Diagnostic Laboratory Immunology, 1*(2), 125–133.

Wybran, J., & Plotnikoff, N. P. (1991). Methionine-enkephalin, a new lymphokine for the treatment of ARC patients. In N. Plotnikoff, A. Murgo, R. Faith, & J. Wybran (Eds.), *Stress and immunity* (pp. 417–432). Boca Raton, FL: CRC Press.

Zakowski, S. G., McAllister, C. G., Deal M., & Baum, A. (1991). Stress, reactivity and immune function in healthy men. *Health Psychology, 11*(4), 223–232.

Zeller, J. M., McCain, N. L., McCann, J. J., Swanson, B., & Colletti, M. A. (1996). Methodological issues in psychoneuroimmunology research. *Nursing Research, 45*(5), 314–318.

5

Chronic Sorrow in Long-Term Illness Across the Life Span

➤ CAROLYN L. LINDGREN

Chronic illness transforms the lives of afflicted individuals and their families. Over a prolonged time, the afflicted lose what their lives had once been. They live with irreversible changes. They must relinquish the physically sound self and learn to function with a less efficient and dependable body. Old ways of functioning must be abandoned. Roles in the family, workplace, and social networks are altered. Independence gives way to varying forms of dependency. Medical regimens and monitoring of symptoms fill time once occupied by more pleasurable and productive activities. Previously held expectations for the future must be reshaped into plans that incorporate the illness.

The demands and effects of chronic illness extend to family members. The interdependent system of the family is emotionally distressed by the suffering and deterioration of their ill member. Role functions previously performed by the ill person are assimilated by other family members. Family operations must be altered to meet the afflicted individual's illness demands. Caregiving is added to the family's activities.

For adults, one family member is usually designated as the primary caregiver. For children, the parents, principally the mother, assume care of the ill child. Unalterable change occurs in these caregivers' lives, and they too experience losses and emotional pain. They must give up other roles and responsibilities to learn and take on the caregiving role. Time and attention to others outside of the caregiving role must be diminished to allow time and energy for the care activities. Caregivers' expectations for the future must be readjusted.

The losses suffered by afflicted individuals and family caregivers instigate a grief process, labeled chronic sorrow, which has been identified in a variety of chronic illness situations at various stages in the life cycle. The purpose of this chapter is to explore the impact of chronic sorrow on chronically ill individuals and their families at different phases of the life span. Nursing-care strategies to facilitate coping in loss and grief and to promote adaptation, health, and well-being are presented.

UNDERSTANDING CHRONIC SORROW

Grief is a normal human response to a significant loss. The death of a family member or friend is considered the ultimate loss (Weenolsen, 1988). Such a loss is obvious and the ensuing grief process is recognized by others with condolences, flowers, and supportive visits. In chronic illness, the losses and ensuing grief may be less obvious, even to healthcare professionals. Therefore the grieved person may receive little or no support from others.

To understand chronic sorrow, it is necessary to understand the nature of grief in general. Grief is a reconstructive process that begins after suffering a loss. Persons suffering a loss must reshape their perceptions of themselves and the world to form new perceptions that incorporate the loss (Parks, 1988). Grief is a painful psychosocial transition. The aggrieved person suffers as he or she is drawn emotionally to, and tries to hang on to, something or someone that is no longer there (Parkes, 1988). The process is characterized by:

- A reaction of numbness and denial to the first realization that a loss has occurred.
- A yearning for the return of the lost object or person and denial of the permanence of the loss.
- Feelings of disorganization, bewilderment, and helplessness. Previously held assumptions about the predictability of the world have been turned around.
- A sense of reorganization or reorder of one's world occurs as the loss is incorporated into new assumptions of one's world.

Throughout this process, emotions vary in their nature and intensity. Feelings experienced in grief are anger, sadness, disbelief, anxiety, fear, loneliness, helplessness, guilt, self-reproach, and depersonalization. Physical symptoms experienced can include tightness in the chest, breathlessness, weakness, fatigue, dry mouth, and hollowness in the stomach.

Chronic sorrow is a continuous grief that occurs in a cyclical pattern of resurging feelings of sorrow interspersed with periods of calmer emotions. The resurging feelings of sorrow can increase in intensity with the accumulation of new losses and remembrance of old losses. This pattern of peaks and valleys in sorrowful feelings does not usually abate (Burke, 1989; Lindgren, 1996; Lindgren, Burke, Hainsworth, & Eakes, 1992). Historically, the term *chronic sorrow* was first used by Olshansky (1962) to describe the resurgence of grief feelings experienced by parents of mentally retarded children. As the children grew and did not meet developmental norms, the parents grieved for each loss of normalcy their child suffered, as an ever-widening gap formed between the child's disability and normative expected performance (Lindgren, 1996).

Just as chronic illness is progressive and permanent, chronic sorrow is also progressive and continuing, albeit periodic, with surges of emotions that can heighten in intensity along a roller-coaster trajectory. Losses that trigger sadness are based on individuals' perceptions of what is meaningful to their world and what has changed in that world. It may be awareness of personal losses such as inability to go to the grocery store unaccompanied or perception of their body as disfigured and unattractive. Triggers to their sorrow can be feelings of disappointment, such as when friends no longer come to share the holidays. The feelings of sorrow may come when they sit and think of the future, fearing the prospect of being incapacitated.

The symptoms of chronic sorrow mirror those of grief caused by a death. At times, the losses may trigger anger. An example is the client with Parkinson's disease (PD), as described by Lindgren (1996), who lamented that she got angry when she sat on the porch and saw all those young people racing down the street in their cars, laughing and having a good time. She could not even get up out of the chair. Feelings of sadness or regret come when losses of what had been are remembered. For example, one woman whose husband had Alzheimer's disease lamented that now her days were spent watching him every minute rather than being at their lakeside cabin enjoying fresh fish dinners from their catch of the day. Feelings of despair may come as the mother of a severely handicapped child with cerebral palsy changes the wet bed twice a night and knows that there is no end in sight.

CHRONIC SORROW WITHIN THE LIFE STAGES

Chronic illness affects the lives of individuals across the life span. The phase of life, or developmental stage, is an influencing factor in the nature and meaning of the losses and grief experienced. The unique meaning of loss and chronic sorrow is examined for young families dealing with a handicapped child, for middle-aged families struck by chronic illness in the productive years, and for elderly couples coping with deteriorating illnesses. Particular strategies for nursing care of persons in these situations are presented.

Chronic Sorrow and Loss in Children and the Young Family

Children live with numerous chronic illnesses such as arthritis, asthma, diabetes, cancer, and conditions such as muscular dystrophy, mental retardation, cerebral palsy, and handicaps resulting from injury and illness. A child is an embodiment of the future, and having an ill child threatened with death or continual physical deterioration is often perceived as an "off-time" loss. Illness and impending death are perceived as happening to older persons who have lived a full life, not to an infant or child (Weenolsen, 1988).

The effect of the illness on the family begins with the diagnosis, the "receiving the news" period, which is usually an intensely painful, emotional crisis. Parents have reported remembering this traumatic time in their lives, even years after the event, with specific details of what the physician said or how it was said (Damrosch & Perry, 1989). Feelings of shock, numbness, and sadness with bouts of denial and disbelief are characteristic as parents attempt to hold on to the normalcy so yearned for (Bristor, 1984; Seideman & Kleine, 1995). Parents lose their image of the "perfect child." They are suddenly bereft of the images of the baby they expected, with cute physical characteristics and predictable delightful behaviors.

To help them cope and recover from the devastation, some parents take an "I-can-take-care-of-this" or "this-loss-is-manageable" attitude and begin searching for answers to their questions and resources to help them. At this phase of life, other family members, such as other children in the family and grandparents, must also learn the diagnosis and grieve. If grandparents are supportive of the parents, they will help them with the grief, but if they are not understanding and cannot accept the diagnosis, the pain for the parents can be that much greater (Seideman & Kleine, 1995).

After initial grasp of the loss, the long quest to incorporate the handicapped child's care into daily family life begins. Previously held perceptions of parenthood must be reshaped. The extent and the meaning of the child's disability will likely become more real as the parents begin interacting with health-care personnel to learn what their child's problems are and how to care for his or her special needs (Seideman & Kleine, 1995). Seideman and Kleine (1995) described this stage as "planning for differences." For example, one mother said that at first she realized that her son was hearing impaired and later came to understand that he was also mentally retarded, even though health professionals working with her son had that realization long before she did. Some parents have described this as steps of realization (Seideman & Kleine, 1995).

Parents realize the losses and cope in different ways. Some may put off accepting the reality of a potential loss. For example, one mother of a retarded daughter accepted the diagnosis of slow learning but was grieved and left the physician's office crying when he told her that the child also had a muscle coordination problem. The mother knew that the toddler had trouble walking but did not want to believe it was really a problem. Some parents consciously put off learning about their child's potential difficulties. For example, parents of a developmentally delayed 2-year-old son decided not to have him tested at a special center to avoid possible labeling of their child (Seideman & Kleine, 1995). Accepting multiple losses one at a time can be considered healthy if it allows the parents time to comprehend and grieve for those losses one at a time and if it does not impede provision of needed health care for the child.

For some, the thought of the child's future may immediately come to mind, bringing waves of grief. For example, a new father called his mother to tell her of her new granddaughter. He was crying and reported that the baby was genetically determined to be a girl but had male and partial female genital characteristics. He was sobbing and questioning how his poor child could go to school without being laughed at. He was already grieved to think that his child might not be able to have children.

The sorrow experienced throughout a child's illness or disability can be triggered by anything that reminds the parents of the losses to their child and them. In the often-complex care process for a handicapped or ill child, numerous experiences can trigger sadness. One mother of a child with muscular dystrophy said that accepting the new braces only brought new waves of sadness to her (Lindgren et al., 1992). Failing to reach developmental milestones, such as being able to wear a backpack and get on the school bus like all the other first graders in the neighborhood, can also trigger chronic sorrow. The parents often suffer in silence as they see those things that remind them of their child's special needs. When the mother of a retarded child heard a coworker telling everyone at work about her child's reading prizes at school, she experienced feelings of sorrow and went to the restroom for a brief cry. She had had a conference that day with her child's teacher concerning her daughter's limitations. Grieving for the child's milestones, as well as social and health shortcomings, is a normal process of adaptation that allows the parents to go on and accept revised goals for their child. The mother described had accepted the fact that her child could not learn, but she had to acknowledge the loss and grieve so that she could go on with revised aims and expectations for the child. However, parents report that each missed milestone needs to be grieved for, and this contributes to the ongoing nature of chronic sorrow. The chronic sorrow often intensifies as the child approaches and enters adulthood and is unable to participate in activities that signify independence and self-sufficiency such as driving or getting a job (Damrosch & Perry, 1989; Lindgren et al., 1992; Seideman & Kleine, 1995; Wikler, Wasow, & Hatfield, 1981).

Mothers and fathers differ in their experiences of sorrow, with mothers usually experiencing more chronic sorrow (Damrosch & Perry, 1989; Hobdell, 1996). Mothers are usually much more involved in the care of handicapped infants, which could account for some of the differences in sorrow between mothers and fathers (Damrosch & Perry, 1989). Parents who are supportive of one another and share their sorrow are likely to fare better. Marital satisfaction and support from a spouse can contribute to the mother's coping more effectively with a handicapped child. A mother's continuous care of a handicapped child is not recognized as a significant societal accomplishment. Such a mother operates on the periphery of societal acceptance, with no expectation of recognition (Damrosch & Perry, 1989; Schilling, Schinke, & Kirkham, 1985).

The stress of an ill or disabled child increases the chance of other losses in the family. Marital discord and dissatisfaction can result in the seemingly healthiest families as a result of the strain of the illness. Parents also lose their sense of normalcy in society, which is replaced by a sense of being different and perhaps stigmatized. In a class on caregiving, one mother reported that, although continually caring for her child who had spina bifida, she was finally able to go to a party. She soon realized that just mentioning that she was caring for a handicapped son caused discomfort in the other party-goers. Her life was so consumed by her responsibilities that she had no time to cultivate any other interests that she could talk about. She left the party feeling dejected and saddened.

A major secondary loss is social contact. Young parents who are totally consumed with the care of their ill child must forgo other social contacts and fun-filled events. Friends may stop coming to visit if the parents do not have any time to devote to them and if they feel awkward around an ill or deformed child. This isolation enhances the parents' sense of loss and grief. Furthermore, it eliminates a very therapeutic element for grief work, support from others. Loss is removal of known elements from one's psychological and physical environment. Support from others seems to fill in some of those gaps. For those who are abandoned by others, even professionals, at this time of greatest need, the suffering can be unbearable.

Practice Implications for Chronic Sorrow in Young Families

The unique grief experience for parents of a chronically ill or handicapped child requires specialized care practices by nurses.

- These parents need recognition of their grief and reassurance that their feelings are legitimate and normal (Copley & Bodensteiner, 1987).
- At diagnosis, parents need information that is not overwhelming, as well as comfort and support. If a physician gives a hurried diagnosis to the parents, it is the nurse's responsibility to be there to answer the parents' questions. The parents need to be allowed to express their feelings of numbness, shock, disbelief, and anger in a private, nonthreatening environment. Parents may displace their anger on health-care professionals. Such displacement should be handled with tact and understanding.
- When care of the child becomes a part of family life, major adjustments and alterations in the family's daily life occurs. The changes and losses in the family's lifestyle can trigger the family's sadness and distress. Specific assessment of the impact and significance of the family's 24-hour home routine is helpful not only to determine ways to help them with the care, but also to allow them to express the meanings of the care and those changes in their life routine.
- The family may need help and support in telling other members of the extended family about their needs and feelings. Families may need counseling to help them learn to negotiate help from family members. For those whose extended families are not emotionally supportive, the situation needs to be assessed and the parents helped with suggestions for responding and accepting their families' lack of support.
- Clinicians need to be aware of the needs of parents throughout the life of the child. It cannot be assumed that parents who are veteran caregivers do not need support and assistance.

➤➤➤ CASE STUDY

Eric was a 14-year-old mentally retarded boy with the intelligence of about a 5-year-old child. He was the son of Jan and David, who also had another son, Mark, who was 9 years old. When Eric was given a diagnosis of retardation in his first year, Jan and David cried and supported one another, relying on their spiritual faith to sustain them. As Eric grew, Jan and David had a very loving, accepting attitude toward him. They laughed and played with him and enjoyed him. They had taken him to special developmental workshops offered by a local university the previous summer. The workshops had helped his eye-hand coordination, and he was a little less clumsy. Only brief episodes of sorrow had been a part of Jan and David's experiences in the years while Eric was growing up. It had been especially tough integrating him with the neighborhood kids, but they had come to accept him. Eric had had a recent growth spurt, and his tibial torsion, combined with the increased length of his feet, made it difficult for him to walk, and he could not run. He was having difficulty getting off the special education school bus. Jan took him to an orthopedic specialist who told her that because Eric was retarded, he could do nothing for him. The frustration of such a pronouncement triggered a profound session of grief for Jan. She was sorrowful that her child had to suffer like this and angry that people like the doctor could not treat him as a human being. It brought fears of the future that she had not had before. What if others treated Eric this way after she and David were not around? Fortunately, she told another mother her story of the doctor's refusal to do anything. This mother knew of a pediatric orthopedic surgeon who had treated developmentally impaired children frequently and with respect. Eric had orthopedic surgery and was able to walk normally after the surgery. The bout of sorrow also prompted Jan to consult with David about active planning for Eric's future.

This case study illustrates:

- The unique aspects of chronic sorrow based on the situation and the family's coping style
- Normality of chronic sorrow in a family that was relatively adaptable and hardy
- Chronic sorrow as a therapeutic emotional process that allowed the family to move on to another phase in the care of their child

Nursing interventions for this self-sufficient family include:

- Counseling, comfort, and understanding of the orthopedic physician's visit
- Counseling about options open to them for planning Eric's future

Chronic Sorrow in the Middle Years

Major devastating illnesses such as multiple sclerosis (MS), amyotrophic lateral sclerosis (ALS), sickle cell disease, cancer, kidney failure, and catastrophic injuries with spinal cord damage can markedly affect individuals in the young to middle productive years. Their unique losses and grief experiences need to be considered. In the middle years, the developmental tasks are geared toward income productivity, raising a family, and achieving aims of self-fulfillment. These are usually considered the pleasurable and rewarding years of life. Grief is often related to missing prime events in life.

Degenerative illnesses such as MS and ALS bring loss of control and predictability about one's life. Previous plans for one's self and family must be forsaken and revised to include the changes caused by illness. Afflicted individuals grieve for the plans they must abandon. For example, Don, who had ALS, lamented over the loss of his plans to teach his daughter to play baseball. He had plans for financial security that included his wife's being able to stay home and not work. Some mornings, when she went off to work, he remarked that he had never meant things to be that way and that it was a sorrow for him.

Because this phase of life is very active, seeing peers participating in rewarding activities triggers sorrow for the afflicted and their caregivers. Being part of an active social group of friends, going out for pizza after a hockey game, taking the kids camping, and fixing up and taking pride in a home are activities that they cannot take part in, and seeing others taking part in them is a reminder of what has been lost. Grieving for changes and then building other meaningful activities are necessary to help the afflicted and their families.

Multiple sclerosis, a degenerating neurological disease, strikes people in the prime of life. The presence and nature of chronic sorrow in persons with MS and their caregiving spouses were described by Hainsworth (1994, 1995). Eight of the 10 afflicted individuals, who ranged in age from 28 to 55 years with illness lasting 4 to 22 years, reported experiencing bouts of sorrow. Their sorrow was related to feelings of loss of control, comparison to healthy peers, remembering how it had been before the illness, and acknowledgment of the control or influence of the MS over their lives. Family members were not always perceived as helpful in coping with the illness because they were also dealing with effects of the illness and not coping effectively themselves.

The caregiving spouse can feel cheated when his or her usual activities are replaced by bedside care. Chronic sorrow can be related to changes in social life, comparisons to healthy others, and anniversaries of stressful events, such as the diagnosis (Hainsworth, 1995). A husband of a woman with MS related to a nurse that he took up modeling as a way to find some self-fulfillment aside from caregiving. After having been involved with the illness for almost 20 years, he was angry when he looked back at all he and his wife had missed. He related that he wanted her to go into a nursing home, but she would have no part of it, even though he was obviously distressed by his caregiving role and the losses the disease had brought. Their daughter had also been found to have MS, and that only increased his desire to separate himself somewhat from the illness. Their social life was lost, and this couple did not seem to enjoy each other's company, either, which added to their agony.

The ill spouse in this example was preoccupied with her illness, which required her full attention and left little energy for consideration of others. In another case study of a client with MS (Hainsworth, Burke, Lindgren, & Eakes, 1993), the client recounted that she encouraged her spouse to take a trip to Florida, but when he phoned her and talked of having fun at Disney World, she felt left out. For the afflicted one, thinking of the responsibility, loss, and pain that the illness has caused a loved one who must assume the role of caregiver may be too painful to contemplate and is therefore suppressed.

The losses for persons in the 20 to 40 age range are dramatic. For the 20-year-old with paraplegia or quadriplegia, grieving for the losses suffered is necessary for the person to go on and build a new life with the abilities remaining. Such illnesses are not necessarily deteriorating, but as life progresses, the disability requires the afflicted and their families to make readjustments and confront losses that the healthy do not encounter.

Although their chronic sorrow has not been empirically documented to any extent, the losses for persons aged 20 to 40 years are blatantly evident. They, along with their family caregivers, must grieve for all that has changed because of the illness. For persons at this age to be suddenly thrust outside the mainstream of society requires acknowledgment of such a change. Removal from the mainstream inherently cuts off the social support needed to handle the distress and grief. The nature and extent of the injury may influence how much the expectations for the future must be readjusted and reshaped.

PRACTICE IMPLICATIONS FOR CHRONIC SORROW IN THE MIDDLE YEARS

- Afflicted individuals and their families should be supported in identifying and expressing the losses and changes they are experiencing and their feelings concerning the losses.
- Listening to the client's expression of grief can be therapeutic in itself. Conveying a sense of understanding to those with sorrow requires the nurse to establish rapport and connect with the client.
- It is important for the afflicted person to recognize that grief can be related to major losses or changes in lifetime aims and goals. Counseling and support are needed to help the individual accept those changes and reconstruct goals and aims that help him or her regain a sense of purpose and hope.
- Support from and interaction with others help the afflicted individual to cope with the emotional suffering of

chronic sorrow. Working to help socially isolated people connect to others is essential. For those who cannot get out of the house, connection to community groups that visit the homebound may be an option, or hook-up to telephone or computer support services run by health agencies may be possible.

• Caregiving spouses need emotional support. Grief expressed by caregivers needs to be accepted by the nurse. The spouse may feel guilty expressing some of his or her feelings, such as anger or frustration. Such feelings need to be legitimatized and reassurance given that such feelings are normal and appropriate. Personal counseling may be indicated for persons who display signs of depression and are not coping well with their emotions or their situation.

➤➤➤ CASE STUDY

Jean was a 42-year-old woman who had been given a diagnosis of MS when she was 18 years old. She had married her high school sweetheart, Jim, who was aware of her illness at the time of the marriage. They had two children, Mary, 23 years old, and Bill, 21 years old. Jean's maiden aunt, Sarah, had come to live with the family over 20 years ago and helped raise the children. Jean was now confined to bed and needed total care. She could feed herself with assistance and, although her speech was dysarthric, she could converse. When the nurse came to visit Jean, she began to cry and said that she was sad because Mary was planning to get married. Jean said that she was thinking about all the things she had missed already in her daughter's life. Now her daughter would no longer be present in the house. Aunt Sarah and Jim had really raised the daughter, and the daughter was pleasant to Jean but did not confide in her. Jim and Aunt Sarah had helped Mary with her homework, bathed her at night when she was little, and took her to school events. Jean felt that she was always an outsider in her daughter's life. She said, weeping, "I was always too weak to be much of a mom. I thought I was being so brave having children, and yet I can't help but think I lost them a long time ago."

This case study illustrates:

• The perpetual nature of chronic sorrow within a chronic illness trajectory
• The high level of intensity of the sorrow many years into the illness
• Yearning for normalcy as a way to ward off or deny that the illness has brought loss

Nursing interventions for Jean's chronic sorrow include:

- Assessing loss and chronic sorrow throughout the illness trajectory
- Actively listening to Jean's grieving experience and offering reassurance that it is normal
- Exploring with Jean the ways in which she could establish some gradual rapport with her daughter
- Reminiscing with Jean about the good things she remembers about her children and their growing up
- Exploring with Jean the contributions she has made by producing two children who have grown into responsible adults

Chronic Sorrow in the Later Years

With advancing age, chronic illnesses are more prevalent. However, technological advances in care and an emphasis on health promotion and prevention have increased long-term survival with these conditions. For elderly persons, chronic conditions bring diminished physical capacities, mental abilities, productivity, self-sufficiency, and social interaction. The older person's social network diminishes as friends and relatives move away and die. Major losses from illnesses common to this age group, such as Alzheimer's disease (AD) and Parkinson's disease (PD), cause chronic sorrow experiences.

Alzheimer's disease is becoming increasingly prevalent as the population ages. Estimates indicate that 5 percent of persons 65 years and older and 47 percent of persons 85 years and older are afflicted to some degree (Matteson, McConnell, & Linton, 1997). The loss and devastation brought about by this illness are experienced mainly by the family members who take on the care demands of their afflicted relatives. They experience significant emotional turmoil, including grief.

Death of the care recipient is the ultimate loss, but grief during the long-term care period of the illness is very much a part of the caregiver's experience (Collins, Liken, King, & Kokinakis, 1993; Theut, Jordan, Ross, & Deutsch, 1991). The deterioration of the ill relative produces gradual loss of his or her personality, ability to converse with others, ability to fulfill role functions within the family, and physical and mental incapacities. For the caregiver, these losses result in the absence of the relative as once known and with whom life was shared (Lindgren, Connelly, & Gaspar, 1996).

The devastation experienced at the time of diagnosis and realization of the disease exert an impact that is reflected in caregivers' perceptions of their grief throughout their experience. Caregivers who experienced feelings such as anger, fear, panic, uncertainty, and sadness at the time of realization have reported anger and hostility, despair, depersonalization, loss of control, and somatization as they were in the midst of caring for their relatives with AD and being reminded daily of their losses. The length of time since diagnosis does not necessarily affect these feelings for caregivers (Lindgren, Connelly, & Gaspar, 1996).

The quality of the previous relationship with the person with AD corresponds with the degree of sorrow experienced. Caregivers who have had happy marriages have reported less sorrowful experiences of anger and hostility and loss of control when dementia strikes a spouse (Lindgren, Connelly, & Gaspar, 1996). Caregivers whose marriages have been less than satisfactory are more likely to be ambivalent and have conflicting emotions such as guilt and anger about the illness, the losses, and the caregiving responsibilities imposed on them. For care-givers with less-than-satisfactory marriages, the illness brings reduced hope that the marriage can ever be better. Such feelings only complicate the losses and grief experienced by the caregivers, just as ambivalence in an affective relationship is a potential cause for difficulty in grief after a death because of unresolved feelings toward the deceased (Worden, 1991).

For caregivers, loss of the future produces grief symptoms (Lindgren, Connelly, & Gaspar, 1996). The plans for the future made before the illness have been lost, and future plans include more illness and the potential death of the care recipient. Looking to the future is a threatening experience for these caregivers.

Another illness that changes the trajectory of elderly persons' lives is PD. With this illness, the afflicted and the caregiver experience numerous losses and resultant grief. PD is a degenerative neurological disease that affects more than 1 million persons older than 50, or about 1 percent of those older than 60 (Cutson, Laub, & Schenkman, 1995). The pathological neurochemical changes of the disease produce bradykinesia, increased muscle tone and rigidity, tremors, motor planning deficits, and autonomic postural instability (Cutson, Laub, & Schenkman, 1995; Kayser-Jones & Jones, 1991). Over the course of the illness, which can last 20 years or more, clients develop inability to rise from a chair or initiate walking. Performing simple motor tasks is hampered by tremors. Postural instability leaves clients susceptible to falls (Cutson, Laub, & Schenkman, 1995; Kayser-Jones & Jones, 1991). About one-third suffer cognitive impairments that limit their function (Mayeux & Stern, 1983). Cognitive deficits include inability to encode, comprehend, and analyze new information; remember recent events; follow instructions; and change behavior to meet a new situation (Cools, Van den Bercken, Horstink, 1984; Kayser-Jones & Jones, 1991). Although progressive dementia occurs in the rates just described, many PD clients endure the physical changes in their bodies with reasonable awareness of what is happening to them. It is not surprising that clinical depression has been found in 30 to 40 percent of PD clients, especially in the early stages of the illness (Cassileth, Lusk, & Strouse, 1984).

Chronic sorrow in persons with PD and their families has been found to be more than an occasional feeling of sadness at the remembrance of how they felt before diagnosis. They are faced with continual reminders of the losses and changes in their lives as they deal with functional restrictions and drug therapy regimens. Such experiences arouse sorrowful expressions of anger, denial, fear, frustration, despair, guilt, and depression that contribute to their sorrow.

For couples coping with PD, a common loss is abandonment of plans for a pleasurable retirement and replacement with monitoring and treatment of the illness and uncertainty about the future. As one wife of a person with PD said, ". . . my husband's retired, I played golf for years, I bowled for years. We were going to do all of those things together, after he retired. Well, it just didn't work that way" (Lindgren, 1996, p. 359).

Another source of shared grief is marital discord resulting from different perceptions of the illness and need for care. Afflicted individuals sometimes perceive their spouse-caregivers as coercive when they try to get them to accept help or use assistive devices such as quad canes or walkers to prevent falls. One person with PD said he wished his wife were not such a bully. From the caregiver's perspective, the care recipient's insistence on doing tasks that he and she is not capable of only increases anger and frustration at the situation (Lindgren, 1996). If the caregiver gets angry with the care recipient, the anger becomes a source of guilt.

For the afflicted and their caregivers, sorrowful situations are reminders of the unrelenting degeneration caused by the illness. One person with PD who was wheelchair-bound related that he became sorrowful when new symptoms developed in spite of his continual hand exercise program with a rubber ball. A spouse-caregiver reported that seeing her husband fall brought intense sorrow, fear, and panic (Lindgren, 1996).

Another loss for the afflicted and their caregivers that triggers sorrow is the necessity to withdraw from social activities such as traveling, doing volunteer work, or dancing at weddings. For the afflicted person, embarrassment or fear of embarrassment in public is cause for sorrow. Fear of falling or falling in public, tipping over water glasses or dishes in restaurants, trouble speaking in public, or not being able to get out of a chair in a restaurant without assistance can trigger sorrow. For caregivers, seeing their partners suffer in public situations can be emotionally painful (Lindgren, 1996). Moreover, as social interactions become restricted to service personnel and health-care professionals associated with the illness needs, caregivers experience a further sense of loss and sorrow.

Adjusting to loss of physical capabilities, social contacts, and attachments is a normal part of the later years. But major illnesses such as AD and PD bring a chronic sorrow that many suffer from alone and without support from others. Such emotional pain only contributes to the devastation these illnesses bring.

Practice Implications for Chronic Sorrow in the Later Years

- The losses of afflicted persons and their families need to be recognized and support provided for their feelings of grief and loss. Just having someone say "I understand" and mean it can be a major help. One of the most difficult things for persons with chronic illness and their caregivers to endure is the indifference of others to what they are going through.
- Emotional support for afflicted persons at the time of diagnosis and crisis is essential. The emotional impact of the diagnosis, which includes feelings of uncertainty, fear, and anger, needs to be recognized, and clients need to be allowed to ventilate and express understanding of those feelings. Denial is more likely in the beginning phase of the illness, and the practitioner must recognize this and support the client and family when that denial falls away and emotional reaction to the impact of the illness is realized (Walker, Pomeroy, McNeil, & Franklin, 1994).
- At the time of diagnosis, supplying information about the illness and resources for help is necessary. The practitioner needs to be sensitive to the learning styles of the afflicted and their caregivers (Walker, Pomeroy, McNeil, & Franklin, 1994). Because of the emotional turmoil of the early phases of the illness, information may not be absorbed and needs to be repeated later and/or provided in amounts that can be understood. Providing information published by health-care organizations such as the Alzheimer's Association and the Parkinson's Disease Foundation can be helpful. Names and telephone numbers of community health agencies that might be helpful to the client should also be provided.
- Referral to a support group can be made after assessing the client's and caregiver's desire for such intervention. For care recipients and caregivers at the diagnostic or early phase of the illness process, suitability of support group intervention needs to be considered before a referral is made. Some Alzheimer's organizations run orientation support groups to allow participants to develop an understanding of support groups, the way in which they operate, and the nature of their content. A beginning

caregiver may be saddened and overwhelmed by a support group in which participants are "veterans" and which describes illness degeneration and demands the beginning caregiver has not yet encountered.

• Facilitating the support between care recipient and family caregiver may be needed. Open communication between them is required for their recognition of each other's grief and to provide comfort and support to each other. As mentioned earlier, the demands of illness and the differing perspectives of the caregiver and care recipient can precipitate marital discord and bring past differences to the surface. Open communication between the afflicted and family members allows for completion of "unfinished business." Professional counseling may be indicated if their interactions only add to the burden of the illness.

• When the afflicted individual changes or suffers another setback, that individual and the caregiver should be allowed to acknowledge the loss and grieve for the experience. Professionals can offer support at the time and allow the individual to ventilate his or her feelings.

• An aim of intervention is life satisfaction for the afflicted and their caregivers in spite of the illness. Interventions for developing the self in rewarding experiences may mean helping afflicted persons to find diversions and hobbies that are within their limitations and give them satisfaction.

• Another way to help caregivers make up for the loss of their partner as an active family member is to facilitate the caregiver's taking on new role functions such as financial management and automobile maintenance. Successfully taking on new role functions can provide caregivers with a sense of accomplishment.

➤➤➤ Case Study

Max was 68 years old and shared his life with Helen, his wife of 44 years. He was given a diagnosis of PD 3 years ago after putting off going to the doctor for several years about his slurred speech and trembling in his leg and arm. The time before the diagnosis had been very upsetting for Helen because she knew that something was wrong and she was taking over more and more activities for Max. His stubbornness and denial of symptoms only made it more difficult for both of them. When the diagnosis was made, Helen was depressed and sorrowful for several weeks as she realized that her life had changed direction. Their retirement plans to live in a cottage by the lake 400 miles from their home and their married children needed to be altered. Max was deteriorating rapidly and was beginning to have memory problems. Her sorrow and sadness would escalate when Max could no longer drive, handle the checkbook, remember how to go around the block, or even button his pants any more. He refused to give her the car keys, and she had to resort to hiding them. For a while Max realized that his mind was slipping, and he became very angry with Helen, blaming it on her and calling her a bully when she encouraged him to use his walker or refused to tell him where the car keys were. Helen had a major bout of crying and sorrow when they returned from the doctor's office after he confirmed Max's dementia.

This case illustrates:

- Chronic sorrow related to the complexity of losses suffered by ill elderly persons
- Chronic sorrow related to loss of the future that had been planned for a number of years before the illness
- Continuous triggers to sadness from the physical changes and care demands of Max
- The emotional crisis of the diagnostic period
- Denial used to ward off confronting the loss
- Denial as harmful when it forestalled treatment for Max

Nursing interventions for Max and Helen's chronic sorrow include:

- Comforting and supporting Helen during her acute chronic sorrow crisis
- Offering counseling to help Helen cope with her caregiving responsibilities
- Providing information about community agencies and services that could be helpful to Helen and Max
- Providing for Helen to receive support and assistance throughout her caregiving experience
- Explaining to Helen how support groups for caregivers of persons with PD operate and referring her to groups in her area that she could choose to attend
- Discussing with Max his feelings about his illness and his relationship with Helen
- Comforting and reassuring Max as he tries to handle his losses with reduced mental resources

SUMMARY

Chronic sorrow is the emotional suffering that is the natural consequence of perceived losses of enduring illness. The nursing supports needed for helping persons cope with this continuous grief process require recognition of the phenomenon and understanding of the unique situational and personal factors affecting the sorrow. Through effective intervention and support to cope with loss and grief, the afflicted and their families can be helped to find more satisfying lives and greater well-being.

REFERENCES

Bowlby, J. (1977). The making and breaking of affectional bonds, I and II. *British Journal of Psychiatry, 130,* 201–210, 421–431.

Bristor, M. W. (1984). The birth of a handicapped child: A wholistic model for grieving. *Family Relations, 33,* 25–32.

Burke, M. L. (1989). Chronic sorrow in mothers of schoolage children with myelomeningocele disability. (Doctoral dissertation, Boston University, 1989) *Dissertation Abstracts International, 50,* 233–234B. (University Microfilms No. 89-20, 093)

Bushkin, E. (1993). Signposts of survivorship. *Oncology Nursing Forum, 20*(6), 869–875.

Cassileth, B. R., Lusk, E. J., & Strouse, T. B. (1984). Psychosocial status in chronic illness: A comparative analysis of six diagnostic groups. *New England Journal of Medicine, 311*(8), 506–511.

Collins, C., Liken, S., King, S., & Kokinakis, C. (1993). Loss and grief among dementia caregivers. *Qualitative Health Research, 3,* 236–253.

Cools, A. R., Van Den Bercken, J. H. L., & Horstink, M. W. I. (1984). Cognitive and motor shifting aptitude disorder in Parkinson's disease. *Journal of Neurological Neurosurgical Psychiatry, 47,* 443–453.

Copley, M. F., & Bodensteiner, J. B. (1987, January). Chronic sorrow in families of disabled children. *Journal of Child Neurology, 2,* 67–70.

Cutson, T. M., Laub, K. C., & Schenkman, M. (1995). Pharmacological and nonpharmacological interventions in the treatment of Parkinson's disease. *Physical Therapy, 75,*(5), 363–373.

Damrosch, S. P., & Perry, L. A. (1989). Self-reported adjustment, chronic sorrow and coping of parents of children with Down syndrome. *Nursing Research, 38*(1), 25–30.

Hainsworth, M. A. (1994). Living with multiple sclerosis: The experience of chronic sorrow. *Journal of Neuroscience Nursing, 26,* 237–240.

Hainsworth, M. A. (1995). Helping spouses with chronic sorrow related to multiple sclerosis. *Journal of Gerontological Nursing, 21*(7), 29–33.

Hainsworth, M. A., Burke, M. L., Lindgren, C. L., & Eakes, G. G. (1993). Chronic sorrow in multiple sclerosis. *Home Healthcare Nurse, 11*(2), 9–13.

Hanson, S. M. H., & Boyd, S. T. (1996). *Family health nursing: Theory, practice, and research.* Philadelphia: FA Davis.

Hobdell, E. F. (1996). Response to "Chronic sorrow in persons with Parkinson's and their spouses." *Scholarly Inquiry for Nursing Practice: An International Journal, 10*(4), 367–370.

Kayser-Jones, J. S., & Jones, T. H. D. (1991). Parkinson's disease. In W. C. Chenitz, J. T. Stone, & S. A. Salisbury (Eds.), *Clinical gerontological nursing: A guide to advanced practice* (pp. 491–505). Philadelphia: WB Saunders.

Kutner, L. (1993, November 25). How youngsters cope with a parent's illness. *New York Times (Late New York Edition).* p. C9.

Lindgren, C. L. (1993). The caregiver career. *IMAGE—Journal of Nursing Scholarship, 25*(3), 214–219.

Lindgren, C. L. (1996). Chronic sorrow in persons with Parkinson's and their spouses. *Scholarly Inquiry for Nursing Practice: An International Journal, 10*(4), 351–366.

Lindgren, C. L., Burke, M. L., Hainsworth, M. A., & Eakes, G. G. (1992). Chronic sorrow: A lifespan concept. *Scholarly Inquiry for Nursing Practice: An International Journal, 6*(1), 27–40.

Lindgren, C. L., Connelly, C., & Gaspar, H. (1996). *Patterns of grief in spouse and children caregivers of dementia patients.* Unpublished manuscript.

Matteson, M. A., McConnell, E. S., & Linton, A. D. (1997). *Gerontological nursing: Concepts and practice* (2nd ed.). Philadelphia: WB Saunders.

Mayeux, R., & Stern, Y (1983). Intellectual dysfunction and dementia in Parkinson's disease. In R. Mayeux & W. G. Rosen (Eds.), *The dementias* (pp. 211–227). New York: Raven Press.

Olshansky, S. (1962). Chronic sorrow: A response to having a mentally defective child. *Social Casework, 43,* 191–193.

Parkes, C. (1988). Bereavement as a psychosocial transition: Process of adaptation to change. *Journal of Social Issues, 44*(3), 53–65.

Schilling, R., Schinke, S., & Kirkham, M. (1985). Coping with a handicap child: Differences between mothers and fathers. *Social Science and Medicine, 21,* 857–863.

Scott, J. P., Roberts, K. A., & Hutton, T. H. (1986). Families of Alzheimer's victims: Family support to the caregivers. *Journal of the American Geriatrics Society, 34,* 348–356.

Seideman, R. Y., & Kleine, P. F. (1995). A theory of transformed parenting: Parenting a child with developmental delay/mental retardation. *Nursing Research, 44*(1), 38–44.

Theut, S. K., Jordan, L., Ross, L. A., & Deutsch, S. I. (1991). Caregiver's anticipatory grief in dementia: A pilot study. *International Journal of Aging and Human Development, 33*(2): 113–118.

Walker, R. J., Pomeroy, E. C., McNeil, J. S., & Franklin, C. (1994). Anticipatory grief and Alzheimer's disease: Strategies for intervention. *Journal of Gerontological Social Work, 22*(3/4), 21–39.

Weenolsen, P. (1988). *Transcendence of loss over the life span.* Washington, D.C.: Hemisphere Publishing.

Wikler, L. M., Wasow, M., & Hatfield, E. (1981). Chronic sorrow revisited: Parents vs. professional depiction of the adjustment of parents of mentally retarded children. *American Journal of Orthopsychiatry, 51*(1), 63–70.

Worden, J. W. (1991). New York: Springer.

6

Courage in Young Adults with Long-Term Health Concerns

➤ Deborah L. Finfgeld

The term *courage* is frequently used in casual conversation when speaking of individuals who have bravely and heroically fought in battle or risked death to save someone else's life. The word is also used to describe how some people manage their lives while struggling with long-term health concerns. Within this context, it has been suggested that the ability to be courageous in the face of health problems enables individuals to live their lives in the best way possible (Shelp, 1984).

The importance of courage to individuals with health problems can be illustrated by juxtaposing the proposed consequences of being courageous with those of being noncourageous. Lack of courage was found by various investigators to result in decreased longevity and proliferation of disease (Maslow, 1970), apathy (Moran, 1945), resignation (Palmour, 1986), mediocrity (Finfgeld, 1997a), depression (Rachman, 1990; Rorty, 1986), despair (Finfgeld, 1992; Rorty, 1986; Tillich, 1952), and despondency (Finfgeld, 1992). In contrast, the outcomes of being courageous have been reported to range from personal growth (Campbell, 1949; Crovitz & Buford, 1978; Haase, 1987; Linderman, 1987; Rorty, 1986; Tillich, 1952) to affirmation of one's self (Haase, 1985; Koestenbaum, 1991; Kohut, 1985; Moran, 1945; Palmour, 1986; Rawnsley, 1994; Servan-Schreiber, 1987; Tillich, 1952). It is also suggested that

145

courageous individuals develop a zest for living (Finfgeld, 1997a), joy (Asarian, 1981; Shelp, 1984; Tillich, 1952), self-confidence, and self-respect (Asarian, 1981; Finfgeld, 1997a; Haase, 1985, 1987). In an attempt to reconcile joy and sorrow, it is thought that individuals who live their lives in a courageous manner develop a sense of satisfaction and equanimity about life (Berman, 1989; Crovitz and Buford, 1978; Finfgeld, 1992, 1997a; Shelp, 1984).

In spite of these assertions, a limited number of research studies (Asarian, 1981; Cuff, 1993; Finfgeld, 1992, 1995, 1997a; Haase, 1985, 1987) have been conducted in which the primary purpose has been to explore the concept of courage and the role it plays in managing one's life with health problems. As such, a greater understanding of courage is needed to give health-care providers a more holistic perspective of the strategies used by individuals to manage long-term health concerns. Thus, the question asked in this study was the following: What role does courage play in the management of persistent health problems among young adults?

BACKGROUND

This is the sixth in a series of studies (Asarian, 1981; Cuff, 1993; Finfgeld, 1992, 1995, 1997a; Haase, 1985, 1987) that have been carried out with the explicit intent to examine the role of courage in the management of long-term health concerns. Asarian (1981) used a phenomenological approach to study courage among three individuals, one of whom was living with terminal cancer. Based on this work, two types of courage were identified. The first, *assertive determined courage,* is characterized by active mobilization of energy, expressed ego strength, and the seeking out of stimulating challenges. The second type of courage, *dignified acceptance,* consists of concerned and sensitive engagement with others, a willingness to take maximum responsibility for one's self, and the ability to gain satisfaction from struggling with challenging situations.

Haase (1985, 1987) also used a phenomenological approach and examined courage among a group of nine chronically ill adolescents. Haase (1985, 1987) assessed that, as a result of their courage, the adolescents in her study experienced a sense of mastery, accomplishment, and competence. In addition, they were able to accept their situations while struggling to maintain, improve, and inspire others. Both Asarian (1981) and Haase (1985, 1987) concluded that courage is learned over time and involves taking responsibility while getting on with life in spite of struggles. Factors such as significant others and hope were identified to help maintain courage, and personal integrity was reported to emerge as courage was sustained.

Cuff (1993) went on to use a combination of qualitative and quantitative approaches to explore courage among 30 individuals who had been victims of sexual assault or who were managing their lives with human immunodeficiency virus, acquired human immunodeficiency syndrome, or severe physical disabilities. Using content analysis and triangulation methods, four themes emerged that characterized courage among the respondents in this study: (1) concern for others, (2) tenaciousness, (3) resilience in the face of loss, and (4) the perception that life is spiritually meaningful. Cuff (1993) concluded that the multistage process of developing courage is fostered by encouragement from others.

On the basis of Haase's (1985, 1987) and Asarian's (1981) suggestion that becoming and being courageous involves a process, Finfgeld (1992, 1995) used grounded theory (Glaser & Strauss, 1967; Strauss & Corbin, 1990) to study this phenomenon among 21 elderly individuals with long-term health concerns. Results from this study suggest that courage is learned over time within the context of threatening experiences that involve a struggle. Problem solving moderated by discernment is evident and results in the transformation of struggles into challenges. Courageous behavior consists of participating in self-care, getting on with life, quiet acceptance, and development of a lifestyle that incorporates these strategies. Factors that help to promote and maintain courage include the expectations of others, role models, values, significant others, hope, and input from health-care providers. Among elderly persons, outcomes of becoming and being courageous include equanimity and personal integrity.

Finfgeld (1997a) went on to develop a substantive grounded theory of courage among 25 middle-aged individuals with persistent health concerns. Within this age group, becoming and being courageous involve an ongoing process of gaining full awareness of and accepting the threat of a long-term health concern, problem solving moderated by discernment, and developing enhanced sensitivities to personal needs and the world in general. Taking responsibility and being productive are courageous behaviors that are promoted by hope, values, role models, and gestures of support. Results of becoming and being courageous among middle-aged individuals with persistent health concerns include thriving in the midst of normality and personal integrity.

Finfgeld's work (1992, 1995, 1997a) offers valuable insights into becoming and being courageous among middle-aged and elderly adults with persistent health problems. As noted by Olshansky (1996), however, conducting only a few grounded theory studies in an area may preclude the possibility of obtaining new insights into other realities. For this reason, it was determined that a theoretical framework of courage among young adults with long-term health problems could offer valuable and unique perspectives. Thus, the purpose of this study was to develop a substantive grounded theory of courage among young adults with persistent health problems.

METHOD

Grounded Theory

Based on the need to develop a substantive theory of courage among young adults and prior evidence (Asarian, 1981; Finfgeld, 1992, 1995, 1997a; Haase, 1985, 1987) that becoming and being courageous involve a process, grounded theory (Glaser & Strauss, 1967; Strauss & Corbin, 1990) was used to conduct this study. Grounded theory is based on the interpretive tradition of symbolic interactionism and provides not only a philosophical perspective but also methodological guidelines for carrying out research investigations (Annells, 1996). The aim of grounded theory research is to explicate common social life patterns (Annells, 1996) while focusing on the "(a) complexities of people undergoing change, (b) influence of social interactions on outcomes, (c) critical junctures that affect processes of adaptation, and (d) ways by which the social environment influences human experiences" (Benoliel, 1996, p. 417).

Sample

Theoretical sampling techniques were used (Glaser & Strauss, 1967), and 21 individuals were invited and agreed to participate. Initially, results from previous research studies (Asarian, 1981; Finfgeld, 1992, 1995, 1997a; Haase, 1985, 1987) were used as sampling criteria. These included dignified acceptance, taking responsibility, and being productive. Later, emergent findings from this project, such as making a positive contribution, were also used to guide the selection process.

Twelve women and nine men, who were 20 to 39 years old and managing their lives with a variety of long-term health concerns, were studied. Their health problems included Crohn's disease, insulin-dependent diabetes, heart disease, paraplegia, quadriplegia, cancer, residual effects from head injuries, and chronic severe abdominal pain of undetermined origin.

Participants were solicited from support groups for persons with spinal cord injury and cancer survivors and from professional colleagues' referrals. The respondents lived in low-, middle-, and upper-income areas of rural or suburban communities in Missouri or Illinois. One individual was Hispanic; the rest were white. All of the respondents had a high school or general equivalency diploma, many were currently attending college, and several held bachelor's or higher degrees. At the time when data were collected, all respondents were managing their health problems at home.

Data Collection and Analysis

As suggested by Olshansky (1996), special precautions need to be taken any time a grounded theory study is conducted in a substantive area that has already been explored among participants in differing conditions or circumstances. To avoid simply verifying and reverifying the same saturated categories among a new sample, the researcher must ensure that the findings are truly grounded in the data. Thus, before launching this study, the investigator reflected on her preconceived notions of courage in an attempt to become acutely aware of biases that could influence the resultant findings. In addition, throughout the data analysis process, attempts were made to remain vigilantly cognizant of negative or alternative cases and to develop sensitivity to their potential meanings among this unique cohort.

The majority of interviews were conducted in private residences ($n = 14$); however, some took place in offices ($n = 6$), and one was completed in a secluded corner of a local rural restaurant. After written consent was acquired from each respondent, audiotaped interviews lasting 1 to 2 hours were carried out using an interview guide that was initially based on findings from prior studies of courage (Asarian, 1981; Finfgeld, 1992, 1995, 1997a; Haase, 1985, 1987). The interview guide was subsequently updated throughout the study based on emergent findings. In general, the interviews focused on respondents' definitions of courage, their perspectives of how courage was developed and demonstrated, factors that helped to promote and maintain courage, and outcomes of being courageous.

The audiotapes were transcribed verbatim, and the data were analyzed using grounded theory methods (Strauss & Corbin, 1990). Textbase Alpha (Sommerlund, 1989) computer software was used to assist with initial open coding. Axial and selective coding were subsequently carried out; and the data were intermittently grouped into subcategories and, later, categories, which had clearly defined characteristics. Throughout this process, the emergent findings were considered within the grounded theory paradigm outlined by Strauss and Corbin (1990), which is composed of casual conditions, context, intervening conditions, action-interaction strategies, and consequences. In order to link various levels of conditions and consequences to the phenomenon under study, the findings were also examined within the conditioned matrix prescribed by Strauss and Corbin (1990). The core category, becoming and being courageous, was continually verified as initial and emergent relationships among and between phenomena were supported or rejected based on the data.

FINDINGS

Overview: Progressive-Regressive Process

Becoming and being courageous among young adults with long-term health concerns involves an ongoing ambiguous process that is learned in a progressive-regressive manner. Progressive-regressive movement occurs on a continuum in which noncourageous behavior is on one end, and courageous behavior is on the other (Fig. 6.1). On the noncourageous end of the continuum, individuals may refuse to participate in their own care or may sabotage others' efforts to help. In addition, they may tend to give up in spite of the potential for a better outcome. In contrast, courageous young adults tend to push themselves beyond the norm and get on with life as much as possible. Coping lies between the two extremes of the continuum and is characterized by meeting basic needs, maintaining the status quo, and doing what is necessary to get by. These sentiments are captured in the words of a participant with brittle diabetes.

> Coping is just kind of getting by with a positive attitude. On the other hand, being courageous involves having the strength to conquer it all. It involves appreciating what I have learned from dealing with this disease, becoming a better person, helping other people, and enjoying life.

Based on the data, courage is learned over time and is developed when individuals must struggle to manage a threat. A young man described how courage emerged for him after a motorcycle accident left him a quadriplegic. "I think courage was something that came out as I dealt with the outcome of my accident. I knew it was in there somewhere; it just took something to grab hold of it and bring it to the outside." The young adults in this investigation struggled with managing the pain and inconvenience of their health problems; altering their goals and plans for the future; losing personal freedom, independence, control, and physical health and abilities; feeling uncertain; and being different than others in their age group. These continual struggles were characterized by intermittent frustration and disappointment; however,

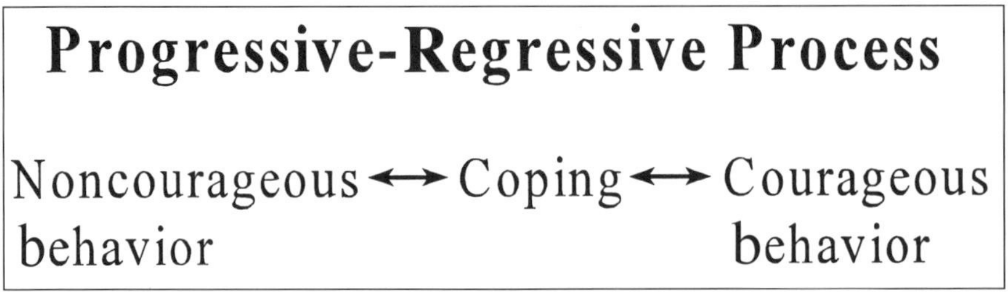

Progressive-Regressive Process

Noncourageous ⟷ Coping ⟷ Courageous
behavior   behavior

FIGURE 6.1 ➤ Progressive-regressive continuum of becoming and being courageous.

when successful management of problems occurred, movement toward becoming and being courageous was promoted.

Varying degrees of courage are needed depending on the circumstantial threats at hand. As suggested by an individual with diabetes, sometimes courage is unnecessary and coping will suffice. "When I'm not having problems, things are hunky-dory—just fine. But when my blood sugar is way out of whack, and I can't get it under control, it takes a hell of a lot to keep going." In other instances, coping is too difficult, and as described by a young woman with paraplegia, noncourageous behavior prevails. "I put my mom through so much. There were days when I crawled into a hole and had my little pity parties. I could just kick myself." For this respondent and others, however, efforts toward courage forced movement in an overall progressive rather than regressive direction. In time, they transcended their health concerns and got on with life in the most optimal way possible.

Courageous Cognition

DISCERNMENT

Courageous cognition among young adults with long-term health concerns is characterized by discernment, or the ability to moderate extremes (Fig. 6.2). For example, efforts are initially made to fully accept reality while handling fear and avoiding denial. These efforts lead to the perception that the struggles accompanying long-term health concerns are manageable challenges instead of inconsequential problems or paralyzing threats. Cognitively framing long-term health concerns in this manner also helps to avoid recklessness or overly conservative management of problems. As described by one respondent with a life-threatening heart problem, excessively conservative perceptions were avoided by thinking of his condition as an "obstacle" rather than a "complete barrier" to maintaining a job and participating in family activities.

Discernment continues to be evident as courageous individuals move beyond the initial stages of accepting their situations as challenges. It is implemented as priorities are balanced between one's own needs and the needs of others; anger is used to motivate rather than enrage or provoke complacency; control is seized when possible and relinquished to others or a higher power when necessary; rigidity and capriciousness are avoided in lieu of adaptive creativity and flexibility; and challenges are approached with realistic persistence rather than shortsightedness or stubbornness. The following excerpt illustrates how an individual with Crohn's disease learned to manage problems using discernment.

> I have realized that situations in which I'm out of control really upset me. But I'm learning that's just the way things are going to be, and it's kind of counterproductive to get too emotionally upset rather than

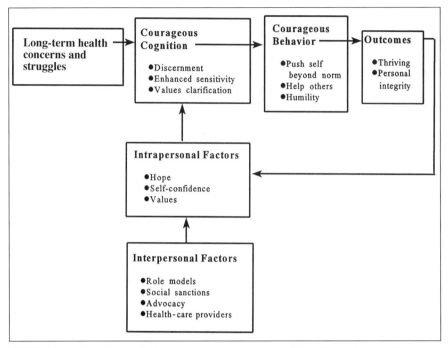

FIGURE 6.2 ➤ Becoming and being courageous among young adults with long-term health concerns.

thinking what would best serve this problem. There's more of an attempt to think rationally and logically.

Enhanced Sensitivity

In spite of the significant negative implications of their long-term health concerns, the courageous young adults in this study appeared to develop a greater cognitive awareness of the positive aspects of their lives. They described an enhanced appreciation of life in general, their remaining health, and future opportunities for fulfillment. There was also a heightened awareness of life's subtleties, God's grace, and the warmth and generosity of others around them. Some went so far as to suggest that their experiences provided them with a wake-up call that forced them to totally re-evaluate how they viewed the world. A female respondent with residual effects from a head injury expressed some of these ideas in the following manner.

> A lot of people take life for granted, and I can't. I can't do that. Since my accident, I have lived each day to its fullest instead of just living each day as if I can't wait for tomorrow. Now I enjoy each day a little

bit more and understand exactly what we're here for. You know, it just lets you appreciate things a little bit more.

VALUES CLARIFICATION

For the young adults in this study, courageously managing their lives with long-term health concerns also meant making adjustments in their value systems. Many values were clarified, whereas others were reformulated or new ones were established. Age-appropriate values such as getting an education, finding a mate, and achieving financial security were clarified and became high priorities if they were not already. Other values, however, such as getting beyond one's own problems, needs, and concerns; helping others; and making a positive impact on the world emerged as new priorities. This new altruistic focus is expressed by a young man with residual effects from a head injury.

> Before all of this I was scum. I mean I just didn't care about others. I only cared about myself. I did whatever I wanted whenever I wanted. Now I try to help other people. I mean people who are troubled and people who are fine. I write letters, poems, songs—everything to brighten up someone's day. Right now, I'm trying to help a girl with a severe problem with self-esteem. She doesn't even eat.

Courageous Behavior

PUSHING BEYOND THE NORM

Over time, courageous cognition results in overt acts of courage. A hallmark of courageous behavior among the respondents in this study was pushing themselves beyond the norm to transcend health problems, strive toward normality, and get on with life versus merely getting by. Courageous respondents reported taking responsibility for their own well-being, engaging in self-care whenever possible, and taking calculated risks. They also emphasized staying involved and being as productive as possible. A woman with brittle diabetes, who is a nurse and regularly checks her blood sugar before driving, explained how she pushes herself.

> I push myself to drive back and forth to work. Once I get there, I know if there's a code, my blood sugar is going to drop, and I better get something in my stomach quick. I also push myself to go hiking, swimming, roller blading, and all kinds of stuff. I lead an exciting life rather than just going to work, coming home, and watching TV.

HELPING OTHERS

In keeping with their emerging altruistic values, courageous young adults push themselves not only for their own betterment but also for the welfare of others. Pushing themselves means helping others in similar situations, making a contribution to society, meeting financial obligations, or, at the very least, avoiding becoming a burden. For example, a quadriplegic described how he tried to maintain some financial independence by pushing himself to be a part-time physical education instructor at a private grade school near his home. He was also completing his 14th year as a volunteer youth minister at his church.

Humility

In spite of being characterized by others as courageous, the participants in this study were humble, unassuming, and somewhat embarrassed when they were referred to as such. Participants made it clear that their actions were not motivated by a desire to solicit attention or accolades. However, they felt comfortable labeling someone else acting in a similar fashion as courageous. A young man who was managing his life with quadriplegia illustrated this point in the following dialogue.

> Respondent: Courage to me would be somebody who goes beyond their capabilities to do normal things. As some people would say, even beyond what's normal. And to set examples for others.
> Interviewer: Do you feel that definition applies to you?
> Respondent: Yes, but I hate to admit it. I have difficulty with the modesty part of this.

Some of the reluctance to identify themselves as courageous also appears to relate, at least in part, to the fact that what started out as challenging for them later became part of their everyday lives. For example, a man with paraplegia described how, over the years, it just seemed natural to rake leaves out of the road ditch while sitting in his wheelchair. He did not recognize this behavior as extraordinary until someone brought it to his attention.

Intrapersonal Factors That Promote and Maintain Courage

Hope

According to the respondents in this study, courage is not limitless and continual renewal is required. Intervening factors that help to promote and maintain courage are interpersonal and intrapersonal in nature. Hope is an example of an intrapersonal factor that is composed of religious faith as well as secular optimism. Secular optimism involves having a positive attitude and perceiving that life is good in spite of challenges. Religious faith offers hope by rendering a sense of security that order will emerge from chaos, and that no matter what happens, an ever-present benevolent higher power has a purposeful grand plan in mind. A young woman with brittle diabetes expressed some of these sentiments in the following manner: "I have hope that people will help me, and that I can make it. I also believe that no matter what the weave on this side of the cloth looks like, God's creating something beautiful on the other side."

SELF-CONFIDENCE

Self-confidence is another intrapersonal factor that tends to promote courage and is characterized by a sense of perceived control that is generated when individuals have an accurate and thorough understanding of their health problems. In addition, successful management of threats in the past leads to the belief that similar success is possible in the future. For example, a young man who was struggling with a life-threatening heart condition described how several years ago he managed to resume walking after a very serious automobile accident and a dismal prognosis. He felt that previous successful efforts to regain his mobility gave him the self-confidence necessary to deal courageously with the current challenges imposed by his cardiac problem.

Having self-confidence also involves feelings of self-worth. For the young adults in this study, having self-worth meant understanding and accepting one's value in spite of differences. Differences that initially diminished feelings of self-worth included strict self-care routines such as insulin administration protocols or bowel maintenance programs; altered mobility; changes in physical appearance caused by chemotherapy, surgery, or trauma; and excessive fatigue. To become and be courageous, individuals needed to perceive that their differences were secondary to their overall potential as human beings. In the following excerpt, a young man with residual effects from a head injury explains how he was able to move toward being courageous after rediscovering a sense of self-worth.

> Early on, I actively tried to commit suicide several times. I walked out in the middle of the highway late at night in black clothes. I also tried jumping off buildings and running into a glass door. I didn't feel like I had a lot to live for. But, eventually, I began to appreciate life more. I began to see that there are other people like me who live valuable lives.

VALUES

Personal values influence the promotion and maintenance of courage by rendering purposeful goals and expectations. Some courageous behavior is based on already established age-appropriate values such as getting an education or becoming financially secure. Emergent values such as altruism, however, also served as primary motivators for the respondents in this study.

In addition to a global sense of altruism, the young adults in this study also felt a specific reciprocal need to be courageous for others who had cared about them or for them. A sense of reciprocal caring was fostered by a desire to diminish any potential distress that significant others might be experiencing in relationship to their long-term concerns. This is illustrated in the words of a young woman who was struggling to do well and complete college in spite of residual effects from a head injury.

> I have tried real hard in rehab and school. I am trying to make it for my parents. They have been very supportive, but they've also had lots of trouble dealing with this. I guess it was just overwhelming for them. And I thought, you know, I can do this. I've got to show them I can.

Interpersonal Factors That Promote and Maintain Courage

ROLE MODELS

Family members, individuals in similar situations, and famous people serve as positive and negative role models, which play an important part in the promotion and maintenance of courage. Positive role models inspire courageous behavior, whereas negative role models do the same by providing contrary examples. Courageous behavior that was emulated included maintaining a positive attitude while continually trying to face adversity and going beyond the norm to help others and/or contribute to society. Noncourageous behavior that was avoided involved being persistently angry and pessimistic, giving up, failing to take the welfare of others into consideration, abusing substances, relinquishing responsibility for self-care, and failing to take calculated risks. A young man who was managing his life with quadriplegia recalled how he was influenced by negative role models in the hospital.

> I met paraplegics who were still able to do things for themselves. They could still get themselves in and out of their chairs and bed. They could dress themselves and everything. But they were so angry, they didn't want to accept any help or try. I didn't want to be like that.

SOCIAL SANCTIONS

Another way in which courage is promoted and maintained is by socially sanctioning courageous behavior and reassuring individuals of their worth in spite of their differences. Respondents reported a sense of worth when others appreciated them and perceived that they could make a valuable contribution. They indicated that feelings of value and worth were communicated through simple gestures of kindness that projected acceptance, love, and caring. Being willing to talk, expressing sensitivity to their situations, including them in activities, sending cards, and praying for them were identified as ways in which feelings of self-worth could be instilled.

Respondents went on to suggest that their courageous behavior was promoted and maintained when it was acknowledged as culturally, morally, and ethically congruent with the predominant mores of the community. Approval of courageous behavior was communicated through simple words of acknowledgment, approval, and admiration. Such expressions of approval are akin to sanctioning individuals as valuable human beings. Although the respondents made it clear that their primary motivation was not to seek accolades, they admitted that positive reinforcement of courageous behavior helped to promote and maintain it. A young man who was challenged with cognitive and motor deficits after a car accident expressed some of these sentiments in the following way: "It really helps when somebody says 'thanks' after I've really tried to do something for them or I get a hug every once in a while."

It should be emphasized that, in spite of the fact that respondents placed considerable importance on doing the *right* thing, this did not preclude them from being assertive when necessary, taking calculated risks, and occasionally pushing their limits. For example, a wheelchair-dependent respondent spent a great deal of time assertively trying to defend the rights of the disabled and eliminating barriers that could impede their mobility. Another individual with limb paralysis water-skied using a custom-made apparatus that he sat in.

ADVOCACY

Being an advocate also helps to promote and maintain courage by providing an environment that is perceived as safe and secure. Respondents suggested that a sense of safety and security exists when there is reason to believe that others have their best interests in mind and are willing to help when necessary. Being an advocate may involve simply being present when case assistance is needed, helping with daily activities, or taking control when individuals are unable to do so for themselves. Advocacy may also include the presence of a higher power who will benevolently assist when others are unable.

Individuals also serve as advocates when they promote normality and avoid pandering. Normality is fostered by diverting attention away from health concerns and expecting as normal participation in life as possible. Advocates tend to frame situations in a positive manner by sharing words of encouragement, using humor, truncating negative talk, and focusing on assets instead of limitations. For example, after learning that she was diabetic, one respondent remembers her mother framing the situation in the following manner.

> You can still do whatever you want to do—tennis, basketball, softball. You might want to take something to eat, and you'll have to be careful, but you aren't limited. Giving yourself insulin will just be a normal part of your routine.

Health-care Providers

The respondents indicated that health-care providers (HCPs) also play an important role in the promotion and maintenance of courage. One way in which they have an impact on the process is by projecting optimism. Using encouraging words, focusing on assets rather than deficits, using humor in a prudent manner to reframe situations, and validating the worth of individuals in spite of their problems were suggested as ways in which optimism can be projected.

Respondents also noted that open communication helps to promote and maintain courage. Open communication occurs when HCPs are accessible; willing to listen; and forthright about discussing problems, frustrations, and feelings. Providing information and teaching patients about their health concerns were noted as important components of this type of communication, along with a sense of empathy. Participants recommended that HCPs project empathy by being sensitive to individual concerns, placing client needs first, and approaching clients in a benevolent, caring, and respectful manner. One respondent described how he became very discouraged one day when an insensitive physician came into his hospital room and glibly announced, "I guess you'll never walk again," and walked out.

Instilling a sense of trust is also important in promoting and maintaining courage. Trust is established when HCPs demonstrate professional competence and provide individualized care. When trust exists, young adults with long-term health concerns feel that they do not need to be concerned about the services they are receiving; their stress level is diminished; and they are free to get on with the task of becoming and being courageous. The distress experienced when HCPs cannot be trusted to do their jobs competently is illustrated by the experiences of a young person with quadriplegia. "I became very upset when the nurses' aides didn't do their jobs well. I hated it when my teeth weren't brushed adequately, or I didn't feel clean. It was hard to concentrate on anything else."

In general, the role that inter*personal* factors play in the promotion and maintenance of courage has a direct impact on intra*personal* factors. For example, when optimism is projected, normality is encouraged, trust is established, advocates are present, and courageous role modeling occurs; hope is generated that optimal results are possible. In addition, when individuals make efforts to project optimism, communicate openly, express empathy and admiration, and function as advocates, feelings of personal worth are enhanced and self-confidence is bolstered. Finally, values are molded by the examples that role models provide and through the sanctioning of socially congruent behaviors.

Outcomes of Becoming and Being Courageous

THRIVING

The courageous individuals in this study developed a sense of thriving and vitality. They felt as if they were involved in life and living it to the fullest. As a young woman with metastatic melanoma stated, "If I didn't fight and take risks, my life would be boring. I wouldn't be fulfilled, and there wouldn't be any enjoyment." Health problems were managed discreetly; and dreams of learning new skills, going to school, getting married, having children, maintaining a job, and being independent were fulfilled to every extent possible. Respondents expressed that personal growth had taken place that would not have occurred without courageously managing their long-term health outcomes. They also suggested that a better self emerged that could look beyond personal concerns and was more responsive to the needs of others. Although their health-care needs sometimes took priority, many of the participants indicated a long-term desire to help others and make a positive contribution to society.

PERSONAL INTEGRITY

Because of the manner in which they had managed their struggles, courageous individuals experienced a sense of personal integrity that was characterized by feelings of dignity, self-satisfaction, and pride. They had gotten on with their lives in a way that allowed them to live without overwhelming regrets, bitterness, or anger, and they were thankful for their enduring personal assets, remaining health, and interpersonal resources. Respondents expressed a healthy respect for the challenges that they had to face, but this was coupled with the knowledge that these struggles could be confronted in a courageous manner. A young man who became a quadriplegic because of a football injury expressed similar sentiments about his situation in the following way: "There's no one to blame. Life's too short to be bitter. I just play the cards I'm dealt each day in the best possible way."

In summary (see Fig. 6.2), the threat of a long-term health concern and the struggles that ensue in managing that threat appear to promote the process of becoming and being courageous among young adults. The greater the severity of the threat and the struggles involved, the more the development of courage is needed. In learning to be courageous, young adults use cognitive thinking strategies that involve discernment, enhanced sensitivity to reality, and clarification of values. Courageous behavior typically includes pushing beyond the norm, helping others, and being humble. The development of courage is progressive-regressive in nature, and there are times when intrapersonal factors (hope, self-confidence, and values) and interpersonal factors (role models, social sanctions, advocacy, and HCPs) are needed to help maintain and promote the process in a positive direction. Outcomes of being courageous include personal integrity and a sense that one is thriving rather than merely getting by. All components of becoming and being courageous, including outcomes, have a simultaneous impact on one another. For this reason, feelings of personal integrity and thriving become additional intrapersonal factors that aid in the promotion and maintenance of courage.

DISCUSSION

Similarities and Differences among Conceptualizations of Courage

Findings from this study and others suggest that courage is learned over time in a progressive-regressive process (Asarian, 1981; Finfgeld, 1992, 1995, 1997a, 1997b; Haase, 1985, 1987) that is elicited by struggles (Asarian, 1981; Crovitz & Buford, 1978; Finfgeld, 1992, 1995, 1997a, 1997b; Haase, 1985, 1987; Kohut, 1985; Leeming, 1981; Rawnsley, 1994; Rorty, 1986; Tillich, 1952; Walton, 1986, 1990). Cognitive aspects of becoming and being courageous are thought to involve accepting reality and transforming threats into challenges (Asarian, 1981; Finfgeld, 1992, 1995, 1997a, 1997b; Haase, 1985, 1987), and courageous behavior appears to include taking responsibility for one's own welfare and unpretentiously getting on with life in spite of difficulties (Asarian, 1981; Finfgeld, 1992, 1995, 1997a; Haase, 1985). Factors that have been reported to promote and/or maintain courage include encouragement from others (Cuff, 1993; Finfgeld, 1997a; Haase, 1985, 1987; Hockenberry-Eaton & Minick, 1994), role models, hope (Asarian, 1981; Finfgeld, 1992, 1995, 1997a, 1997b; Haase, 1985, 1987), and being courageous for the sake of others who may be experiencing distress (Asarian, 1981; Cuff, 1993; Dollard, 1944; Finfgeld, 1992, 1995, 1997a, 1997b; Haase, 1985, 1987; Linderman, 1987; Shelp, 1983, 1984). In addition, findings from all age groups (Finfgeld, 1992, 1995, 1997a; Haase, 1985, 1987) support the notion that HCPs can play an important role in promoting and sustaining courage. Finally, a sense of equanimity and personal integrity have consistently been reported to be outcomes of this process (Asarian, 1981; Finfgeld, 1992, 1995, 1997a, 1997b; Haase, 1985, 1987).

Although similarities exist among findings from investigations of courage, differences can also be identified. Unlike the findings from this study and others (Asarian, 1981; Finfgeld, 1992, 1995, 1997a, 1997b), discernment can be inferred but not clearly identified to be an overt characteristic of courageous cognition among adolescents (Haase, 1985, 1987). Finfgeld (1997a) noted that this may be due to the fact that discernment is a cognitive skill that adolescents have not fully acquired. Another possibility is that because Haase's (1985, 1987) respondents were interviewed while hospitalized, their ability to make decisions using discernment may not have been of great importance. Instead, these individuals were probably more focused on simply getting through diagnostic tests, therapeutic treatments, surgery, and hospital routines (Finfgeld, 1997a).

Another notable discrepancy between the findings in this work and others is Asarian's (1981) and Haase's conclusion (1985, 1987) that creativity is a component of becoming and being courageous that results in enhanced perceptions. Although data from this work and Finfgeld's (1997a) lend credibility to the notion that individuals experience enhanced sensitivities, there is no indication that creativity precedes this experience. As noted by Finfgeld (1997a), this discrepancy may relate to the manner in which the terms *creativity* and *problem solving* have been used by the researchers.

In keeping with age-appropriate tasks for young adults, the respondents in this study indicated that throughout the process of becoming and being courageous, they tended to clarify their value systems, which up to that point had been somewhat vague. This finding is in harmony with Haase's (1985, 1987) conclusion that values do not appear to play a significant role in the development and maintenance of courage among adolescents, and Finfgeld's (1992, 1995, 1997a) finding that values appear to play a more significant role in the process of becoming and being courageous among middle-aged and older individuals. There appears to be a developmental progression of values clarification that influences the emergence of courage. Nurses may need to focus on assisting adolescents and young adults with their ongoing struggle to clarify values so that they can move toward dealing with their situations in a courageous manner.

In contrast to Finfgeld's (1992, 1995) and Haase's (1985, 1987) findings among elderly individuals and adolescents respectively, thriving appears to be a significant outcome of becoming and being courageous among middle-aged (Finfgeld, 1997a) and young adults. Older individuals have already slowed down and do not experience feelings of vitality and thriving to the same extent that young and middle-aged adults do.

A possible explanation for the absence of feelings of zest and vitality among the adolescents in Haase's (1985, 1987) investigation may have been the setting in which data were collected. The adolescents in Haase's study were hospitalized; thus, the immediate challenges of that environment may have precluded a sense of thriving (Finfgeld, 1997a).

Research Implications

With rare exceptions (e.g., Hockenberry-Eaton & Minick, 1994), courage has not been examined among children with long-term health concerns and rarely, if ever, has it been the primary focus of an investigation of this age group. Although this is an area that needs to be explored, respondents who have not reached adolescence may represent special challenges to researchers because their verbal and cognitive skills are not fully developed and their understanding of the concept of courage may vary widely (Szagun, 1992). Thus, investigators who are interested in studying courage among children are recommended to have specialized interviewing skills and insight into interpreting the meanings of their responses. In spite of these challenges, becoming and being courageous needs to be more thoroughly examined among this age group, particularly because courage is apparently learned over the entire life span (Finfgeld, 1992, 1995).

As indicated by Strauss and Corbin (1990), a grounded theory should be considered within various levels of contextual conditions that may relate to the phenomenon under investigation. Based on the contextual value systems of the Midwesterners in rural and suburban communities who took part in this study, there was a strong commitment to be courageous in order to help others and avoid being a burden. Additional research needs to be carried out to investigate how differing societal and cultural values may alter the development and manifestation of courage.

Consideration also needs to be given to conclusions that can be collectively drawn from the numerous studies of courage that have been carried out among individuals with long-term health concerns. Finfgeld (1997b) has set a precedent for synthesizing findings from several studies of courage; however, additional work needs to be completed in light of the results of this study and others (e.g., Cuff, 1993; Finfgeld, 1997a; Hockenberry-Eaton & Minick, 1994; Kahn, Steeves, & Benoliel, 1994; Rawnsley, 1994).

REFERENCES

Annells, M. (1996). Grounded theory method: Philosophical perspectives, paradigm of inquiry, and postmodernism. *Qualitative Health Research, 6,* 379–393.

Asarian, R. D. (1981). The psychology of courage: A human scientific investigation. *Dissertation Abstracts International, 42,* 2023B. (University Microfilms No. 8121943)

Benoliel, J. Q. (1996). Grounded theory and nursing knowledge. *Qualitative Health Research, 6,* 406–428.

Berman, P. L. (1989). *The courage to grow old.* New York: Ballantine Books.

Campbell, J. (1949). *The hero with a thousand faces.* Princeton: Princeton University Press.

Crovitz, E., & Buford, E. (1978). *Courage knows no sex.* North Quincy, MA: Christopher Publishing.

Cuff, W. T. (1993). The experience of courage and the characteristics of courageous people (Life trauma response) (*Doctoral dissertation, University of Minnesota, 1993*). *Dissertation Abstracts International, 54,* 5408B.

Dollard, J. (1944). *Fear in battle.* Ann Arbor: University Microfilms.

Finfgeld, D. L. (1992). Courage in the chronically-ill elderly: A grounded theory study. *Dissertation Abstracts International, 53,* 1783B. (University Microfilms No. DA9225575)

Finfgeld, D. L. (1995). Becoming and being courageous in the chronically ill elderly. *Issues in Mental Health Nursing, 16,* 1–11.

Finfgeld, D. L. (1997a). *Courage in middle-aged adults with long-term health concerns.* Manuscript submitted for publication.

Finfgeld, D. L. (1997b). *Development of an emergent grounded theory of courage using meta-interpretation.* Manuscript submitted for publication.

Glaser, B. G., & Strauss, A. L. (1967). *The discovery of grounded theory: Strategies for qualitative research.* New York: Aldine de Gruyter.

Haase, J. E. (1985). The components of courage in chronically ill adolescents: A phenomenological study. *Dissertation Abstracts International, 46,* 1869B. (University Microfilms No. 8516721)

Haase, J. E. (1987). Components of courage in chronically ill adolescents: A phenomenological study. *Advances in Nursing Science, 9,* 64–80.

Hockenberry-Eaton, M., & Minick, P. (1994). Living with cancer: Children with extraordinary courage. *Oncology Nursing Forum, 21,* 1025–1031.

Kahn, D. L., Steeves, R. H., & Benoliel, J. Q. (1994). Nurses' views of the coping of patients. *Social Science and Medicine, 38,* 1423–1430.

Koestenbaum, P. (1991). *Leadership: The inner side of greatness.* San Francisco: Jossey-Bass.

Kohut, H. (1985). *Self psychology and the humanities.* New York: WW Norton.

Leeming, D. A. (1981). *Mythology: The voyage of the hero.* New York: Harper & Row.

Linderman, G. F. (1987). *Embattled course: The experience of combat in the American Civil War.* New York: Free Press.

Maslow, A. H. (1970). *Motivation and personality.* New York: Harper & Row.

Moran, L. (1945). *The anatomy of courage.* London: Chiswick Press.

Olshansky, E. F. (1996). Theoretical issues in building a grounded theory: Application of an example of a program of research on infertility. *Qualitative Health Research, 6,* 394–405.

Palmour, J. (1986). *On moral character: A practical guide to Aristotle's virtues and vices.* Washington, DC: The Archon Institute for Leadership Development.

Rachman, S. J. (1990). *Fear and courage* (2nd ed.). New York: WH Freeman.

Rawnsley, M. M. (1994). Recurrence of cancer: A crisis of courage. *Cancer Nursing, 17,* 342–347.

Rorty, A. O. (1986). The two faces of courage. *Philosophy, 61,* 151–171.

Servan-Schreiber, J. L. (1987). *The return of course.* Reading: Addison-Wesley.

Shelp, E. E. (1983). Courage and tragedy in clinical medicine. *Journal of Medicine and Philosophy, 8,* 417–429.

Shelp, E. E. (1984). Courage: A neglected virtue in the patient-physician relationship. *Social Science and Medicine, 18,* 351–360.

Sommerlund, B. (1989). Textbase Alpha [Computer software]. Desert Hot Springs, CA: Qualitative Research Management.

Strauss, A., & Corbin, J. (1990). *Basics of qualitative research: Grounded theory procedures and techniques.* Newbury Park: Sage.

Szagun, G. (1992). Age-related changes in children's understanding of courage. *Journal of Genetic Psychology, 153,* 405–420.

Tillich, P. (1952). *The courage to be.* New Haven: Yale University Press.

Walton, D. N. (1986). *Courage: A philosophical investigation.* Berkeley: University of California Press.

Walton, D. N. (1990). Courage, relativism, and practical reasoning. *Philosophia, 20,* 227–240.

7

Middlescent Obese Women: Overcoming Powerlessness

> Judith Fitzgerald Miller

Middlescent individuals who have never been concerned about controlling food intake and balancing dietary discretion with adequate energy expenditure are likely to be either obese (weighing 20 percent more than their ideal body weight) or overweight (weighing less than 20 percent more than ideal body weight). One-third of middle-aged Americans are 20 percent overweight, and the majority of these are women. At least one of every five Americans is overweight. It is a discouraging fact that most obese persons will not remain in treatment. Of those who remain in treatment, most will not lose much weight, and of those who do lose weight, most will regain it (Stunkard, 1972). The efficient health professional is frustrated by not having fast, accurate answers to a problem that seems to have a simple treatment, having persons stop eating an excess amount of food. Nonetheless, this problem is complex.

Very little is known about self-control and eating behaviors. Theories have been proposed by both obese subjects and scientists, such as carbohydrate intolerance (the belief that when some persons eat a carbohydrate, they cannot stop) (Edelstein, 1977); appestat dysfunction, in which the satiety center that acts like a thermostat may be set higher than normal; underactivity (Mayer, 1968); obese eating behaviors learned as a child from obese or nonobese parents; and parents' giving food to children as a reward, a means of comfort during anxiety, or a relief from depression.

This chapter examines yet another combination of factors that influences obesity in middle-aged women: powerlessness and a developmental vulnerability to obesity. The main thrust is to present a variety of strategies that may be used to enable obese women to control food intake. Assessing obesity is the first consideration.

Obesity is determined in a number of ways. A simple measure is to look at a person's physical appearance. A woman 5 feet 3 inches tall who weighs 180 pounds looks obese. An approximate ideal body weight can be calculated by the use of the following formula (Mahoney & Mahoney, 1976):

Approximate ideal weight for women = (height in inches × 3.5) − 110

Approximate ideal weight for men = (height in inches × 4) − 130

Factors not considered in this formula include whether the body frame is large, medium, or small, and the muscle content of the body. (Athletes weigh more, but this is due to increased muscle mass.) Measuring skinfold thickness is an accurate determination of body fat. The triceps skinfold is measured at a midpoint between the elbow and shoulder. A man between the ages of 35 and 50 years should have a triceps skinfold of less than 23 mm, and a woman between the ages of 35 and 40 years should have a measurement of less than 30 mm (Mayer, 1968). Any larger measurement indicates that the body mass contains more than 39 percent fat. Height and age charts according to body frame (Table 7.1) are also used as an ideal weight index.

DEVELOPMENTAL VULNERABILITY

Obesity in Women

There are specific developmental vulnerabilities to obesity that occur during infancy, adolescence, pregnancy, the middle years, and menopause. During these phases, the individual or parent must be aware of the tendency to gain weight and must exercise restraint in overeating or overfeeding.

During infancy, the number of adipose cells increases (hyperplasia) as a result of overeating. The increased number of cells stays with the individual for life, causing an extreme lifelong risk of obesity. Obesity that occurs during adolescence and adulthood results in hypertrophy of existing cells and is a less resistant form of obesity. After infancy, the developmental hazards are unique to women.

During adolescence, the growth spurt stops; however, the estrogen levels in girls continue to rise and promote fat formation. Fat is laid down in the breasts and hips and will continue unchecked if eating is

Table 7.1 ➤ **DESIRABLE WEIGHTS (IN POUNDS)***

MEN OF AGE 25 AND OVER

Height with Shoes 1-in Heel	Small Frame	Medium Frame	Large Frame
5 ft 2 in	112–120	118–129	126–141
5 ft 3 in	115–123	121–133	129–144
5 ft 4 in	118–126	124–136	132–148
5 ft 5 in	121–129	127–139	135–152
5 ft 6 in	124–133	130–143	138–156
5 ft 7 in	128–137	134–147	142–161
5 ft 8 in	132–141	138–152	147–166
5 ft 9 in	136–145	142–156	151–170
5 ft 10 in	140–150	146–160	155–174
5 ft 11 in	144–154	150–165	159–179
6 ft 0 in	148–158	154–170	164–184
6 ft 1 in	152–162	158–175	168–189
6 ft 2 in	156–167	162–180	173–194
6 ft 3 in	160–171	167–185	178–199
6 ft 4 in	164–175	172–190	182–204

WOMEN OF AGE 25 AND OVER

Height with Shoes 2-in heel	Small Frame	Medium Frame	Large Frame
4 ft 10 in	92–98	96–107	104–119
4 ft 11 in	94–101	98–110	106–122
5 ft 0 in	96–104	101–113	109–125
5 ft 1 in	99–107	104–116	112–128
5 ft 2 in	102–110	107–119	115–131
5 ft 3 in	105–113	110–122	118–134
5 ft 4 in	108–116	113–126	121–138
5 ft 5 in	111–119	116–130	125–142
5 ft 6 in	114–123	120–135	129–146
5 ft 7 in	118–127	124–139	133–150
5 ft 8 in	122–131	128–143	137–154
5 ft 9 in	126–135	132–147	141–158
5 ft 10 in	130–140	136–151	145–163
5 ft 11 in	134–144	140–155	149–168
6 ft 0 in	138–148	144–159	153–173

*Derived from Metropolitan Life Insurance Co. (1959) Build and Blood Pressure Study, Society of Actuaries, and from Bray, G. (1980). *Obesity: Comparative methods of weight control* (p. 3). Westport, CT: Technomic Publishing.

not controlled. Girls gain weight during adolescence, whereas boys lose weight during this time.

Pregnancy is the most vulnerable time for permanent weight gain (Edelstein, 1977). One-third of obese women became obese during pregnancy (Kemp, 1972). The increased appetite may remain with the woman after delivery, and breastfeeding mothers may overindulge during a time when excess calories are allowed. Once a woman is 10 percent heavier than her ideal body weight, she has the lifelong potential for becoming obese and must be constantly on guard against that predicament.

During middle age (35 to 55 years old), physiological changes occur. Muscle tone and skin tone diminish, and basal metabolic rate (BMR) decreases. Aging causes the BMR to decrease approximately 5 percent; so for every 30 years after age 25, the caloric intake should be decreased by 7.5 percent (Williams, 1996).

During the middle years, life events that were previously controlled and that provided security and comfort may now be a source of anxiety and grief, for example, role reversal (middle-aged child caring for elderly, dying parents), young adult children leaving home and entering lifestyles disapproved of by parents, adolescent children experiencing developmental crises, marital strain, uncertainty of future, and feeling of unproductivity. Overeating may be the individual's means of coping with these stressors of middle years. Rosenfield and Stevenson (1988) found that both "normal" and alcoholic middle-aged women increased their food intake on stressful days.

Weight gain from overeating may be insidious. Increasing food intake by 100 calories a day without increasing exercise will result in a 10-pound weight gain in 1 year (Mahoney & Mahoney, 1976). A woman's attitude may be, "I've had three children; what do you expect my figure to look like?" This type of passive resistance blocks success in a weight-control program.

Weight gain may increase in women at menopause. At this phase of development, the obesity has been attributed to hormonal changes and decreased activity, as well as to depression (Diekelmann, 1977). In addition to developmental vulnerability to weight gain, powerlessness is a factor in obesity.

POWERLESSNESS AND OBESITY

Powerlessness (the perception that individual behavior will not affect outcomes) is a prevalent theme in obesity in two dimensions:

1. Powerlessness results when weight loss does not occur after attempts at dieting.
2. Powerlessness is a factor that contributes to overeating.

With regard to the first dimension, powerlessness is a perception that is confirmed in obese individuals after bingeing on "forbidden foods" or having lost no weight after a week without desserts. The lack of positive reinforcement of immediate weight loss as a result of what the obese person perceives to be a drastic change in eating behaviors contributes to powerlessness. The feeling that nothing the individual does will result in weight loss causes a feeling of helplessness (powerlessness). The prevailing feeling of powerlessness causes the individual to stop trying and to return to overeating, feeling guilt and a sense of no control. Thus the cycle (Fig. 7.1) has been completed.

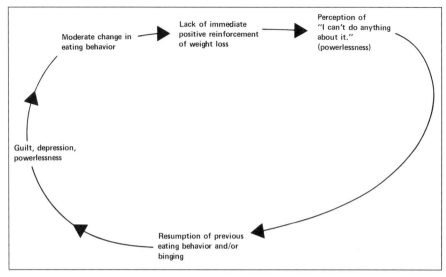

FIGURE 7.1 ➤ Powerlessness obesity cycle.

The key to breaking the cycle may lie in the nurse's providing re-inforcement for slightly altered behavior patterns and not focusing on weight loss. The client needs to set realistic weight loss goals—no more than an average of 2.5-pound loss per week. Helping the client feel some sense of accomplishment in having changed the bedtime snack from an ice cream sundae to a more acceptable, lower-calorie treat is an example of positive feedback without anxiously waiting for the scale to record a 2-pound loss after 2 days of slight diet modification.

Powerlessness may not only result from weight loss failure but may also contribute to obesity in the first place. Individuals may have a life-long pattern of behaviors resulting from powerlessness contingencies. "Powerlessness contingencies" refer to those psychosocial states that stem from a long-term perception of being unable to influence outcomes. The psychosocial states prompt a behavior pattern that may result in overeating and little energy expenditure through exercise. These power-lessness contingencies may be categorized as self-induced and other-induced. Select contingencies of powerlessness and the resulting be-havior pattern related to obesity are presented in Table 7.2. The self-induced contingencies are low tension tolerance, inability to in-crease activity, inability to accurately identify and express emotions, self-deprecation, unconscious positive meanings of fatness, lack of in-sight into eating behavior, uninvolvement in caring for self, and lack of self-confidence. Examples of other-induced powerlessness contingencies are family interactions, parents' use of food as a reward, and stigmatiz-ing reactions of persons in the social network. Although each powerless-

Table 7.2 ➤ POWERLESSNESS CONTINGENCIES AND CONSEQUENCES

Powerlessness Contingencies	Behavior Pattern	Consequence
Self-induced		
Low tension tolerance	Recognizes or develops few or no alternatives for tension release	Overeating
Lacks ability to mobilize self to exercise	Moves as little as possible in daily activities. No exercise routine	Imbalance of energy intake and expenditure
Lacks ability to identify and express emotions (anger, unhappiness, frustration)	Short circuiting vague feelings without clear identification of feelings. Interprets as a need for food*	Overeating
Self-deprecation	Feelings of low self-esteem, depression	Overeating
Perceives fat as positive	Feeling comfort in being obese as a protection from sexual exploitation; keeping part of their mother; and/or protection of husband's fears and jealousy of slimmer, shapely wife†	Overeating
Lacks self-insight, awareness	Unaware of eating behavior—quantity consumed, internal cues of hunger and satiation. Unaware of mood states	Overeating
Uninvolved in caring for self	Detaches own behavior from outcomes—"can do nothing about it" attitude. "Whatever happens is beyond my control"	Overeating
Lacks self-confidence	Unusual dependence on other persons or things for self-satisfaction	Overeating
Other-induced		
Family and society influences	Use of food as rewards, overfeeding children, clean-the-plate syndrome from childhood. Use of alcohol and food to provide an unguarded, comfortable milieu in social encounters	Overeating
Stigmatizing reaction of persons in social network	Withdrawal, reinforcement of poor self-concept	Overeating

*McCall and Siderits (1977).
†Orbach (1997).

ness contingency results in a unique behavior pattern, the consequence is the same—overeating and underexercising. Powerlessness contingencies contribute to maladaptive behavior patterns that are so ingrained that changing them may be difficult, if not impossible. The ultimate consequence is obesity.

Some research findings reinforce the fact that powerlessness is a problem in obesity. McCall (1973) noted that 169 refractorily obese women differed on the Minnesota Multiphasic Personality Inventory from the 181 Take Off Pounds Sensibly members who were successful with their weight-reduction program and who kept their weight within 5 percent of ideal body weight for 6 months. Women who were resistive to weight loss were found to have more:

- Feminine dependence
- Touchiness
- Body overconcern
- Psychic hurting
- Somatization
- Rebelliousness
- Compulsive and ruminative tendencies
- Bizarre or confused thinking

Although the findings of dependence lend some support to the powerlessness theory proposed in this chapter, McCall is quick to point out that we cannot determine whether the degrees of psychological disturbance present in refractorily obese persons are antecedent or consequent to the obesity.

Powerlessness in obese individuals is reinforced by the stigmatizing behaviors of others. Obese people are automatically categorized as sloppy, weak willed (Peternelj-Taylor, 1989), nonproductive, lazy, slow paced, easygoing, jolly, unattractive (Clayson & Klassen, 1989), and obsessed with oral gratification. Employers may view obese employees as a liability because of health risks (missed work days, insurance payments) as well as portrayal of a poor company image. In the American culture, obese persons are characterized as immature, passive, dependent, low in self-esteem, and responsible for their fatness.

"Cultural contempt" and psychological prejudice against obesity exist (Radvila, 1989; Wadden & Stunkard, 1987; Wright & Whitehead, 1987). Besides body image disturbances (Brodie & Slade, 1988; Gardner, Martinez, Espinoza, & Gallegos, 1988) and social discrimination, obese persons suffer no greater psychological problems than normal-weight individuals (Radvila, 1989).

Obese persons do not appear to be assuming responsibility for adherence to prescribed weight-reduction programs. Physicians and nurses were found to have negative attitudes toward obese individuals (Maddox & Liederman, 1969; Peternelj-Taylor, 1989), which contributed to the dropout rate in weight-reduction programs. The obese subjects suffer shame and self-derogation when returning to the physician after failing to lose weight (Stunkard & Mendelson, 1967). Thin people generally do not like obese people, and obese people do not like other obese people (Sundberg, 1978).

Reactions to condemnation by others lead the obese subject to conclude, "No one would want to be associated with me or seen in public with me." This negative self-talk reinforces individuals' perceptions that they are powerless even in maintaining close personal relationships. Stunkard and Mendelson (1967) found through interviews with 74 obese subjects that obese persons experienced two behavior disorders. First, they overate. Second, they experienced a disturbance in body image; that is, they felt their bodies were grotesque, loathsome, and viewed by others with contempt.

Eating behaviors of obese individuals may indicate no control. The fact that the obese have particular vulnerabilities and unique eating styles has been supported (Bruch, 1979; Bruno, 1972; McDonald, 1977; Stunkard & Kaplan, 1977) and refuted (Adams, Ferguson, Stunkard, & Agras, 1978; Mahoney, 1975). Because eating behavior may be drastically altered both in experimental conditions and when the subjects are eating in public, eating-style studies must be evaluated carefully. Obese persons overeat in privacy but seldom do so in public (Sundberg, 1978). The obese person's susceptibility to food cues includes environmental stimuli of food sights, smells, familiar binging places, and time of day without regard to internal cues of hunger and satiety as signaled by blood sugar levels, gastric motility, and gastric stretch receptors.

Binge eating is sporadic, seemingly uncontrolled eating of large quantities of food associated with agitation and self-condemnation (Straw & Sonne, 1979). Orbach (1997) described characteristics of obese persons who eat compulsively (binge) as eating when not physically hungry, feeling out of control around food, feeling awful about self because of being out of control, spending time thinking and worrying about food and fatness, scouting latest diets for new information, and feeling awful about their bodies. Eating is done quickly and usually furtively during bingeing.

Bruch (1979) described obese individuals not only as being unable to control eating but as having the feeling that other forces are in control of their life situation. Bruch went on to state that obese persons do not correctly identify hunger or differentiate emotional feelings from hunger. A significant relationship between control and social responsibility and weight loss was found by Hartz, Kalkoff, Rimm, & McCall (1979). Women with low control and low social responsibility scores were less successful in weight control than were women with high control and high social responsibility. Rodin (1977) found obese persons were more dependent on others and more persuadable than were persons of normal weight.

Persons who believed that they were responsible for their being overweight rather than blaming fate or others lost weight at a significantly faster rate than those who did not hold this belief (Rodin, 1977).

Eating styles of thin persons do not have characteristics of no control. Thin persons generally do not eat very quickly, nor do they take large bites without stopping to taste the food. Lifestyles and eating behaviors of thin persons need careful scrutiny so that the skills they have used to remain thin can be applied in therapy for obese persons. Sundberg (1978) determined that thin persons' skills included ability to balance exercise with energy intake, to discriminate between adequate and excessive food intake, to adhere to regular meal patterns and control snacking (keeping frequency and type of snack food controlled), to adapt to negative emotions by means other than using food, to accurately perceive how others view them, to obtain sexual satisfaction, and to make a conscious successful effort to control weight through understanding the impact of indiscriminate eating and drinking.

Summary of Powerlessness and Obesity

Powerlessness is a factor in causing obesity, and powerlessness is a problem that results when individuals feel they have failed in a weight-loss program. Lack of control is also evident in the obese individual's eating style (vulnerability to food cues and so forth). The powerlessness contingencies presented provide an analysis of the etiology of overeating (see Table 7.2). The research base on powerlessness and obesity is almost nonexistent. Studies need to be done to develop the nursing diagnostic category of powerlessness and to determine the relationship between powerlessness and obesity.

The terms *obese, fat,* and *corpulent* all have negative connotations and prompt a reaction of reproach from others. Bruch (1979) described obese persons as being under the influence of others and not in control of their bodies. Some fat people talk about their bodies as being external to themselves; some do not feel identified with the bothersome ugly physical thing. The excuses obese people use for not being able to lose weight also point to their feeling powerless, not only in having gotten fat, but also in recovering from obesity.

MIDDLESCENT OBESE WOMEN
Stressors Confronting Middle-aged Women

Most middlescent obese women became obese before reaching their middle years and the obese state is either maintained or escalated during the middle years. The stresses of middle years (ages 35 to 55 years) contribute to maladaptive behavior or successful coping. [For a thorough analysis of the middle years, see Stevenson, J. (1977). *Issues and crises during middlescence.* New York: Appleton-Century-Crofts.] Stressors are those stimuli requiring adaptation. In middle-aged women, stressors may include caring for aging parents and parents-in-law; dealing with children becoming independent; having to resolve that previous nurturing patterns are no longer needed; feeling unproductive—handling new freedom without learning new skills; experiencing role conflicts from various factors such as social pressures for liberation; dealing with changing marital intimacy; managing physical changes that result in worry and preoccupation with health; and grieving over loss of youth. Each stressor is discussed briefly (Fig. 7.2).

The role reversal of the middle-aged daughter now having to assume responsibility for care of aging parents creates stress; affects fam-

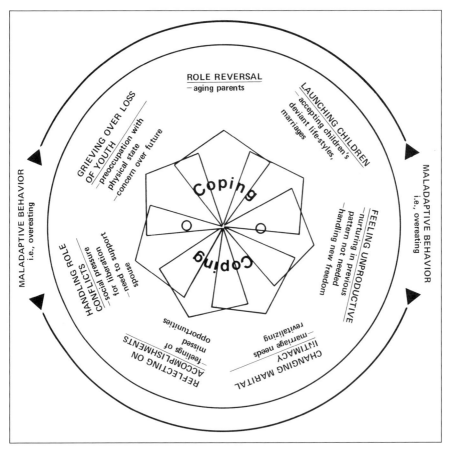

FIGURE 7.2 ➤ Stressors of middle-aged women.

ily harmony; and may cause feelings of resentment, guilt, or despair. In some instances, an ill single parent is displayed into the daughter's home or into a nursing home. Disrupted family systems, conflicts, and emotional energy expenditure take place in either instance.

At the same time, young adult children may be leaving home and beginning marriages, careers, and lifestyles that parents may oppose. The mother fully realizes that previous patterns of nurturing not only are no longer needed but also may be shunned by her offspring. New ways of finding satisfaction from mothering need to be learned. Obese middle-aged women who had no children may need to resolve a sense of loss over a missed opportunity to bear children.

Unless a woman has planned for and developed productive skills throughout her life, she may find herself feeling unneeded, unproductive, and unsure of her identity. Prock (1975) described the need for women to develop multiple anchors so that when one anchor (e.g., a dependent child) is gone, other anchors still provide a sense of stability and self-worth. These anchors prevent women from feeling adrift without direction. Examples of anchors may include having a job, maintaining developed social activities, and doing volunteer work.

Marital intimacy and the source of strength that was once present in the marital bond may be waning during the middle years. As a result of schedules, communication between husband and wife may be decreasing. Husbands may have well-established patterns of confiding in business associates or fellow workers, and wives may be caught up in activities they consider of no particular interest to men—planning to advance their careers or talking about returning to school. Feelings are not shared, and sexual relationships become dull. New sources of conflict may arise, such as disagreement over each other's goals. Confirmation of affection may have disappeared from a humdrum marriage. Unless time and effort are spent to develop and share interests, few common interests will remain. The full-blown feeling of disenchantment after 20 years of marriage, although insidious in coming, has arrived. Eating may soothe the need for affection.

Coping with physical changes may precipitate a preoccupation with health. The changes may be anything from changes in the oral cavity (receding gum line) to graying of the hair to pathological conditions such as hypertension. These changes emphasize the realization that youth is lost.

The liberation of women in our society creates new pressures for women. Women may no longer reap self-satisfaction from supporting husbands in their successful careers. Women no longer move from school to higher education to home for child rearing, and then to low-paying jobs reserved for women when they are more stable in the workforce (after childbearing years). Now women move from higher education to professions and child rearing, and remain in the productive workforce. Multiple role expectations—raising children, pursuing career, taking care of spouse, and so forth—all create role strain. Women who have not been engaged in professions may feel a more intense pressure to be productive without having developed skills.

Although there may be a wide variety of responses to these stressors, one response is overeating. Obese individuals respond to stress by overeating, whereas thin people do not; on the contrary, a thin person's behavior during stress may be to eat less.

Being fat is a stressor in and of itself. Orbach (1997) recorded her observations resulting from leading a therapeutic diet group with various women participants for 5 years. Some of the connotations fat had for these obese women included:

- To be fat means to compare yourself to every other woman, looking for the ones whose own fat can make you relax
- To be fat means to be excluded from contemporary mass culture, fashion, sports, and the outdoor life
- To be fat means to worry every time a camera is in view
- To be fat means having to feel ashamed for existing
- To be fat means having to wait until you are thin to live
- To be fat means to have no needs
- To be fat means to be constantly trying to lose weight
- To be fat means never saying "no"
- To be fat means to have an excuse for failure
- To be fat means to wait for the man who will love you despite that fat—the man who will fight through the layers

Other life circumstances of middle-aged women may influence eating. There may be a change in exercise, with little physical energy expenditure taking place. The physical demands of a young family are gone. Boredom may result, with concomitant overeating. In a routinized marriage, there may be little motivation to maintain a sexually attractive appearance. There may also be misconceptions that interfere with weight loss, such as believing that losing weight may increase vulnerability to cancer and communicable diseases. A healthy appetite may be equated with general health, and quick complete satisfaction of appetite is needed to stay healthy. Frank rationalizations for overeating are used by some obese persons. Such rationalizations are described by Orbach (1997) and include:

- Fear that food will not be available later so I must overeat now to tide me over
- Need to have something in my mouth

- Had a bad day so need to cheer up by noshing a pan of brownies
- Had a great day so I deserve one lemon pie
- Eating because it is the only way I know to give myself pleasure
- Nothing else to do in the evening

Themes of using food to alleviate boredom and as a tranquilizer, reward, and means of oral gratification are noted in the foregoing client comments.

Uniqueness of Obesity in Women

Women are the fatter sex. Edelstein (1977) explained that men burn twice as many calories as women do for the same amount of exertion. A man's body contains more muscle mass than a woman's body. Muscle requires five more calories per pound to maintain itself than fat or connective tissue. However, even though the woman's body requires half as many calories as a man's, the woman's appetite is the same as a man's (Edelstein, 1977). The fat pad is necessary as a mechanism for food storage and heat protection for the fetus during pregnancy. Unfortunately, the extra fat is always with the woman, pregnant or not. Female hormones, estrogen and progesterone, are fat producing and fat hoarding.

Generally, women have more exposure to food stimuli than men. In most households, women are responsible for planning appealing menus and spend a good deal of their time shopping for and preparing food and cleaning up leftovers.

Obese women are more stigmatized than obese men. Fat men may be viewed as having authority and substance, whereas fat women are viewed as undisciplined (Edelstein, 1977).

In Orbach's (1997) feminist viewpoint on obesity, she proposed three explanations for overeating in women: (1) women with children are constantly giving to others, feeding the world, and feeling everyone else's needs are to be met first; the mother uses food as a means of replenishing herself; (2) becoming fat is a rebellion against pressure to look and act shapely and be sexually attractive to men; fat is a protection from sexual exploitation; (3) conflicts and ambivalences in mother-daughter relationships express themselves in fat. Eating serves as a source of love, comfort, and warmth, which may have been missing in the mother-daughter relationship. Fat may be viewed by some women as taking part of their mothers with them.

In our society, it may be more difficult for women than men to express anger in socially acceptable ways (McCall & Siderits, 1977).

Women have also been taught to be less assertive (Orbach, 1977). Women feel safer using their mouths to feed themselves rather than to talk assertively and thus satisfy internal frustration.

The female giving of self is equated with food (McBride, 1988). Some women equate their role as good mother with the ability to provide delicious baked goodies ready to satisfy an adolescent's never-ending appetite. Efforts to maintain good communication with adolescents take place, and mother's sharing the goodies is an example of spending time trying to show interest in, understand, and communicate with the child; at the same time, this extra effort is deleterious to ideal body weight.

The yo-yo effect of losing weight, gaining it back, losing and gaining leads to giving up. The giving-up phenomenon can be avoided if the refractory nature of weight loss is understood by clients and health workers. The BMR decreases by as much as 20 percent after a month of dieting (Straw & Stone, 1979). Fewer calories are used to maintain the body's metabolic function. For example, an obese woman whose daily caloric intake is 2000 calories and whose BMR is 1400 calories with 600 calories activity expenditure is maintaining her obese state. If she goes on a 1000-calorie-a-day diet, she will have lost approximately 1 kg a week. The BMR adapts to a change in caloric intake and decreases by 20 percent, so after 1 month, the BMR is not 1400 calories but 1100. If the woman's activity level decreases, despite strict adherence to the 1000-calorie-a-day diet, weight loss will not continue (Straw & Stone, 1979).

Still another reason for failure of dieting may be patients' lack of understanding that relatively unorthodox eating styles are the cause of obesity. For example, night eaters consume excessive calories from dinner time until bedtime and have morning anorexia. They take pride in not eating throughout the day but eat excessively at night. The sudden glucose load is quickly absorbed and converted to fat. Caloric intake should remain moderate and be spread throughout the day. A daily exercise routine is of paramount importance. Consuming all 1400 calories at once most likely will result in weight gain.

Whatever the underlying etiology, middle-aged obese women must struggle against weight gain and fight for control to maintain any weight loss achieved; weight control must continue for the rest of life.

Powerlessness has been described as one component contributing to obesity that results from aborted attempts at weight reduction. The first goal should be to help the obese individual feel less powerless. Empowerment strategies nurses can use to help obese women are discussed in terms of behavior therapy, physical activity, dietary counseling, assertiveness, and rational emotive therapy to handle the stressors of middle years.

NURSING STRATEGIES: EMPOWERMENT OF THE OBESE WOMAN

Behavior Therapy

Behavior therapy means helping the individual to change an undesirable behavior to a desirable behavior. In obese persons, the undesirable behavior is overeating. There is no emphasis on uncovering intrapsychic conflicts or changing the personality structure. The focus is on changing the maladaptive behavior. Teaching the client self-application of techniques to change behavior enables the client to be in control.

Behavior is influenced by its consequences. Brightwell, Lemon, and Sloan (1975) summarized the learning of specific behaviors through the sequence of stimulus, behavior, event, or reward reinforcement. The sequence of eating behavior is summarized in Figure 7.3. The components of behavior therapy proposed for obesity control include obtaining an obesity profile, patient self-monitoring, environmental management, self-reinforcement, and contracts.

OBESITY PROFILE

Obtaining a comprehensive understanding of the individual's eating behaviors, including the stimuli that prompt eating, is the first step in developing client and nurse insight into the unique patient situation. An obesity profile contains the following components: history of obesity, eating style, client's social network, client's knowledge, motivation, developmental stressors present, concept of self, need satisfaction and appropriate reward system, and analysis of assigned patient tasks (Fig. 7.4).

Stimulus ⟶	Behavior ⟶	Response
Desire to eat	Eating	Relief of hunger
Boredom, anger, anxiety	Eating	Relief of negative emotions
Depression	Eating	Alleviation of depression
Joy, elation	Eating	Continued pleasure
Food cues, sights, smells, environment	Eating	Relief of desire to eat

FIGURE 7.3 ➤ Sequence of learning eating behavior.

A. History
1. When did you become overweight (obese)?
2. Can you recall gaining weight associated with any particular event or period of development?
3. Family history of obesity—parents, siblings, children, spouse?
4. Health problems present (thyroid dysfunction, diabetes, hypertension, coronary artery disease).

B. Eating style
1. At what time/times during the 24-hour day are you more likely to overeat?
   When is your appetite the strongest?
   When is your temptation tolerance to food cues the lowest?
2. What types of stimuli prompt eating?
3. Are you aware of your own eating behaviors:
   Amounts of food consumed, size of bites, speed of eating; automatically take seconds?
4. Do you eat until you feel full?
5. Where are you located when eating your meals?

C. Social network
1. Who prepares meals?
2. Number of family members eating meals together or separately in the same home?
3. Are your significant others a help or deterrent to weight control?
4. Relationship with spouse?

D. Knowledge
1. What are the basic food groups?
2. What are your dietary excesses and deficits?
3. Do you understand the calorie restriction according to food exchange lists?
4. Awareness of caloric value of foods routinely and occasionally consumed?
5. What are the health hazards of obesity?

E. Motivation
1. Whose idea was it to begin a weight-control program?
2. What has been your previous involvement with weight-control programs?

3. How long did you persist in trying to be successful in previous weight-control programs?
4. OBSERVATION—Does the client present a package of excuses for not losing weight in the past as well as how any new approach will not work?
5. What do you expect to accomplish in this weight-reduction program?

F. Developmental and life stressors
1. What have been your most stressful events during the past year?
2. How do you respond, cope with stress?
3. Developmental needs—adjustment.

G. Concept of self
1. Does the client use negative self-talk?
2. How would you describe your physical appearance?
3. Do you see yourself as being fat, slightly overweight, grossly overweight, obese?
4. Do you feel you are able to influence what happens to your weight?
5. OBSERVATION—Does client behavior indicate high or low self-esteem?

H. Need satisfaction and reward system
1. Do you have a need for immediate satisfaction of needs and desires in all facets of life?
2. Do you find it necessary to satisfy hunger immediately?
3. What would be a positive reward for yourself when you have done a good job? (Preferably not food.)

I. Analyses of assigned client tasks
1. Explain self-monitoring and record keeping.
2. At later sessions review diet diary (food intake, moods, times, places) for each 24-hour period. The number of days of self-recording depends upon how beneficial this direct feedback is to the client.
3. Provide appropriate feedback on analyses of client self-monitoring.

FIGURE 7.4 ➤ Obesity profile.

Self-Monitoring

The obese individual needs to be involved in analyzing the data gathered in the obesity profile. The goal is to begin to sensitize the client to her eating style. The client should develop an awareness of amounts and types of foods eaten, how food is eaten and in response to what stimuli, and the time of the day when the client is increasingly vulnerable to food cues and has an excessive appetite. When the appetite becomes excessive, as during the afternoon and evening, a plan for engaging in substitute activities needs to be made. For example, food preparation can take place in the early afternoon so that the woman is not exposed to food cues during the vulnerable time of day. An exercise routine can be employed during the vulnerable time. In discussing this with the woman, determine various substitute activities that are meaningful to her, for example, practicing the piano, doing the correspondence, gardening, and doing library work. Physical activity decreases appetite, so substituting such an activity would be beneficial.

Date	Time	Food eaten, amounts	Calories	Place	Stimulus prompted eating	Related feelings before eating	Feelings after eating	Type and duration of exercise

FIGURE 7.5 ➤ Diet and activity diary.

Teaching the client record keeping is a good means of self-monitoring. The record, or diet diary, helps clients become aware of their behavior; it also helps control food intake because whatever clients put into their mouths is recorded on paper for themselves and others to review. A variety of diary formats can be used. An example is given in Figure 7.5.

ENVIRONMENT MANAGEMENT

Restricting food cues that signal eating is another aspect of behavior therapy (Stunkard & Penick, 1979). This includes avoidance of fast foods, potato chips, candy, and ice cream by not having them in the house or easily accessible. Whenever possible, places and situations contiguous with eating are to be avoided. For example, the client should be advised not to take a coffee break in the snack room where workers share home-baked treats daily.

Having the client examine what prompts eating is helpful for developing insight. This includes becoming aware of whether eating occurs in response to the time of day, seeing other people eat, smells, low blood sugar, or increased peristalsis. Clients also need to know what prompts them to stop eating, such as an extremely full feeling, having eaten all food, or seeing that eating companions have finished.

Other environmental management, or cue-suppression techniques, include eating in the same room at home, using the same dishes and place mats, doing nothing else while eating, shopping from a list, setting the fork down between bites, using a smaller plate, eating with someone, and saving one item from a meal to eat later (Stuart, 1971). Eating with the nondominant hand and swallowing each bite before eating another are other techniques to help the overeater slow down. The goals of environmental management are to increase cues that support discretionary eating patterns and to decrease cues that lead to overeating.

Mahoney and Mahoney (1976) include responding to friends and family as social environment management. Significant others may be the least supportive. Mahoney and Mahoney described four harmful patterns of reactions from loved ones:

1. Teasing about weight and size and severely criticizing eating
2. Open sabotage by offering high-calorie foods
3. Ignoring dieter's efforts
4. Giving verbal support, yet demanding that high-calorie treats be on hand in the house

Another harmful reaction is hypervigilant scale watching by a domineering spouse.

Nurses can help family members become sensitive to their influence on obese loved ones. Because their behavior can facilitate success or failure, family members must cooperate. The assistance may include avoidance of any jokes and derogatory comments such as, "Not another diet." Family members must not offer food and eat empty calories (to be avoided by the dieter) in front of the overweight person. In some instances, open communication needs to be promoted so that food is not viewed as a display of affection. (I show my love for my husband by concocting luscious desserts.) The husband who is anxiety ridden about his wife's weight, expecting reports of foods consumed and daily weigh-in quotas while giving criticism or verbal abuse, is supporting weight gain and may be the cause of overeating in the first place. His perceptions and anxiety state need to be reviewed by the nurse.

SELF-REINFORCEMENT

To maintain accurate monitoring and changes in behavior, a method of self-rewards should be determined. Types of rewards are endless, including enjoying solitude while listening to a favorite symphony, making a phone call to a friend, spending time at a hobby, or spending extra time relaxing in a bubble bath before dinner. One client would walk to the newsstand to buy an evening paper on the days when she was exceptionally good with her prescribed diet and exercise routine. Involving significant others in rewards may be very helpful. For example, a husband may participate more in unpleasant household chores, such as scrubbing floors. Another self-reinforcement technique is having clients list adverse consequences of overeating and review this list. Reviewing the adverse outcomes helps counteract the pleasure of eating.

CONTRACTS

For some, reinforcement that is formally specified in a written contract is effective. An example of using a contract is described by Harris and Hallbauer (1973). Subjects were to decide on a reasonable amount of weight they would lose in 12 weeks and deposit a sum of money for each pound lost. Whatever amount the subject determined was acceptable. The money was refunded to the subject the week after the weight loss, providing the weight loss was maintained. The contract specified that any money remaining for failure to lose weight or dropping from the program was automatically forfeited. The forfeited money was equally divided among remaining group participants at the end of 12 weeks. Three groups with three conditions for weight control were compared after 12 weeks. Group 1 used a contract and was given information regarding diet; group 2 was given a contract and was counseled on diet and exercise; group 3 was a control group and met to discuss dieting problems. Group 2 experienced the most weight loss. The nonparticipants (dropouts) achieved significantly less weight loss than all three types of participants (Harris & Hallbauer, 1973). The contract approach weeds out obese persons who are not seriously motivated to lose weight.

Physical Activity

Routine physical activities need to be reviewed by the obese woman, and a means of increasing caloric expenditure through daily exercise needs to be adopted. Obese individuals tend to expend less energy than thin persons during routine activities; that is, they move as little as possible. The mother may become aware that she is requesting the children to change the channel on the TV, bring a glass of water to her in the living room, walk to the mailbox, and so forth. The first step to increase activity is to simply move about more in daily routines. The next step is to deliberately park two blocks away from the destination, take the stairs instead of using the elevator, and incorporate some enjoyable physical outlet into the daily routine. Unless the new exercise is viewed as pleasurable, it will not be continued. The exercise must not be contradictory to the person's health state. The routine may become more firmly established if the exercise is combined with performing other roles, such as bike riding with the children to spend time with them and get exercise at the same time. Other examples include walking, running the dog, and renewing or establishing mutual interests with a spouse by taking up tennis or some other form of exercise of common interest. This may be the beginning of a new communication pattern for the couple and may help resolve one of the stressors of middle-aged women as identified in Figure 7.2. Estimated energy expenditure for selected physical activities is presented in Table 7.3 and also in Chapter 11, Table 11.2.

Dietary Counseling

Clients need a basic understanding of nutritional values of foods, for example, how fats, proteins, and carbohydrates differ in caloric values. One gram of protein equals 4 calories, 1 gram of carbohydrates equals 4 calories, and 1 gram of fat equals 9 calories. One gram of alco-

Table 7.3 ➤ **ENERGY EQUIVALENTS OF FOOD CALORIES EXPRESSED IN MINUTES OF ACTIVITY***

Food	Calories	*Minutes of Activity*				
		Walking†	Riding Bicycle‡	Swimming§	Running¶	Reclining**
Apple, large	101	19	12	9	5	78
Bacon, 2 strips	96	18	12	9	5	74
Banana, small	88	17	11	8	4	68
Beans, green, 1 c	27	5	3	2	1	21
Beer, 1 glass	114	22	14	10	6	88
Bread and butter	78	15	10	7	4	60
Cake, 2-layer, 1/12	356	68	43	32	18	274
Carbonated beverage, 1 glass	106	20	13	9	5	82
Carrot, raw	42	8	5	4	2	32
Cereal, dry, ½ c with milk, sugar	200	38	24	18	10	154
Cheese, cottage, 1 tbsp	27	5	3	2	1	21
Cheese, cheddar, 1 oz	111	21	14	10	6	85
Chicken, fried, ½ breast	232	45	28	21	12	178
Chicken, TV dinner	542	104	66	48	28	417
Cookie, plain	15	3	2	1	1	12
Cookie, chocolate chip	51	10	6	5	3	39
Doughnut	151	29	18	13	8	116
Egg, fried	110	21	13	10	6	85
Egg, boiled	77	15	9	7	4	59
French dressing, 1 tbsp	59	11	7	5	3	45
Halibut steak, ¼ lb	205	39	25	18	11	158
Ham, 2 slices	167	32	20	15	9	128
Ice cream, ⅙ qt	193	37	24	17	10	148
Ice cream soda	255	49	31	23	13	196
Ice milk, ⅙ qt	144	28	18	13	7	111
Gelatin, with cream	117	23	14	10	6	90
Malted milk shake	502	97	61	45	26	386
Mayonnaise, 1 tbsp	92	18	11	8	5	71
Milk, 1 glass	166	32	20	15	9	128
Milk, skim, 1 glass	81	16	10	7	4	62
Milk shake	421	81	51	38	22	324
Orange, medium	68	13	8	6	4	52
Orange juice, 1 glass	120	23	15	11	6	92
Pancake with syrup	124	24	15	11	6	95
Peach, medium	46	9	6	4	2	35
Peas, green, ½ c	56	11	7	5	3	43
Pie, apple, ⅙	377	73	46	34	19	290
Pie, raisin, ⅙	437	84	53	39	23	336
Pizza, cheese, ⅛	180	35	22	16	9	138
Pork chop, loin	314	60	38	28	16	242
Potato chips, 1 serving	108	21	13	10	6	83
Sandwiches:						
Club	590	113	72	53	30	454
Hamburger	350	67	43	31	18	269
Roast beef with gravy	430	83	52	38	22	331
Tuna fish salad	278	53	34	25	14	214

Table 7.3 ➤ **ENERGY EQUIVALENTS OF FOOD CALORIES EXPRESSED IN MINUTES OF ACTIVITY* (Continued)**

		Minutes of Activity				
Food	Calories	Walk-ing[†]	Riding Bicycle[‡]	Swim-ming[§]	Running[¶]	Reclin-ing[**]
Sherbet, ⅙ qt	177	34	22	16	9	136
Shrimp, french fried	180	35	22	16	9	138
Spaghetti, 1 serving	396	76	48	35	20	305
Steak, T-bone	235	45	29	21	12	181
Strawberry shortcake	400	77	49	36	21	308

*Reprinted with permission from Konishi, F. (1965). Food energy equivalents of various activities. *Journal American Dietary Association, 46,* 186.
[†]Energy cost of walking for 150-pound individual = 5.2 calories per minute at 3.5 miles per hour.
[‡]Energy cost of riding bicycle = 8.2 calories per minute.
[§]Energy cost of swimming = 11.2 calories per minute.
[¶]Energy cost of running = 19.4 calories per minute.
[**]Energy cost of reclining = 1.3 calories per minute.

hol contains 7 calories. Realizing how their own diets have deviated from required nutritional intake provides an initial insight. Edelstein (1977) suggested the following dietary changes: (1) Obese women without other pathology need to eat 1000 calories a day to lose weight. (2) Spreading calories throughout the day is important because more weight will be gained if 800 calories are consumed at dinner and 200 calories are eaten in the morning. Edelstein recommended the following breakdown: breakfast—250 calories, lunch—250 calories, and dinner—500 calories. (3) Approximately 40 to 50 percent of the caloric intake should be protein.

Some clients tolerate dietary change and are more adherent in the long run when changes occur gradually. One major problem may have to be eliminated each week, such as omitting the ice cream at bedtime and substituting a lower-calorie carbohydrate food such as a graham cracker.

The prescribed diet and environmental management techniques need to be given to the client in writing. The American Dietetic Association exchange list is a most effective means of teaching diet and ensuring variety in the diet. Consultation with a dietitian is needed so that an individual's calorie-restricted diet will incorporate nutritional requirements of the basic four food groups and will be individually tailored to the client's likes and dislikes.

Consuming preloads of food works for some people to decrease volume of food consumed at a subsequent meal. The preload, taken approximately 30 minutes before eating, should be low in calories and high in volume, for example, two or three glasses of water or diet soda or raw vegetables (Mahoney & Mahoney, 1976).

Other strategies to control food intake may be helpful to some individuals. Have the obese client eat in front of a full-view mirror, paying attention to body size, double chin, rotund appearance, and so forth. Frustration tolerance needs to be developed so that the need for immediate satisfaction is eliminated. Teach the client that instead of gratifying a perceived need for between-meal snacks by eating, she should set a timer for 10 or 15 minutes. When the timer rings, if the snack is absolutely necessary, she can have it—ideally, a food permitted on the diet and preferably something saved from a previous meal. Creating a different response to the stimulus to eat is helpful. In response to a need to have baked goodies, the obese client could bake a favorite dessert and give it away (Bruno, 1972). Leaving a bit of each type of food on the plate helps to eliminate the clean plate signal to stop eating. However, this strategy is unacceptable to individuals who are conscious of food costs.

Assertiveness

Assertiveness can be developed and used as a means of achieving control over life situations in general, thereby enhancing control over eating. "Assertion is any open expression in word or deed that leads others to consider seriously your desires. Assertive behavior is emotionally honest, direct, self-enhancing, and expressive" (Stuart, 1978, pp. 126–127). Assertive behavior leads to self-respect and respect from others. Open, genuine, direct means of expressing self are characteristics of assertiveness. A goal of developing assertiveness is to enhance self-worth (Gareri, 1979) to eliminate indirect, self-denying, and dishonest communication. The emotional reactions concomitant with low self-assertion are destructive to self-worth. Feelings of anxiety, anger, frustration, and guilt lead to generalized powerlessness, and the behavioral consequence may be overeating. Quereshi and Soat (1976) found that persons addicted to alcohol were low in self-assertiveness. Self-assertion needs to be studied in persons addicted to food. Obese individuals cannot afford to be passive when others are suggesting and offering forbidden foods.

The four components of teaching assertiveness as identified by Lange and Jakubowski (1976) are a useful guide in developing assertiveness in the obese individual. The components include:

1. Helping individuals identify needs and their rights as well as the rights of others
2. Helping individuals differentiate among assertive, aggressive, and passive behaviors
3. Decreasing obstacles to assertive behavior—previous communication patterns learned throughout development—anxiety, guilt, low self-worth

4. Trying out assertive behaviors in controlled-environment group practice

To be successful with these components, individuals need to begin to think and talk positively about themselves. "When nonassertive behavior is practiced, high anxiety and low self-esteem are the result for all participants in the interaction" (Herman, 1978, p. 129). It is hoped that obese individuals will cope with life situations by self-assertion and not by overeating.

McBride (1988) proposed that in a holistic approach to weight loss for women, multiple criteria for success be used beyond focusing on the number of pounds lost. Success may include adopting improved grooming habits, deciding not to fixate on insurance companies' weight charts, losing inches by improving muscle tone, being able to wear smaller-sized clothing, increasing energy, and eating a nutritious diet.

Rational Emotive Therapy and Stressors of Middle Age

The ability to accurately recognize thoughts related to events helps one to control feelings resulting from the event. The identified stressors of middle years stimulate thoughts, feelings, and coping behaviors. Rational emotive therapy (RET) is effective in dealing with the stressors of middle years. If each stressor is rationally analyzed, the overeater's maladaptive behavior may be avoided.

The basis for RET is the assumption that control of emotions lies in the individual's thoughts about the precipitating event (Ellis, 1979). A goal of RET is to help clients think rationally, developing a realistic but not self-defeating outlook regarding the event; subsequently, coping behaviors will not be self-destructive or maladaptive as in overeating. Consider a stressor of middle years as an example:

A. (Event) Children leaving home.
B. (Thoughts) "Isn't this awful?"
C. (Feelings) Anxiety, depression, guilt over missed opportunities while children were home and dependent.

The cycle continues with the symptoms being the event:

A. (Event) Anxiety, depression, guilt.
B. (Thoughts) "This is awful; I can't stand these feelings. This must stop."
C. (Feelings) Deepened depression, increased anxiety, and increased guilt.

The cycle may seem to be made temporarily tolerable to the individual by overeating (or using some other maladaptive behavior). Ellis (1973) added two more stages to RET with which the nurse can instrumentally help the client: (1) disputing the irrational thoughts and (2) analyzing effects of the disputed thoughts.

    D. Disputing or challenging irrational thoughts and beliefs. Continuing with the above example: Why is this awful? Why can't I stand this change? In what way does this normal developmental progression affect my own growth?

    E. Analyzing the effects of disputing the thoughts and beliefs.

       1. It is not awful for young adult children to move out on their own.

       2. This change is a mark of maturity and independence in normal young adults.

       3. Love bonds are maintained and continue to be expressed.

       4. "This developmental progression marks new opportunities for me." This is the substituted self-talk.

Each stressor of middle-aged women can be confronted using RET. The desired end is abatement of overeating, a maladaptation to the stressors of middle years.

SUMMARY

Physiological hazards of obesity have been well documented in the literature, as have some psychosocial characteristics of obese individuals. This chapter proposes another variable—powerlessness—to be considered in analyzing the etiology and response pattern of obese persons. It also proposes that a plan of empowerment strategies be designed and implemented as a weight-control program. The dimensions of this empowerment program for obese individuals include behavior therapy (use of obesity profile, self-monitoring, environment management, self-reinforcement, and contracts), physical activity prescriptions, dietary counseling, assertiveness training, and rational emotive therapy (RET). The goal is to have clients realize that they are their own best therapists. They have the ability to control food intake and to exercise as well as to control many other aspects of their lives. Rodin et al. (1977) state that believing that the individual is in control has proved beneficial in achieving significant weight loss.

REFERENCES

Adams, N., Ferguson, J., Stunkard, A., & Agras, S. (1978). The eating behavior of obese and nonobese women. *Behavior Research and Therapy, 16,* 225–232.

Brightwell, D., Lemon, F., & Sloan, C. (1975). *New eating behavior: Practical management of obesity.* New York: Penwalt.

Brodie, D. A., & Slade, P. D. (1988). The relationship between body-image and body-fat in adult women. *Psychological Medicine, 18,* 623–631.

Bruch, H. (1979). *Eating disorders.* New York: Basic Books.

Bruno, F. J. (1972). *Think yourself thin.* Los Angeles: Nash Publishing.

Clayson, D. E., & Klassen, M. L. (1989). Perception of attractiveness by obesity and hair color. *Perceptual and Motor Skills, 68,* 199–202.

Diekelmann, N. (1977). *Primary health care of the well adult.* New York: McGraw-Hill.

Edelstein, B. (1977). *The woman doctor's diet for women.* New York: Ballantine Books.

Ellis, A. (1973). *Humanistic psychotherapy: The rational emotive approach.* New York: Julian Press.

Ellis, A. (1979). Rational-emotive therapy, in R. Corsini (Ed.), *Current psychotherapies* (pp. 185–229). Itasca, IL: FE Peacock Publishers.

Gardner, R. M., Martinez, R., Espinoza, T., & Gallegos, V. (1988). Distortion of body image in the obese: A sensory phenomenon. *Psychological Medicine, 18,* 633–641.

Gareri, E. (1979). Assertiveness training for alcoholics. *Journal of Psychiatric Nursing and Mental Health Services, 17,* 31–36.

Harris, M., & Hallbauer, E. (1973). Self-directed weight control through eating and exercise. *Behavior Research and Therapy, 11,* 523–529.

Hartz, A., Kalkoff, R., Rimm, A., & McCall, R. (1979). A study of factors associated with the ability to maintain weight loss. *Preventive Medicine, 8,* 471–483.

Herman, S. (1978). *Becoming assertive.* New York: D Van Nostrand.

Kemp, R. (1972). The overall picture of obesity. *Practitioner, 209,* 654–660.

Konishi, F. (1965). Food energy equivalents of various activities. *Journal of the American Dietetic Association, 46,* 186.

Lange, A. J., & Jakubowski, P. (1976). *Responsible assertive behavior: Cognitive behavioral procedures for trainers.* Champaign, IL: Research Press.

Maddox, G. L., & Liederman, V. R. (1969). Overweight as a social disability with medical implications. *Journal of Medical Education, 44,* 214.

Mahan, K. (1979). Sensible approach to the obese patient. *Nursing Clinics of North America, 14,* 229–245.

Mahoney, M. J. (1975). Fat fiction. *Behavior Therapy, 6,* 416–421.

Mahoney, M., & Mahoney, K. (1976). *Permanent weight control: A total solution to the dieter's dilemma.* New York: WW Norton.

Mayer, J. (1968). *Overweight: Causes, Cost and Control.* Englewood Cliffs, NJ: Prentice-Hall.

McBride, A. B. (1988). Fat: A women's issue in search of a holistic approach to treatment. *Holistic Nursing Practice, 3,* 9–15.

McCall, R. (1973). MMPI factors that differentiate remediably from irremediably obese women. *Journal of Community Psychology, 1,* 34–36.

McCall, R., & Siderits, M. A. (1977). *Becoming a graceful loser: Psychological factors in weight control.* Milwaukee, WI: TOPS Club.

McDonald, M. C. (1977). Obesity: Why a losing fight? *Psychiatric News, 12,* 27.

Orbach, S. (1997). *Fat is a feminist issue.* New York: Galahad Books.

Peternelj-Taylor, C. A. (1989). The effects of patient weight and sex on nurses' perceptions: A proposed model of nurse withdrawal. *Journal of Advanced Nursing, 14,* 744–754.

Prock, V. (1975). The mid-stage woman. *American Journal of Nursing, 75,* 1019–1022.

Quereshi, M., & Soat, D. (1976). Perception of self and significant others by alcoholics and nonalcoholics. *Journal of Clinical Psychology, 32,* 189–194.

Radvila, A. (1989). Psychosocial aspects of obesity. *Therapeutische Umschau, 46,* 291–296.

Rodin, J. (1977). Research on eating behavior and obesity, where does it fit in personality and social psychology? *Personality and Social Psychology Bulletin, 3,* 333–335.

Rodin, J., Atkinson, R., Dahms, W., Greenway, F., Hamilton, K., & Molitch, M. (1977). Predictors of successful weight loss in an outpatient obesity clinic. *International Journal of Obesity, 1,* 1.

Rosenfield, S. N., & Stevenson, J. S. (1988). Perception of daily stress and oral coping behaviors in normal, overweight and recovering alcoholic women. *Research in Nursing and Health, 11,* 165–174.

Straw, W., & Sonne, A. (1979). The obese patient. *Journal of Family Practice, 9,* 317–323.

Stuart, R. (1971). A three-dimensional program for the treatment of obesity. *Behavior Research and Therapy, 9,* 177–180.

Stuart, R. (1978). *Act thin, stay thin.* New York: WW Norton.

Stunkard, A. (1972). Preface. In R. Stuart & B. Davis (Eds.), *Slim chance in a fat world.* Champaign, IL: Research Press.

Stunkard, A., & Kaplan, D. (1977). Eating in public places: A review of reports of direct observation of eating behavior. *International Journal of Obesity, 1,* 1.

Stunkard, A., & Mendelson, M. (1967). Obesity and the body image: Characteristics of disturbances in the body image of some obese persons. *American Journal of Psychiatry, 123,* 1296–1300.

Stunkard, A., & Penick, S. (1979). Behavior modification in the treatment of obesity. *Archives of General Psychiatry, 36,* 801–896.

Sundberg, M. (1978). Framework of nursing intervention in the treatment of obesity. *Issues in Mental Health Nursing, 1,* 25–44.

Wadden, T. A., & Stunkard, A. (1987). Psychopathology and obesity. *Annals of the New York Academy of Sciences, 499,* 55–65.

Williams, S. (1996). *Basic nutrition and diet therapy.* St. Louis: CV Mosby.

Wright, E. J., & Whitehead, T. L. (1987). Perceptions of body size and obesity: A selected review of the literature. *Journal of Community Health, 12,* 117–129.

8

Powerlessness in Elderly Persons: Preventing Hopelessness

► JUDITH FITZGERALD MILLER •
CHRISTINE BOHM OERTEL

Aging is a process that is basic to the human experience. There has been a 900 percent increase in the number of Americans over age 65 (from 3 to 27 million) since 1900, with the fastest-growing group being over 85 years (Russell, 1989). The losses and stresses experienced by elderly persons make them vulnerable to powerlessness (Fuller, 1978; Teitelman, 1982). The increased vulnerability of elderly persons is related to their having fewer intact resources than individuals in the middle years or young adulthood. For example, elderly persons may have less physical strength and reserve and diminished social support network; lower self-esteem; decreased energy; and in some instances, less motivation to improve their health or adhere to medical prescriptions. (See client power resources model, Fig. 1.1.) Coping resources of elderly persons are challenged by sociological, physiological, and psychological stressors. For example, financial management is a stress because many elderly persons exist near poverty levels on fixed incomes through inflationary periods—approximately 18 percent of persons over age 65 are living below the poverty level (Kalish, 1975). Maintaining adequate housing may be difficult. Other sociological stressors include maintaining social contacts, getting to and depending on public transportation, gaining access to continuous health care, maintaining nutrition, and combating stereotypes and myths imposed by a youth-oriented society (Aguilera, 1980; Lancaster, 1981).

Psychological stressors include demands to adapt to rapid change inherent in our Western society (Eisdorfer & Wildie, 1977). In addition to the stress of living in a "fast-paced" society, elderly persons have to deal with changes resulting from unexpected losses such as deaths, retirement, and relocation (a move to a different city, to retirement complexes, or to nursing homes). Decreased sensory acuity may lead to misinterpretation of stimuli, suspicion, and withdrawal (Lancaster, 1981), especially after relocation. Maintaining protection from victimization through crime (Robb, 1989) and dealing with other fears, such as personal injury from falls or accidents, are other psychological threats.

Physiological stressors include adapting to multiple structural and functional losses. Physiological changes of aging are highlighted later as a cause of perceived powerlessness in elderly persons.

The purpose of this chapter is to examine powerlessness as a behavioral variable in the aging person threatened by chronic illness and hospitalization. A case study is included to depict situational powerlessness in elderly persons and to portray the devastating consequence of uncontrolled powerlessness. When powerlessness is not contained, a self-destructive cycle of powerlessness-depression-hopelessness occurs, which may hasten death (Seligman, 1975). The powerlessness-hopelessness cycle is illustrated in Figure 19.3. Identifying powerlessness in elderly clients in order to intervene and prevent hopelessness is of critical importance for nurses. Being able to identify clients' perceived situational powerlessness is the first step. The initial development of a behavioral assessment tool to identify powerlessness in hospitalized elderly clients is included in this chapter. It is beyond the scope of this chapter to present analyses of biological, psychological, and sociological theories of aging.

DEVELOPMENTAL VULNERABILITY

Powerlessness in Elderly Persons

Various factors cause powerlessness in elderly persons. Langer and Benevento (1978) classified contextual events that may render a person "helpless," including (1) being assigned a label that connotes inferiority in relation to other persons, (2) engaging in a consensually demeaning task, and (3) no longer engaging in a previously reinforcing, valued task. When applied to elderly persons, examples of each contextual event easily come to mind. Elderly persons are the targets of many false labels, myths, and stereotypes (Matteson & McConnell, 1988). They are regarded as rigid, inflexible, and intolerant (Butler, 1975). Other myths that aging is a decremental process rendering elderly persons unteachable, asexual, less than beautiful, and unable to actively participate in their own health care (Atchley, 1981), as well as unable to grow emotionally (Lancaster, 1981), destroy self-esteem (Rodin & Langer, 1980), cause inferiority, and induce powerlessness. Many elderly persons internalize these beliefs imposed by others in their social spheres.

When assigned a consensually demeaning task, as may occur when elderly persons live with offspring or in nursing homes, the elderly individual erroneously infers self-incompetence. If a task of sealing envelopes is viewed as unimportant, elderly persons could conclude that they are incapable of doing anything more important. If elderly persons living with offspring are included in household activities only by being asked to make their own bed, when in fact they are capable of much more, feelings of incompetence and helplessness may result.

The individual may not be able to make a transition from a work-centered role to a leisure-centered role (Robinson, 1981) and still maintain a feeling of self-worth and importance to others. No longer engaging in tasks that are reinforcing to the individual may be detrimental.

Chronic illness in elderly persons is another cause of powerlessness. Kalish (1975) stated that 85 percent of persons over age 65 report at least one chronic illness, and about 50 percent of these report limitation of desired activity because of chronic health problems.

Roy (1976) described elderly persons as having a constricted sphere of influence and control that increases powerlessness. "Independence, or the ability to provide for one's needs, is the most important aim of the majority of the elderly regardless of their state of health" (Culbert & Kos, 1971, p. 607). When this goal is fulfilled, a sense of control, or powerfulness, can result. Frustration of this goal leads to powerlessness. Powerlessness is frequently experienced by aging persons in our culture and is a prominent nursing diagnosis of elderly persons admitted to acute-care facilities. The aging person is vulnerable to powerlessness because of physiological and psychosocial changes inherent in the aging process.

Overview of Physiological and Psychosocial Changes of Aging

Aging is a time marked by multiple losses and multiple changes. The onset of these losses varies from individual to individual and is not correlated with any specific chronological age. There seems to be a reduction in the reserve capacity for the aged person to adapt to changes and to stress. This reduction occurs at a time when there is a corresponding increase in the number and intensity of stressors in the person's life. The changes accompanying aging demand an adaptive response and represent a potential source of powerlessness. Because the changes are multiple, only a limited overview is provided in this chapter.

As humans age, sensory changes occur. Changes in vision include decreased peripheral vision, decreased color perception, increased threshold for light stimulation, increased intraocular pressure, and presbyopia. There is a decreased pupil accommodation and diminished pupil size. Changes in hearing include lessened ability to hear high tones and to differentiate sounds. Aging also results in a marked decrease in the sense of taste. By age 75, there is a 64 percent loss of taste buds (Hayter, 1974). Taste buds that detect bitter and sour remain intact (Shore, 1976). This increased sensitivity to bitterness and decreased sensitivity to sweetness and saltiness may account for some dietary indiscretion in elderly persons; however, further research is needed. Although there are reports of a marked decrease in the sense of smell, there is wide variation from person to person (Hayter, 1974; Yurick, 1989). Olfactory acuity is influenced by environmental toxins and occupational odors that have been present throughout the individual's life. The sense of touch also becomes less acute, with a steady loss of peripheral pain perception. Cataracts, glaucoma, and hearing loss increase with age (Matteson & McConnell, 1988).

The aging person must cope with an altered body image. The person in the mirror, as well as the person trying to fit into clothes, may not be the person the individual expects. It is not uncommon for older persons to remark that they still feel like 35 until they look in the mirror or attempt to do what they were able to do at age 35. The alteration of body image results from changes such as loss of subcutaneous tissues, atrophy of muscle, skin dryness, decreased skin elasticity and thickness, decreased number of sweat glands, atrophy of hair follicles with hair loss, loss of pigment in hair and skin, increased angularity of the body, degenerative joint changes, and a shortening or stooping posture related to the narrowing of the vertebral disks. The loss of subcutaneous fat accounts for the elderly person's sensitivity to cold (Matteson & McConnell, 1988). If tooth loss occurs, it is usually a result of change in supportive structures, that is, gingival recession and osteoporosis, not tooth decay (Rossman, 1988).

Important physiological changes occur in the cardiovascular system. As aging occurs, there is a decrease in cardiac efficiency despite a lack of change in heart size. Heart valves become thick, rigid, and less effective. The cardiac rate at rest may be similar to that of a younger adult, but under stress it does not increase as much and takes longer to return to normal. Arterial changes include elongation, fibrosis, and calcification. There can be a decreased blood flow to organs such as the kidney, liver, heart, and brain because of arterial changes. Blood pressure may have a higher normal value resulting from increased arterial resistance.

The lung tissue of the older person becomes less elastic. This results in about a 40 percent decline in the mechanical efficiency of air exchange (Culbert & Kos, 1971). There is also a decreased capacity for oxygen uptake by the red blood cells. Respirations are further compromised by limited lung expansion related to musculoskeletal changes and resulting posture change—stooping.

The reabsorptive and excretory abilities of the kidneys decrease. The kidneys are less able to concentrate urine and thus prevent dehydration. There is a slowed compensatory response to acid-base shifts and altered chemical composition of the blood.

The individual's homeostatic mechanisms become less effective with age. Imbalances tend to develop more easily. A longer period is needed to restore equilibrium. A greater degree of deviation can result from a much lesser provocation with less tolerance. There is a diminished reserve capacity of organs and tissues.

The accumulative effect of these physiological changes can mean decreased functional ability, diminished energy stores, and an overall lessening of speed and efficiency. Because these changes occur gradually, the individual is usually able to adapt to them, maintaining a sense of powerlessness. When these changes are complicated by the presence of one or more chronic pathological conditions, the individual's ability to adapt successfully may be impaired.

Although statistics vary from source to source, the percentages of persons over 65 years having the following chronic health problems are arthritis (65%), hypertension (42%), hearing impairment (40%), cardiac conditions (34%), cataracts (23%), and vision impairment (14%). The top three leading causes of death are heart disease, cancer, and cerebrovascular disease (Christ & Hohloch, 1988).

Loss of control or an inadequate knowledge base regarding health changes increases the aging individual's vulnerability to powerlessness. One author described old age as "a time for savoring life, the world, and all that is in it. It is a time for making peace with oneself and the universe" (Hayter, 1974, p. 307). In reality, for many, aging may not result in such a beautiful experience.

Aging can threaten one's self-concept. The restrictions imposed by the social and cultural environment may deny the individual prestige and authority. Security may be bought at the price of loneliness and inactivity. According to Rynerson (1972), lower-level needs for food and safety may be met, while higher needs for affection, social recognition, and a role in society in which dignity, self-worth, and self-satisfaction are maintained may be neglected. Enhancing self-esteem would mean generating attitudes that lead to one's feeling of being useful and necessary in the world. Maintaining self-esteem in elderly persons combats despair and promotes successful attainment of the developmental task of ego integrity versus despair (Erikson, 1975).

Psychosocial losses of aging may include loss of former roles and status, loss of family members and friends, loss of economic security, and loss of familiar surroundings. Financial strain increases with age and contributes to depression in the elderly (Krause, 1987). In addition, there may be loss of health and function. The number of significant others in the older person's life may be reduced, compromising the individual's loving support system. Death of a spouse may result in a 50 percent decrease in social contacts for the remaining partner (Rathbone-McCuen & Hashimi, 1982). Diminished physiological reserves may force the individual into social isolation. The elderly person may be forced to face fears, dependency, chronic illness, and death alone and may respond to these overwhelming odds with perceived powerlessness and eventual despair.

As persons become more dependent on outside agencies for assistance, the individual's decision-making role and personal control are usurped (Angrosino, 1976). The stressors that alter the elderly person's perceived control are specifically pertinent for this chapter. The following discussion is limited to the perceived control in elderly subjects.

RESEARCH ON CONTROL AND ELDERLY PERSONS

Schultz (1976) studied the effect of increased predictability and control on physical and psychological well-being of 40 elderly subjects living in a retirement home. Subjects were randomly assigned to one of the following four conditions for visitation from college students: (1) subjects were in control of frequency and duration of visits; (2) subjects were informed when they would be visited and how long the visit would last (subjects in this group could predict this event); (3) subjects experienced a random visit schedule; and (4) subjects were not visited. Subjects in the predictable and control-visit groups had significantly higher levels of hope, less lonely time, less bored time, greater zest for life, and greater happiness, usefulness, and activity level than subjects in the no-treatment and random-visit groups. Schultz concluded that the decline in physical and psychological status associated with aging may be inhibited or reserved by providing residents with predictable or controllable positive events. Schultz and Hanusa (1978) did a follow-up study on these same subjects. Data on physical and psychological status were collected 24, 30, and 42 months after completion of the 1976 study. No positive long-term effects attributable to the interventions were found. Instead, those persons who initially benefited from the interventions exhibited precipitous declines after the study was terminated, and those subjects who showed no improvement in the original study remained stable in physical and psychological functioning over time. Schultz and Hanusa (1978) warned other researchers engaged in similar field studies to provide substitute predictable and controllable events after treatment conditions of control are terminated.

The effects of enhanced personal responsibility and choice on alertness, activity participation, and overall sense of well-being were studied in 91 ambulatory nursing home residents (Langer & Rodin, 1976). Subjects were assigned to two treatment groups. The first group was given a communication by the nursing home director emphasizing self-responsibility and decision making regarding their environment and activities. Subjects in this group were given a plant they selected and were then responsible for the plant's care. Subjects in the other treatment group were given a message that emphasized the staff's responsibility for them. These subjects were given a plant that the staff tended. Subjects in the responsibility-induced group were significantly more active, alert, happy, and generally improved. The improvement rating was determined by nurses' blind ratings. No significant difference was found on the perceived-control measure between the two treatment groups.

Rodin and Langer (1977) did an 18-month follow-up study on 26 of the subjects from Langer's 1976 study. Those subjects in the control-induced group had sustained beneficial effects. Mortality showed a striking difference in that only 7 (15 percent) of the 47 subjects in the responsibility-induced group had died during the 18 months, whereas 13 (30 percent) of the 54 subjects of the comparison (staff-controlled) group died. Significant difference was noted at the .01 level.

A study of 50 residents in a home for elderly persons was done to determine predictors of resident's self-reported morale (Fuller, 1978). Variables considered were the resident's perceived degree of choice in moving to the home, perceived degree of choice while living in the home, and amount of time spent in social interactions weekly, as well as age, income, recent loss of a significant other, and length of time at the home. The only significant predictors of morale were perceived choice within the home and amount of time spent in social interactions each week. Those residents who perceived greater choice and who spent more time in social interactions reported higher levels of morale. Fuller emphasized that current opportunity to make choices is predictive of well-being. Opportunities for resident decision making can be provided by nurses.

Chang (1978a) found that of 30 nursing home residents studied, those who perceived themselves in control of their immediate situations as determined by the Situational Control of Daily Activities scale had higher morale scores regardless of their internal and external personality orientations. Self-determination (person's own control of daily activities) resulted in a higher morale for subjects with both internal and external locus-of-control orientations. In a similar study, Chang (1980) examined congruence of locus of control and the client's perceived situational control with morale in 39 clients in skilled nursing facilities. All subjects completed a self-rating of their health. Internals who rated their health as "fair" and whose locus of control was congruent with their perception of having situational control had high morale compared with the incongruent group ($p = .04$). No significant differences were found in subjects with health ratings other than "fair." Of the externals with "fair" health ratings, incongruent subjects had low morale more frequently than did the congruent subjects ($p = .03$). No differences were found in terms of comparisons of race or sex. Chang also found a strong correlation between internal locus of control and high morale (.05 level of significance).

In other studies of locus of control and elderly persons, external locus of control correlated with depression (Hanes & Wild, 1977), and internal locus of control correlated with a positive self-concept (Reid, Haas, & Hawkins, 1977). Ziegler and Reid (1979) confirmed that desired control is related to psychological adjustment. Desired control was significantly negatively correlated with depression and positively correlated with health, knowledge of services for elderly persons, and use of services for elderly persons in 88 elderly community residents. The researchers also studied 77 elderly men in a chronic-care hospital ward. Desired control was significantly positively correlated with life satisfaction, self-concept, tranquility, and subject senescence.

Bradley (1976) studied locus of control in 306 subjects whose ages ranged from 19 to 90 years. Locus of control in three areas of activity—intellectual, social, and physical—was studied. Bradley found that subjects over age 60 perceived themselves as having less control in the social area than did subjects in the 35- to 50-year-old age group.

Powerlessness-Hopelessness-Death

Loss of hope can have catastrophic consequences such as hastening death (Seligman, 1975). Seligman reviewed studies of death from helplessness and hopelessness in humans. Death was documented to have occurred in humans soon after the death of a spouse, parent, or other loved one; after loss of status; and during times of extreme threat. In all instances, the subjects were described as helpless. Seligman warned that loss of control that accompanies hospitalization further weakens a sick person and may cause death. "We should expect that when we remove the vestiges of control over the environment of an already weakened human being, we may well kill him" (p. 186).

Rowland (1977) completed a review of literature to determine the effect of the environmental events on death of elderly persons. The three events were (1) death of significant others, (2) relocation, and (3) retirement. The research reports reviewed suggest that death of a significant other and relocation may predict death for elderly persons under certain circumstances. Relocation predicted death for elderly persons who were in poor physical health, which may or may not have been accompanied by poor mental health. Forced relocation may remove the last perceived control elderly persons had over situations and events. Death of a significant other seems to predict death under certain conditions. The risk of death is greatest during the first year of bereavement, and Rowland's summary suggests the risk is higher for men than for women. The suggestion that elderly persons who have few contacts with others may be more likely to die needs investigation. No conclusive evidence existed regarding retirement as a predictor of death in the studies reviewed by Rowland (1977).

NURSING IMPLICATIONS

Any action that promotes elderly persons' maximum control over their lives will maintain or improve their overall well-being (Fuller, 1978) and may have an effect on life expectancy. Simple measures to enhance perceived control in a nursing home might include providing the resident with food selection alternatives, having the resident decide on the schedule for hair appointments, or enabling the resident to request specific library books. Meaningful control measures can be assumed by residents of nursing homes according to their own desires but should not be of a temporary nature serving someone else's best interest. Meaningful activities could include:

- Caring for plants
- Surveying residents for activity choices or other needs
- Providing scheduled companionship time with more disabled residents
- Delivering mail and reading it to visually impaired residents
- Organizing a monthly newsletter
- Recognizing residents' birthdays by planning specific events or surprises
- Sharing favorite recipes
- Conducting musical evenings (playing "old favorites" on records or piano)
- Helping others with correspondence
- Organizing discussions after and about the national news on television
- Planning field trips

The residents themselves could devise creative activity lists based on their own talents and interests. Hutchison, Carstensen, & Silberman (1983) found that nursing home residents wanted input regarding increasing their activities and access to such activities, food selection, and resident meetings. The use of councils with residents as members enhances control for nursing home residents (Ryden, 1985).

The elderly person can be helped to realize retirement is a fulfilling, self-enriching time to "savor life." Without some specific preparation for retirement, the newly found freedom may fade into disenchantment and depression (Robinson, 1981). Nurses in all practice settings, especially community agencies, may have specific responsibilities for promoting elderly persons' health through satisfying use of leisure time, helping persons recognize leisure as a "personally significant" self-actualizing activity. Community health nurses also help elderly persons take advantage of resources geared to them, for example, senior citizen centers, meal programs for elderly persons, and special transportation services. Elderly persons are to be provided with the options for decision making for various needs, such as using resources, engaging in activities, and relocating or modifying living environments. The emphasis is on allowing the elderly person to make the decisions.

Aging persons may need to look beyond self to find meaning and order in their lives and to resolve fears of death. To meet this need, religion may take on new importance (Brown, 1980; Moberg, 1980). The nurse can discuss spiritual well-being and ways appropriate for individuals to attain this well-being (Prayer, meditation, religious rituals, reading the Bible and/or religious writings, listening to tape recordings on faith, and so forth). Despair is incongruent with spiritual well-being and having a relationship with God combats loneliness (McCreary, 1980).

Assessment of manifestations of powerlessness in the elderly is important so that early and accurate nursing diagnoses can be made and appropriate interventions can be implemented. Roy (1976) stated that the indicators of powerlessness include apathy, withdrawal, resignation, fatalism, malleability, anxiety, restlessness, sleeplessness, wandering, aimlessness, and lack of decision making. Because these behaviors could be indicative of many nursing diagnoses, validation of the nurses' clinical impressions by using a valid, reliable tool is desirable.

PERCEIVED CONTROL ASSESSMENT
TOOLS FOR ELDERLY PERSONS

Specific tools to measure situational control in the elderly have been developed (Chang, 1978b; Reid, Haas, & Hawkings, 1977). Chang's (1978b) tool was developed to measure elderly subjects' situational control in institutional settings. Situational control refers to the perception that either the individual or others determine the use of time, space, and resources in daily activities (Chang, 1978b). The Situational Control of Daily Activities scale has two factors: (1) control of socializing and privacy, and (2) control of physical care. Test-retest reliability was

0.96. Subjects respond to questions about eight activities in terms of whether they themselves or others control the activities. The activities include ambulating, dressing, eating, grooming, socializing in a group, socializing in a twosome, using the toilet, and performing solitary activities. This is a valuable tool for nurses to use in validating the elderly person's perceived situational control.

A General Health Status (GHS) scale for elderly persons was developed by Haney, Stephens, Cooper, Oser, & Blau (1981) and its validity and reliability have been established. The tool was correlated with a detailed valid Physician Assessment of Health Status scale. The GHS is a simply constructed tool in which subjects respond to 27 questions indicating whether they have trouble with the item by marking "yes," "no," or "don't know." There are 11 items related to day-to-day activities, such as "putting on or tying shoes," "going up stairs," "remembering things," "bathing," and "preparing meals." There are 16 items dealing with health problems, for example, "cannot sleep through the night," "trouble seeing," "trouble starting or stopping urine," and "swollen feet." The 11 items about daily activities are helpful in alerting the nurse to problems of control for the elderly individual.

Reid, Haas, and Hawkings (1977) developed a tool to measure locus of desire and expectancy for control in elderly persons. The tool was situationally specific (instead of measuring an enduring personality trait of locus of control) and considered the immediate environment as well as desires and interests of the subjects. Subjects rated each of 14 items on a Likert-type scale. For example, "How desirable or important is it for you to be able to decide on your own daily activities?" is an item on the interest and/or desires component of the tool. Subjects rated the item as (1) not important/desirable, (2) somewhat important/desirable, (3) generally important/desirable, or (4) very important/desirable. The same question is rephrased on the expectancy component of the tool: "How often can you decide what your daily activities are going to be?" Subjects respond by answering (1) never, (2) sometimes, (3) quite often, or (4) always.

In studies of institutionalized elderly persons, internality correlated positively with nurses' ratings of subjects' happiness, and with subjects' self-ratings of contentment and happiness. Negative correlations were found between internality and length of residency in the nursing home and age (Reid, Haas, & Hawkings, 1977).

Ziegler and Reid (1979), using the desired-locus-of-control scale, confirmed that desired expectancy for control is related to psychological adjustment in their studies of 88 elderly community residents and 77 elderly residents in a chronic-care hospital ward.

As a result of the clinical study presented later in this chapter and a comprehensive review of the literature, a powerlessness behavioral assessment tool (Fig. 8.1) was developed. This tool is an observational

		Nurse Rating of Behaviors			
		1 Never	2 Occasionally	3 Frequently	4 Always
VERBAL RESPONSE	Verbal expressions of lack of control over what is happening.				
	Verbal expressions of doubt that self-care measures can affect outcome.				
	Verbal expressions of giving up.				
	Verbal expressions of fatalism.				
EMOTIONAL RESPONSE	Withdrawal.				
	Pessimism.				
	Undifferentiated anger.				
	Diminished patient-initiated interaction.				
	Submissiveness.				
PARTICIPATION IN ACTIVITIES OF DAILY LIVING	Nonparticipation in daily personal hygiene.				
	Noninterest in treatments.				
	Refusal to take food or fluids.				
	Inability to set goals.				
	Lack of decision making when opportunities are provided.				
	Dependency on others for activities of daily living.				
INVOLVEMENT IN LEARNING ABOUT CARE RESPONSIBILITIES	Lack of questioning concerning illness.				
	Low level of knowledge of illness after being given information.				
	Lack of knowledge related to treatment.				
	Lack of motivation to learn.				

FIGURE 8.1 ➤ Powerlessness behavioral assessment tool.

guide for nurses to use in diagnosing powerlessness. The tool contains four categories of assessment data: verbal response, emotional response, participation in activities of daily living, and involvement in learning about care responsibilities. Nurses rate client behaviors for each item on the tool using a four-point scale: (1) client never manifests this behavior, (2) client occasionally manifests this behavior, (3) client frequently manifests this behavior, (4) client always manifests this behavior.

➤➤➤ **CASE STUDY**

PREVENTING HOPELESSNESS

Mrs. B. was a 71-year-old married woman with five children, two of whom lived in town. Her husband was an active 77-year-old man with no major health problems. The couple lived in a low-rent townhouse during the summer and spent their winters in Florida in a trailer home they owned. Before her hospitalization, Mrs. B. had managed to maintain a high level of independence, in spite of a progressive deterioration of her right hip joint.

About 3 years before this hospitalization, Mrs. B. had sustained a subcapital fracture of her right leg, which had been pinned. Within 1½ years, she began experiencing progressive pain in her right hip joint, causing ambulatory difficulty that necessitated the use of a walker. Radiologic examination revealed deterioration of the right hip joint. After more than a year and a half of continued pain and disability, Mrs. B. was admitted to the hospital for an elective total hip replacement. At the time of her admission, her health history revealed no significant findings. There was no evidence of any other chronic disease.

Upon admission Mrs. B. presented herself as an energetic person. She detailed how she and her husband were able to maintain their two homes. She did not seek outside help, expressing a perceived sense of control over most of the circumstances of her life. She demonstrated a high degree of knowledge related to the hip deterioration and the planned total hip replacement. She was able to describe the planned surgery in basic terms. Her expectation of her hospitalization was a stay of about 3 weeks.

Mrs. B. underwent surgery for the total hip replacement on May 21. For the first week, her postoperative course was uneventful. She maintained a positive, goal-oriented approach to her convalescence, participating in her care, seeking information, and complying with all that she perceived would enhance her return to health. On May 30, Mrs. B. became dyspneic and cyanotic and complained of chest pain. Diagnostic examination revealed multiple pulmonary emboli. She was transferred to the intensive-care unit and started on anticoagulant therapy. The expected response to the anticoagulant therapy was not achieved. Further testing revealed that Mrs. B. had a serum factor that caused platelets to aggregate in contact with heparin. On June 6, Mrs. B. developed a deep iliofemoral thrombosis of the right leg with marked edema and discoloration of the lower portion of the leg. A venous thrombectomy was performed the next day. Subsequently, gangrene of the right foot developed from the impairment of circulation with ischemic changes. The right foot was treated conservatively, using pHisoHex soaks. Pulmonary status returned to normal. Mrs. B. remained hospitalized for the treatment of her right foot. Most of this time was spent on the rehabilitation unit.

During the acute crisis, Mrs. B. became withdrawn, interacting less with the persons in her environment. Her appetite decreased. She expressed a sense of being overwhelmed by her circumstances, stating, "I'm not sure what is happening to me." She also expressed a lack of previous experience to provide her with needed coping mechanisms stating, "I've never been through anything like this before." Much of the time she was quiet.

Mrs. B. returned to the surgical unit on July 18 for debridement of the lesion on her right foot and a possible transmetatarsal amputation. When she returned to the surgical unit, Mrs. B. was in a state of depression, expressing resistance to the amputation and using denial. She stated that she did not know who she was anymore and desired to go home to "find herself." In contrast to her knowledge of the original surgery, Mrs. B. had a low level of knowledge about this surgery and expressed a lack of desire to know anything about it. A transmetatarsal amputation of the right foot was performed on July 19.

Her first postoperative day was uneventful. On her second postoperative day, Mrs. B. began to exhibit acute anxiety behavior. She referred to this as her "nerves being so uptight." In her interaction with her husband, she was slightly hostile and withdrawn. The focal stimulus of her anxious behavior was the pending dressing change on her foot that had been spoken of by the surgical team during morning rounds. There was a delay of several hours before the dressing change was actually done. She stated that she wished that she "could tell them what to do and when to do it." She referred to the surgical team as "the Gestapo" and felt that no matter what she did she was "at their mercy." Her expectations of the dressing change were all negative. She perceived that it would be extremely painful, that she would not be medicated in time, and that the pain medication would not be effective. Mrs. B. also expressed concern that she would not be able to control her own reactions to the dressing change.

Mrs. B.'s behaviors at this point demonstrated a high degree of perceived powerlessness (Fig. 8.2). The first step in intervention was to recognize the existing state of powerlessness and then to help Mrs. B. recognize her sense of powerlessness. This was done by identifying the behaviors and interpreting them to Mrs. B. An attempt was then made to reduce her global sense of helplessness to a more specific focus. This involved separating things Mrs. B. could control from things she could not control. For example, Mrs. B. could control the extent of the pain that occurred during the dressing change by requesting and receiving pain medication and by learning relaxation and refocusing techniques. She could also control the extent of the pain by using the presence of a support person in the environment. She could not control the fact that

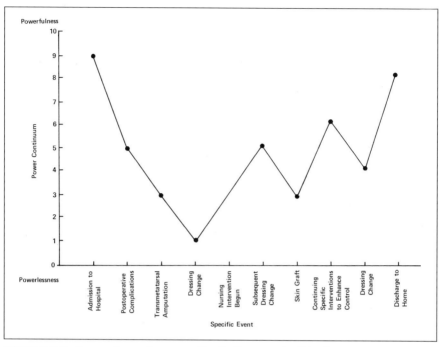

FIGURE 8.2 ➤ Degree of powerlessness and health-illness events of Mrs. B.

the procedure would involve pain. She also could not control the time that the surgical team would do the procedure.

As a result of these interventions, the client became more relaxed. Her body position showed less tension. She was able to sleep for short intervals. Her verbalization was increasingly goal directed in terms of stating that perhaps she could control the amount of pain she would experience. Although the actual dressing change was a difficult experience for Mrs. B., her sense of powerlessness was reduced. This was demonstrated in her comments the next day regarding further dressing changes: "I really screamed yesterday when they took that dressing off, but it wasn't so bad this morning when the nurses did it." Her other comments during the day revealed a much more positive, goal-oriented, hopeful approach to her circumstances. She stated that her foot was less painful, that she had decided to walk again, and that she felt like eating. She also had begun to take an active interest in herself, using part of her time in the morning to set her hair.

Because of the changes in her behavior, time was spent reinforcing her increased sense of powerfulness. Mrs. B. was helped to identify those events in her current situation that indicated improvement. These included the need for less pain medication, the discontinuation of intravenous therapy, and her increased interest in food. This nursing intervention was effective in increasing Mrs. B.'s level of hopefulness by refocusing her attention away from the series of complications that had induced the sense of powerlessness within her and toward attending to signs of improvement.

Mrs. B. continued to move from powerlessness to powerfulness. She began to exert more control over her immediate environment, although she remained on bedrest. She began deciding where things should be kept and directed her caregivers accordingly. The nursing staff reinforced this behavior by allowing Mrs. B. to decide when she wanted to have her bath or have a procedure done. She began to express future-oriented thinking, planning for things she would do after her discharge. Mrs. B. also began to seek information about the effects of the amputation on her ability to walk. Her anxiety was markedly decreased, and previous signs of withdrawal and depression were absent.

Mrs. B.'s return to powerfulness was threatened when she was informed that she would need a skin graft at the amputation site. Her perception of this proposed treatment was that she was not improving. This perception reinforced her former negative expectations. She began to express uncertainty about returning home, frustration over not receiving information from her attending physicians, and reluctance to have further anesthesia. Her perceived powerlessness increased, having a more global, all-encompassing effect this time. She demonstrated anxiety toward trying something new, such as using the walker. She said, "Please don't let go of me. I can't walk alone with this thing." Despair was noted in Mrs. B.'s responses, "What's the use? There have been so many setbacks."

Mrs. B.'s increased sense of powerlessness was also due to her inability to obtain answers from the surgical team to her questions about the planned skin graft ("they don't stay long enough to ask questions"). She felt a perceived loss of control in the area of decision making related to her body. She had not received sufficient information to even agree to have the skin graft. Her powerlessness resulted from a lack of knowledge about the procedure, the rationale for doing it, the time when it would occur, and the expected outcome.

Again, nursing intervention began by recognizing that a state of powerlessness existed. Mrs. B. was helped to recognize her feelings of powerlessness. To increase her sense of powerfulness, the focus of her greatest concern regarding the skin graft was identified. Her identified concern was that the physicians would not give her needed information. Her right to ask questions was reinforced. A strategy was developed to obtain information from the surgical team. Mrs. B. identified specific questions she wanted answered and then set a goal to get them answered. As she focused on this task, her anxiety behaviors decreased. Her verbal comments changed from fear and depression to references to specific things she could do. Mrs. B. was able to achieve her goal, which enhanced her sense of power.

During the days before the skin graft procedure, Mrs. B. vacillated between a sense of powerfulness and powerlessness. She demonstrated a heightened anxiety level but was more realistic in approaching the problem than she had been previously. Her anxiety was not accompanied by apathy, depression, withdrawal, or pessimism. She continued to maintain control over her immediate environment and directed nursing care. She also continued her goal of walking with the walker.

Nursing interventions at this time focused on reinforcing Mrs. B.'s sense of powerfulness by supplying her with needed realistic information and encouraging her to make decisions related to her care. Anxiety was kept within limits by means Mrs. B. determined, for example, planning for physician's rounds by writing down questions and using television soap operas as a distraction from her own plight. She expressed relief to know that it was all right to feel some anxiety.

Her powerlessness increased after the skin graft at the time of the first dressing change. This was manifested by a high degree of anxiety, a lack of goal orientation, and verbalization of negative expectations. She became very angry with the surgical team during the procedure. This anger seemed to indicate her growing realization that she had a right to have control over her circumstances. She expressed her sense of the discrepancy between the words and the actions of the surgical team: "You can't trust them at all. They said that they would soak the dressing off, but instead they rush in and rip it off. They lie to you every chance they get."

During the subsequent days of hospitalization, Mrs. B.'s physical status continued to improve. Nursing interventions were directed toward helping Mrs. B. identify specific indicators of physical improvement. These included the progressive healing of the skin graft and her increased ambulation. Mrs. B. responded with increased hopefulness and futuristic, goal-oriented thinking. She became involved in activities of daily living and in her dressing changes. Her anxiety level related to the dressing changes became markedly reduced. She no longer viewed these as potential complications but as routine procedures. She retained a sense of powerlessness in response to the surgical team, commenting on their tendency to do whatever they pleased.

At the time of her discharge, Mrs. B. was ambulating well with a walker. Her foot was healed. She was doing her own dressing changes with assistance from her husband. She had begun to plan how they would manage activities of daily living at home in spite of alterations in her health. She expressed confidence in her ability to work this out. Her increased self-esteem, goal-oriented behavior, and positive responses to her situation indicated that powerlessness had been resolved and she was returning to a functional state of powerfulness.

Mrs. B. entered the powerlessness cycle at the time when multiple complications to her recovery began to occur. Within her frame of reference, these complications were seen as being outside her control. This perception led to immobilization. Her growing sense of powerlessness was reinforced by the actions of medical and nursing staffs. Their lack of perception of Mrs. B.'s need to be incorporated into decision making enhanced her perception of powerlessness. Nursing interventions that recognized Mrs. B.'s state of powerlessness and assisted her to learn new methods of control proved effective in returning Mrs. B. to a state of powerfulness. The events, with hypothetical degrees of powerlessness for Mrs. B., are depicted in Figure 8.2. No quantitative powerlessness scores were used to validate the clinical impressions depicted in Figures 8.1 and 8.2.

Discussion

As demonstrated in the case study, powerlessness has serious nursing implications. Powerlessness affects a person's behavioral responses. In the individual experiencing powerlessness, learning or goal achievement is not seen as helpful in affecting an outcome. "Acquisition of knowledge or goal-directive behavior is simply irrelevant or unnecessary when the individual does not perceive that future events can be controlled by his own actions" (Johnson, 1967). Knowledge or goal-directive behavior can mean the difference between successful or unsuccessful adaptation to illness. The aging client is more vulnerable to powerlessness because of the aging process itself. In facing powerlessness, the elderly client is less able to cope because of diminished psychosocial reserve capacity.

Powerlessness can be prevented. In the case presented, hospitalization meant some degree of loss of control, which the client was able to limit through her expectations of a limited hospital stay. Complications in recovery precipitated a lack of fulfillment of these expectations, leading to some degree of immobilization. These complications also produced increased physical powerlessness. This individual viewed the complications as being outside her sphere of control.

A second factor that contributed to the development of powerlessness in this individual was the tendency of both medical and nursing staffs to dehumanize. There was a failure to recognize the individual's right and need to be incorporated into the decision-making process, as well as failure to note special adaptive needs and limited coping capacity of the elderly person. Information was not supplied fully to the individual. Decisions were made without consulting the individual. No alternatives were presented.

Because of these factors, nursing strategies for preventing powerlessness need to be aimed at preventing loss of involvement and supplying the client with an adequate knowledge base. Preventive strategies would include involving aging individuals in planning their own care, enhancing their self-esteem by referring decisions directly to them, supplying them with cognitive control through helping them anticipate events and outcomes, and giving them time to adjust to changes. Strategies also need to be developed to help individuals understand complications that occur, bringing them into a framework that diminishes the sense of loss of control.

SUMMARY

As demonstrated in the case study, powerlessness can lead to hopelessness. Hopelessness was an accurate indicator of suicide ideation in a study of 120 depressed elderly (Hill, Gallagher, Thompson, & Ishida, 1988). Depression was more predictive of suicide ideation than hopelessness, however. Even without persistent physical decline caused by illness, if hopelessness becomes a reality, suicide may result. Powerlessness affects a person's behavioral responses. When apathy and depression are pronounced, routine teaching and refocusing on goal achievement may be inadequate. Very specific concrete interventions based on individual clinical events to enable accurate and optimistic interpretations of events may be needed. Strategies to enhance elderly persons' control have been suggested by Teitelman and Priddy (1988). These have been modified here to include:

1. Promoting choice and predictability. This includes adhering to mutually determined schedules.
2. Eliminating helplessness-engendering stereotypes such as "being old means being unable to participate in care." Use of negative labels needs to be avoided.
3. Avoiding severe self-blame for events. Promoting a sense of responsibility for participating in health care.
4. Promoting a feeling of success in goal accomplishment.
5. Modifying unrealistic expectations without destroying generalized hope.
6. Using control-enhancing communication. The interpersonal relationship is the nurses' vehicle for care and needs to be characterized by respect, genuineness, individuation, and skill in uncovering and reviewing the elderly person's unique assets.

For the client profiled in this chapter, it was essential to foster decisional involvement because she wanted and expected it. On the other hand, nurses need to refrain from requiring decision making by persons who cannot cope with what they may interpret as added stress (Dennis, 1987). The aging client needs more time, consistent trusting support, and repeated explanations to facilitate control. Alternative decisions with potential consequences need to be reviewed with clients using careful deliberation.

Reed's (1983) work prompts nurses to think about combating a mechanistic developmental view of aging as decline and substituting a view of aging as transformation to a more specialized integrated complex human being. Life-span scientists pose a development theory that focuses on interaction between organismic and environmental factors. Throughout life, conflicts are encountered between the person and the environment, but new energy is obtained from each successful encounter (Reed, 1983).

Russell (1989) also counters views of aging as decline. Attention must be given to the richness of being old, that is, having a wealth of life's experiences that fosters wisdom and enhances inner (not outer) direction and autonomy. Results of analysis of work by life-span developmentalists disclose select themes of aging such as "self-acceptance, positive relationships with others, autonomy, environmental mastery, purpose in life and personal growth." The elderly person's personality does not shift from optimism to pessimism; however, poor health does threaten the elderly person's overall sense of well-being (Russell, 1989).

Powerlessness is not synonymous with aging. Membership in organizations such as the Grey Panthers and American Association for Retired Persons may provide specific empowerment for some elderly persons. Age gives a person assets with which to assess life positively (Russell, 1989). Elderly persons have a broad range of success in changing conflicts into meaningful life experiences and thus avoiding powerlessness and hopelessness. During illness, nurses can facilitate the elderly person's review of life successes.

REFERENCES

Aguilera, D. (1980). Stressors in late adulthood. *Family and Community Health, 2,* 61–69.

Angrosino, M. (1976). Anthropology and the aging: A preliminary community study. *Gerontologist, 16,* 174–180.

Atchley, R. (1981). Common misconceptions about aging. *Health Values: Achieving High Level Wellness, 5,* 7–10.

Bradley, R. (1976). Age-related differences in locus of control orientation in three-behavior domains. *Human Development, 19,* 49–55.

Brown, P. (1980). Religious needs of older persons. In J. Thorson & T. Cook (Eds.), *Spiritual well-being of the elderly* (pp. 76–82). Springfield, IL: Charles C Thomas.

Butler, R. (1975). *Why survive?* New York: Harper & Row.

Chang, B. (1978a). Generalized expectancy, situational perception and morale among the institutionalized aged. *Nursing Research, 27,* 316–323.

Chang, B. (1978b). Perceived situational control of daily activities: A new tool. *Research in Nursing and Health, 1,* 181–188.

Chang, B. (1980). Black and white elderly: Morale and perception of control. *Western Journal of Nursing Research, 2,* 371–387.

Christ, M. A., & Hohloch, F. (1988). *Gerontologic nursing.* Springhouse, PA: Springhouse.

Culbert, P., & Kos, B. (1971). Aging: Considerations for health teaching. *Nursing Clinics of North America, 6,* 605–614.

Dennis, K. (1987). Dimensions of client control. *Nursing Research, 36,* 151–156.

Eisdorfer, C., & Wildie, R. (1977). Stress, disease, aging and behavior. In J. E. Birren & J. W. Shaie (Eds.), *Handbook of the psychology of aging* (pp. 251–275). New York: Van Nostrand Reinhold.

Erikson, E. (1975). Eight ages of man. In F. Rebelsky (Ed.), *Life the continuous process, readings in human development* (pp. 23–38). New York: Alfred A. Knopf.

Fuller, S. (1978). Inhibiting helplessness in elderly people. *Journal of Gerontological Nursing, 4,* 18–22.

Hanes, C., & Wild, B. (1977). Locus of control and depression among noninstitutionalized elderly persons. *Psychological Reports, 41,* 581–582.

Haney, C. A., Stephens, R. C., Cooper, H. P., Oser, G. T., & Blau, Z. S. (1981). A measure of health status in an elderly population. *Health Values: Achieving High Level Wellness, 5,* 61–66.

Hayter, J. (1974). Biologic changes of aging. *Nursing Forum, 13,* 289–308.

Hill, R., Gallagher, D., Thompson, L., & Ishida, T. (1988). Hopelessness as a measure of suicidal intent in the depressed elderly. *Psychology and Aging, 3,* 230–232.

Hutchison, W., Carstensen, L., & Silberman, D. (1983). Generalized effects of increasing personal control of residents in a nursing facility. *International Journal of Behavioral Geriatrics, 1,* 21–32.

Johnson, D. (1967). Powerlessness: A significant determinant in patient behaviors. *Journal of Nursing Education, 6,* 40.

Kalish, R. (1975). *Late adulthood: Perspectives on human development.* Monterey, CA: Brooks/Cole.

Krause, N. (1987). Chronic strain, locus of control, and distress in older adults. *Psychology and Aging, 2,* 375–382.

Lancaster, J. (1981). Maximizing psychological adaptation in an aging population. *Topics in Clinical Nursing, 3,* 31–43.

Langer, E., & Benevento, A. (1978). Self-induced dependence. *Journal of Personality and Social Psychology, 36,* 886–893.

Langer, E., & Rodin, J. (1976). The effects of choice and enhanced personal responsibility for the aged: A field experiment in an institutionalized setting. *Journal of Personality and Social Psychology, 35,* 897–902.

Matteson, M. A., & McConnell, E. (1988). *Gerontological nursing: Concepts and practice.* Philadelphia: WB Saunders.

McCreary, W. (1980). Creative transformation and the theological resources for loneliness. In J. Thorson & T. Cook (Eds.), *Spiritual well-being of the elderly* (pp. 108–112). Springfield, IL: Charles C Thomas.

Moberg, D. (1980). Social indicators of spiritual well-being in the elderly. In J. Thorson & T. Cook (Eds.), *Spiritual well-being of the elderly* (pp. 20–37). Springfield, IL: Charles C Thomas.

Rathbone-McCuen, E., & Hashimi, J. (1982). *Isolated elders.* Rockville, MD: Aspen.

Reed, P. (1983). Implications of the life-span developmental framework for well-being in adulthood and aging. *Advances in Nursing Science, 6,* 18–25.

Reid, D., Haas, D., & Hawkings, D. (1977). Locus of desired control and positive self-concept of the elderly. *Journal of Gerontology, 32,* 441–450.

Robb, S. (1989). Resources in the environment of the aged. In A. Yuric, B. Spier, S. Robb, & N. Ebert (Eds.), *The aged person and the nursing process* (3rd ed.). Norwalk, CT: Appleton & Lange.

Robinson, F. (1981). Leisure well-being for longer living people. *Health Values: Achieving High Level Wellness, 5,* 55–60.

Rodin, J., & Langer, E. (1977). Long term effects of a control-relevant intervention with the institutionalized aged. *Journal of Personality and Social Psychology, 35,* 897–902.

Rodin, J., & Langer, E. (1980). Aging labels: The decline of control and the fall of self-esteem. *Journal of Social Issues, 36,* 12–29.

Rossman, I. (1988). Human aging changes. In I. M. Burnside (Ed.), *Nursing and the aged* (3rd ed.). New York: McGraw-Hill.

Rowland, K. (1977). Environmental events predicting death for the elderly. *Psychological Bulletin, 84,* 349–372.

Roy, C. (1976). *Introduction to nursing: An adaptation model.* Englewood Cliffs, NJ: Prentice-Hall.

Russell, C. (1989). *Good news about aging.* New York: John Wiley & Sons.

Ryden, M. (1985). Environmental support for autonomy in the institutionalized elderly. *Research in Nursing and Health, 8,* 363–371.

Rynerson, B. (1972). Need for self-esteem in the aged: A literature review. *Journal of Psychiatric Nursing, 10,* 22–25.

Schultz, R. (1976). Effects of control and predictability on the physical and psychological well-being of the institutionalized aged. *Journal of Personality and Social Psychology, 33,* 563–573.

Schultz, R., & Hanusa, B. (1978). Long-term effects of control and predictability-enhancing interventions: Findings and ethical issues. *Journal of Personality and Social Psychology, 36,* 1194–1201.

Seligman, M. (1975). *Helplessness: On depression, development and death.* San Francisco: WH Freeman.

Shore, H. (1976). Designing a training program for understanding sensory loss in aging. *Gerontologist, 16,* 157.

Teitelman, J. (1982). Eliminating learned helplessness in older rehabilitation patients. *Physical and Occupational Therapy in Geriatrics, 1,* 3–10.

Teitelman, J., & Priddy, J. (1988). From psychological theory to practice: Improving frail elders' quality of life through control-enhancing interventions. *The Journal of Applied Gerontology, 7,* 198–315.

Yurik, A. (1989). Sensory experiences of the elderly persons. In A. Yurik, B. Spier, S. Robb, & N. Ebert (Eds.), *The aged person and the nursing process* (3rd ed., pp. 438–461). Norwalk, CT: Appleton & Lange.

Ziegler, M., & Reid, D. (1979). Correlates of locus of desired control in two samples of elderly persons: Community residents and hospitalized patients. *Journal of Consulting and Clinical Psychology, 47,* 977–979.

PART III

Coping with Specific Chronic Health Problems

➤ Stressors and coping responses of persons to specific prototypical chronic health problems are identified in this part. Particular emphases are given to etiologies of powerlessness in persons with end-stage renal disease (Chap. 9); profiles of control and coping typologies in persons with peripheral vascular disease (Chap. 10); energy deficits, a prevalent diagnosis in persons with arthritis (Chap. 11); pathophysiology, coping, and nursing care of persons with multiple sclerosis (Chap. 12); chronic lung disease (Chap. 13); and persons with acquired immunodeficiency syndrome (AIDS) (Chap. 14). Detailed clinical examples are presented.

Hastings presents a model depicting holistic assessment, stressors, and coping resources as an overall framework for nursing care of persons with multiple sclerosis. Her research on hope, social support, and adaptation is presented in Chapter 12.

McMahon analyzes four dimensions of quality of life in persons with chronic lung disease: illness phenomena; client perceptions, functional capacity, and personal resources in Chapter 13. Detailed nursing strategies are presented. Complex challenges of managing persons with AIDS are reviewed in Chapter 14.

9

Powerlessness in Persons with End-Stage Renal Disease

➤ Susan Stapleton

Multiple stressors confront persons with end-stage renal disease (ESRD), also referred to in this chapter as chronic renal failure (CRF). Stressors can be categorized as physiological, psychological, role disturbance, and life change stressors. The purpose of this chapter is to present a review of these stressors, as well as to report observations of powerlessness in clients with CRF. Interventions to alleviate powerlessness are included.

STRESSORS IN END-STAGE RENAL DISEASE

Physiological Stressors

The toxic effects of uremia are manifested in virtually every body system. The pathophysiological effects can be categorized as (1) disturbances in body biochemistry (altered body water homeostasis; metabolic acidosis; and elevation of serum potassium, sodium, phosphorus, calcium, magnesium, creatinine, and uric acid) and (2) organ systems disturbances (hypertension, heart failure, anemia, gastrointestinal irritation, osteodystrophy, soft-tissue calcification, clotting deficiencies, altered endocrine function, and neuropathy) (Baldree, Murphy, & Powers, 1982; Czaczkes & DeNour, 1978; Harrington & Brenner, 1973; Lancaster, 1984; Stegman, Duncan, Pohren, & Sandstrom, 1985; Ulrich, 1989). Decreased energy, impaired concentration, insomnia, weight loss, and restricted use of the extremity with the fistula contribute to stress of persons on chronic dialysis (Wright, Sand, & Goodhue, 1966). Cummings (1970) reported that the mechanisms of attention and concentration are among the first cognitive skills affected by azotemia of ESRD, impairing higher intellectual functions (e.g., abstraction, generalization). Individuals lack control over the physical changes and the course of the illness and may not be able to predict or control how they will feel and function from day to day.

Psychological Stressors

Body Image

A psychological stressor related to the changes in appearance and function of the body is alteration in self-concept (specifically body image). Clients on dialysis come to perceive themselves as part of the machine, or endow the machine with human qualities (DeNour & Czaczkes, 1974). Abram (1969) related that clients incorporate the machines upon which they are dependent for life into their body images. Clients unconsciously think of themselves as not entirely human and therefore "freakish" (Abram, 1969). The individual may experience a temporary loss of body part of each dialysis in that blood is viewed flowing outside of the body and into the machine. This visual experience can contribute to a disturbance in body image.

Frustration in Basic Drives

A second type of psychological stressor is the frustration of basic drives, including aggression, satisfaction of hunger and thirst, and sexual expression. Halper (1971) discussed the limitations placed on normal outlets for aggression. Persons with ESRD cannot compete as successfully at work, and their capacity to participate in physical activities and athletics is limited.

Another basic drive that is frustrated in the person with ESRD is satisfaction of hunger and thirst. Eating is a satisfying and pleasurable experience, and therefore clients have difficulty complying with dietary and fluid restrictions (Anger, 1975).

The person with ESRD frequently experiences frustration of the basic sexual drive in that there is a marked deterioration in sexual interest and/or performance (O'Brien, 1983). Levy (1973) found that hemodialysis clients of both sexes, but particularly male clients as well as male transplant recipients, had substantial deterioration in sexual functioning. Levy, as well as Abram, Moore, and Westervelt (1975), found a further decrease in sexual performance in about 35 percent of the clients after the initiation of dialysis. Some degree of sexual dysfunction contributes to client and spouse depression and marital discord in most couples (Davison, 1986; Finkelstein, Finkelstein, & Steele, 1976; Shambaugh, Hampers, Bailey, Snyder, & Merrill, 1967). Marital discord was judged to be moderate or severe in 53 percent of the couples studied. Frustration of basic drives is beyond the individual's control and may be seen as contributing to powerlessness.

Fear of Death, Fear of Life

Beard (1969) labeled another psychological stressor "fear of death and fear of life." It is essential to keep in mind that the prolongation of life involves not only adding to the length of life but also the quality and worthwhileness of the life that is prolonged. Individuals with ESRD fear that their lives will be cut short, yet at the same time they fear that their lives may not be acceptable. In a study of life satisfaction of clients on dialysis, Jackle (1974) reported that these clients rated their present lives as slightly less satisfactory than did the normative group. They rated their past lives, however, near the top of the life satisfaction scale. There is also a strong fear that something will go wrong during dialysis—events such as hypovolemic shock, ruptured dialyzer, or separation of tubing connections. Individuals frequently feel that they are at the mercy of the machine and are powerless to control it. One client stated that the machine "maintains a powerful hold on my life—I find it impossible to make friends with the monster" (Abram, 1968). However, the contrast of dialysis or death is a powerful one (Plough, 1986).

Dependence-Independence Conflict

A dependence-independence conflict confronts the person with ESRD. The client is expected to comply with the treatment regimen, which requires dependent behavior; however, the client is also told to remain independent and live a "normal life," including meeting family, job, and social obligations. Reischman and Levy (1972) stated that the major feeling experienced by clients is one of helplessness. They feel trapped between the wish to be passive and dependent on the one hand and the expectation of health personnel that they be active and independent on the other. The degree of the dependence-independence conflict experienced is related to the individual's predialysis personality in that subjects who were dependent before dialysis had fewer dependence-independence conflicts after beginning dialysis; those subjects who were independent had greater dependence-independence conflicts after beginning dialysis (DeNour & Czaczkes, 1974; Reischman & Levy, 1972).

Role Disturbances

Role disturbances are closely related to both physiological and psychological stressors. Because of the illness, the client may be forced to eliminate social, family, and occupational roles that are important to self-concept. Loss of membership in groups and loss of job or occupation are stressors identified by persons with ESRD (Wright, Sand, & Goodhue, 1966). These losses result in feelings of isolation and disengagement. In a study of the family unit's response to dialysis, Maurin and Schenkel (1976) described a withdrawal of the entire family from social life into an existence focused on the family and, in some instances, focused only on the client.

Role reversal within the family is common (Anger, 1975). Three types of roles may be vulnerable in the person with ESRD: breadwinner, disciplinarian, and decision maker (Cumming, 1970). The individual may experience guilt over being unable to fulfill role expectations. This inability to perform expected role behaviors is a great threat to the individual's self-esteem (O'Brien, 1983; Ulrich, 1980) and may well contribute to powerlessness.

Lifestyle Changes

All the previously mentioned factors contribute to lifestyle changes in the individual with ESRD. Loss of financial security is a major stress (Anger, 1975; Cummings, 1970; Levy, 1973; Wright, Sand, & Goodhue, 1966). Loss of income due to loss of jobs with a decreased standard of living is a problem.

Uncertainty regarding future plans affects lifestyle. Uncertainty over the future was identified as a stressor by Baldree, Murphy, and Powers (1982) in a study of 35 persons on hemodialysis. Clients plan on a day-to-day basis, with future planning being related to transplantation. Clients describe being unable to plan for vacations, a new home, or their children's education because of the uncertainty related to illness (Wright, Sand, & Goodhue, 1966). The time required for the dialysis treatment interferes with other desirable life activities and roles. Uncertainty and ambivalence were two major problems for persons awaiting renal cadaveric transplants (Weems & Patterson, 1989).

Measurement of Hemodialysis Stressors

The Hemodialysis Stressor Scale (Baldree, Murphy, & Powers, 1982) is a 29-item instrument to measure incidence and severity of stressors associated with hemodialysis. The paper-and-pencil test has a five-point response format, with 0 = "not at all" and 4 = "a great deal," with a possible range of scores from 0 to 116. A higher score indicates more stress. The internal consistency alpha coefficient for the total score is .89, indicating good internal reliability. Factor analysis resulted in a three-factor solution with items characterized as psychobiological, psychosocial, and dependency-restriction stressors (Murphy, Powers, & Jalowiec, 1985). The instrument has been used in subsequent studies of persons on hemodialysis by Baker (1987); Bihl, Ferrans, and Powers (1988); Eichel (1986); and Gurklis and Menke (1988). Baker (1987) found that limitation in activity, itching, fluid restriction, and muscle cramps were the most frequently identified stressors in 81 persons with ESRD. A negative relationship existed between stress and hope and between stress and self-esteem in Baker's sample. That is, the greater the patient's stress, the lower the hope and the self-esteem. Stressors reported by both hemodialysis and continuous ambulatory peritoneal dialysis (CAPD) clients included fatigue, limitation in physical activity, muscle cramps, change in body appearance, itching, and problems with work role (Eichel, 1986). The most frequent stressors reported by hemodialysis clients in decreasing order were fluid restriction, muscle cramps, fatigue, and uncertainty over the future (a stressor not identified by the CAPD subjects) (Baldree, Murphy, & Powers, 1982).

Gurklis and Menke (1988) found that physiological stressors were more troublesome than the psychosocial stressors in the 68 hemodialysis clients studied. These clients used problem-oriented coping strategies more often than affective strategies to deal with stress. Coping methods used by the 35 persons in the Baldree et al. (1982) study included *maintaining some control,* hope, prayer, trust in God, and looking at the problem objectively. Similar coping strategies were found in the Eichel (1986) study of persons on CAPD.

Summary of Stressors

Table 9.1 summarizes stressors of ESRD. It is evident that illness and its management have widespread effects on the individual's life. Many of these stressors may contribute to a feeling of powerlessness. Learned helplessness and powerlessness were identified as nursing diagnoses in persons on hemodialysis (Burns, 1983; Frank, 1988; Fuchs, 1987; O'Brien, 1983). Frank (1988) reviewed the use of Roy's (1989) adaptation model for nursing care of the hemodialysis client. Nursing diagnoses generated for the interdependence adaptive mode included powerlessness.

With increasing years on dialysis, persons reported better adjustment. As the number of hours spent on dialysis increased, client hardiness decreased (Goodwin, 1988). The feeling of diminishing control seemed to affect the state of hardiness and resilience to life's stress. In a

Table 9.1 ➤ **SUMMARY OF STRESSORS IN END-STAGE RENAL DISEASE**

Physiological	Psychological	Role Disturbances	Lifestyle Changes
Body biochemistry changes	Alterations in body image:	Loss of group membership	Loss of financial security
Effects of uremia on organ systems	Inability to control body functioning	Loss of job or occupation	Forced acceptance of government assistance
Lack of control over symptoms	Body does not function normally	Role reversal with spouse	Time required for dialysis
Progression of illness trajectory	Incorporation of dialysis machine into body image	Decreased ability to fulfill role expectations	Limitation of activity
	Loss of body part, blood, kidneys	Marital discord and family tension	Failure of future plans
	Change in body structure—shunt or fistula		Uncertainty
	Frustration of basic drives:		
	Inability to express aggression		
	Dietary and fluid restrictions		
	Decreased sexual drive and/or performance		
	Fear of death and fear of life:		
	Uncertain life expectancy		
	Fear of death due to illness		
	Fear of death due to malfunction of dialysis machine		
	Decreased life satisfaction		
	Fear that life will not be acceptable		
	Dependence-independence conflict:		
	Expected compliance with treatment regimen		
	Dependence on others and machine for satisfaction of needs		
	Subconscious desire for dependence		
	Societal expectations for independence		

meta-analysis of 40 studies of persons with ESRD, personality factors were the strongest predictors of adjustment. Internal control was positively related to adjustment (Olsen, 1983).

CLINICAL DATA

Six clients with ESRD on hemodialysis were studied using a participant-observer method for a period varying from 3 to 6 months. Factors causing powerlessness and the clients' responses were identified. General indicators of powerlessness manifested in the clients were lack of information seeking, failure to share relevant health information, decreased willingness to make decisions, expression of loss of hope, crying and depression, and verbal expression of loss of control.

Specific factors that contributed to the powerlessness state in these clients were the disease process, hospitalization, relationship with health-care personnel, the dialysis procedure and medical regimen, changes in family relationships, and employment and financial concerns. Each factor contributing to powerlessness and examples of client responses are included in the following discussion.

Disease Process of Chronic Renal Failure

The disease process itself is a factor over which the individual feels little control. The symptoms of CRF are quite uncomfortable and have a marked impact on the individual's lifestyle. Fatigue and weakness are very disturbing symptoms and curtail the individual's activities a great deal. Comments such as "I'm always so tired—I can never get anything done" and "I'll never get this house painted if I can only do this much without getting exhausted" indicate how incapacitating the fatigue can be. The unpredictability of the energy level also contributes to feelings of powerlessness. Mrs. F. described this: "Maybe the next day you'll have a good day and be able to get something done, and maybe not. You never know." This unpredictability makes it difficult for the individual to make plans for activities and may greatly decrease social life. Mrs. M. stated, "After a while you just stop associating with other people. You lose a lot of friends. You just don't have the energy." Although the individual may desire to participate in certain activities, the physiological status prevents the client from doing so.

Other central nervous system manifestations of CRF include decreased alertness, memory loss, and impaired thought processes. Mrs. M. described the frustrations of these symptoms. "People think you're crazy or something is wrong with you mentally. You feel so dull, aren't interested in others, and can't carry on a conversation. You forget what you wanted to say."

The general downward course of the illness causes many individuals with CRF to feel powerless. Mrs. F. stated, "It's like dying slowly when you're on dialysis. Every day you know that you're going downhill, but what can you do?" Mr. O. described himself as "feeling like I'm in a car going downhill and the brakes don't work."

Even when a client has a kidney transplant, the inability to control or predict the outcome of the transplant is a real cause of feelings of powerlessness in the postoperative transplant client. This is often expressed verbally with statements such as "It's really hard not knowing what's going to happen" and "I wish I could do something to be sure the kidney keeps working." The realization that the outcome of the surgery is out of one's control may cause severe depression. Mrs. B. cried, "It's not fair! I did everything just the way I was supposed to and I still rejected the kidney." Most clients finally resign themselves to this and make comments such as, "I guess you have to get used to the idea that you really don't have much control over what happens with the transplant."

Severe pain, which may occur postoperatively as a result of the surgery or complications, may cause feelings of powerlessness. Anxiety, depression, and prolonged pain often decrease the individual's ability to control the response to pain. Mr. F. experienced severe bladder spasms postoperatively and stated, "They come so suddenly that I don't have time to get ready for them. It's all I can do to keep from screaming." When the cause of the pain is unknown, the feelings of powerlessness are even more acute.

Hospitalization

Hospitalization automatically results in a tremendous loss of control for an individual. Decisions such as when to eat, sleep, exercise, and bathe are made for the client, sometimes with little consultation. As a result of client role expectations, individuals who are hospitalized may demonstrate passive behavior, follow staff directions without comment or question, and have difficulty making small decisions when given the opportunity to do so. These behaviors are all indicative of a feeling of loss of control, or powerlessness. Even individuals who have previously managed their medical regimens alone without difficulty suddenly have them managed by others. Nurses administer medications, which the client may take without knowing or asking what they are. The dietitian calculates the client's diet, and other staff members weigh the client and record intake and output.

One aspect of this management by others that contributed to feelings of powerlessness in Mrs. M. was her dependence on the nurses for pain medication. She often had to wait longer than she felt was necessary, and she expressed the feeling that the staff was "taking advantage of me because I'm so helpless." This feeling was strengthened when Mrs. M. was told by a nurse, "Your imagination can make you think that you're having pain."

Frequently, hospital routines and efficiency are given higher priority than client needs, resulting in client feelings of powerlessness. A nurse on the renal transplant unit told Mr. F., "You'll have to eat breakfast and wash up later. Radiation therapy is ready to do your treatment now." Mr. F. started to protest, "But I'm hungry . . .," then shrugged his shoulders and walked over to the wheelchair. When Mrs. Z. was told that she had to move to a different room because her private room was needed for another client, she said, "I'm low man on the totem pole, so I don't have anything to say about whether or not I move." She was told to hurry her packing so the room could be cleaned, and then she sat in the lounge for 6 hours because no one was available to clean rooms. Mrs. Z. merely accepted this passively and said, "I'm being evicted."

Because of a malfunctioning machine, Mr. F. experienced a long wait in the x-ray department while he was in severe pain. He was not told the cause for the delay, and he worried, "Waiting this long makes you worry that they've forgotten you and you'll end up sitting here all day before someone notices you." Although he made this statement to the author upon her arrival in the department, he had not attempted to ask any x-ray personnel the reason for the delay or to remind them of his presence.

Hospitalized clients, as well as those on dialysis, often exhibit behaviors indicative of powerlessness that can affect their ability to learn. Individuals who feel powerless often demonstrate a marked failure to seek information about their health status. They seem to think that any action they might take based on such information will not influence what happens to them, and therefore the information seems useless. Although Mr. O. had kept careful records of his weight and blood pressure before starting dialysis, he never asked what they were before or after dialysis runs. The staff contributed to this by failing to volunteer this information to him. At times, hospitalized individuals do not ask questions of health-care professionals, even though they do not understand something about the management of their illness.

In addition to lack of information seeking, the individual who feels powerless often displays a lack of information sharing. When Mrs. M. was reprimanded because she had gained too much weight between dialysis runs and was told to weigh herself at home daily, she did not inform the nurse that she had no scale. Miss L. allowed the medical staff to proceed with the scheduling of pretransplant tests without telling them that she had serious reservations about having a transplant. When the physician and social worker informed Mr. O. that he was to be transferred to another dialysis center, he was quite unhappy, but he did not discuss this with them or tell them that going to the proposed center would present difficult travel problems for him. When the author asked him why he had not discussed this with the physician, Mr. O. responded, "It wouldn't do any good. If they want me to go there, then I'll have to go."

Client-Staff Relationships

Interactions with the staff and routines of the hospital or dialysis unit play a large role in causing powerlessness. One client expressed frustration and a feeling of lack of control over the scheduling of appointments in the outpatient department: "They just tell me when to come in, and since the doctors are only here on certain days, it doesn't matter whether the day is convenient for me." The client's options are limited, because survival depends on compliance with the health-care system demands.

The fact that the health-care personnel have more knowledge than the client about CRF and its management can contribute to feelings of powerlessness in the client. Clients feel that they must depend on the personnel to tell them what to do. A dialysis client with diabetes stated, "I just do what they tell me. I don't even try to adjust my insulin dose the way I used to."

Just before the institution of dialysis, Mr. O. expressed anxiety about the level of competence of the dialysis staff. He stated, "But I guess I'll just have to trust them since I don't know enough to tell if they're competent or not. And I can't request only the good ones anyway."

This feeling that the staff is in control may make the individual reluctant to express anger. Mr. F. reported, "You have to be nice to them—can't get along without them." After three unsuccessful attempts had been made to insert a needle for dialysis, Mr. O. said angrily, "This is your last chance." Then he said, "Oh, I guess I can't say that, can I? I have to have this." Even when the individual attempts to express anger, the staff may not acknowledge it, thus subtly telling the client that this expression is not appropriate.

Health-care personnel may increase the individual's feelings of powerlessness by comments that accentuate the control they have over the client. A dietitian teased Mr. F as she helped him fill out his menu, "You're lucky you have that kidney, or I'd never let you order those tomatoes."

Dialysis Procedure

The individual often feels controlled not only by the dialysis and hospital staff, but by the dialysis machine, too. People on dialysis commonly refer to the machine as "the monster" or "that thing." One client stated, "It's scary to think of being attached to that thing—to be at its mercy." He joked about needing a screwdriver "to take the machine apart if I want to, so I can stay in control." His wife gave him a tiny screwdriver, which he wore on a chain around his neck, and he often brought it out when the alarm sounded on the dialysis machine.

The immobility imposed by dialysis contributes to a loss of control by preventing individuals from meeting some of their own needs for several hours. They must ask to have their food cut up, their beds lowered, or a blanket put over them. Mr. O. expressed frustration when trying to eat or hold a book while on dialysis. "You're so doggone helpless when you're hooked up to that thing!"

Once dialysis is begun, the individual has little power to stop it. Mrs. M. cried before and during dialysis, "I don't want to do this. I want to leave." Individuals sometimes experience uncomfortable symptoms during dialysis, such as leg cramps, weakness, and nausea. But no matter how uncomfortable or inconvenient dialysis is, if an individual wants to live, then he or she is dependent upon a machine. Most clients on dialysis are acutely aware of this dependency. As Mrs. A. stated, "You can't get very far from a dialysis machine or stay for very long. It's like there's a chain tying you to that machine." Mr. O. said resignedly, "I guess I'll just have to get used to this (dialysis). I really have no choice." The feeling of having no choice about the institution of dialysis is a common one, and individuals often express the feeling that "things are moving too fast." This is particularly true if the individual was too ill to participate in the decision to start dialysis.

Medical Regimen

Aspects of the medical regimen other than dialysis may also contribute to the individual's feelings of powerlessness. Although following the regimen may provide some feeling of power by helping with symptom control, there is still the knowledge that the regimen is necessary for life. Most individuals seem to feel that they have no choice as to whether or not they will follow the regimen.

Dietary management, in particular, poses many difficulties, and feelings of dissatisfaction are often expressed. Mrs. F. cried, "They say I can live a normal life, but I can't. I won't be able to eat or drink what I want and join in the fun." Mrs. Z. reported, "We've stopped eating out completely, and we really miss it. But it was just too hard to stick to my diet." The desire to eat or drink favorite foods and beverages is sometimes overwhelming. Mrs. S. repeatedly exceeded her fluid limitation in spite of severe discomfort from fluid overload. She expressed the feeling that she was unable to control her fluid intake. "I try not to drink too much—I swell up so bad—but it's really hard. I'm thirsty all the time."

Family Relationships

In addition to factors directly related to the illness and its treatment, the individual with CRF often experiences changes in family relationships that contribute to feelings of powerlessness. Role reversal commonly occurs, with the spouse and children taking on many of the individual's previous role tasks. At the same time, the client takes on a more dependent role in the family.

The individual often expresses guilt at being unable to fulfill previous role obligations. As Mrs. O. reported, "I can't pull my share of the weight at home." Dependency on one's children seems to produce particularly strong feelings. Mrs. Z. said, "My daughter had to wash my hair when I had the shunt. Isn't that a terrible thing to put that job on a 12-year-old for a whole year? But I had no choice." Many of these individuals express the fear that they have become, or will become, a "burden" to their families.

In spite of the guilt, however, the individual usually recognizes the need for dependence on others. Mrs. S. said, "You can't complain. After all, you're lucky to have someone to help you." This comment was made after Mrs. S. had expressed frustration that her housework was not being done as well as she would like.

The central nervous system manifestations of CRF produce irritability and mood changes that can also influence family relationships. Mr. O. reported, "I get so depressed and irritable. It bothers me a lot, but I can't control it."

The individual's symptoms and treatment regimen also frequently prevent participation in enjoyable family activities. Camping and hiking with his family had been an important part of Mr. O.'s life, and he became very depressed when he was unable to continue these activities. Mrs. S. cried over her inability to join in physical activities previously enjoyed with her daughters. "I used to skate and swim with my daughters, but now I'm a real dud. All I can do is sit. I told them, 'If I can't keep up, please understand.'" Mr. O. regretted having missed some of the family activities on vacation because of dialysis. "I was stuck with that machine while they were out sightseeing. Then after I'd finished, they'd already seen everything and didn't want to go back."

The incidence of impotence in men and decreased libido in both men and women with CRF interferes with sexual intimacy and provokes marital strain.

All of these examples indicate that the individual with CRF has less control over family relationships and activities than before the illness. Because of the value most individuals place on family relationships, this is an important factor contributing to an overall sense of powerlessness.

Employment and Financial Concerns

The individual with CRF may experience changes in work role and resulting financial concerns, which contribute to feelings of powerlessness. Time is often lost from work because of physician's appointments and dialysis. Mr. O. expressed fear that his employer would eventually tire of these absences. "They're agreeable now, but I don't know how much longer they'll put up with me missing so much work." This fear, combined with a feeling that his job performance had decreased, caused much anxiety about his job security. He stated, "I'm losing my creativity. I feel thick-headed. I forget things all the time." Although he was unhappy with his job, he also feared losing it. He lamented, "I'm stuck here. I could never get another job with my kidney disease and my age. I'm lucky to have this one, but sometimes I feel like I'm trapped." One indication of Mr. O's feelings of powerlessness is his failure to make an effort to plan for the institution of dialysis with his employer, even though this scheduling was a great source of anxiety to him.

Mr. F. expressed frustration that he was no longer able to work and "support my family the way I'm supposed to." When his wife went to the welfare department to apply for assistance and was treated rudely, Mr. F. expressed extreme anger at his lack of control. "I'm stuck here (in the hospital) and can't do a damn thing about it! I'd like to go down there and just start punching." Job loss, or fear of job loss, and extraordinary expenses are significant factors contributing to feelings of powerlessness in individuals with CRF. The factors causing powerlessness in patients with CRF are summarized in Table 9.2.

INTERVENTIONS

Nursing interventions to enhance control in persons with CRF on dialysis may include modifying the environment, setting realistic goals, increasing client and family knowledge, enhancing the health team's sensitivity to potential causes of powerlessness, and facilitating verbalization of feelings.

Modifying the Environment

Modifying the environment may include, for example, supporting the client's control of interruptions during rest periods at home by having him or her post a sign on the house door indicating when visitors could be received. A note pad for messages could also be attached. Other control measures that need to be addressed to enhance the comfort of the psychological environment relate to clients' feelings of deference and inferiority within the health-care system and communicating with

Table 9.2 ➤	FACTORS CAUSING POWERLESSNESS IN END-STAGE RENAL DISEASE

Factor Category	Example of Specific Causes
Disease process	Uncertainty over relief of symptoms. Fatigue, mental changes. Multiple body systems involved. Decreased sexual functioning.
Hospitalization	Basic decisions are made for the client, that is, when to perform ADLs. Routines imposed on the client without negotiation—timing of medications and treatments. Loss of control over privacy.
Client-staff relationships	Client acknowledges staff has more control than she does so fears expressing anger in order to avoid being shunned by the staff. Staff knows more about the client's pathology. Clients not introduced to staff and other clients who occupy the same room. Verbalizations by staff that they are making the decisions regarding room assignments, fluid restriction, and so forth. Client not informed about progress, weight, or laboratory values.
Dialysis procedure	Venipunctures are painful, unavoidable. Unpleasant side effects after dialysis may prevent functioning (headaches, dizziness). During procedure, client is immobilized. Client is dependent on others for all needs during dialysis.
Medical regimen	Lack of client involvement and tailoring the regimen to client's needs beyond the pathology (scheduling dialysis procedure during work time).
Family relationships	Role reversal. Spouse assuming breadwinner and/or household-manager roles. Increased dependence on family for needs. Lack of full participation with family during special events.
Employment and financial concerns	Client may miss work because of symptoms and/or treatment. Client feels loss of job security due to illness. Job performance may be decreased or job may be lost. Perceived inability to support family.

physicians. Nurses can reinforce with clients the idea that their needs are the first priority of the health team. Specific interventions include reviewing with the client specific medical concerns before the physician visit, helping clients to prepare for getting the most out of the physician-client contact by formulating questions and writing them down, and reassuring the client of the health team's commitment to meeting his or her needs.

Setting Realistic Goals

Individuals who can set realistic goals feel less powerless as the goals are achieved. Chronically ill individuals often need assistance in setting realistic goals and in rehearsing possible outcomes. Depression and feelings of hopelessness may inhibit clients from setting goals at all. Lack of information about illness or use of denial as a coping mechanism may lead clients to set goals they are unable to achieve. Never achieving goals reinforces powerlessness.

Clients should be given the opportunity to participate in their total plan of care by mutually identifying goals with the nurse, validating assessment of self-care skills, and confirming with the nurse that they do have unique strengths that empower them to assume responsibility to achieve desired outcomes. Nurse-client collaborative decisions increase perceived control (Fuchs, 1987).

Laborde and Powers (1980) compared 20 clients with osteoarthritis and 20 clients undergoing hemodialysis on their ratings of past, present, and future life satisfaction using the Cantril Self-Anchoring Life Satisfaction Scale. No differences were found on past and future ratings; however, the clients on dialysis had significantly higher present life satisfaction scores (at the .05 level). Considering the extensive body-system involvement with multiple symptoms in CRF, this finding is surprising. The dialysis procedure provides a predictable outcome of temporary alleviation of symptoms. Clients on dialysis may have been helped to set realistic expectations of dialysis as an extension of life and a provider of temporary relief of symptoms. For some clients on dialysis, the relief of symptoms gave them a "new lease on life" compared with predialysis states. The pain experienced by clients with arthritis so interfered with present quality of life that their scores were significantly lower than those of the clients on dialysis. Nurses can use specific verbal reinforcers with the client on dialysis to decrease powerlessness, such as "the dialysis will control symptoms by restoring fluid and electrolyte balance and eliminate wastes." Careful explanation of the desired therapeutic effects of the medical regimen, which helps the client have realistic expectations from the treatment, will enhance control.

The following is an example of helping the individual develop pacing behaviors to cope with the fatigue of CRF. Mrs. A. expressed feelings of powerlessness from fatigue that interfered with her ability to do her housework. She was asked to keep a list of her activities and her required rest periods for 1 week. At the same time, Mrs. A. made a list of the things she wanted to do in order of their importance to her. Using these lists, Mrs. A. was assisted in evaluating her tolerance of specific activities and planning her activities according to her energy level. For example, she discovered that she could perform only one major task each day, such as grocery shopping or vacuuming. She planned her weekly schedule so that these especially tiring tasks were done, one each day, on the days after dialysis, when her energy level was highest. This was a more realistic goal than trying to do several major tasks in one day, and Mrs. A.'s feeling of powerlessness decreased when she was able to reach this goal. At the same time, Mr. A. suggested that his wife plan her arrival from the grocery store to coincide with his arrival home from work so that he could carry the bags of groceries into the house. This decreased her energy expenditure so that she was still able to participate in family activities that evening. The list of activities according to priority also enabled her to determine which activities she could delegate to other family members, or eliminate completely, without damaging her self-esteem. A goal for increasing physical activity may be appropriate. Improving physical fitness through regular exercise programs has helped increase energy levels and self-satisfaction in persons with ESRD (Jagusch & Butchart, 1989; Snyder, 1989).

Increasing Knowledge

Knowledge is a power resource. Control in a given situation increases with increasing knowledge about the situation. When individuals experience powerlessness, they may subsequently fail to seek information about their situations, further increasing feelings of powerlessness. Chronically ill individuals need knowledge about their illness and its management so that they can make decisions and take actions relative to the illness. This ability to make decisions and act on them gives individuals some control over what happens to them, thereby decreasing powerlessness. Being informed of physiological changes, positive responses to therapy, and expected results from therapy increases the perception of control. Nurses need to assume major responsibility for increasing clients' knowledge.

Devins' (1989) study confirmed that higher levels of ESRD-relevant information are significantly associated with increased levels of perceived control over nonillness aspects of life. He also recommended forewarning clients about impending changes in treatment to control powerlessness and decrease uncertainty. Knowledge about selected coping strategies such as relaxation and guided imagery is another type of information to be given (Horsburgh & Robinson, 1989).

Increasing the Sensitivity of Health Teams and Significant Others to Imposed Powerlessness

Factors within the health-care system itself are often the most significant causes of powerlessness in the chronically ill. These include unexplained delays and waiting in various hospital departments (e.g., x-ray) and brisk, insensitive verbal interaction by admitting clerks, out-patient receptionists, or home health aides. The sterile environment of a hospital with clearly identified boundaries promotes powerlessness (e.g., the nurses' station is off limits for clients; clients cannot review their records without obtaining special permissions as established by hospital policy). Health-care professionals need to develop sensitivity to these and other causes of powerlessness. Efforts need to be made to be humanistic and to avoid depersonalizing clients.

Health-care workers may need to review principles of therapeutic communication in addition to simply remembering to introduce themselves to the client. Personnel need to wear name tags on which their titles are clearly indicated. Acute-care nurses often describe persons with ESRD as presenting difficult care challenges, creating a tendency in some nurses to avoid these clients (Wolfsen, 1989).

For clients to monitor physiological progress, having access to the dialysis record on which weight, vital signs, and laboratory values are recorded is important. Some clients achieve control by keeping detailed records and graphs of blood chemistry values. By noting a controlled creatinine level and having a visual representation of the creatinine level over time on a graph, the client realizes that no physiological deterioration is occurring. This is a positive feedback mechanism for the client to continue to engage in the present therapeutic plan as well as a sign of physiological control. Teaching the client the significance of the laboratory values must be included in this control strategy.

Increasing the sensitivity of persons at home, at work, and in social settings is important to decreasing powerlessness in the client. Dimond (1979) found a positive correlation between the hemodialysis client's morale and the presence of social support (family environment, spouse support, and the presence of a confidant). A negative correlation was found between the family cohesion (one aspect of family environment), presence of a confidant, and the amount of change in social functioning in adjusting to the chronic illness. Social changes since beginning dialysis were fewer if the client had family cohesiveness and a confidant available. The nurse can work with families to help them realize how significantly they can influence adaptation and control in their ill family member. The greater the family cohesiveness and open expression, the higher the client's morale and the fewer medical problems occurred. Nurses can help families improve communication, increase expressions and types of support, and demonstrate caring and affection. Nurses can also devise specific mechanisms the family can use to increase the client's perceived and/or actual control. Decisions can be referred to the client; the family can encourage the client's resumption of family maintenance tasks, such as paying the bills. The task of planning for maximal use of leisure time and family togetherness activities can be assumed by the ill family member (in this case the client on dialysis).

Social support has been identified as a resource for chronically ill clients and contributes to psychological well-being in persons with ESRD (Christensen, Turner, Slaughter, & Holman, 1989; Dimond, 1979; Muthny, 1984; Siegal, Calsyn, & Cuddihee, 1987). Reviewing with family members the important sustaining role they play may help them enhance client well-being and control.

Verbalization of Feelings

When the chronically ill individual is able to verbalize feelings of powerlessness, a basis for beginning problem solving to increase feelings of control is established. The client may be able to identify factors contributing to the present state and pose alternative solutions. Through discussion, feedback is solicited from the nurse. The verbalization is a sharing of feelings and provides the nurse with an opportunity to demonstrate understanding.

When powerlessness is caused by deteriorating health that cannot be controlled, discussion of these feelings enables the nurse to share them, lessening the client's burden. When clients hear their feelings verbalized, the distortion that occurs through mental rumination about the situation is controlled—feelings and concerns are brought into perspective. Reactions from others and empathy are solicited and alternative solutions to problems are generated as a result of verbalization.

DEVELOPING A PLAN TO DECREASE POWERLESSNESS

In using these strategies to decrease powerlessness in the chronically ill individual, the nurse must carefully develop strategies specific to each individual. The first steps are to recognize client indicators of powerlessness and to identify the factor(s) causing powerlessness. Specific strategies can then be developed to decrease powerlessness. Criteria for evaluation of the strategies are specific client behaviors that can be expected to occur if the strategies are to be effective.

The care plan in Table 9.3 contains examples of strategies used in working with individuals with CRF who were experiencing powerlessness. Some dealt with situations that occurred once; others dealt with broader, recurring factors that caused powerlessness. The stressors or factors causing powerlessness in CRF clients provide the basis for the plan. The types of factors promoting powerlessness included in the care plan are client-staff relationships, disease process, family relationships, and employment. Although the strategies on the care plan are specific to the client's situation or specific precipitant of powerlessness, the types of strategies used can be classified as (1) modifying the environment, (2) helping the client set realistic goals, (3) increasing the client's

(text continues on page 243)

Table 9.3 ➤ PLAN OF CARE TO ALLEVIATE POWERLESSNESS IN CLIENTS WITH CHRONIC RENAL FAILURE

Situation or Factor Causing Powerlessness	Client Indicators of Powerlessness	Strategies to Decrease Powerlessness	Criteria for Evaluation
		CLIENT-STAFF RELATIONSHIPS	
Appointments in outpatient department: a. Long waits before seeing physician b. Difficulty in obtaining desired information from physician	1. Verbalizes the feeling that client cannot control when client sees physician and that client's time is not seen as important 2. States, "The doctor never tells me anything, I can't get him to answer my questions."	1. Meet client in clinic waiting room before each appointment. 2. Help client to formulate a list of specific questions for the physician for that visit. 3. If necessary, see physician with the client to assist client in asking questions. 4. Suggest that client take the list of questions out of pocket and refer to it while talking with the physician.	1. States that the time in waiting room is spent productively 2. Appears calm while waiting: no pacing, tapping fingers, picking at nails 3. Makes list of questions and uses list while talking with physician 4. Verbalizes satisfaction with the amount of information received from the physician about illness and treatment
Enforced dependence during dialysis and dependence on dialysis staff and machine for life. Health-care personnel have a much greater knowledge about CRF and its management than client. Staff expression of anger toward the client; client unable to show anger in return.	1. Expresses fear that some dialysis staff members are less competent than others and that client cannot judge them 2. Jokes that client wants a screwdriver "so I can take the machine apart if I want to and stay in control" 3. Expresses the feeling that client is at the "mercy" of the dialysis machine and staff 4. Refers to dialysis machine as "the monster" 5. States that client cannot get	1. Provide organized, individualized teaching program that includes the following content: normal kidney function, basic CRF pathophysiology, laboratory values and their significance, purpose of dialysis, dialysis procedure, diet, medications. 2. Explain and demonstrate alarm system on machines. 3. Arrange for client to meet some of the other clients to discuss dialysis from client's point of view. 4. Arrange for clients to observe the start and ending of dialysis on	1. Correctly explains dialysis to someone else in simple terms 2. Remains calm when alarm on machine goes off 3. Demonstrates confidence in dialysis staff 4. Asks questions when client does not know something about CEF and its management 5. States present weight and range of blood pressure

Table 9.3 ➤ PLAN OF CARE TO ALLEVIATE POWERLESSNESS IN CLIENTS WITH CHRONIC RENAL FAILURE (*Continued*)

Situation or Factor Causing Powerlessness	Client Indicators of Powerlessness	Strategies to Decrease Powerlessness	Criteria for Evaluation
	CLIENT-STAFF RELATIONSHIPS		
	angry at the staff because "I can't get along without them"	another patient (movie or in person) before beginning dialysis.	6. Asks for weight, blood pressure, and lab values
		5. As dialysis is started, explain each step and reinforce prior teaching. Continue to provide opportunities for questions as they occur to patient and family.	7. Assists with some aspects of dialysis
		6. Use primary nursing or assign client to the same one or two people for the first few weeks.	8. Freely expresses anger toward staff when appropriate and in an appropriate way
		7. Give client a screwdriver on the day dialysis starts.	
		8. Keep client informed of progress during dialysis—weight, lab values, blood pressure—and explain their significance.	
		9. Encourage client participation in dialysis as client is ready—holding tubings, applying pressure to puncture sites, taking pulse.	
		10. Give client as much responsibility as patient is ready for—bringing any medications to be taken while on dialysis, arranging own transportation (including driving self), explaining dialysis to own family or new clients.	
		11. Encourage client to keep own record of blood pressure and predialysis and postdialysis weight.	

12. Encourage verbalization of feelings about dialysis machine and staff and client's dependence on them.
13. Allow for joking or expression of anger during dialysis as a means of maintaining some control.
14. Avoid ignoring client's expressions of anger or responding with anger in return. Use accepting manner.
15. Avoid comments by staff, even joking ones, that emphasize the control staff has over client during dialysis.

1. Assist client in weighing the pros and cons of each center.
2. Serve as a liaison in planning a visit to the other center to meet the staff and discuss routines.
3. Support the client in decision to agree or disagree with the physician's decision.
4. Serve as client advocate, if needed, in explaining client's decision to physician.

1. States the advantages and disadvantages of each center for client
2. Visits the other dialysis center and asks questions there to obtain the information needed to make a decision about the two centers
3. Questions the physician as to the rationale for switching to the other center
4. Determines, on the basis of all the previous information, which dialysis center is better for client
5. Discusses the decision with the physician, explaining the reasons for choice

1. Verbalizes feelings of not having control over where client will go for dialysis
2. Does not tell physician that the planned dialysis center is very inconvenient for client

Physician tells client that client will be transferred to a different dialysis center without asking client's approval.

Table 9.3 ➤ PLAN OF CARE TO ALLEVIATE POWERLESSNESS IN CLIENTS WITH CHRONIC RENAL FAILURE (*Continued*)

Situation or Factor Causing Powerlessness	Client Indicators of Powerlessness	Strategies to Decrease Powerlessness	Criteria for Evaluation
		CLIENT-STAFF RELATIONSHIPS	
Client is severely reprimanded because client gained too much weight between dialysis runs.	1. Accepts reprimand and anger from staff without comment—hangs head and looks at floor 2. Later remarks that "they're always yelling at me, but I can't afford to yell back" 3. When told to weigh self daily at home, did not inform staff that client has no scale 4. States, "I try to follow my diet and not drink too much, but I'm always so thirsty. I just can't help myself"	1. State amount of weight gain in a matter-of-fact, nonscolding manner. 2. Explore with client possible reasons for excess weight gain. 3. Ask client to keep a list of everything eaten and drunk for 1 wk—including time of day, amounts, what client was doing at the time, and how client felt at the time. 4. Explore with client the meaning of food and drink to client. 5. Assist client to identify own eating and drinking patterns. 6. Teach basic pathophysiology of CRF and the physiological effects of excess fluid retention if client does not already know this. 7. Suggest that client weigh self daily at home, keep record of weights and bring this to dialysis. Help client get scale. 8. Assist client to correlate weight changes with food and fluid intake. 9. Assist client to identify how client feels when client has excess fluid retention.	1. Explains, in simple terms, basic CRF pathophysiology and the effects of fluid retention on the body 2. Identifies various reasons for eating and drinking patterns: hunger, thirst, tension, boredom 3. Verbalizes what food and drink mean to self and own feelings about food and fluid restrictions 4. Keeps record of daily weights and brings to dialysis 5. Correlates changes in weight with food and fluid intake 6. Identifies how it feels to have excess fluid retention 7. Actively participates in development of a diet pattern 8. Reports that new diet pattern is more acceptable and there is more success in complying with it

9. Practices, on a regular basis, some type of relaxation technique

10. Work with client, dietitian, and physician to develop diet pattern that is most acceptable to client, considering previous patterns, and meets the criteria of the medical treatment plan.

11. If client eats or drinks in response to stimuli other than hunger or thirst (e.g., tension or boredom), teach other methods of coping with these feelings (e.g., relaxation techniques, self-hypnosis, physical activities).

DISEASE PROCESS

1. Looks at shunt
2. Asks questions when some aspect of the care of the shunt is unknown
3. Correctly describes actions to be taken if shunt comes apart and teaches this to significant other
5. Reports ability to cope with stares and questions of others about the shunt

Client expected to take care of her AV shunt before feeling ready.

1. Cries and states, "I don't want to do this" while shunt care is done, but does not refuse to do it if staff insists
2. Asks no questions about shunt

1. Assess client's stage in the grieving process and in adaptation to an altered body image.
2. Explore with client the meaning of the shunt to self.
3. Observe for verbal and behavioral clues that client is ready to learn shunt care—looking at shunt, asking questions, watching while care is done.
4. Follow this sequence to develop self-care: Explain care as done, client assists with care, client describes procedure verbally, client performs care with help, client performs care with observation by nurse, client takes full responsibility for care.
5. Assist client in explaining procedure to significant other—especially what to do if shunt comes apart.

Table 9.3 ➤ **PLAN OF CARE TO ALLEVIATE POWERLESSNESS IN CLIENTS WITH CHRONIC RENAL FAILURE** (*Continued*)			
Situation or Factor Causing Powerlessness	**Client Indicators of Powerlessness**	**Strategies to Decrease Powerlessness**	**Criteria for Evaluation**
		DISEASE PROCESS	
		6. Encourage client to verbalize feelings and fears regarding shunt and its care.	
		7. Discuss ways of covering the shunt.	
		8. Role-play with client the explanation of the shunt to a friend.	
		9. Role-play dealing with questions from a curious stranger.	
Irritability from the central nervous system manifestations of azotemia.	1. States an inability to control moods as easily as before illness with family	1. Discuss the etiology of the irritability with client and significant others.	1. Correctly explains, in simple terms, the physiological basis for the irritability
Client feels weak and tired constantly; must take frequent naps.	2. Expresses guilt about irritability with family	2. Explore with client effective ways of dealing with anger and depression without damaging relationships with family members.	2. Practices some form of relaxation technique on a regular basis
Client cannot plan activities because of uncertainty of symptoms.	3. Says, "I'm always tired. I can't get anything done"	3. Allow verbalization of feelings of guilt about irritability.	3. Significant others explain physiological basis for client's irritability
Client cannot see printed instructions on diet, kidney disease, dialysis.	4. Reports decrease in social activities, never being able to plan ahead	4. Teach specific activities to relieve tension and help deal with stress.	4. Significant others describe ways in which they provide for meeting their own needs
	5. States, "How can I help myself, I cannot even see the instructions?"	5. Support family members in understanding and dealing with client's mood changes.	5. Adheres to specific sleep-rest pattern throughout the day
		6. Assist family members in identifying sources and effects of stress on each of them, and explore ways of meeting the needs of each family member.	

		Nursing Interventions	Expected Outcomes
		7. Plan for balancing energy expenditure with energy conservation. 8. Set priorities; engage in activities that confirm self-worth, and have the highest value for the client. 9. Provide with large print, magnifying glass, and verbal reinforcement of instructions.	6. Verbalizes understanding; asks appropriate questions
Inability to predict or control the outcome of renal transplantation.	1. States, "I guess you just have to get used to the idea that you really don't have much control over how the surgery turns out" 2. Does not ask questions about present health state 3. States, "It's not fair—I did everything I was told and I still rejected the kidney"	1. Provide client with as much data as possible about client's level of physiological control (lab values, weight, vital signs, results of diagnostic tests). 2. Allow client to verbalize feelings about lack of control of the outcome of the surgery. 3. Explore with client the meaning of the kidney transplant to self. 4. Assist client in recognizing and dealing with any incongruences between expectations and the actual results of surgery.	1. Demonstrates an interest in present health state by asking for information such as test results, urine output, vital signs, weight 2. Verbalizes realistic expectations about how the transplant will affect own life 3. Indicates an ability to cope satisfactorily with the possibility of rejection and the uncertainty of prognosis 4. Expresses a sense of hope in relation to the prognosis

FAMILY RELATIONSHIPS

		Nursing Interventions	Expected Outcomes
Decreased ability to participate in social activities with family and friends. Client missed part of family vacation because of dialysis.	1. Expresses guilt and regret over inability to participate in activities with family: "I used to skate with my daughters, but now I'm a real dud—all I can do is sit" 2. "I was stuck with that machine while they were out sightseeing."	1. Ask client to make a list of previous activities and their importance to client. 2. Assist client in setting priorities regarding those activities that client would most like to continue. 3. Explore with client the meaning to	1. Lists activities in which participation is desired according to priority 2. Identifies which activities are most important and why they are important

Table 9.3 ➤ PLAN OF CARE TO ALLEVIATE POWERLESSNESS IN CLIENTS WITH CHRONIC RENAL FAILURE (Continued)

Situation or Factor Causing Powerlessness	Client Indicators of Powerlessness	Strategies to Decrease Powerlessness	Criteria for Evaluation
		FAMILY RELATIONSHIPS	
Spouse repeatedly reminds client to rest and not to do any strenuous activities. Role reversal: Spouse takes over many of the patient's roles—paying bills, shopping, yard work.	Then after I'd finished, they'd already seen everything and didn't want to go back" 3. States, "Sometimes I feel like doing something, but she gets upset, so it's easier just to do nothing"	self of participation in family activities. 4. Assist patient and family in realistically evaluating the client's abilities and limitations. 5. Encourage spouse to avoid unnecessarily restricting client's activities. 6. Explore with spouse feelings and fear that cause spouse to "shelter" the client. 7. Assist client in developing new interests and/or modifying previous activities according to present abilities and limitations. 8. Assist client and family in developing new ways of interacting that are compatible with the client's limitations. 9. Encourage family members to continue their own activities and interests as much as possible, and allow for the expression of any guilt that may be associated with these activities. 10. Provide family members with a safe outlet for the expression of any anger that might be felt toward the client.	3. Realistically identifies own abilities and limitations 4. Uses the above information to decide which activities will be continued 5. Significant others realistically identify client's abilities and limitations and encourage client to continue activities client can tolerate 6. Modifies activities as necessary to accommodate any changes in health 7. Significant others continue with some activities that meet their own needs, even if client is unable to participate 8. Expresses the feeling that client is coping satisfactorily with any changes in activities and roles required by illness

11. Allow for the expression of any feelings of anger or resentment the client may have toward family members as they continue with activities in which client cannot participate.
12. Encourage verbalization about feelings related to role reversal; determine significance of previous role expectations.

EMPLOYMENT

Effect of dialysis on ability to retain job. Effect of CRF symptoms on job performance. Inability to work requires family to apply for public assistance.	1. Verbalizes fear of inability to continue working after starting dialysis. 2. Does not like job, but also fears loss of job; states, "I'm stuck here. I can never get another job with my age and kidney disease. I'm lucky to even have this one, but sometimes I feel like I'm trapped" 3. Feels that job performance has decreased. States, "I'm losing my creativity. I feel thick-headed. I forget things all the time" 4. Has made no effort to plan for dialysis with employer, even though this is a source of great anxiety for client	1. Provide client with specific information about dialysis: number of times a week, number of hours for each dialysis run, tentative day and time. 2. Assist client in making plans with employer for when dialysis starts. 3. Explore meaning of job with client and encourage verbalization of fears about being unable to continue working. 4. Ask if client would like the nurse to talk with personnel at company (supervisor or company nurse) to communicate information about dialysis schedule, symptoms of CRF, client's health-care needs, client's concern about retaining job. 5. Support the client in obtaining feedback from employer about his job performance (e.g., role-play	1. Makes specific plans with employer about fitting dialysis into work schedule 2. Indicates a decrease in anxiety level about continuing to work after starting dialysis 3. Identifies why job is important to self 4. Discusses job performance with supervisor and obtains feedback as to own performance 5. Begins to consider alternative ways of meeting needs now met by job in the event that it will be difficult to continue working 6. Identifies the effects that being unemployed

Table 9.3 ➤ PLAN OF CARE TO ALLEVIATE POWERLESSNESS IN CLIENTS WITH CHRONIC RENAL FAILURE (*Continued*)		
Situation or Factor Causing Powerlessness	**Client Indicators of Powerlessness**	**Strategies to Decrease Powerlessness**	**Criteria for Evaluation**

		EMPLOYMENT	
		how client will approach supervisor, suggest that client do own evaluation first).	have had on self-esteem
		6. Explore with client the effects of being unemployed on self-esteem.	7. Explores alternative ways of enhancing self-esteem—what client can do to feel better about self
		7. Allow client to verbalize feelings regarding inability to support family.	
		8. Allow client and family to verbalize feelings about receiving public assistance.	
		9. Explore with client and significant others alternate ways of enhancing client's self-esteem (other than functioning as breadwinner in the family).	
		10. Assist client in identifying own strengths and provide positive reinforcement to enhance self-esteem.	

Table 9.4 ➤ **EMPOWERMENT STRATEGIES**
Client education
Individual approach to the client and client teaching
Assessment of and emphasis on each person's uniqueness
Emphasis on self-care assets and personal strengths
Setting realistic goals
Behavior modification
Environment modification
Removal of barriers to client control
Involvement of significant others
Sensitizing clients to importance of their reactions
Helping clients devise means of permitting client control
Facilitating verbalization of feelings
Eliminating misperceptions
Developing coping skills

knowledge, (4) increasing the sensitivity of health-team members and significant others to the imposed powerlessness, and (5) encouraging verbalization of feelings. Lack of personal control over health and non-illness aspects of life has a negative impact on psychosocial well-being (Devins, 1989). A negative relationship was noted between hope and stress of 81 persons with ESRD (Baker, 1987), adding yet another challenge for nurses to inspire hope and control stress.

Although the strategies discussed in this chapter were developed specifically for individuals with CRF, they provide a prototype for health professionals and significant others working with individuals with any chronic illness. The strategies to decrease powerlessness in clients with CRF described in this chapter are collectively labeled *empowerment strategies* and are summarized in Table 9.4. These strategies are specific for strengthening the power resources of psychological stamina and social support network, motivation, and knowledge. (Refer to the power resource model in Chap. 1.)

REFERENCES

Abram, H. (1968). The psychiatrist, the treatment of chronic renal failure and the prolongation of life. *American Journal of Psychiatry, 124,* 1351–1357.

Abram, H. (1969). The psychiatrist, the treatment of chronic renal failure and the prolongation of life—Part II. *American Journal of Psychiatry, 126,* 157–167.

Abram, H., Moore, G., & Westervelt, F. (1975). Suicidal behavior in chronic dialysis patients. *Journal of Nervous and Mental Diseases, 160,* 220–226.

Anger, D. (1975). The psychologic stress of chronic renal failure and long-term hemodialysis. *Nursing Clinics of North America, 10,* 449–459.

Baker, L. (1987). *Relationship among hope, self-esteem and stress of hemodialysis in persons with end stage renal disease.* Unpublished master's thesis, Marquette University, Milwaukee.

Baldree, K., Murphy, S., & Powers, M. (1982). Stress identification and coping patterns in patients on hemodialysis. *Nursing Research, 31,* 107–112.

Beard, B. (1969). Fear of death and fear of life. *Archives of General Psychiatry, 21,* 373–380.

Bihl, M. A., Ferrans, C. E., & Powers, M. J. (1988). Comparing stressors and quality of life of dialysis patients. *ANNA Journal, 15,* 33–36.

Burns, P. (1983). Learned helplessness in the renal patient. *Nephrology Nurse, 4,* 14–16.

Christensen, A., Turner, C., Slaughter, J., & Holman, J. (1989). Perceived family support as a moderator of psychological well-being in end-stage renal disease. *Journal of Behavioral Medicine, 12,* 249–265.

Cummings, J. (1970). Hemodialysis: Feelings, facts and fantasies. *American Journal of Nursing, 70,* 70–73.

Czaczkes, J. W., & DeNour, A. K. (1978). *Chronic hemodialysis as a way of life.* New York: Brunner/Mazel.

Davison, N. (1986). Mourning the loss of sexuality. In M. Hardy et al. (Eds.), *Positive approaches to living with end stage renal disease: Psychosocial and thanatologic aspects* (pp. 142–151). New York: Praeger.

DeNour, A., & Czaczkes, J. W. (1974). Personality and adjustment to chronic hemodialysis. In N. B. Levy (Ed.), *Living or dying: Adaptation to hemodialysis* (pp. 102–126). Springfield, IL: Charles C Thomas.

Devins, G. (1989). Enhancing personal control and minimizing illness intrusiveness. In N. Kutner, D. Gardenas, & J. Bower (Eds.), *Maximizing rehabilitation in chronic renal disease* (pp. 109–136). New York: PMA Publishing.

Dimond, M. (1979). Social support and adaptation to chronic illness: The case of maintenance hemodialysis. *Research in Nursing and Health, 2,* 101–108.

Eichel, C. J. (1986). Stress and coping in patients on CAPD compared to hemodialysis patients. *ANNA Journal, 13,* 9–13.

Finkelstein, F., Finkelstein, S., & Steele, T. (1976). Assessment of marital relationships of hemodialysis patients. *American Journal of Medical Science, 271,* 21–27.

Frank, D. (1988). Psychosocial assessment of renal dialysis patients. *ANNA Journal, 15,* 207–210, 232.

Fuchs, J. (1987). Use of decisional control to combat powerlessness. *American Nephrology Nurses Association Journal, 14,* 11–13, 56.

Goodwin, S. (1988). Hardiness and psychosocial adjustment in hemodialysis clients. *ANNA Journal, 15,* 211–216.

Gurklis, J., & Menke, E. (1988). Identification of stressors and use of coping methods in chronic hemodialysis patients. *Nursing Research, 37,* 236–239, 248.

Halper, I. (1971). Psychiatric observations in a chronic hemodialysis program. *Medical Clinics of North America, 55,* 177–190.

Harrington, J., & Brenner, E. (1973). *Patient care in renal failure.* Philadelphia: WB Saunders.

Horsburgh, M., & Robinson, J. (1989). Relaxation therapy and guided imagery in ESRD. *ANNA Journal, 16,* 11–14, 19.

Jackle, M. (1974). Life satisfaction and kidney dialysis. *Nursing Forum, 13,* 360–370.

Jagusch, W., & Butchart, B. (1989). A conducted exercise program for the ESRD patient at an outpatient dialysis center. In N. Kutner, D. Gardenas, & J. Bower (Eds.), *Maximizing rehabilitation in chronic renal disease* (pp. 79–86). New York: PMA Publishing.

Jones, K. (1987). Policy and research in end stage renal disease. *Image: Journal of Nursing Scholarship, 19,* 126–129.

Laborde J., & Powers, M. (1980). Satisfaction with life for patients undergoing hemodialysis and patients suffering from osteoarthritis. *Research in Nursing and Health, 3,* 19–24.

Lancaster, L. (1984). *The patient with end stage renal disease.* New York: John Wiley & Sons.

Levy, N. (1973). Sexual adjustment to maintenance hemodialysis and renal transplantation. *Transactions of the American Society for Artificial Internal Organs, 18,* 138–142.

Maurin, J., & Schenkel, J. (1976). A study of the family unit's response to hemodialysis. *Journal of Psychosomatic Research, 20,* 163–168.

Murphy, S., Powers, M., & Jalowiec, A. (1985). Psychometric evaluation of the Hemodialysis Stressor Scale. *Nursing Research, 34,* 368–371.

Muthny, F. A. (1984). Postoperative course of patients during hospitalization following renal transplantation. *Psychotherapy and Psychosomatics, 42,* 133–142.

O'Brien, M. E. (1983). *The courage to survive: The life career of the chronic dialysis patient.* New York: Grune & Stratton.

Olsen, C. A. (1983). A statistical review of variables predictive of adjustment in hemodialysis patients. *Nephrology Nurse, 6,* 16–26.

Plough, A. (1986). *Borrowed time: Artificial organs and the politics of extending lives.* Philadelphia: Temple University Press.

Reischman, F., & Levy, N. (1972). Problems in adaptation to maintenance dialysis. *Archives of Internal Medicine, 130,* 859–865.

Roy, C. (1984). *Introduction to nursing: An adaptation model.* Englewood Cliffs, NJ: Prentice-Hall.

Shambaugh, P., Hampers, C., Bailey, G., Snyder, D., & Merrill, J. (1967). Hemodialysis in the home: Emotional impact on the spouse. *Transaction of the American Society for Artificial Internal Organs, 13,* 41–45.

Siegal, B. R., Calsyn, R. T., & Cuddihee, R. M. (1987). The relationship of social support to psychological adjustment in end stage renal disease patients. *Journal of Chronic Disease, 40,* 337–344.

Snyder, B. (1989). An exercise program. *American Journal of Nursing, 89,* 362–364.

Stegman, M. R., Duncan, K., Pohren, E., & Sandstrom, R. (1985). Quality of life: A patient's perspective. *American Nephrology Nurses Association Journal, 12,* 244–264.

Ulrich, B. T. (1980). Psychological adaptation of end stage renal disease: A review and a proposed new model. *Nephrology Nurse, 2,* 48–52.

Ulrich, B. T. (1989). *Nephrology nursing: Concepts and strategies.* Norwalk, CT: Appleton & Lange.

Weems, J., & Patterson, E. (1989). Coping with uncertainty and ambivalence while awaiting cadaveric renal transplant. *ANNA Journal, 16,* 27–31.

Wolfsen, C. (1989). Acute care nurses' perceptions of hemodialysis patients. *ANNA Journal, 16,* 329–336.

Wright, R., Sand, P., & Goodhue, L. (1966). Psychological stress during hemodialysis for chronic renal failure. *Annals of Internal Medicine, 64,* 611–621.

10

Profiles of Locus of Control and Coping in Persons with Peripheral Vascular Disease

➤ Patricia S. Schroeder • Judith Fitzgerald Miller

Individuals with altered health states have been described as experiencing powerlessness. Because circumstances and events appear to be beyond the ill person's control, powerlessness is situationally determined. The chronically ill person's powerlessness may be caused by many factors—including illness-related changes, the health-care environment, and the health team's interactions with the ill individual. In addition to this situationally determined powerlessness, a personality trait (locus of control) influences the chronically ill client's response to the health problem. Locus of control refers to the individual's perception of whether rewards are dependent on the individual's own behavior or are dependent on forces external to the individual. If outcomes (rewards) are perceived to be contingent on the individual's own behavior, the individual is said to have an internal locus of control. If events are perceived to be contingent upon external forces of fate, chance, or powerful others, the individual has an external locus of control (Rotter,

1966, 1975). (To avoid cumbersome phrases, such individuals are referred to as "internals" and "externals" throughout this chapter.)

The purpose of this chapter is to describe behavioral indices of locus of control derived from the qualitative study of six clients with peripheral vascular disease (PVD). Knowing the client's locus-of-control tendency enables the nurse to anticipate:

- How independent the client will seek to become
- How anxiety provoking the situational powerlessness will be for individuals (internals may have more anxiety in powerlessness situations than externals)
- The importance of mastering control-relevant health information for internals

It is also important for nurses to understand how coping strategies vary: internals use approach and direct confrontation strategies, and externals use withdrawal, hostility, and aggression (Anderson, 1977). Understanding the client's locus-of-control tendencies enables the nurse to have a more holistic approach to the client.

LITERATURE REVIEW OF LOCUS OF CONTROL

Locus of control has been measured by using objective tests such as Rotter's Social Attitude Survey or the I-E (Internal-External) Scale (Rotter, 1966), the Health Locus of Control Scale (Wallston, Wallston, Kaplan, & Maides, 1976), or the Multidimensional Health Locus of Control (Wallston, Wallston, & DeVellis, 1978). Validation studies using cluster analysis have resulted in six clusters depicting variations in locus of control: (1) pure internals, (2) double externals, (3) pure chance, (4) yea sayers, (5) nay sayers, and (6) believers in control (Rock, Meyerowitz, Maisto, & Wallston, 1987). The advantages of using a quantitative approach to such a concept are obvious. Data are gathered by scales with established validity and reliability, and the score is a clear, definitive indication of the subject's locus-of-control tendency. However, administering written psychological tests could be cumbersome and impractical for nurses. Traditionally, nurses have not used quantitative measures to validate clinical impressions. This type of validation will become a routine component of practice as more valid and reliable tools to measure selected client phenomena are developed.

Even though quantitative measures are not always feasible, nurses can use observational skills to note behavioral indices of locus-of-control tendencies. This chapter presents the initial progress in developing a behavioral observation index for nurses to use in assessing locus-of-control tendencies.

A participant-observer methodology was used to determine the client's locus of control and individual coping strategies. The eight subjects studied were hospitalized for evaluation and treatment of PVD. The process of participant-observer research is well defined by Byerly (1969) as involving

> . . . a sensitive awareness of the behaviors of the persons being observed, similar insight into the investigators' actions and reactions, a careful and complete recording of these events, and retrospective evaluation and analysis of data (p. 236).

Research findings on various characteristics of internals and externals provided the framework for making behavioral observations. Seeman (1963) and Seeman and Evans (1962) found that internals readily mastered control-relevant information. Lefcourt (1976) concluded from a review of literature on locus of control and cognitive activity that internals are more perceptive to, and ready to learn about, their surroundings. They are more inquisitive, curious, and efficient in processing information than are externals. Internals with high health values sought more information about a threat to health—hypertension—than did externals or the internals with low health values (Wallston, Maides, & Wallston, 1976). Fish and Karabenick (1971) studied self-esteem and locus of control in college freshmen. Their findings suggest that persons with an internal locus of control exhibit higher self-esteem.

The necessity of congruency between an individual's actual environment and locus of control was discussed by Watson and Baumal (1967). An incongruency is bound to produce anxiety. That is, a person with an external locus of control placed in a nonstructured environment and required to do a task that necessitates more self-direction will experience more anxiety than if placed in an authoritative, structured situation (Watson & Baumal, 1967). Likewise, persons with spinal cord injuries who have high preference for control have low depression when perceiving they do indeed have control in situations of importance to them (Ferrington, 1986).

Williams, Poon, and Burdette (1977) studied the effect of the cardiovascular response on 29 subjects during sensory processing, using forearm blood flow to determine response to sensory intake and sensory rejection. Forearm blood flow increased in externals but remained the same in internals during sensory intake. It was thought that the smaller forearm blood flow could be associated with active vasoconstriction during sensory intake. In accord with other research, Williams et al. found that the sensory intake of internals reflected a greater involvement in the task at hand than that of externals and that vascular resistance occurred in internals. The vasomotor response could be considered a means of physiological coping. Lack of vascular resistance in externals may be significant. A number of questions can be raised, such as: Do the personality characteristics of internals serve as a prerequisite for developing vascular disease or other diseases that may have a psychosomatic component? What other psychosocial factors are involved in developing cardiovascular disease?

Lowery and DuCette (1976) found that internals with long-term diabetes were less compliant than externals with long-term diabetes. Internals were more active information seekers early in the course of their disease. Internality is also related to preventive actions such as wearing seat belts and using preventive dental care (Williams, 1972).

Health promotion and community health models emphasize personal responsibility for health (Jordan-Marsh & Neutra, 1985; Pender, 1996; Saltzer & Saltzer, 1987). Persons who used preventive health behavior had significantly lower chance locus-of-control scores than persons who did not (Zindler-Wernet & Weiss, 1987). Internal health locus of control, low chance locus of control, and high self-esteem were related to a health promotion lifestyle in 262 women (Duffy, 1988). Although internality has been related to greater health, experience or lack of experience with the problem influences expectations about control (Saltzer & Saltzer, 1987).

Benefits of internality have been supported. Ehlke (1988) found a negative relationship between symptom distress and internal locus of control beliefs in 107 women receiving chemotherapy for breast cancer. That is, the greater the internality, the less distressing symptoms from chemotherapy were experienced (i.e., reported). Internally oriented persons were more likely to quit smoking after the release of the surgeon general's report in the 1960s than externally oriented persons (James, Woodruff, & Werner, 1965). Internals were more likely than externals to complete a weight-control program (Balch & Ross, 1975).

Arakelian (1980) proposed that exposure to planned programs can modify locus-of-control beliefs. Internal locus of control was increased by a selected intervention of relaxation training in persons with hypertension (Pender, 1985).

Although the health locus-of-control research reviewed supports a health advantage for persons with an internal control tendency, caution must be used in judging this as the goal for all persons. For persons with a chronic health problem, assistance in accepting the situation without striving for absolute control over it may be necessary.

PERIPHERAL VASCULAR DISEASE

Peripheral vascular disease includes conditions of the arteries (arterial occlusive disease due to atherosclerosis), veins (venous insufficiency or incompetency of venous valves), and lymph vessels (lymphedema due to inadequate lymph transport) (Wagner, 1986; Wheeler & Brenner, 1995). All clinical profiles presented in this chapter are of persons having arterial occlusive disease due to atheromatous plaques on the intimal vessel surface.

Clinical Data

In this study, hospitalized clients were provided with professional nursing care by the registered nurse investigator, with careful documentation of the indicators of internal and external locus of control in a clinical journal. The following are profiles of six subjects and their feelings of control, as well as coping behaviors observed by the investigator. Three subjects were classified as having an internal locus-of-control tendency, and three were considered to have an external locus-of-control tendency. A behavioral assessment tool of locus of control is also presented.

➤➤➤ **CLINICAL PROFILES: INTERNALS**

MR. K.

Mr. K. is a 53-year-old engineer with an 8-year history of PVD for which he has had 10 operations, including lower-limb bypass grafts and embolectomies, before having one leg amputated above the knee. He was independent and strong-willed and had a well-developed self-care agency. His behaviors and conversations centered on how he could regain complete independence and autonomy, not just when discharged to his home but during his hospitalization. His internal locus of control was also demonstrated by statements he made during interviews:

- "I am responsible for the loss of my leg. I have continued to smoke cigarettes. If I wouldn't have gone back to work so fast after my other surgeries, maybe they could have saved it."
- "A person is only a cripple if he lets himself be one, and I won't."
- "I've been a professional person all my life, and I know that sometimes professionals can be stupid too, so I won't let my doctors railroad me. I let them know how I feel about what they're doing."
- "It's up to me to follow through on the therapy so I can get out of here (hospital)."

These statements are presented out of context, but Mr. K.'s attitudes and behaviors were compatible with the description of an internal locus of control as noted in the literature.

Mr. K. exhibited coping strategies that one would expect of a person with an internal locus of control. He read a great deal to be current and knowledgeable about his pathology, thereby enhancing his control. He actively participated in self-care and worked to be autonomous. He planned aspects of his care, such as routines to care for his remaining foot, and took special vitamins (including vitamin E) that he perceived as vital in maintaining his health. When he had nothing to do, he would daydream about inventions he could develop for amputees: "It would take someone creative and with my background to think this stuff up." Toward the end of his hospitalization, he began to act out sexually. Playful propositions to nurses and therapists, jokes about sex, and a flirtatious attitude could be interpreted as evidence of his altered body image and masculinity; by using this behavior, he was able to cope with the situation and demonstrate his virility. He expressed the idea that he was still sexually potent in spite of his impaired circulation. It seemed important to him that he reinforce the nurses' understanding of this fact.

MRS. L.

Mrs. L. is a 50-year-old housewife with a 9-year history of PVD and arteriosclerotic heart disease. Like Mr. K., she has had several lower-limb bypass grafts, both aortoiliac and femoral-popliteal. Unlike him, she has not had an amputation. Mrs. L. is strong-willed and takes pride that she was able to walk unassisted in the intensive-care unit after her aortoiliac bypass surgery. Even during exacerbations of her illness, she continued to exhibit a strong self-care agency and internal locus of control. Some of the following statements show further indications:

- "I'm the strong one in my family."
- "You've got to help yourself get better around here. No one can do it but you."
- "God can give me strength and courage to do anything, even to quit smoking."
- "What I do to take care of myself will make the difference; it's not up to the nurses."

Mrs. L. coped by striving for autonomy and using self-care practices. She had a daily routine of walking the halls and sitting in the lounges so that she could meet new friends, and through her encouragement to them, she herself became encouraged. She was very aware of her health regimen and felt she was more in control if she knew what was going on. Prayer and religion were very important to her and were a source of strength. In regard to her family supports, she stated that she had to support her husband and children whenever she was hospitalized because "I am the strong one."

MRS. B.

Mrs. B. is a 46-year-old housewife who has a medical history of two myocardial infarctions within the previous 2 years and began to develop intermittent claudication at the same time. She had several lower-limb bypass grafts on both legs, and because the grafts failed, she had a left above-knee amputation after a prolonged hospitalization in attempts to save the leg.

Mrs. B. speaks freely about her pathologies and hospitalizations; although she has a limited vocabulary, she uses all the appropriate medical terminology with obvious understanding. She, too, has a very strong self-care agency and works to do as much for herself as possible. She maintains control of her environment by being up in her wheelchair whenever possible. She is assertive. For example, when the medical team told her they wanted to attempt another bypass graft, she stated she would not sign the permit until her husband came. She informed them that when her husband arrived, she would page the doctors to return and have them provide her and her husband with information needed to make an informed decision.

In coping with her chronic illness, Mrs. B.'s basic strategy was to be knowledgeable about her disease and treatment. This allowed her to relate better to her caretakers and to take a more active role in decision making. She stated that when she felt "blue," she would call her husband to cry or complain, and he would be able to support her enough to allow her to regain control of herself and her surroundings. When she felt stressed, Mrs. B. would increase her smoking. Although alternate methods of tension control were encouraged, Mrs. B. stated that she has decided it was "too late" to quit smoking. She also devised ways of adapting her environment to her chronic illness, such as developing a makeshift waist restraint "in case I fall asleep in my chair." She organized her belongings within easy reach from her sitting position.

▶▶▶ CLINICAL PROFILES: EXTERNALS

MRS. E.

Mrs. E. is s 56-year-old woman who exhibits an external locus of control. She has diabetes and reportedly did not take her hypoglycemic medications for 4 years because of the cost. She also reports that because of poor heating in her home, she wore boots for several months without caring for her feet. On admission, she had a large necrotic area on the inner aspect of her right foot, probably caused by the boots, and subsequently had a below-knee amputation of the right leg.

Mrs. E. is hesitant to do anything for herself and feels hopeless. Although she is not "submissive" to authority, she relies on persons in authority to make all decisions. Her physical condition improved greatly after admission, and psychologically she became more pleasant and has learned a small amount about diabetes. When asked her attitude about herself, she replies:

- "I know I'm helpless, and I'll always be helpless."
- "My husband won't wait on me when I get home, so I don't know what I'll do."

- "I lost my leg because my husband didn't repair the furnace."
- "Do you think my wearing boots for those months made my foot bad, or do you think it was the diabetes?"

Mrs. E. exhibits behaviors that, in general, demonstrate a very dependent role. Initially, Mrs. E. coped by exhibiting noncompliance and demonstrating total immobility and dependence. She was disinterested in learning self-care practices and refused to attempt them. She was withdrawn and depressed. Later she became more responsive to teaching but remained far from becoming an information seeker. She socialized minimally but did follow directions. She had no helping relationships with any supportive significant others in her life.

MRS. K.

Mrs. K. is a 48-year-old woman who has had PVD for 2 years and had a femoral-popliteal bypass on the left leg. Her disease had increasingly limited her activity, and she was hospitalized to be evaluated for a graft on the right leg. Although she had much pain, she did not elect to have surgery at that time because of the uncertainty of its long-range success.

Mrs. K. lacked knowledge of her disease and the treatments. She was unsure why these painful tests were being performed, yet she consented to them. She stated that there was nothing she could do to "alter the course of her fate" and prayed that medical science would find a cure for diabetes and her vascular problems. Her conversations were laced with statements such as "You can't win—there's no way you can come out on top with this (disease)." She took all her medications at home but was unable to identify their names or actions. When discussing her plan of care, she stated, "You have to do what they say."

The coping behaviors Mrs. K. used appear to be based heavily on denial and expressions of guilt. She did not look for ways in which she could function maximally despite her disease, but instead focused on praying for a cure and expressing much guilt at her inability to fulfill her roles within the home. She used religion in a basically unrealistic way. She avoided confronting the realities of her situation.

MRS. T.

Mrs. T. is a 61-year-old widow who lives with her daughter and family. She has had PVD for 3 years and had a femoral-popliteal bypass graft on the left leg approximately 1 year ago. She has now been hospitalized for the same procedure on her right leg.

Mrs. T. is a very passive woman who generally agrees with anything that is said, even if it is contradictory. When asked how she felt about impending surgery, she stated, "I don't know. You've got to do what they say." Although her surgery was canceled three times because of laboratory tests not being completed or scheduling difficulties, she never became overtly angry. Postoperatively, she participated little in self-care, even to the day of discharge.

Mrs. T. used religion as a coping strategy. She would pray for relief of pain and strength to handle it, which was quite realistic. When Mrs. T. was stressed, she closed her eyes and turned her head away as if to block out the undesired stimuli. Her coping reflected nonverbal avoidance. She remained dependent and tolerant of everything because "you have to go along with it."

Behavioral Indicators of Locus of Control

In examining these data as a whole, commonalities specific for internals and externals were noted. Based on the review of research on locus of control, client behaviors were categorized as indicating an internal or external control tendency. Two nurse-educators who had knowledge of locus-of-control research and had conducted locus-of-control studies independently rated the behaviors. Only those behaviors for which there was 100 percent agreement were included on the assessment tool. Items that prompted a discrepancy between the raters were omitted. The assessment tool provides a framework for the organization of observations of behavioral indices of internal and external locus-of-control tendencies (Table 10.1).

Clients may not exhibit behaviors related to each category noted in Table 10.1, as was true of the client examples presented in this chapter;

Table 10.1 ➤ **BEHAVIORAL INDICATORS OF LOCUS OF CONTROL**		
	Internals	**Externals**
Role definition and satisfaction	More clearly defined, more satisfying	Less clearly defined, less satisfying
Relating to authority	Peerlike interactions	Passivelike interactions
Self-esteem	Higher or more stable self-esteem	Lower or less stable self-esteem
Responsibility for self-care	Active knowledge-seeking behavior	Do not actively seek information, accept what is given
Compliance with health-care regimen	Manipulate regimen	Compliant
Confidence in abilities	Self-confident	Lack self-confidence
Problem-solving abilities	More successful	Less successful
Goal-setting behavior	Realistic in goals set	Unrealistic
Level of motivation	Motivation	Tend toward helplessness at times
Involvement in decision making	More involvement	Less involvement

however, through observation of some of these behaviors, a general tendency toward internal or external control can be discovered.

Caution needs to be used to avoid rigidly categorizing clients as being at one or the other extreme of locus of control. Locus of control is to be viewed as a continuum, with most persons falling somewhere between the extremes. Although quick interpretation of Table 10.1 may lead nurses to believe that externality is negative, this may not be the case in terms of clients' experiences of anxiety, recovery rates, and select client outcomes after illness episodes. Too little data exist to draw conclusions at this point. Strickland (1979) suggested that type A patients with cardiovascular disease may be extremely internally oriented. Increasing internality in the type A person may increase personal striving, stress, and eventually maladaptation (Wallston, Wallston, & DeVellis, 1978).

In a review of literature on locus of control and health, Wallston, Wallston, and DeVellis (1978) concluded that although internals seemed to engage in more positive health- and sick-role behaviors than externals did, findings are contradictory, and in some instances it is more functional to hold external beliefs. In general, internals were more positive in seeking health information, adhering to prescribed medications, keeping physician appointments, maintaining a diet, and giving up smoking. Lack of consistency in findings may stem from use of Rotter's I-E Scale without validating findings using other locus-of-control measures as well as not using convenience samples and not controlling samples' variance in terms of severity and length of illness (Arakelian, 1980).

Careful study is needed to determine the desirability of internality training and the circumstances that warrant strategies to develop clients' internality. Arakelian (1980) reviewed literature on locus of control and suggested means of internalization. Three types of internalization strategies include (1) reconstruction of stimuli—helping clients change their perceptions of stimuli (reinterpretation of stimuli); (2) action orientation—helping clients learn problem-solving techniques and eliminate self-defeating behaviors; and (3) counseling—helping clients recognize contingencies between their own behavior and outcomes.

Coping Behaviors

The case examples in this chapter suggest that the coping strategies used by internals and externals differ. Internals obtained strength from maintaining control over their environment, if only through their knowledge of what was occurring. This knowledge provided internals with the opportunity to make informed choices and accept, reject, or supplement their therapy. Internals also worked to develop self-care abilities. Religion or spouses were frequent sources of support that were generally aimed at returning the client's strength to handle the situation rather than removing the situation.

Externals more frequently coped through the use of denial or expression of guilt feelings, which was not followed by actions to alter the situation. They were passively accepting and did little to increase their own self-care abilities. Religion was used by some externals but was directed at unrealistic goals such as a "cure" for their chronic disease or a return of an amputated part. In general, the externals' coping strategies did not deal directly with the situation. The use of denial did seem to decrease anxiety for the externals.

Similar findings of coping behaviors of internals and externals were found by Ewig (1979) who used two quantitative locus-of-control measures. Ewig studied coping behaviors of clients who had chronic pain to determine differences in coping between internals and externals. Subjects were classified as internal or external based on both a modified Rotter scale (Seeman & Evans, 1962) and the original Rotter scale (Rotter, 1966). Ewig's findings support the descriptive research presented in this chapter. Externals used passive coping behaviors (withdrawal, lack of goal setting, lack of self-care involvement, denial, lack of information seeking). Internals used active coping behaviors (initiation of action based on self-care knowledge and skills, goal setting, use of appropriate decision-making strategies, purposeful use of relaxation and/or distraction, pride in self-care strides, and information seeking). A comparison of the coping behaviors of internals and externals is presented in Table 10.2.

Nursing Implications

Because of the uncertain course of PVD, as with any chronic illness, clients are placed in "uncontrollable" situations. How chronically ill clients react to their health problem is very individual. This chapter has reinforced the idea that knowledge about clients' locus of control is important in understanding clients' behavioral response. Knowledge of a client's locus-of-control tendency can give direction for appropriate nursing approaches. For example, in interpersonal relationships, persons with an internal locus of control might best respond to "one-to-one" collaborative planning with the nurse in which maximum involvement of the client is encouraged. Persons with a more external locus of control might be more responsive to an "authority-to-subordinate" approach, as this is in accord with their perceived view of success in interaction with authority figures. The nurse would need to demonstrate competence and knowledge and share experience so that the client can surrender planning and involvement and look to the nurse as the authority.

Table 10.2 ➤ **COPING BEHAVIORS OF INTERNALS AND EXTERNALS**

Internals	Externals
Active in self-care	Passive dependence
Helped others recognize self-care strides, boasted of ability	Sleeping
Planned for care needs, made suggestions to health worker	Lack of self-care skills
	Disinterested
Social interaction	Social isolation
Active interest in others, helped them solve problems	Withdrawn
	Focused on unrealistic cures
Set goals	
Modified environment, planned for safety needs	Refused therapies that increase mobility (physical therapy)
Used problem solving	
	Verbal expressions such as there is nothing more to be done
Information seeking	
Asked specific, relevant questions	
Read about condition	
Shared perceptions of self as being important	
Described positive role as strong person in family	
Deliberate use of prayer to provide strength	
Purposeful distraction	

Internals may be more capable of dealing with situations that affect their concepts of themselves. They may be able to preserve a positive self-concept in the face of chronic illness, whereas externals may be in greater need of nursing interventions to maintain a positive self-concept. Externals perceive physical disorders as more disabling than mental disorders, and internals perceive mental disorders as more disabling than physical disorders (MacDonald & Hall, 1971). Likewise, self-esteem of externals may be more vulnerable to physical health changes than is the self-esteem of internals.

Responsibility for self-care is a major area with divergent approaches based on the client's locus of control. Internally oriented persons might be eager to receive as much information as possible about their health and plan of care. They could then approach prescribed regimens with confidence and enthusiasm and feel better able to deal with unforeseen situations. Much of the health education could be unstructured or self-directed. Externally oriented persons, however, might be best approached by a structured teaching plan including only the information that is absolutely necessary for safely implementing self-care. Externally oriented persons can be anticipated to be initially unsure of abilities, to need more direction in assuming self-care responsibilities, and to have potentially greater difficulty in problem solving in un-planned situations.

The amount of structure and self-direction did influence internals' and externals' success in a weight-control program (Wallston et al., 1976). Wallston et al. found that externals lost more weight in a group-structured, externally controlled program, whereas internals lost more weight in a self-directed, internally oriented program.

Goal-setting behaviors of internally oriented persons are generally more realistic, requiring an honest and supportive approach by the nurse. Throughout the problem-solving process, the client would benefit optimally from being the focal point of decision making. Because of a higher level of motivation, internals have a good chance of achieving re-alistic goals that tend to be self-determined. Externals can be expected to be responsive to having some decisions made for them. Because of ex-ternals' tendency to set unrealistic goals, they may need more assis-tance in identifying achievable outcomes and support in believing that the goals are actually attainable.

Locus of control is a fertile area for research and is relevant for nursing. Controversy exists over appropriate means of measuring locus of control and the desirability of internal versus external tendencies. Both qualitative and quantitative studies are needed on locus of control in the chronically ill. Knowledge of locus of control needs to be devel-oped through research questions such as "Do internals display apathy and giving-up behavior more readily than externals when placed in powerless situations?" Valuable studies could include how individuals' locus-of-control tendencies influence compliance, help seeking, anxiety levels, health-maintenance behaviors, perceived vulnerability to dis-eases, and other sick-role behavior.

Although specific care plans are not the focus of this chapter, prev-alent nursing diagnoses are outlined. Herman (1986) identified nurs-ing diagnoses for each of the following functional patterns of Gordon (1994).

1. Nutrition-metabolic pattern
   a. Impaired skin integrity
2. Activity-exercise pattern
   a. Activity intolerance
   b. Alteration in tissue perfusion
3. Cognitive-perceptual pattern
   a. Alteration in comfort
   b. Pain self-management deficit
   c. Knowledge deficit
4. Self-perception self-concept pattern
   a. Anxiety

      b. Reactive depression
      c. Powerlessness
      d. Body image disturbance
   5. Coping-stress tolerance pattern
      a. Ineffective coping
   6. Health-perception health-management pattern
      a. Noncompliance
      b. Health-management deficit

Nursing care for clients with PVD may include interventions directed at risk modification and prevention. These include reduction of hypercholesterolemia through diet, exercise, and weight control; blood pressure control; smoking cessation; and anxiety reduction. Client teaching includes information about medication regimens (vasodilators), monitoring exercise tolerance, foot care, and control of related health problems such as diabetes (Beaver, 1986; Cookingham, 1995; Turner, 1986). Avoidance of trauma to legs and feet by avoiding use of warming devices (heating pads), changing elastic stocking daily, inspecting skin for breakdown, and examining calves of legs for tenderness caused by thrombophlebitis all need nursing emphasis. Client's altered comfort state needs to be managed with medications and/or adjunctive modalities (distraction, imagery, relaxation). A drug used when claudication is a problem is Trental (pentoxifylline). This is a rheologic agent that increases the red blood cells' flexibility and decreases platelet aggregation and blood viscosity. Microcirculation is improved with use of pentoxifylline) (Turner, 1986). Surgical treatment modalities include the use of laser surgery (Cox & Jacobs, 1987; Webber & Jenkins, 1988).

SUMMARY

Emphasis in this chapter is on analysis of clinical data of six clients with PVD on their control tendencies. For a summary of nursing assessment, diagnostic testing, and therapies, refer to Doyle (1986), Ekers (1986), Fahey (1987), Herman (1986), Krenzer (1995), and Massey (1986).

Planning and providing care appropriately designed for the individual client's unique needs and personality are dependent on understanding the client's control tendency. By developing sensitivity to their own locus-of-control tendencies, nurses will not expect similar control behaviors in their patients. It is possible that an astute practitioner may be routinely assessing clients' locus of control and coping behavior; however, few nurses choose to organize care plans considering the locus-of-control variable. Omitting locus-of-control data in the assessment may lead to inappropriate nursing approaches that are incongruent with the client's unique control tendency. The client's behavior may be one of noncompliance unless effort is made to tailor nursing approaches congruent with the client's control tendencies.

REFERENCES

Anderson, C. (1977). Locus of control, coping behaviors and performance in a stress setting: A longitudinal study. *Journal of Applied Psychology, 62,* 446–451.

Arakelian, M. (1980). An assessment and nursing application of the concept of locus of control. *Advances in Nursing Science, 3,* 25–42.

Balch, P., & Ross, W. (1975). Predicting success in weight reduction as a function of locus of control. A unidimensional approach. *Journal of Consulting and Clinical Psychology, 43,* 119.

Beaver, B. M. (1986). Health education and the patient with peripheral vascular disease. *Nursing Clinics of North America, 21,* 265–272.

Byerly, E. (1969). The nurse researcher as participant-observer in a nursing setting. *Nursing Research, 18,* 230–236.

Cookingham, A. (1995). Peripheral vascular disease: Educational concerns for patients with a chronic disease in a changing health-care environment. *AACN Clinical Issues, 6,* 670–676.

Cox, J., & Jacobs, C. P. (1987). Laser-assisted angioplasty. *AORN Journal, 46,* 835–846.

Doyle, J. (1986). Treatment modalities in peripheral vascular disease. *Nursing Clinics of North America, 21,* 241–253.

Duffy, M. (1988). Determinants of health promotion in midlife women. *Nursing Research, 37,* 358–362.

Ehlke, G. (1988). Symptom distress in breast cancer patients receiving chemotherapy in the outpatient setting. *Oncology Nursing Forum, 15,* 343–346.

Ekers, M. A. (1986). Psychosocial considerations in peripheral vascular disease. *Nursing Clinics of North America, 21,* 255–263.

Ewig, J. (1979). *The relationship between locus of control and pain coping style.* Unpublished master's thesis, Marquette University, Milwaukee.

Fahey, V. (1987). *Vascular nursing.* Philadelphia: WB Saunders.

Ferrington, F. (1986). Personal control and coping effectiveness in spinal cord injured persons. *Research in Nursing and Health, 9,* 257–265.

Fish, B., & Karabenick, S. A. (1971). Relationship between self-esteem and locus of control. *Psychological Reports, 29,* 784.

Gordon, M. (1994). *Nursing diagnoses: Process and application* (3rd ed.). New York: McGraw-Hill.

Herman, J. A. (1986). Nursing assessment and nursing diagnosis in patients with peripheral vascular disease. *Nursing Clinics of North America, 21,* 219–231.

James, W., Woodruff, A. B., & Werner, W. (1965). Effect of internal and external control upon changes in smoking behavior. *Journal of Consulting Psychology, 29,* 184–186.

Jordan-Marsh, M., & Neutra, R. (1985). Relationship of health locus of control to lifestyle change programs. *Research in Nursing and Health, 8,* 3–11.

Krenzer, M. (1995). Peripheral vascular assessment: Finding your way through arteries and veins. *AACN Clinical Issues, 6,* 631–644.

Lefcourt, H. (1976). *Locus of control: Current trends in theory and research.* Hillsdale, NJ: Lawrence Erlbaum Associates.

Lowery, B., & DuCette, J. P. (1976). Disease-related learning and disease control in diabetics as a function of locus of control. *Nursing Research, 25,* 358–362.

MacDonald, A. P., & Hall, J. (1971). Internal-external locus of control and perception of disability. *Journal of Consulting and Clinical Psychology, 36,* 338–343.

Massey, J. (1986). Diagnostic testing for peripheral vascular disease. *Nursing Clinics of North America, 21,* 207–218.

Pender, N. (1985). Effects of progressive muscle relaxation training on anxiety and health locus of control among hypertensive adults. *Research in Nursing and Health, 8,* 67–72.

Pender, N. (1996). *Health promotion in nursing practice* (3rd ed.). Norwalk, CT: Appleton-Lange.

Rock, D., Meyerowitz, B., Maisto, S., & Wallston, K. (1987). The derivation and validation of six multidimensional health locus of control scale clusters. *Research in Nursing and Health, 10,* 185–195.

Rotter, J. B. (1966). Generalized expectancies for internal versus external control of reinforcement. *Journal of Consulting and Clinical Psychology, 21,* 56–67.

Rotter, J. B. (1975). Some problems and misconceptions related to the construct of internal versus external control of reinforcement. *Journal of Consulting and Clinical Psychology, 43,* 56–57.

Saltzer, E., & Saltzer, E. (1987). Internal control and health: Which comes first? *Western Journal of Nursing Research, 9,* 542–554.

Seeman, M. (1963). Alienation and social learning in a reformatory. *American Journal of Sociology, 69,* 270.

Seeman, M., & Evans, J. (1962). Alienation and learning in a hospital setting. *American Sociological Review, 27,* 772–782.

Strickland, V. R. (1979). IE and cardiovascular functioning. In L. C. Perlmutter and R. A. Monty (Eds.), *Choice and Perceived Control* (pp. 221–231). Hillsdale, NJ: Lawrence Erlbaum Associates.

Turner, J. A. (1986). Nursing intervention in patients with peripheral vascular disease. *Nursing Clinics of North America, 21,* 233–240.

Wagner, M. (1986). Pathophysiology related to peripheral vascular disease. *Nursing Clinics of North America, 21,* 195–206.

Wallston, B. S., Wallston, K. A., Kaplan, C. D., & Maides, S. A. (1976). Development and validation of the Health Locus of Control (HLC) Scale. *Journal of Consulting Clinical Psychology, 44,* 580–585.

Wallston, K. A., Maides, S., & Wallston, B. S. (1976). Health-related information seeking as a function of health-related locus of control and health value. *Journal of Research and Personality, 10,* 215–222.

Wallston, K. A., Wallston, B. S., & DeVellis, R. (1978). Development of the Multidimensional Health Locus of Control (MHLC) Scales. *Health Education Monographs, 6,* 160–170.

Watson, D., & Baumal, E. (1967). Effects of locus of control and expectations of future control upon present performance. *Journal of Personality and Social Psychology, 6,* 212–215.

Webber, M., & Jenkins, N. (1988). Laser treatment of peripheral vascular disease: Implications for nursing care. *Progress in Cardiovascular Nursing, 3,* 81–88.

Wheeler, E., & Brenner, Z. (1995). Peripheral vascular anatomy, physiology, and pathophysiology. *AACN Clinical Issues, 6,* 505–514.

Williams, A. F. (1972). Personality characteristics associated with preventive dental health practices. *Journal of the American College of Dentistry, 39,* 225–234.

Williams, R. B., Poon, L., & Burdette, L. (1977). Locus of control and vasomotor response to sensory processing. *Psychosomatic Medicine, 39,* 127–133.

Zindler-Wernet, P., & Weiss, S. (1987). Health locus of control and preventive health behavior. *Western Journal of Nursing Research, 9,* 160–179.

11

Energy Deficits in Chronically Ill Persons with Arthritis: Fatigue

➤ JUDITH FITZGERALD MILLER

Energy is the capacity to do work. Within the complexity of the human system, work takes place on a variety of planes. In a biological sense, energy is a requirement for cell metabolism. Energy is needed for mobilizing psychological defense mechanisms. Cognitively, energy is needed for learning, generating ideas, solving problems, and striving for goal attainment. Social energy includes being able to interact with others as members of family and community systems. Social energy is needed for interacting with persons for whom the individual has a cathexis as well as with persons for whom there is no attachment.

ENERGY AS A POWER RESOURCE

Energy is viewed as a power resource because of the vastly important role it plays biologically, psychologically, cognitively, and socially. Energy provides power in the following ways: It is a resource for mobility (Fagerhaugh, 1984), a factor in promoting well-being and a feeling of physical reserve, a means of providing confidence in task accomplishment, and a means of responding to unexpected stress. An energy deficit contributes to powerlessness. When the capacity to do work is lacking, powerlessness exists. The term *entropy* is used to describe disorganization resulting from energy loss (Putt, 1978). When a state of entropy exists, the organism is powerless. Energy deficits are a common problem in chronically ill clients.

In nursing care of chronically ill clients, helping the client to become aware of energy resources and to manage energy deficits is an empowerment strategy. Specific aspects of energy as a power resource will be examined closely.

Energy Is a Basic Mobility Resource

Fagerhaugh (1984) described energy, time, and money as basic mobility resources. Individuals draw on basic mobility resources for physical mobility and sociability. The individual's needs for physical mobility and sociability are easily met during various states of health, if adequate financial resources are present. However, basic mobility resources are decreased and continue to dwindle in persons with chronic health problems. Persons who have low energy resources but sufficient money resources can purchase the basic mobility resources of another. Mobility assistants can be hired (Fagerhaugh, 1984) to help with various living tasks—cleaning, cooking, transportation, and so forth.

Typically, the chronically ill person suffers from a deficit of energy—the basic mobility resource. Furthermore, when the ill person also lacks sufficient financial resources, the only remaining basic mobility resource is time. Having all the time available that is needed, the client will spend it to accomplish the mobility task. For example, the client with emphysema may require the entire morning to get dressed and perform normal morning hygiene activities. The same client may also spend twice as much time performing routine errands such as walking to the store, because the client may have to stop to "catch a breath" at puffing stations along the way. Figuring out which route has the least resistance (terrain not requiring walking uphill) and allowing sufficient time to avoid the routes with difficult terrain are ways of using time as a basic mobility resource (Fagerhaugh, 1984).

Energy Promotes Well-Being

A sense of self-satisfaction and well-being is felt when energy is present. The individual can control interactions with the environment and engage in meaningful activities, which provide positive feedback about self and a sense of joy. Exercise enhances well-being; however, lack of energy may prohibit this.

Energy Enables Task Accomplishment and Ability to Respond to Needs

Energy is a basic necessity for task accomplishment. Whether the tasks are providing self-care, learning new skills, working on the job, performing other roles, or responding to unexpected stress, energy gives the individual confidence in being able to complete the task successfully. Fatigue is the physical and psychological manifestation of energy deficits; it is a subjective feeling of tiredness that is influenced by circadian rhythm and varies in unpleasantness, duration, and intensity (Piper, 1993). There is a progression from tiredness to fatigue to exhaustion, a totally decompensated state (Rhoten, 1982). Fatigue interferes with coping, optimal participation in treatment programs, social activities that are important for positive feedback about self, role performance, and sexual activities.

Etiologies for fatigue are classified by Rhoten (1982) as (1) physical—posture, sedentary life; (2) mental—monotony or boredom; (3) environmental—noise, temperature; (4) emotional—anxiety, frustration, depression, conflicts; (5) physiological—nutritional deficits, sleep-rest disturbance, select medications, and (6) pathological—inflammation, disease processes.

Fatigue has been identified as a prevalent response to varied chronic health problems including cancer (Kaempfer & Lindsey, 1986; Kobashi-Schoot, Hanewald, Van Dam, & Bruning, 1985; Haylock & Hart, 1979; Jamar, 1989), multiple sclerosis (Hart, 1978), cardiac problems (Hertanu, Davis, & Focseneanu, 1986; Winslow, Lane, & Gaffney, 1985), end-stage renal disease (Baldree, Murphy, & Powers, 1982; Eichel, 1986; Srivastava, 1989), and respiratory problems. Analysis of the energy state of the chronically ill is important.

ENERGY-ANALYSIS FORMAT

Energy Sources and Transformation

Ryden (1977) presented a comprehensive format to examine energy. Three constructs proposed in Ryden's energy utilization model are (1) energy sources, (2) energy transformation, and (3) energy expenditure or storage. Energy sources include nutrients, oxygen, and water; other sources are rest and motivation. Motivation promotes perseverance, interest, and determination. These, as well as pleasure and satisfaction derived from an activity or task, serve to counteract fatigue (Hart & Freel, 1982). Energy transformation refers to the body's physiological processing and distribution of energy sources (Ryden, 1977). In chronically ill persons, energy is affected by pathophysiological changes that may interfere with digestion, circulation, respiration, endocrine bal-

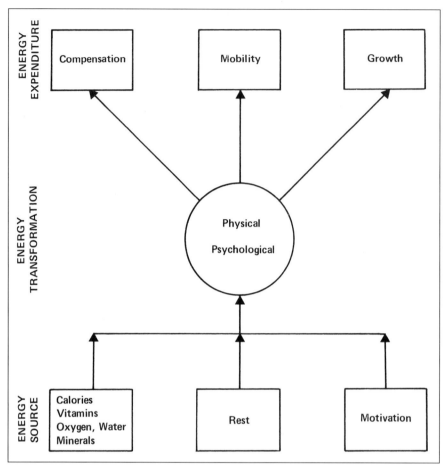

FIGURE 11.1 ➤ Knoebel's interpretation of Ryden energy source-utilization model.

ance, and cellular metabolism. The third construct is energy expenditure. According to Ryden, energy expenditure takes place on three levels: compensation, mobility, and growth. At the compensation level, energy is used for restoration of physical and psychological equilibrium. At the mobility level, energy is spent in work, hobbies, and dealing with the external environment. At the growth level, energy is spent in learning. Figure 11.1 contains Knoebel's interpretation (1978) of Ryden's model (1977).

Energy Requirements in Chronically Ill Persons

To understand the energy deficits in chronically ill persons, a more specific analysis of energy requirements is needed. Energy requirements are discussed in terms of restoration of physical integrity; role expansion and coping with the effects of illness; daily activities that cannot be omitted; and activities that provide social stimulation, recreation, exercise, and learning. In this light, energy requirements include specific energy needs above and beyond that energy needed for basal metabolism. The model presented in Figure 11.2 is the basis for discussion throughout this chapter.

Restoration of physical integrity refers to wound healing (soft tissue and bones), recovering from inflammatory processes, achieving a metabolic balance (as between nutrients, insulin level, and exercise), generating new cells after cell destruction from medical therapy (chemotherapy and radiation therapy), and participating in physical therapy regimens to restore muscle strength. Pathophysiological and therapy demands create a compromised energy state in chronically ill persons.

Role expansion and coping with the effects of illness require energy. Illness demands the individual learn new self-care practices, monitor self-response to therapy, and become sensitive to cues that need action to avert a crisis. Role expansion includes learning the goals, behaviors, and sentiments of the new role. For chronically ill clients, the new role is self-care agent. A self-care agent is the individual (or designate) who carries out self-care practices to meet requisites presented to the individual. Such requisites arise from therapies, developmental needs, and universal needs (Orem, 1985). The role of self-care agent includes varied activities, for example, administering prescribed medications or irrigating a wound.

The new role expectations of the self-care agent are beyond the continuing roles and role expectations. These continuing roles may include mother, housewife, participant in children's school events, member of

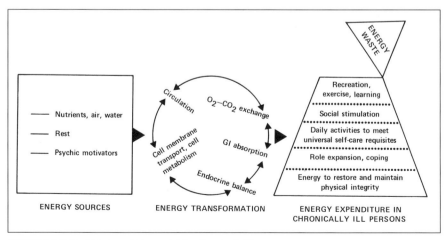

FIGURE 11.2 ➤ Energy analysis model for chronically ill persons.

the symphony women's league, and part-time teacher of an adult art education course. The role expansion increases energy demands, adding new time pressures, problem solving, and anxieties because of role insufficiency. Role insufficiency is any difficulty in learning and/or performing new role behavior.

Coping with the tasks of a chronic illness requires energy. Coping is discussed in detail in Chapter 2, and only examples of energy depletion and coping are presented here; these examples are those that do not require extreme physical exertion such as jogging. Coping strategies such as self-disclosure, examining feelings, developing insights, and relating feelings to behaviors are challenging and energy draining. Other preferred verbal modes of expression used as coping mechanisms—such as laughing, crying, and singing—may be especially taxing to a person with a chronic condition such as severe pulmonary emphysema. The coping tasks of chronic illness identified in Chapter 2 and the psychosocial challenges of illness discussed later in this chapter all require energy.

Energy is required for daily activities that satisfy basic needs. These can be considered synonymous with the universal self-care requisites proposed by Orem (1985), including air, water, food, elimination, activity and rest, solitude and social interaction, and protection from harm. Maintaining personal hygiene and getting dressed are other examples of activities of daily living.

Activities that may not be required daily but are essential to preventing loneliness, low self-esteem, or distorted self-concept are those that provide social interaction. The indirect result of communication is feedback about one's self. The person may think, "I was successful in relating to another; she seemed to enjoy my company; I was able to be of assistance to another; and I received positive feedback about how I am doing." Recreation, exercise, and learning are essential for enjoying life. Adequate energy sources are needed for all three activities to take place.

Energy Wasters

Although energy expenditure in the above categories is required, energy is depleted or wasted in many ways in chronically ill persons.

Preventing energy depletion by eliminating energy waste is a responsibility of nursing. Energy is wasted through physical means, lack of environmental management, and unchanneled psychological reactions and feelings (Table 11.1). Nursing interventions can be directed toward alleviating physical discomforts that waste energy, including inadequate pain management, anorexia, fever, infection, diarrhea, and interrupted sleep. Forced immobility, which occurs when clients are in traction or casts or on bedrest, causes diminished muscle strength and muscle atrophy. Lack of environmental management by poor planning—

Table 11.1 ➤ **ENERGY DEPLETION FROM WASTE**

Physical	Lack of Environmental Management	Psychological
Pain—inadequate pain-management resources	Uncoordinated efforts directed at a variety of tasks to be accomplished	Uncontrolled anxiety
Anorexia		Unexpressed anger, hostility
Fever	Lack of planning before engaging in physical activities	Unresolved grief
Infection	No priorities identified so as to eliminate frustration when least important tasks are not accomplished	
Diarrhea		
Interrupted sleep		
Forced immobility—traction, casts, bedrest	Procrastination; working at avoiding getting started	
	Giving up quickly, necessitating repetitious starting over in task-accomplishment efforts	

for example, by making unnecessary trips up and down stairs—or by lack of priority setting in undertaking the day's activities can be alleviated by the nurse. Nurses can help clients gain insight into their behavior and recognize specific ways their environment can be managed to eliminate energy waste. Psychological energy wasters may include uncontrolled anxiety, unexpressed anger, and unresolved grief. Identifying the client's energy wasters is an important component of the energy-analysis format (see Fig. 11.1). It is nursing's responsibility to assess energy sources, transformation, and expenditure. Specific nursing diagnoses describing energy deficits can be identified.

Nursing Diagnoses and Client-Identified Dilemmas

Specific descriptive nursing diagnostic statements related to energy can be made as a result of the energy analysis, for example:

- Guilt due to an inability to fulfill expected roles according to personally established criteria
- Anxiety due to lack of knowledge regarding the meaning of energy depletion
- Unpredictable daily work-rest patterns due to changing energy availability
- Inability to recognize depleted energy states due to lack of internal awareness

- Helplessness due to a perceived lack of control over energy expenditure
- Frustration related to inability to complete desired tasks within a specified time

Although it is easy to empathize with clients who may have to curtail activities because of energy deficits, the real impact of energy dilemmas can be felt and expressed only by the clients themselves. Consider the following abbreviated descriptions of dilemmas that occur in clients with rheumatoid arthritis.

A 56-year-old woman described the difficulty she felt when she could not even plan ahead during a day. A friend called her at 9 AM and suggested that they meet for lunch. Because the client was feeling stiff, with increased pain and fatigue, at that particular time, she refused lunch, only to be symptom free by noon. The client described the inability to predict how she would feel or how much energy she would have, being unable to plan ahead, feeling somewhat embarrassed over having misjudged her status, and being unable to explain the dilemma to her healthy friend. She regretted needlessly missing an opportunity to alleviate her loneliness (she lived in a rural area, her husband was at work all day, and there were no neighbors who dropped by). She was hesitant, therefore, to initiate social plans with others because of her uncertainty in being able to carry out the plans.

A middle-aged woman who had studied music enjoyed playing classical music on the piano, but was forced to give it up because of lack of strength and dexterity and increased pain in her hands. For someone who had taught music and interpretation of musical works, this posed a difficult problem. She had to refrain from playing for months at a time during arthritic changes to protect her joints and provide them with rest. Absence of this important part of her life caused her real grief.

Another woman expressed role insufficiency because of the weakness and fatigue caused by her arthritis. She stated, "Now that I finally have grandchildren, I am unable to enjoy them. With my arthritis, I'm afraid I will drop the baby. I looked forward to running in the backyard with them; by the time they're old enough to run, I'll be lucky if I'm able to get myself to the table to eat." She expressed feeling deprived of a role that belonged to her and foresaw a future filled with disability and dependence.

A middle-aged factory worker had newly diagnosed rheumatoid arthritis. For a number of years, he and his fellow workers played cards during breaks and lunch hour, keeping a running tally of wins and losses. Now, instead of playing cards, he uses the time to rest and relax in a lounge chair within view of the card playing. He feels that his buddies resent his behavior and view it as an abnormal withdrawal. He feels that it is impossible to convince the other men of his necessity to rest so he can complete his 8-hour shift. The fellow workers have commented to him, "You're making too much of this arthritis thing. You don't look any different than you ever did." He feels socially isolated at work as a result of his careful use of time to restore energy.

A grade-school teacher in her 30s discovered that standing outside for playground duty in the morning and at noon precipitated pain and unnecessarily depleted energy. She felt guilty trying to be excused from this duty even though she could exchange this activity with lunchroom monitoring. She felt it was a reflection that she was inadequate as a teacher.

The feelings of being a burden are readily described by a woman with rheumatoid arthritis. Since her disease has progressively worsened, she has been unable to keep up her own apartment. "Now I have to live with my son, daughter-in-law, and their family. They don't like it any more than I do. I feel in the way, so always present—someone extra who is monitoring their fights and their times of intimacy."

The defining characteristics of energy-deficit diagnoses identified by Pinekenstein (1979) in her study of clients with cancer have relevance for analysis of energy states in general. Two categories of defining characteristics of the nursing diagnosis "energy deficits" were client verbalizations and nonverbal responses. Clients' verbalizations of actual or perceived changes in energy level included references to past energy: "I used to be able to work all day, make supper, and attend an evening class. Now it's difficult to set the table." Clients' references to present energy level may include, "I'm weak, just don't have any strength." Clients may verbalize hopelessness by stating, "I'm just the same, as weak as ever, despite the physical therapy. It's no use."

The nonverbal responses to energy changes include decreased social involvement (irritability, use of frequent rest periods, decreased socialization with family and friends), weight loss and muscle wasting, decreased activity tolerance, excessive use of routine patterns, and use of others' basic mobility resources.

Analysis of energy in clients with rheumatoid arthritis serves as a prototype for energy analysis in chronically ill persons. The unique problems of clients with arthritis are discussed.

Nursing Diagnoses and Etiologies

The American Nurses' Association and Arthritis Health Professions Association have developed Outcome Standards for Rheumatology Nursing Practice (1983). The nursing diagnoses that provide the framework for the standards are as follows:

- Pain management deficit
- Alteration in comfort: stiffness

- Alteration in energy level: fatigue
- Self-care deficit
- Knowledge deficit regarding physical mobility (ambulation)
- Knowledge deficit regarding self-management decisions
- Ineffective individual or family coping
- Disturbance in self-concept

The rationales for each diagnosis, outcome statement, and outcome criterion have been described in detail (ANA, 1983; Pigg & Schroeder, 1984). For example, the outcome statement for the energy alteration diagnosis is "the individual incorporates as part of daily activities, those measures necessary to modify fatigue" (ANA, 1983, p. 5).

ENERGY DEPLETION IN CLIENTS WITH ARTHRITIS

Arthritis afflicts more than 31 million Americans, and 6.5 million of these have rheumatoid arthritis (National Center for Health Statistics, 1989). Rheumatoid arthritis is a systemic autoimmune disease that affects joints and connective tissue. The effects of the disease can be widespread and completely debilitating. The outstanding client challenges are to maintain comfort, preserve joint mobility and function, protect joints during exacerbations, complete prescribed exercise routines to maintain muscle strength and joint function, adhere to medicine regimens, pace activities to conserve energy, and obtain emotional and systemic rest. Because of these challenges, the client with arthritis is described as a prototype for understanding energy deficits in chronically ill clients. Etiologies for fatigue in persons with arthritis may include:

- Anemia
- Increased physical exertion
- Increased disease activity
- Muscle atrophy
- Pain
- Emotional stress
- Inadequate nighttime rest
- Lack of knowledge (about importance of rest, ways to rest, pacing, joint protection, and medication regimen) (Pigg, Driscoll, & Caniff, 1985)

Energy depletion in clients with arthritis results from physiological and psychological processes.

Physiological Energy Depletion

Physiologically, energy depletion in arthritis is caused by inflammation, metabolic changes, and pain. The connective tissue and joint become inflamed. The resultant swelling, stiffness, and muscle spasm cause pain that depletes energy. In rheumatoid arthritis, metabolic changes occur, such as synovial membrane hypertrophy, articular cartilage destruction, and invasion of pannus into the bone. Other systemic effects of the disease include muscle atrophy, myositis, fever, anorexia, and malaise. The inflammatory process can be widespread, as in arteritis, iritis, pneumonitis, and carditis (Groer & Shekleton, 1983). Anemia contributes to poor energy reserve in clients with arthritis and results from the blockage of iron release from the reticuloendothelial cells to the erythropoietic cells (Tobe, 1978).

Joint protection and work simplification directed at reducing stress and pain in affected joints result in decreased inflammation and ultimately in less energy loss. Joint protection includes resting painful swollen joints, balanced body mechanics, avoidance of excess loads, frequent change in body position, and proper use of prescribed corrective devices (Wegener & Kulp, 1988).

Although evening exercise has proved effective in decreasing the arthritis client's morning joint stiffness and immobility (Byers, 1985), changes in fatigue states due to this or other interventions have not been systematically studied. Pain-coping studies have indicated that active pain-coping behaviors correlated with less pain, whereas passive pain coping is related to greater pain (Brown & Nicassio, 1987). Again, fatigue was not a variable included in the pain studies.

Because arthritic pain is chronic, the client cannot anticipate an end to it. The kind of relief experienced in the healing of a surgical incision or the birth of a baby would be a pleasant outcome. However, as Swartz (1970) puts it, "Arthritis is so damned daily."

Effect of Psychological State on Energy

The psychological and social processes and characteristics that accompany chronic illness deplete energy. Psychological characteristics of individuals with chronic illness and those specifically prevalent in clients with arthritis may include anger, contained hostility, depression, hypochondriasis, hysteria, and mourning (Spergel, Ehrlich, & Glass, 1978; Zeitlin, 1977). Energy is wasted in anxiety. Clients have anxiety over uncertainty of energy availability from day to day. Anxiety is also present in pain control and sleep interference. Clients ask themselves, "Where will it hit next? How bad will it be? What residual weakness and deformity will I suffer?"

Fatigue is one manifestation of depression related to learned help-lessness of chronic illness (Potempa, Lopez, Reid, & Lawson, 1986). Potempa et al. suggested that fatigue may be combated in part by perceived self-efficacy, that is, a conviction that one can successfully produce outcomes for oneself (Bandura, 1977). Persons with low self-efficacy have less coping ability and have exaggerated perceptions of fatigue.

Burckhardt (1985) found that positive self-esteem, internal control over health, perceived support, and low negative illness attitude contribute directly to a higher quality of life in persons with arthritis. Persons with osteoarthritis have lower life satisfaction than persons on chronic hemodialysis (LaBorde & Powers, 1980). Chronic pain, social isolation, and preoccupation with illness were posed as factors explaining low life satisfaction of persons with arthritis. Likewise, Bradbury and Catanzaro (1989) found that internal control over health and low negative illness attitude correlated with quality of life in men with arthritis. Loneliness was a predictor of pain in persons with arthritis (DeVellis, DeVellis, Sauter, Harring, & Cohen, 1986). Psychosocial factors in adapting to physical disability are said to include social support, positive self-concept, internal health control, and hardiness (Swanson, Cronin-Stubbs, & Sheldon, 1989). Lambert, Lambert, Klippler, and Mewshaw (1989) confirmed that social support and hardiness were significant predictors of psychological well-being in 122 women with arthritis.

Psychosocial tasks of persons with rheumatoid arthritis include managing role change, lack of control, poor self-esteem, hopelessness, altered body image, and challenged coping ability (Ignatavicius, 1987). Use of "wish-fulfilling fantasy" was noted to be a prevalent coping strategy of 84 persons with rheumatoid arthritis (Parker et al., 1988). This strategy was associated with higher levels of depression, helplessness, and more daily stress. The tendency to use self-blame was also associated with greater psychological distress (Parker et al., 1988).

Understandably, behaviors of anger, frustration, anxiety, and depression result from the symptoms and disability of the disease. There are some unique differences in responses between clients with arthritis and clients with other health problems. Clients with rheumatoid arthritis anticipate the course of their disease to get worse, whereas clients with peptic ulcers do not believe this is the future course for the illness (Williams & Krasnoff, 1964).

Disabling Themes in Arthritis

The diagnosis of rheumatoid arthritis is accompanied by disabling themes in that the client fears becoming crippled, being perceived as being old and nonproductive, and not being understood by loved ones—being unable to obtain empathy from significant others. Mayville (1979) proposed reasons some clients with newly diagnosed rheumatoid arthritis display disabled behaviors after the diagnosis although they had not experienced changes in gait, posture, pace of movement, or joint dexterity before diagnosis. She states that their behaviors are due to previous knowledge of arthritis and associations with others who have the disease, client efforts to reduce joint movement to control pain, low energy levels, joint stiffness, self-concept change of perceiving self as being old and disabled, and acting out a need for empathy as a signal to others to try to understand their plight. Some of the identified responses may be a positive means of coping and a way of decreasing joint aggravation. Other behavior reflecting a distorted self-image may need nursing intervention.

NORMALIZING

The client endeavors to normalize the expending of energy (described as a coping task in Chap. 2). Wiener (1975) described the components of this behavior, which she identified in a study of 21 subjects with rheumatoid arthritis. Normalizing refers to behaviors an individual uses to continue what the individual perceives to be a normal life. The categories of normalizing identified by Wiener were covering up, keeping up, justifying inaction, pacing, eliciting help, and balancing the options.

Covering up allows clients with arthritis to view themselves as they would prefer to be viewed by others. It includes keeping the signs and symptoms of the disease (assistive devices, slowed gait, painful expressions) out of view of others.

Keeping up refers to carrying on with the same schedule one kept before the diagnosis, resulting in exhaustion, excessive time for rest to restore energy, and, in some cases, exacerbation of symptoms and fever. Wiener (1975) identified a paradox in clients who cover up and keep up. These clients long for understanding and sensitivity. They verbalize, "Nobody really knows how bad it is," yet state, "If I acted the way I feel, nobody would want to be around me." The clients use energy in wishing for caring and empathy and at the same time use additional energy to guard against alienating family and friends.

Justifying inaction includes providing rationale to others for not being able to engage in activities or meet their expectations. Justifying inaction may be necessary when pain, stiffness, and uncertainty accompany the illness. However, justifying inaction becomes especially problematic after a history of covering up and keeping up. Imagine the dilemma of the woman who in the morning refused an afternoon bridge club engagement and then is seen shopping later in the afternoon. With the uncertainty of severity of symptoms, with increased morning stiffness on this particular day—"one of her bad days"—the client's worry about being able to cover up and keep up during the social event caused her to refuse the social activity. Yet, when symptoms subsided and she faced real demands of household management, she proceeded to do her grocery shopping.

Pacing is the balancing of activities of "keeping up" with rest. This is the desired normalizing strategy and one with which nurses can help clients. Pacing is an energy conservation behavior. Clients can be helped to analyze their daily activities, to provide for complete rest of all joints at some point during the day, and to get 8 to 10 hours of sleep at night.

Balancing the options available to the client requires energy. Balancing the options includes deciding "whether to keep up and suffer the increased pain and fatigue; whether to cover up and risk inability to justify inaction when needed; whether to elicit help and risk loss of normalizing . . ." (Wiener, 1975, p. 102).

CLINICAL DATA AND NURSING INTERVENTIONS FOR ENERGY CONSERVATION AND RESTORATION

The modified Ryden model provides a framework for nursing intervention for clients with energy deficits. Energy sources can be restored, problems in transformation can be referred for medical therapy, and energy expenditure can be managed (see Fig. 11.2). A client example will be used to demonstrate nursing care.

Mrs. S. is a 54-year-old Hispanic woman with an 18-year history of rheumatoid arthritis. Her ankles, knees, hands, wrists, and shoulders are the most seriously involved joints. Mrs. S. weighs 205 pounds and is 5 feet 4 inches tall. Her most recent contact with the ambulatory arthritis center resulted in intervention and support related to rest and weight reduction, and the fitting of hand-wrist splints for nighttime use. Mrs. S. resides with her Hispanic husband, two or more teenage grandchildren, and nieces and nephews. The exact number of household occupants had been changing from week to week. Neither Mr. S. nor Mrs. S. was employed outside of the home, but Mrs. S. cared for three infant and toddler grandchildren (all in diapers) while their parents worked. This work was physically taxing and frustrating because Mrs. S. could not easily manipulate diaper changes and the other routine child care demands.

Analysis of Energy Sources

NUTRIENTS

Mrs. S.'s energy sources were inadequate. Despite her obesity, she was malnourished. Her intake of milk, fruit, vegetables, and lean protein was lacking. Dietary counseling with her cultural needs in mind enhanced her understanding but did not change her pattern of overeating.

REST

Mrs. S. was not able to obtain any rest during the day in her current home situation; at night her sleep was interrupted by what Mrs. S. described as "the same old pains and worry." In completing a sleep history, data regarding time of retiring, bedtime rituals, sleep environment, and the client's perception of sleep disturbance were obtained. Mrs. S. described her worries as interfering with her sleep.

Mrs. S.'s psychic state served as an energy depleter rather than an energy source. She was filled with anxiety over the care of her many grandchildren and in anticipating how to inform her children that she could no longer keep up the pace the grandchildren demanded. She resented her husband's seeming lack of understanding of her pain, fatigue, and slow mobility; his lack of productivity; and his lack of help with the children. Mrs. S. was worried about their finances. Their gas had already been turned off on one previous occasion.

Mrs. S.'s psychological state accounts for her difficulties with energy sources in all three categories (nutrients, rest, and psychic energizers). To help with underlying anxieties about finances, Mrs. S. was referred to a social worker. The nurse acted as a liaison and accompanied Mrs. S. to the first social-work interview. Mobilizing social-services resources was an initial step in alleviating the financial worries.

Mrs. S.'s concept of self as having been a source of strength within the family (maintaining the family network) was enhanced by enabling her to discuss her perceptions of her role and receiving honest praise for a job well done.

Helping Mrs. S. give up her role of care provider for the babies (her final decision after difficult deliberation) was important for Mrs. S. to rest and alleviate her guilt over her grandchildren's care. Mrs. S. needed help with eliminating role strain by reviewing the alternatives and making a decision. She determined that giving up the role of care provider would help her obtain needed rest during the day and would alleviate her guilt over not being able to manage the children adequately. Her role transition was helped by having her rehearse how she would inform her daughters and by giving her a mental picture of what her day would be like without this responsibility (Meleis & Swendsen, 1978).

Family counseling was begun. This therapy helped increase Mr. S.'s participation in household tasks and increased his empathy for his wife. The teenage grandchildren, who had been truant, are less of a behavior problem because their parents and grandparents became more sensitive to the teenagers' needs and demonstrated interest in them and their school activities.

Now that Mrs. S. is less anxious, data obtained in the sleep history can be used to plan strategies to promote sleep. She needed help in re-establishing a bedtime routine. Her pain management at bedtime needed improvement—to take the prescribed sulindac (Clinoril) and aspirin in the evening. Mrs. S. assumed that these contributed to her wakefulness. She was taught progressive relaxation through autosuggestion (Benson, 1975), which promoted rest and well-being and conserved energy.

Because pain-control strategies conserve energy, other means of helping Mrs. S. were to identify and attempt to eliminate the pain promoters that were part of her routine. For example, she was encouraged to avoid extended exposure to cold weather, such as she experienced standing outside waiting for public transportation. She was taught principles of joint protection and to avoid joint strain during routines, that is, to avoid struggling to open screw-top jars and to seek assistance from Mr. S. The necessity of complying with wearing night splints for joint alignment was reinforced.

As the psychosocial energy expenditure was controlled, Mrs. S. was more motivated to improve her nutritional energy source and to lose weight, thereby further alleviating joint strain caused by excessive weight.

Energy Transformation

Although there was no real energy transformation problem with Mrs. S., the excessive intake of calories needed to be controlled. There was no other pathological problem requiring medical intervention.

Energy Expenditure

ENERGY TO RESTORE AND MAINTAIN PHYSICAL INTEGRITY

Although Mrs. S. was extremely anxious about her arthritis and life circumstances, she had been noncompliant with the night splints, diet, and follow-up clinic visits. Now that her psychological stresses were less, she completed her prescribed exercise routine twice daily and followed through with other therapeutic requirements. Less energy was wasted when she was compliant.

ROLE EXPANSION AND COPING

Mrs. S.'s role expansion (learning self-care practices) was accompanied by role contraction—giving up the child care and related pressures. She was also receiving more attention from her husband, which was a psychic energizer for Mrs. S. Her means of coping was through prayer. Although she no longer attended Mass daily, her active prayer life contributed to her energy source. The positive effect of prayer was emphasized.

DAILY ACTIVITIES TO MEET UNIVERSAL SELF-CARE REQUIREMENTS

Mrs. S. was taught to use her present energy efficiently by planning for what she would be doing and where she would be and collecting what she needed in one trip. For example, she was encouraged to complete her personal hygiene and loosening-up exercises in the warm shower in the morning before descending the stairs to make breakfast. (The bedrooms and bathtub are on the second floor.) She was instructed to plan ahead and take downstairs in the morning what she would need for the rest of the day. When she was working in the kitchen, she was taught ways of supporting her joints and reminded to sit down while working whenever possible. Good body mechanics for proper joint alignment were reviewed.

SOCIAL STIMULATION

Many of Mrs. S.'s neighborhood friends were members of the Hispanic culture. These women provide a support group for one another through weekly meetings at each other's houses. Mrs. S. was encouraged to tell them of her uncertainty of being with them for every get-together. The social and morale benefits of this group of friends were reviewed with Mrs. S., and it was determined that the energy expenditure was worthwhile. She received feedback from the group members about being a worthwhile person. She was also able to express her concerns to people of her own culture and felt truly understood by them. When Mrs. S. is in an energy-depleted state, expenditure in this category could be restricted or eliminated.

RECREATION, EXERCISE, AND LEARNING

Mrs. S. used little, if any, energy for recreation, exercise, and learning. Her sole recreation was watching television. Her exercise was necessarily confined to her prescribed routine of range-of-motion exercises to maintain joint mobility. Developing new enjoyable outlets would assist her psychological well-being, which might include singing in the church choir, participating in the weekly bible study class, and corresponding with residents in her native Mexican village.

ENERGY WASTE

Mrs. S. wasted energy through anxiety and immobilized problem solving. Ways to handle anxiety (practicing relaxation exercises, verbalizing feelings to nurse, taking problems one at a time) were discussed.

Mrs. S. was helped to feel self-confident and to have increased self-esteem so that she could resume family decision-making responsibilities. During periods of disease exacerbations, the increased pain and occasional fever wasted energy. Eliminating routine exercises and increasing rest and analgesics during exacerbations helped conserve energy.

Although not needed for Mrs. S., other nursing strategies can be used to conserve energy for clients with arthritis.

GENERAL NURSING INTERVENTIONS FOR ENERGY CONSERVATION AND RESTORATION

A comprehensive nursing approach to conserving and restoring energy includes restoring energy sources, helping the client evaluate energy expenditure, increase energy reserve, and eliminate energy waste.

The energy sources of nutrients (food, vitamins, minerals, and water) have been discussed in relation to Mrs. S. Clients need to be advised of the necessity to make diet adjustments because of deficiencies or excesses of certain foods. Maintaining intact, healthy autoimmune systems to prevent infections and therefore prevent energy waste depends in part on adequate nutrition. The energy sources of sleep-rest have also been described in relation to Mrs. S. Using a sleep history, promoting relaxation at bedtime, and helping the client establish a bedtime routine are helpful nursing activities.

The role of psychic energizers in restoration of energy states needs further emphasis. Energy is obtained through psychic renewal. Psychic renewal takes place through meditation (prayerful or other), routine progressive relaxation, creative imagery, and autogenic suggestion.

Physiological changes during meditation that indicate a calming effect are decreased respiratory and heart rates, decreased oxygen consumption, lowered or stabilized blood pressure, and decreased skin conductivity (Pelletier, 1977). Autogenic training is a self-induced meditation-relaxation procedure (Luthe, 1969). Briefly, the procedure has six stages. During the first stage, the individual focuses "passive attention" (Pelletier, 1977) on each limb, while repeating, "My right arm feels heavy," and progressing throughout the body—all limbs, torso, neck, jaw, forehead. In the next stage, the same progression of limbs is used to review warmth: "My right arm feels warm." In the third stage, the individual is to emphasize, "My heartbeat is calm and regular." Focusing on depth and ease of respiration takes place in the fourth stage, while the individual repeats the phrase, "It breathes me." During the fifth stage, the individual focuses on warmth in the upper abdomen (solar plexus), stating, "My solar plexus is warm." Instructions for the last stage are to repeat, "My forehead is cool." Pelletier stated that after practice ranging from 2 months to 1 year, the entire series of six stages can be completed in 2 to 4 minutes.

Progressive relaxation, in which the person is taught to focus on the extremes of muscle tenseness and complete relaxation of the same muscle group, is another relaxation method.

Mental imagery is a device for promoting calmness and well-being (see Chap. 16). By creating tranquil images in the mind, mind-body pathways extend this feeling from a mental state to an actual physical state. For example, the client with arthritis may visualize lying on a warm, sunny beach at the ocean. The patient pictures the warm sun and sand easing out the joint stiffness and imagines the ocean waves washing in and out, washing away the pain. The patient feels the body to be very light, agile, and floating. The outcome should be deep relaxation and renewed energy. The autosuggestion may have improved the comfort state as well.

Facilitating psychic energizers includes helping patients with motivation. Their eagerness to accomplish something to establish goals and to anticipate desired outcomes is a psychic energizer.

Any discussion on restoration of energy would be incomplete without referring to the work of Krieger (1979). Krieger's premise is that energy from one human being (healer) can be transferred through touch to another (healee). Energy from the healer helps "repattern the patient's energy level to a state that is comparable to that of the healer" (Krieger, Pepper, & Ancoli, 1979). Although countless cases of improved health after therapeutic touch have been documented, the only quantifiable variable that increases significantly at the .01 level of significance after treatment with therapeutic touch is hemoglobin (Krieger, 1979). The group receiving therapeutic touch had significantly higher hemoglobin than the control no-touch group. Perhaps what was once a maneuver to comfort, share an experience, and reassure that dependence is allowed through touch can now be viewed as a powerful transfer and repatterning of energy from someone who is healthy to someone who is ill. The healing act of touch is not understood scientifically, and no attempt will be made to speculate about what actually happens. For a description of the technique, readers are referred to *The Therapeutic Touch* (Krieger, 1979).

Enabling the Client to Evaluate Energy Expenditure

Helping clients plan more precisely for energy use in various activities is now possible through use of METs. MET refers to metabolic equivalents, the amount of oxygen used per minute per kilogram of body weight. One MET equals 3.5 mL oxygen per kilogram of body weight per minute. Table 11.2 contains a list of activities and their approximate energy expenditure in METs.

Table 11.2 ➤ APPROXIMATE ENERGY EXPENDITURE IN METS (ACTIVITIES OF 70-KG INDIVIDUAL)						
Category of Activity	**Light (1–3 METs)**		**Moderate (3.5–6 METs)**		**Heavy (7+ METs)**	
	Rest	1	Showering	3.5	Ambulation with braces or crutches	6.5
	Sitting	1	Using bedpan	4.0	Walking upstairs with 17-lb load	7.5
	Standing (relaxed)	1	Walking downstairs	4.5		
	Eating	1	Conditioning exercises	4.5		
Personal care activities	Conversation	2	Walking 3.5 mph	5.5		
	Dressing-undressing	2				
	Wash hands, face	2				
	Propelling wheelchair	2				
	Shaving	2.8				
	Bedside commode	3				
	Walking 2.5 mph	3				
	Walking level, slowly, 1 mph	1.2	Walking level 3 mph	3.5	Tennis	6.0
	Painting, sitting	1.5	Bowling	3.5	Trotting horse	6.5
	Playing piano	2.0	Cycling 5.5 mph	3.5	Spading	7.0
	Driving	2.0	Badminton	3.5	Jogging level 5 mph	7.5
	Canoeing 2.5 mph	2.5	Canoeing, sailing	3.5	Skiing	8.0

Category	Activity	Value	Activity	Value	Activity	Value
Recreational activities	Horseback riding, slow	2.5	Golfing	4.0	Squash	8.5
	Volleyball	2.5	Swimming	4.0	Basketball	8.5
			Dancing	4.5	Tennis	8.5
			Gardening	4.5	Cycling 13 mph	9.0
					Gymnastics	10.0
					Football competition	10.0
Housework activities	Hand sewing	1.0	Ironing, standing	3.5	Mowing lawn with nonpower mower	6.5
	Sweeping floor	1.5	Scrubbing floors	3.5	Shoveling	7.0
	Machine sewing	1.5	Hanging wash	3.5	Ascending stairs with 17-lb load	7.5
	Polishing furniture	2.0	Cleaning windows	3.5	Planting	7.5
	Peeling potatoes	2.5	Beating carpets	4.0	Construction physical work	6.5
	Washing small clothes	2.5	Plowing with tractor	4.5	Pick-and-shovel work	8.0
	Kneading dough	2.5	Lifting, carrying 20–44 lb	4.5	Splitting wood with axe	10.0
	Cleaning windows	3.0	Carpentry	5.5		
	Making beds	3.0	Using pneumatic tools	6.0		
	Desk work	1.2				
	Typing (electric)	1.2				
	Radio-TV repair	1.2				
	Draftsman work	1.8				

Source: Adapted from Clark (1992); Krusen, Kottke, and Ellwood (1971); and Karvonen and Barry (1967).

Although MET assignment has been used as a specific energy pre-scription for clients with cardiac disease, specific energy expenditure analysis using METs is helpful for all clients striving to understand energy use and planning for bursts of energy expenditure. Planning includes providing for extra rest and avoiding excessive MET expenditure in a 24-hour period. The anxious client uses more METs per activity than the individual who is not anxious.

Increasing Energy Reserve and Decreasing Energy Waste

Energy reserve is increased through physical conditioning. A regular exercise program strengthens muscles (increases muscle fiber size, endurance, and flexibility); burns calories; improves lung aerobic capacity; and affects fat metabolism by increasing high-density lipoproteins, which is helpful in ridding harmful very-low-density lipoprotein from the body. Exercise increases strength of cardiac contraction and decreases blood pressure and heart rate. In addition, exercise promotes a feeling of well-being. For some, physical exercise not only builds up energy reserve but also decreases an energy waster—anxiety.

Eliminating energy waste as summarized in Table 11.1 in the areas of physical waste, or environmental management, and psychological waste is a nursing responsibility. For clients with arthritis, pain is a typical energy waster. Eliminating pain promoters, such as joint strain, damp environment, inadequate rest, and ineffective analgesic schedules, eliminates energy waste due to pain.

Establishing avenues for self-expression and ventilation of hostility may help alleviate psychological energy wasters—anxiety, anger, and unresolved grief or guilt. Eliminating disabling themes (person's self-perception of being old, crippled, and dependent) will also eliminate some psychic energy waste.

Fatigue may be lessened by selected energy conservation methods: rest, planning for activities and priority setting, pacing, and using splints and assistive devices. Pain management, adequate nutrition, and controlling other means of energy waste are important. Anxiety may be controlled by expanding the client's coping skills. Adherence to medical regimen is necessary to control the disease process (increased disease activity is related to increased fatigue).

Furst, Gerber, Smith, Fisher, and Shulman (1987) proposed an energy conservation program that included teaching persons about predisposing factors for energy loss, developing new skills, and reinforcing these learned behaviors. Predisposing factors include developing knowledge about arthritis and the benefits of balancing rest and activity. Attitudes about possible behavior changes are reviewed with emphasis on personal ability to change behaviors. Enabling skills include developing ability to (1) analyze activities in terms of energy expenditure, (2) identify activity related to pain and fatigue, (3) understand desired good posture and body mechanics, and (4) use joint protection measures. Reinforcement includes helping family and clients recognize behavior changes as positive (Furst, Gerber, & Smith, 1985; Furst, Gerber, Smith, Fisher, et al., 1987).

Fatigue Assessment

Instruments to measure fatigue have been developed. The Piper Fatigue Self Report Scale is a 69-item visual analog scale designed to measure patterns of fatigue including temporal, intensity-severity, affective, sensory, evaluative, associated symptom relief, and fatigue relief (Piper, Lindsey, Dodd, Ferketich, Paul, & Weller, 1989). Other fatigue scales include the Fatigue Symptom Checklist (Yoshitake, 1978) and the fatigue subscale for the Profile of Mood States (McNair, Lorr, & Droppleman, 1971). The Pearson Byars Fatigue Feeling checklist consists of a list of 10 adjective phrases describing fatigue. Clinical assessment of fatigue can be completed by observing appearance, communications, activity, and attitude as well as using a 10-point response format on a single line (visual analog scale) with 0 indicating not tired, full of energy, peppy to 10 indicating total exhaustion (Rhoten, 1982).

Other related instruments specific for the chronically ill or persons with arthritis are listed for the reader's further review and critique before use in research. The Arthritis Helplessness Index (AHI) is a 15-item instrument measuring perceived control (Nicassio, Wallston, Callahan, Herbert, & Pincus, 1985; Stein, Wallston, & Nicassio, 1988; Stein, Wallston, Nicassio, & Castner, 1988). The AHI has a modest internal consistency alpha of .69. Construct validity tests reveal negative correlations between high helplessness and self-esteem and negative correlations between helplessness and internal locus of control (Nicassio et al., 1985). Examples of items include "Arthritis is controlling my life" and "I can do a lot of things to cope with my arthritis" (Nicassio et al., 1985, p. 463). The AHI was modified slightly by removing the term "arthritis" from the items and renaming the scale Rheumatology Attitudes Index (RAI) (Callahan, Brooks, & Pincus, 1988). Criterion validity of the RAI was established by significant correlations with activities of daily living (ADLs), disease activity, and physical function measures. Again, only a modest internal consistency of 0.68 was obtained.

Perhaps the most widely used arthritis functional assessment tool is the Arthritis Impact Measurement Scale (AIMS) (Meenan, Gertman, & Mason, 1980). The AIMS evaluates functional status in terms of physical activity, mobility, ADLs, household activity, and manual dexterity. The AIMS also measures psychological well-being, depression, and anxiety.

Lorig, Chastain, Ung, Shoor, and Holman (1989) developed a scale to measure perceived self-efficacy in persons with arthritis. It is based upon Bandura's (1977) theory that persons' beliefs in their ability to perform tasks or behaviors positively influence their performance. Continued refinement and psychometric review of this scale may be of benefit for nursing research.

SUMMARY

Energy is a power resource. A deficit in energy is often present in individuals with chronic health problems. Analysis of energy states can be guided by using the modified Ryden model (1977), in which energy sources, transformation, and expenditure are determined. Nursing diagnoses are identified, and strategies to alleviate the diagnoses are carried out. Alleviation of energy deficits results in alleviation of a degree of powerlessness. The client with arthritis is described in this chapter as a specific prototype in applying the energy-analysis model summarized in Figure 11.2.

REFERENCES

American Nurses' Association and Arthritis Health Professions Associations (1983). *Outcome standards for rheumatology nursing practice.* Kansas City, MO: American Nurses' Association.

Baldree, K. S., Murphy, S. P., & Powers, M. J. (1982). Stress identification and coping patterns in patients on hemodialysis. *Nursing Research, 31,* 107–113.

Bandura, A. (1977). Toward a unifying theory of behavioral change. *Psychological Review, 84,* 191–215.

Benson, H. (1992). *The relaxation response.* New York: Random House.

Bradbury, V. L., & Catanzaro, M. L. (1989). The quality of life in a male population suffering from arthritis. *Rehabilitation Nursing, 14,* 187–190.

Brown, G., & Nicassio, P. (1987). Development of a questionnaire for the assessment of active and passive coping strategies in chronic pain patients. *Pain, 31,* 53–64.

Burckhardt, C. (1985). The impact of arthritis on quality of life. *Nursing Research, 34,* 11–16.

Byers, R. (1985). Effect of exercise on morning stiffness and mobility in patients with rheumatoid arthritis. *Research in Nursing and Health, 8,* 275–281.

Callahan, L., Brooks, R., & Pincus, T. (1988). Further analysis of learned helplessness in rheumatoid arthritis using a Rheumatology Attitudes Index. *Journal of Rheumatology, 15,* 418–426.

Clark, N. F. (1992). Disturbances in the blood pumping mechanism. In D. Jones, C. F. Dunbar, & M. M. Jirovec (Eds.), *Medical-surgical nursing: A conceptual approach* (2nd ed., pp. 813–839). New York: McGraw-Hill.

DeVellis, R. F., DeVellis, B. M., Sauter, S. V., Harring, K., & Cohen, J. L. (1986). Predictors of pain and functioning in arthritis. *Health Education Research, 1,* 61–67.

Eichel, C. J. (1986). Stress and coping in patients on CAPD compared to hemodialysis patients. *ANNA Journal, 13,* 9–13.

Fagerhaugh, S. (1984). Getting around with emphysema. In A. Strauss (Ed.), *Chronic illness and the quality of life* (2nd ed., pp. 99–107). St. Louis: CV Mosby.

Furst, G., Gerber, L., & Smith, C. (1985). *Rehabilitation through learning: Energy conservation and joint protection: A workbook for persons with rheumatoid arthritis.* Bethesda, MD: U.S. Department of Health and Human Services, National Institutes of Health Publication No. 85–2743.

Furst, G., Gerber, L., Smith, C., Fisher, S., & Shulman, B. (1987). A program for improving energy conservation behaviors in adults with rheumatoid arthritis. *American Journal of Occupational Therapy, 41,* 102–111.

Groer, M., & Shekleton, M. (1983). *Basic pathophysiology: A conceptual approach* (2nd ed.). St. Louis: CV Mosby.

Hart, L. (1978). Fatigue in the patient with multiple sclerosis. *Research in Nursing and Health, 1,* 147–157.

Hart, L., & Freel, M. (1982). Fatigue. In C. Norris (Ed.), *Concept clarification in nursing* (pp. 251–261). Rockville, MD: Aspen Systems.

Haylock, P., & Hart, L. (1979). Fatigue in patients receiving localized radiation. *Cancer Nursing, 2,* 461–467.

Hertanu, J. S., Davis, L., & Focseneanu, M. (1986). Cardiac rehabilitation exercise programs: Outcome assessment. *Archives of Physical Medicine and Rehabilitation, 67,* 431–435.

Ignatavicius, D. (1987). Meeting the psychosocial needs of patients with rheumatoid arthritis. *Orthopaedic Nursing, 6,* 16–21.

Jamar, S. C. (1989). Fatigue in women receiving chemotherapy for ovarian cancer. In S. Funk, E. Tornquist, M. Champagne, L. A. Copp, & R. Wiese (Eds.), *Key aspects of comfort: Management of pain, fatigue, and nausea* (pp. 224–233). New York: Springer.

Kaempfer, S. H., & Lindsey, A. (1986). Energy expenditure in cancer: A review. *Cancer Nursing, 9,* 194–199.

Karvonen, M., & Barry A. (1967). *Physical activity and the heart: Proceedings of a symposium, Helsinki, Finland.* Springfield, IL: Thomas Publishers.

Knoebel, P. (1978). An analysis of energy utilization through the implementation of the Ryden Model. Unpublished paper. Marquette University, Milwaukee, WI.

Kobashi-Schoot, J., Hanewald, G., Van Dam, F., & Bruning, P. (1985). Assessment of malaise in cancer patients treated with radiotherapy. *Cancer Nursing, 8,* 306–313.

Krieger, D. (1979). *The therapeutic touch.* Englewood Cliffs, NJ: Prentice-Hall.

Krieger, D., Pepper, E., & Ancoli, S. (1979). Therapeutic touch: Searching for evidence of physiological change. *American Journal of Nursing, 79,* 660–662.

Krusen, F., Kottke, F., & Ellwood, P. (1971). *Handbook of physical medicine and rehabilitation.* Philadelphia: WB Saunders.

LaBorde, J., & Powers, M. (1980). Satisfaction with life for patients undergoing hemodialysis and patients suffering from osteoarthritis. *Research in Nursing and Health, 3,* 19–24.

Lambert, V., Lambert, C., Klipple, G., & Mewshaw, E. (1989). Social support, hardiness and psychological well-being in women with arthritis. *Image: Journal of Nursing Scholarship, 21,* 128–131.

Lorig, K., Chastain, R., Ung, E., Shoor, S., & Holman, H. (1989). Development and evaluation of a scale to measure perceived self-efficacy in people with arthritis. *Arthritis and Rheumatism, 32,* 37–44.

Luthe, W. (1969). *Autogenic therapy.* New York: Grune & Stratton.

Mayville, K. (1979). The significance of crippling response to rheumatoid arthritis. Unpublished master's thesis. Marquette University, Milwaukee, WI.

McNair, D. M., Lorr, M., & Droppleman, L. F. (1971). *POMS: Manual for Profile of Mood States.* San Diego: Educational and Industrial Testing Service.

Meenan, R. F., Gertman, P. M., & Mason, J. H. (1980). Measuring health status in arthritis: Arthritis Impact Measurement Scales. *Arthritis and Rheumatism, 23,* 146–152.

Meleis, A. I., & Swendsen, L. A. (1978). Role supplementation: An empirical test of a nursing intervention. *Nursing Research, 27,* 11–18.

National Center for Health Statistics. (1989). *Vital and Health Statistics Series 10: Data from the National Survey.* Bethesda, MD: U.S. Public Health Service Publication No. 173.

Nicassio, P., Wallston, K., Callahan, L., Herbert, M., & Pincus, T. (1985). The measurement of helplessness in rheumatoid arthritis: The development of the Arthritis Helplessness Index. *Journal of Rheumatology, 12,* 462–467.

Orem, D. (1985). *Nursing: Concepts of practice* (3rd ed.). New York: McGraw-Hill.

Parker, J., McRae, C., Smarr, K., Beck, N., Frank, R., Anderson, S., & Walker, S. (1988). Coping strategies in rheumatoid arthritis. *Journal of Rheumatology, 15,* 1376–1383.

Pelletier, K. (1977). *Mind as healer, mind as slayer.* New York: Dell Publishing.

Pigg, J. S., Driscoll, P. W., & Caniff, R. (1985). *Rheumatology Nursing: A problems-oriented approach.* New York: John Wiley & Sons.

Pigg, J. S., & Schroeder, P. S. (1984). Frequently occurring problems of patients with rheumatic diseases. *Nursing Clinics of North America, 19,* 697–708.

Pinekenstein, B. (1979). Energy alterations in: Deficiencies, identification and comparison of defining characteristics in five hospitalized clients. Unpublished master's essay, Marquette University, Milwaukee, WI.

Piper, B. (1993). Fatigue. In V. Carrieri, A. Lindsey, & C. West (Eds.), *Pathophysiological phenomena in nursing: Human responses to illness* (2nd ed., pp. 219–234). Philadelphia: WB Saunders.

Piper, B., Lindsey, A., Dodd, M., Ferketich, S., Paul, S., & Weller, S. (1989). The development of an instrument to measure the subjective dimension of fatigue. In S. Funk, E. Tornquist, M. Champagne, L. A. Copp, & R. Wiese (Eds.), *Key aspects of comfort: Management of pain, fatigue and nausea* (pp. 199–208). New York: Springer.

Potempa, K., Lopez, M., Reid, C., & Lawson, L. (1986). Chronic fatigue. *Image: Journal of Nursing Scholarship, 18,* 165–169.

Putt, A. (1978). *General systems theory applied to nursing.* Boston: Little Brown.

Rhoten, D. (1982). Fatigue and the postsurgical patient. In C. Norris (Ed.), *Concept clarification in nursing* (pp. 277–300). Rockville, MD: Aspen Systems.

Ryden, M. (1977). Energy: A crucial consideration in the nursing process. *Nursing Forum, 16,* 71–82.

Spergel, P., Ehrlich, G., & Glass, D. (1978). The rheumatic arthritic personality: A psychodiagnostic myth. *Psychosomatics, 19,* 79–86.

Srivastava, R. H. (1989). Fatigue in end-stage renal disease. In S. Funk, E. Tornquist, M. Champagne, L. A. Copp, & R. Wiese (Eds.), *Key aspects of comfort: Management of pain, fatigue and nausea* (pp. 217–284). New York: Springer.

Stein, M., Wallston, K., & Nicassio, P. (1988). Factor structure of the Arthritis Helplessness Index. *Journal of Rheumatology, 15,* 427–432.

Stein, M., Wallston, K., Nicassio, P., & Castner, N. (1988). Correlates of a clinical classification schema for the arthritis helplessness subscale. *Arthritis and Rheumatism, 31,* 876–881.

Swanson, B., Cronin-Stubbs, D., & Sheldon, J. (1989). The impact of psychosocial factors on adapting to physical disability: A review of the research literature. *Rehabilitation Nursing, 14,* 64–68.

Swartz, F. (1970). The rehabilitation process as viewed from the inside. *Rehabilitation Literature, 31,* 203–204.

Tobe, R. (1978). Anemia. In C. Leitch, & R. Tinker (Eds.), *Primary care.* Philadelphia: FA Davis.

Wegener, S., & Kulp, C. S. (1988). Fatigue and sleep disturbance in arthritis. In J. Sands & J. Matthews (Eds.), *A guide to arthritis home health care* (pp. 185–205). New York: John Wiley & Sons.

Wiener, C. (1975). The burden of rheumatoid arthritis: Tolerating the uncertainty. *Social Science and Medicine, 9,* 97–104.

Williams, R. L., & Krasnoff, A. G. (1964). Body image and physiological patterns in patients with peptic ulcers and rheumatoid arthritis. *Psychosomatic Medicine, 26,* 708.

Winslow, E. H., Lane, L. D., & Gaffney, F. A. (1985). Oxygen uptake and cardiovascular responses in control adults and acute myocardial infarction patients during bathing. *Nursing Research, 34,* 164–169.

Yoshitake, H. (1978). Three characteristic patterns of subjective fatigue symptoms. *Ergonomics, 14,* 175–186.

Zeitlin, D. (1977). Psychological issues in the management of rheumatoid arthritis. *Psychosomatics, 18,* 7–14.

12

Adjustment, Coping Resources, and Care of the Client with Multiple Sclerosis

➤ DEBRA HASTINGS

Multiple sclerosis (MS) is the most predominant of the human demyelinating diseases. It is the most common severe neurological disease of young adults, attacking men and women in their productive years while they are planning for and participating in activities involving the major aspects of their present and future lives such as the selection of their life work and the consideration of marriage and family planning. It is a chronic degenerative demyelinating disease that is sometimes progressive and oftentimes unpredictable in its course. It attacks the central nervous system (CNS) and can have crippling effects upon such vital functions as mobility and balance, vision, speech, coordination, cognitive and emotional abilities, and bowel and bladder control. Like many other chronic diseases, it is characterized by periods of remissions and exacerbations.

Because of increased technology and better supportive care, persons with MS now live longer than before, and individuals in the community and long-term care facilities may cope with the effects of this chronic illness for 30 years or more (Kelly & Mahon, 1988). Therefore,

nurses in a variety of clinical settings may come in contact with individuals afflicted with MS. Because MS strikes during the productive years and can be expected to continue over the course of a lifetime, a special challenge is presented to nurses in all settings. The chronic aspects of this disease stress the need for care that cuts across varied settings and includes the maintenance of physical, psychological, social (Catanzaro, 1980), and spiritual health. Symptom evaluation and management with appropriate referrals are needs of the chronically ill. The physiological, social, spiritual, and behavioral responses to the illness are essential components of nursing care.

This chapter is presented in three sections. An overview of MS is included in Section 1. In Section 2, adjustment to chronic illness and related research, including the results of this author's study on adjustment to MS, are discussed. A case study along with appropriate nursing diagnoses and interventions, using the Neuman Systems Model (Neuman, 1994), is described in Section 3. Neuman's model is a comprehensive systems-based conceptual framework for nursing.

SECTION 1: AN OVERVIEW OF MULTIPLE SCLEROSIS

Pathology

Multiple sclerosis is a disease of inflammation and degeneration of myelin with relative sparing of the axon. Myelin, which is derived from oligodendroglia that surround nerve axons in a winding process, functions to control the passage of ions on which the transmission of nerve impulses depend and also serves as insulation. Therefore, myelin is responsible for the speed of nerve impulse conduction. Demyelination is responsible for the conduction failure representative of MS. Complete conduction failure is related to severe demyelination, whereas slow and intermittent conduction indicates less complete destruction of myelin.

The characteristic pathological feature of MS is the occurrence of irregularly shaped plaques of demyelination, both active and sclerotic, in the cerebellum, white matter of the brain, cranial nerves and spinal cord, the optic nerves, and around the third and fourth ventricles. Recent lesions show partial or complete degeneration of myelin and perivascular infiltration with lymphocytes and other mononuclear cells, suggestive of the inflammatory process. Areas of inflammation that interrupt the myelin occur in unpredictable patchy distributions, which can be as tiny as a pinpoint. Brief exacerbations followed by complete remissions in 2 or 3 weeks are thought to indicate early inflammatory depression of neurotransmission without irreversible myelin destruction.

Long-standing lesions, caused by repeated and progressive attacks and the resultant inflammation, are hard, sclerotic plaques that exhibit no inflammatory reaction. Chronic lesions appear gray and shrunken,

and myelin has been removed by phagocytosis, with the degree of myelin loss being dependent upon severity of the inflammation. Axis cylinders are lessened in number, and there is a lack of cellularity and a marked gliosis.

Although the axons are usually preserved, especially in the early stages of the disease, there may be some axonal degeneration in severe, long-standing MS. When axons do become involved, secondary degeneration of the wallerian type takes place in the long tracts of the spinal cord (Pallett & O'Brien, 1985; Schneitzer, 1978; Slater & Yearwood, 1980; Sutherland, 1986).

Incidence and Prevalence

Multiple sclerosis occurs most frequently in people between the ages of 15 and 50 years, with its onset generally occurring between the ages of 20 and 40 years (Holland, McDonnell, & Wiesel-Levison, 1981; Slater & Yearwood, 1980). According to Kritchevsky (1988) the mean age of onset is 33 years with the mean age of diagnosis being 37 years. The disease rarely appears before the age of 10, and approximately 10 percent of cases begin after the age of 50.

While the disease strikes both sexes, females may be affected as often as two times that of males, while whites are affected twice as often as blacks, with an insignificant distribution among other racial groups. Individuals of northern European ancestry are at greater risk of contracting MS, possibly due to immunogenetic factors (Holland, Wiesel-Levison, & Madonna, 1984; Slater & Yearwood, 1980).

One of the more puzzling aspects of MS is its uneven geographic distribution, as there is a wide prevalence of MS (30 to 80 cases per 100,000 population) in the northern, temperate zones in North America and Europe, especially above the 40th north parallel, as well as in the southern portions of New Zealand and Australia. It occurs less frequently in countries near the equator (Franklin & Burks, 1985; Whitaker, 1983). It is believed that geographic locale is significant until age 15 years. Movement after this age does not alter the risk factors (Holland, McDonnell, & Wiesel-Levison, 1981).

Etiology

Although the specific cause of MS is not known, there are several schools of thought as to why an individual develops the disease. One theory is that MS is caused by a slow viral infection acquired in late childhood or early adolescence, with a long interval or latency period before clinical symptoms manifest themselves. Exposure to this viral agent in early life leads to the formation of protective antibodies and immunity. The resultant reinfection or infection in adult life depends

upon genetic vulnerability or the possibility of exposure to an overwhelming infection (Schneitzer, 1978; Sutherland, 1986; Whittington, 1983).

Although MS is neither contagious nor hereditary, a familial tendency to develop MS has been noted, without the confirmation of any true genetic pattern. Although there is a 12- to 20-fold increase in the frequency of MS among first-degree relatives of persons with MS, the genetic effect manifests itself as one that will increase the predisposition for acquisition rather than supporting a definite pattern of inheritance. It is believed that this predisposition may indicate exposure to shared environmental factors. In addition, recent studies of the distribution of histocompatibility antigen (HLA) genetic marker in persons with MS disclosed an overrepresentation of A3, B7, and Dw2 types. In Europe, North America, and Australia HLA-A3 and HLA-B7 and related antigens Dw2 and DR2 occur in a large proportion of persons with MS and their relatives, whereas the frequency of HLA-Dw2 and DR2 types is much less common in a control population and in ethnic groups in whom MS is less common. However, the exact relationship of these factors to the etiology of the illness is not as yet known (Holland et al., 1981; Kritchevsky, 1988; Pallett & O'Brien, 1985; Sutherland, 1986; Whitaker, 1983).

Immune and autoimmune responses are being explored as illness etiologies. It is believed that the disease process may result from an antigen-antibody reaction, immune response to a previous illness, or an immune process (Holland et al., 1981). Sutherland (1986) noted that an abnormality of cerebrospinal fluid (CSF) immunoglobulins has been found in the majority of MS patients. Gamma globulin is increased, while the proportion of the total protein that consists of immunoglobulin G (IgG) is increased. After electrophoresis, diffuse protein bands (the oligoclonal pattern) occur in the gamma globulin region. However, investigation of the general immune status of persons with MS has not shown a consistent blood abnormality, although when more sensitive tests are used, regulatory lymphocytes (cells that promote an immune response or suppress it) have been found to be abnormal (Whitaker, 1983).

According to Morgante, Madonna, and Pokoluk (1989), research has implicated a retrovirus in the disease process, precisely, human T-cell lymphotropic virus type I (HTLV-I). However, they state that further study is needed to substantiate this finding, which may some day facilitate an effective treatment for the illness.

Diagnosis

A medical diagnosis of MS is usually based on the presenting history and physical examination because there is no specific diagnostic test for MS. The physician usually makes the diagnosis when there is

evidence of multiple lesions in time and space. Table 12.1 presents formal diagnostic criteria that have been proposed to aid in establishing a diagnosis of MS. However, the vast symptomatology exhibited by individuals who present for diagnosis makes it necessary to first rule out various other neurological disorders such as tumors and vascular and degenerative diseases.

Establishing a diagnosis can be both difficult and frustrating for the client and clinician. In the early stages of the disease, symptoms are often transient, lasting not just hours or days, but sometimes only minutes. They may be bizarre and are often dismissed as irrelevant by both the patient and physician.

Some clients do not exhibit symptoms that meet the diagnostic criteria, and for others, symptoms may be obvious but neurological deficits minimal. Diagnostic testing for these individuals may be helpful. According to Franklin and Burks (1985) the tests that most often serve as important diagnostic adjuncts are evoked potential testing and CSF evaluation. Clients are frequently given a lumbar puncture to obtain spinal fluid, as almost all people with MS exhibit an increase in antibody (IgG). Eighty-five percent of clients with clinically definite MS have abnormal oligoclonal bands in the IgG zone on CSF electrophoresis (Davison, 1982; Kritchevsky, 1988). Other CSF abnormalities include (1) an elevated total protein, (2) increased white blood cells, (3) an abnormal colloidal gold curve, and (4) the presence of immunoglobulin M (Fischbach, 1995; Holland et al., 1981; Thompson, McFarland, Hirsch, Tucker, & Bowers, 1989).

Evoked potentials are computer-averaged electrical impulses that permit measurement of the rate of nerve impulse transmission through the CNS. Slowed conduction in the visual, auditory, or somatosensory pathway is evidence for the presence of demyelination in that tract even without the presence of associated symptomatology. For example, the

---

Table 12.1 ➤ **PROPOSED DIAGNOSTIC CRITERIA FOR THE DIAGNOSIS OF MULTIPLE SCLEROSIS**

1. Neurological examination must reveal objective abnormalities that can be attributed to dysfunction of the CNS.
2. Examination or case history must supply evidence that two or more parts of the CNS are involved.
3. Evidence of CNS disease must predominantly reflect involvement of white matter.
4. Involvement of the neuraxis must have followed one of two time patterns:
   (a) Two or more episodes of worsening, each lasting 24 hours or more, and each a month or more apart
   (b) Slow or stepwise progression of signs and symptoms over at least 6 months
5. At onset, the client must be from 10 to 50 years old.
6. A physician competent in clinical neurology should decide that the client's condition could not be better explained on the basis of some other disease.

Source: Adapted from Holland et al. (1981); Poser (1983); and Schneitzer (1978).

evoked visual response tests the rate of the visual signal from eye to brain. An abnormal finding would be a delayed blink reflex. The test is most valuable in identifying clinically silent lesions. If all three tests are performed, nearly 80 to 85 percent of clients with a clinically definite diagnosis will have an abnormality on at least one of the tests (Franklin & Burks, 1985; Kritchevsky, 1988; Slater & Yearwood, 1980).

Other diagnostic tools include the use of computed tomography (CT) scan and magnetic resonance imaging (MRI). CT scanning displays a sectional x-ray of the brain tissue, and increased concentrations of the contrast medium used for the test appear in the areas of demyelination. The test may show ventricular enlargement and cerebral atrophy with long-term disease, and areas of low attenuation around cerebral ventricles. However, this test does not provide information about the cause of the lesions, and only 20 percent of clients with clinically definite disease will have CT scan abnormalities (Kritchevsky, 1988; Whittington, 1983; Wierenga, 1993).

Magnetic resonance imaging of the brain and spinal cord may be especially valuable as unsuspected abnormalities can be detected, especially those in the periventricular area and the brainstem, and other CNS disease disorders that may mimic MS can be excluded. The test frequently showed characteristic MS lesions within the white matter of the CNS and may demonstrate a second lesion, making MS the probable diagnosis (Davison, 1982; Kritchevsky, 1988).

Signs and Symptoms

The signs and symptoms of MS are related to the areas of demyelination and duration of the lesion, and because demyelination may occur anywhere in the CNS, the client may manifest a variety of signs and symptoms. The lesions of MS may be located almost anywhere in the white matter of the CNS neuraxis, which includes the white matter of the cerebral hemispheres, optic nerves, brainstem, cerebellum, and spinal cord. The symptoms of MS can mimic those of stroke or tumors, and the sometimes bizarre and transient nature of the symptoms may be mistaken for a psychiatric disorder. Although some individuals present with evidence of wide-spread disease from the onset, others may present with isolated focal involvement (Kritchevsky, 1988).

According to Gulick (1989), signs of the illness have been categorized into eight neurological functional systems. Table 12.2 presents these signs and symptoms.

Clinical Course and Prognosis

Multiple sclerosis in and of itself is almost never a cause of death. On the average, those individuals with MS survive for 35 years after the

Table 12.2 ➤	**EIGHT CATEGORIES OF NEUROLOGIC FUNCTIONAL SYSTEMS AND THEIR RELATED SIGNS AND SYMPTOMS**
System	**Signs and Symptoms**
Pyramidal	Positive Babinski, paralysis of one or more limbs, stiffness, weakness, paralysis, fatigue
Cerebellar	Intention tremor, hypotonia in any limb with truncal ataxia and broad-based gait, dizziness, clumsiness, slurred speech
Brainstem and cranial nerves III to XII	Weakness in facial structures, nystagmus, diplopia, scanning speech
Sensory	Disruptions in touch, vibratory, and position sense including numbness, tingling, pins and needles
Bowel/bladder	Hesitancy, urgency, frequency, urinary and/or bowel retention
Visual/optic	Blurred vision and visual field defects as central or paracentral scotoma (Pallett & O'Brien, 1985)
Mental/cerebral	Depression, memory loss, disorientation
Miscellaneous	Includes those not mentioned above such as seizures, aphasias, spasticity

Source: Adapted from Gulick (1989).

onset of illness. Although the course of the disease can be unpredictable, there are certain patterns in which the course of the disease can fit. About 20 percent of the cases fall into the *benign* form, which is characterized by few, mild, early attacks and complete or nearly complete clearing. Twenty-five percent of the cases are classified as *exacerbating-remitting,* which exhibit more frequent early attacks with less complete clearing. Roughly 40 percent of the cases are of the *chronic-relapsing* type, characterized by fewer and less complete remissions after attacks and by disability that is cumulative and more significant than the other types mentioned previously. The *chronic-progressive* form has a more insidious onset with a course that is slowly progressive without remissions and that is seen in about 15 percent of the cases. A small proportion of clients with MS develop an acute form of the illness that progresses rapidly with incomplete remissions of short duration. This type of MS can be fatal within a few months or years, and it is mainly a result of severe brainstem disease, especially pertaining to the medulla (Scheinberg, 1983; Wierenga, 1993).

Although 50 percent of those with MS will be employed 10 years after diagnosis, by 20 years after diagnosis, only 30 percent will remain employed (Slater & Yearwood, 1980). If the disease shortens the life span, it is usually a result of infection affecting the lungs, urinary tract, or skin due to the paralyzed state (Pallett & O'Brien, 1985; Scheinberg, 1983).

Treatment Modalities

There is no specific preventive or curative treatment for MS, so efforts must focus on supportive therapeutic measures (Slater & Yearwood, 1980). Like the disease itself, treatment efforts are very frustrating because the cause of MS is not known, and one can only guess as to the mechanism of tissue damage. There are, however, various treatment modalities that may be used to ease the symptoms or shorten an exacerbation. All the treatment approaches center around an attempt to stabilize the client with MS who is advancing through different manifestations of the ongoing disease process (Holland et al., 1981).

Scheinberg and Geisser (1983) divided treatment regimens into four categories:

1. Pharmacological: Includes the use of steroids and corticotropin, thought to be useful in decreasing the severity and duration of exacerbations in certain cases. Used only on a short-term basis because of their potent side effects, they do not seem to have an effect on long-term outcome (Franklin & Burks, 1985). Immunosuppressive medications such as azathioprine (Imuran) and cyclophosphamide (Cytoxan) are another mode of treatment, but they cause side effects such as bone marrow depression, bleeding from reduced platelet counts, and various gastrointestinal problems (Whittington, 1983). Other medications used to treat the various symptoms of MS include baclofen (Lioresal) and diazepam (Valium) for spasticity; oxybutynin (Ditropan) and propantheline (Pro-Banthine) for bladder dysfunction; and tricyclic antidepressants such as amitriptyline (Elavil) for depression.
2. Surgical treatment: May consist of cutting nerves or tendons to decrease spasticity.
3. Physical therapy: To maintain muscle tone and strength.
4. Psychological treatment: Includes individual counseling, support group membership, and peer support.

Nursing Diagnoses

Using grounded theory methodology, Gould (1983) discovered that the most frequently occurring nursing diagnosis in 15 persons with MS was self-esteem disturbance related to altered body image (occurring in seven subjects in the sample). Other frequently occurring diagnoses were (1) self-care deficit level I: bathing, (2) social isolation related to impaired mobility, (3) potential ineffective family coping, and (4) sleep pattern disturbance related to anticipatory grieving.

Kelly and Mahon (1988) identified a variety of nursing diagnoses based upon the pathophysiology and psychosocial ramifications of the illness, which include (1) impaired physical mobility related to muscle weakness, (2) alterations in comfort related to physical pain, (3) bowel and bladder incontinence and sexual dysfunction all related to altered nerve innervation, and (4) potential for alterations in individual coping related to multiple stressors.

In addition to a nursing diagnosis framework, two other authors offer different approaches to the care of the client with MS. Cantanzaro (1980) discussed the care of the patient with MS in terms of the American Nurses' Association (ANA) Standards of Nursing Practice as they provide criteria for evaluating the quality of care, regardless of the setting. Gulick (1984) used Orem's self-care model as an organizing framework for a case study of an MS client with the progressive form of the illness, which illustrates a number of self-care deficits typically experienced by clients with MS and their families.

Further explication of nursing diagnoses along with appropriate interventions and outcomes specific to the client with MS, organized by a systems nursing framework, are explored in the case study presented in Section 3 of this chapter.

The next section of this chapter explores the concepts of psychosocial adjustment to chronic illness, and more specifically, adjustment to MS. Because of the unpredictability of MS, including (1) the potential for remissions and exacerbations, (2) variability in symptomatology, (3) the lack of a known cause, and (4) the disturbing knowledge that there is no cure, adaptation to MS can be difficult and frustrating. A working knowledge of these phenomena is important for the nursing practitioner who is responsible for providing professional care in conjunction with the planning and implementation of appropriate and strategic nursing interventions.

SECTION 2: ADAPTATION TO CHRONIC ILLNESS

When individuals are diagnosed as having a chronic and/or disabling illness, they go through a process of adapting to a disease that can be fraught with unpredictability, remissions, and exacerbations. Adaptation is a complex process that varies from one illness to another and is influenced by both internal and external factors ranging across the biological, psychological, interpersonal, and sociocultural spheres of life. Although life demands for the chronically ill remain the same, or are greater than before the onset of the illness, the capacity to respond in a satisfying way is often diminished (Dimond, 1979, 1983; Pollock, 1986).

Various definitions or conceptualizations of adaptation are noted in the literature (Derogatis & Lopez, 1983; Mechanic, 1977). The following conceptualization offered by Feldman (1974) (referred to as *readaptation*) is appropriate for nursing's holistic focus. Readaptation presupposes the ability of the individual to reach a high level of wellness through the use of positive dependency, that is, relying upon others appropriately while honestly accepting one's differences and the special needs and conditions the illness imposes:

> . . . coming to terms existentially with the reality of chronic illness as a state of being, discarding both false hope and destructive hopelessness, restructuring the environment in which one must now function. Most importantly, readaptation demands the reorganization and acceptance of the self so that there is a meaning and purpose to living that transcends the limitations imposed by the illness. (p. 290)

The intrusion of a chronic and disabling illness is a significant life crisis, posing a major challenge (Feldman, 1974). The salient features of chronic illness, including its long-term nature, uncertainty, expense, and the proportionately greater efforts at palliation; the associated problem such as symptom control, preventing and/or living with social isolation, and the prevention and management of medical crises, in addition to the unpredictable dilemmas of symptom exacerbation, failure of therapy, and physical deterioration despite adherence to the prescribed regimen, result in a lack of control in all its aspects. These factors counteract successful adaptation to illness (Miller, 1992; Strauss et al., 1984).

Individuals with MS may experience feelings of powerlessness caused by any of these factors in addition to (1) multiple and unpredictable symptomatology, (2) inability to perform own self-care, (3) forced dependency on others, (4) difficulty in establishing a definitive diagnosis, including anxiety related to the diagnostic process, and (5) the possibility of giving up a career.

The factors that may precipitate powerlessness among persons with MS, along with other attributes of the disease, can also potentiate poor illness adjustment. Difficulty with adjustment to MS has been substantiated. Surridge (1969) found 25 percent of a sample of 108 persons with MS to be depressed. In a sample of 30 persons with MS, Whitlock and Siskind (1980) noted that these subjects manifested more depression before and since their illness onset as compared with a group of 30 subjects experiencing other neurological afflictions with a similar degree of disability. Gould (1983) also noted the existence of emotional disturbances in 15 persons with MS, whereas Hart (1978) found that in samples of 335 subjects with MS and 39 healthy subjects, a greater percentage of the MS group experienced anxiety, nervousness, and emotional stress. Harper, Harper, Chambers, Cino, and Singer (1986) noted that a sample of 301 persons with MS had significantly lower states of health than comparison groups in terms of (1) physical activity, (2) social health, (3) emotional health, and (4) perceived quality of life. Tan

(1986) found that 37 adults with MS had difficulties in emotional and interpersonal adjustment and in overall psychosocial functioning as compared with 68 adults with epilepsy and 42 healthy adults.

Models of Adaptation to Multiple Sclerosis

It is apparent that adapting to and living with MS can be difficult. As with any of the chronic illnesses, the adjustment process itself can be lengthy, perhaps compounded by the psychological implications of the disease. Matson and Brooks (1977) developed a model of adaptation to MS based upon their study of the social-psychological adjustment of 174 persons with MS. The stages of adaptation included (1) denial, (2) resistance, (3) affirmation, and (4) integration. In the stage of *integration,* which is lengthy and must be reestablished with each exacerbation, the client is spending energy on matters other than health and can find certain beneficial aspects of the situation, such as a deeper sensitivity to life's experience.

LaRocca, Kalb, and Kaplan (1983) outlined four stages that clients with MS follow in the process of adjustment. The first stage is that of *uncertainty,* which may predominate after the symptoms first appear and before a diagnosis is made. The person may feel nervous and confused, and because establishing a diagnosis may take an indefinite time, this stage can be lengthy. However, because of the nature of the illness, uncertainty never ends. Once the diagnosis has been made, the client will go through the stage of *acceptance,* when feelings such as shock, disbelief, denial, and confusion may be experienced. Acceptance is difficult because it means coming to grips with forced change due to loss, which is both painful and upsetting. Once acceptance has begun, and some degree of change has started to take place, *adaptation* will begin. Reactions may include shifts in self-concept and body image, anger, and depression. The task of this stage is the preservation of one's quality of life while being able to incorporate the physical, psychological, and social changes brought about by the illness into everyday life. The client tackles the most critical emotional task involved in adjustment: grieving, such as for lost abilities and experiences. Eventually the disease is successfully woven into the facets of everyday life. Once the necessary adjustments take place, *emergence* can begin where there is a lessening of nervousness and anger and a widening of perspective. The major task to be accomplished is to place the illness in perspective as one carries on with everyday life. The physical, emotional, and social changes that have been required have been met and integrated as much as possible into the person's lifestyle. Adaptation is ongoing and lifelong, requiring constant investments of energy to keep life changes and a sense of self intact.

Coping Resources: Factors Influencing Adaptation to Chronic Illness

Adaptation to MS has been shown to be influenced by such factors as duration of disease (Matson & Brooks, 1977), physical dysfunction, stressful life events, and marital status (Zeldow & Pavlou, 1984). Coping resources are important to a person's response to the diagnosis of a chronic illness and its subsequent treatment. Three coping resources that have been noted in the literature to have a significant impact on adjustment to chronic illness and are congruent with nursing's holistic framework are spirituality, hope, and social support.

SPIRITUALITY

Colliton (1981) defined spirituality as "the life principle that pervades a person's entire being, including volitional, emotional, moral-ethical, intellectual, and physical dimensions, and generates a capacity for transcendent values" (p. 492). It can be perceived in terms of personal views and behaviors that signify a sense of relatedness to a transcendent dimension or to something greater than oneself. Spiritual transcendence emphasizes an openness to a perceived environment that goes beyond its spatial and temporal boundaries (Reed, 1987).

Although spirituality can be viewed as a human need defined in terms of a search for meaning and purpose in life (Sims, 1987), it also encompasses the need for love and relatedness and the need for forgiveness (Shelly & Fish, 1988). According to Shelly and Fish (1988):

> . . . a person who knows God's forgiveness can be at peace with God, himself and other people. He has a new awareness of God as his Father who gives life meaning and purpose. He can also experience God's love, which will in turn enable him to love God, himself and others. (p. 53)

Spirituality goes beyond the boundaries of organized religion. However, according to Ruffing-Rahal (1984), religion is the principal aspect of spiritual experience and is "an institutional haven of strength, serenity, and faith against life crises" (p. 12). O'Brien (1982b) stated that most of humankind has had spiritual needs met through the functions of organized religion.

According to Soeken and Carson (1987), nursing's holistic perspective views the client as a balance of mind, body, and spirit, with each dimension affecting or being affected by the others. The spiritual dimension can be viewed as the unifying force that integrates all the other dimensions of the human. The crises brought on by chronic illness may cause impaired functioning of mind-body-spirit systems (Miller, 1985;

Soeken & Carson, 1987). The impaired functioning of these integrated systems can result in spiritual distress, a disruption of one's spiritual well-being.

As the wholeness of body or mind can be considered a state of well-being, the wholeness of one's spirit can then be considered spiritual well-being (Soeken & Carson, 1987). Spiritual well-being is a "sense of harmonious interconnectedness between self, others, nature, and Ultimate Other, which exists throughout and beyond time and space" (Hungelmann, Kenkel-Rossi, Klassen, & Stollenwerk, 1989, p. 394). Spiritual well-being has been viewed as the cornerstone of health that enables holistic integration of a person's inner resources (Stuart, Deckro, & Mandle, 1989). Persons who have spiritual health have (1) an inner state of peace and joy, (2) freedom from abnormal anxiety and guilt, and (3) a sense of security and direction in the quest for life's goals and activities (O'Brien, 1982b).

Although there has been little research in the area of spirituality and spiritual well-being and adjustment as it relates to chronic illness, several studies attest to the importance of this relationship. O'Brien (1982a) found religious faith to be a variable of importance to illness-related and treatment-related adjustment in a sample of 126 chronically ill clients on dialysis, whereas Miller (see Chap. 2) found prayer and faith to be the second most frequent coping strategy used by a sample of 56 chronically ill adults. Thirty-one women receiving their initial chemotherapy course for breast cancer were studied by Brandt (1987), who found a statistically significant negative relationship between hopelessness and religious beliefs. Those women who perceived their spiritual beliefs as helpful in coping tended to have lower levels of hopelessness. Sodestrom and Martinson (1987) interviewed 25 nurses and 25 oncology clients to ascertain their perspectives on clients' spiritual strategies and found that of 96 percent of clients who professed a religious affiliation, 88 percent found their meaning and purpose in life through their belief in and relationship with God. A significant relationship between hope and coping in 120 adults with cancer was found by Herth (1989), who also found that strength of religious convictions was significantly related to the variables of hope and coping.

Only one MS adjustment study discussed spirituality and adjustment to MS (Matson & Brooks, 1977). In a sample of 174 adults with MS, religion was found to be a highly rated coping strategy, and several subjects gave several insightful comments such as, "God will not give us a cross heavier than we can bear. Either you survive or you succumb. If you survive, you profit from the experience" (p. 248). The researchers concluded that using religion was a common and effective way of adjusting to the disease and that the illness had afforded some subjects the time to get in touch with the more essential values.

HOPE

Slater and Yearwood (1980) stated that because of the complex elements in the coping process of clients with MS, health professionals must be able to thwart a natural tendency toward depression and negativism in clients and families. Optimizing the belief that someone cares and that there is *hope* for a return of self-esteem and self-control is fundamental to the management of MS.

Hope is an essentially positive phenomenon necessary for healthy coping whose key purpose is the avoidance of despair (Korner, 1970). It can be thought of as a complex human experience; a mixture of feelings and thoughts that center on the fundamental belief that there are solutions to important human needs and problems (Lange, 1978). The opposite end of the hope continuum is hopelessness. It is a sense of the impossible; what one wants to do is beyond reach. There are feelings that life is too much to handle, and a person may feel a sense of overwhelming defeat or loss of control over oneself. There may also be feelings of intense despair and futility (Lange, 1978; Roberts, 1978; Schneider, 1980).

To inspire hope is an acknowledged part of nursing care. Stoner (1982) stated that nursing authors have written more about hope and have possibly done more to describe and define hope than have other health professionals.

Craig and Edwards (1983) noted that the preservation of a sense of hope is essential for the chronically ill in the face of an uncertain future, and Miller in Chapter 2 classified the maintenance of hope despite uncertainty or a downward illness course as a coping task or challenge. Although illness can be viewed as a crisis situation leading to a state of despair, the situation can also provide conditions for hope. Hope nurtures a person's transition from being weak and vulnerable to that of functioning or living as fully as possible. Hope allows a person to use a crisis as an opportunity for growth (Miller, 1992).

A relationship between health and/or illness and hope has been noted in the literature. Forsyth, Delaney, and Greshman (1984) interviewed 50 hospitalized chronically ill adults and found that they fought to maintain hope and the feeling that they were winning over the disease by adopting specific attitudes that convinced them that they were not helpless victims of the illness. Rideout and Montemuro (1986) studied 23 persons with congestive heart failure and found that those individuals who were more hopeful maintained their involvement with life. Baldree, Murphy, and Powers (1982) and Gurklis and Menke (1988) found hope to be a highly rated coping strategy used by two samples of clients on hemodialysis, and Brockopp, Hayko, Davenport, and Winscott (1989) found significant correlations between perceived level of control and eight issues related to hope and information seeking in 56 adults with cancer. There were no studies found in the literature that examined hope and adjustment in relation to MS.

SOCIAL SUPPORT

Interest in social support has escalated since the 1970s as noted by the increased amount of research and the number of disciplines studying the concept. Several reasons for this interest are (1) its possible role in the etiology of disease and illness, (2) the role it may play in the rehabilitation and treatment of illness, and (3) the function it may have in helping with the conceptual integration of the literature regarding psychosocial factors and illness (Cohen & Syme, 1985).

Social support is actually a set of concepts or a multidimensional construct. It can be viewed as "resources provided by others" (Cohen & Syme, 1985, p. 4) or individuals as interpersonal resources who provide gratification of basic human needs in relationships (Hubbard, Muhlenkamp, & Brown, 1984). Weiss (1974) conceptualized social support as six categories of relational provisions: (1) attachment, (2) social integration, (3) opportunity for nurturance, (4) reassurance of worth, (5) a sense of reliable alliance, and (6) obtaining of guidance.

Sources of support can be formal or informal. Formal sources include professional helpers, and informal sources consist of those such as spouses, friends, and relatives (Tilden, 1986).

Social networks can be defined as the number and types of ties one maintains with others (Gottlieb & Green, 1984), or a subset of persons upon whom one relies for socioemotional, instrumental, or informational aid (Hibbard, 1985). Social networks are viewed from two perspectives: structural, which refers to network links, and functional, which refers to the quality and nature of the links. The structural properties of social networks most appropriate to social support are (1) size, (2) strength of ties, (3) density, (4) homogeneity of membership, (5) dispersion of membership, (6) frequency of contact, (7) multiplexity, (8) ratio of kin to nonkin, and (9) reciprocity of links (Dimond & Jones, 1983).

According to Cohen and Syme (1985), there are two main hypotheses of interest regarding social support and its relationship to health. The buffering hypothesis states that social support protects individuals from the harmful effects of stress. It is thought that increases in the amount of stress place people at risk for illness but that the presence of adequate levels of support should buffer this stress.

The second hypothesis states that support enhances health regardless of the level of stress (Cohen & Syme, 1985). According to Hibbard (1985), social support may actually lessen the likelihood of exposure to stressful events, for example, through group norms and feedback. Individuals with adequate support are more apt to practice positive health behaviors as they receive encouragement or pressure to do so from within their network (Tilden, 1986).

Although previous research has shown an association between social support and adjustment to chronic illness (Corbin & Strauss, 1988; Northouse, 1988), several studies have also indicated that a significant relationship exists between social support and adjustment to MS. Crawford and McIvor (1985) studied the benefits of group psychotherapy for persons with MS in terms of illness adjustment. Based upon a battery of test results examining depression, anxiety, locus of control, and self-esteem, 41 subjects were placed in one of the three following groups: (1) insight oriented, (2) current events, or (3) control. After 50 sessions, the results indicated that those individuals in the insight-oriented group demonstrated significantly less depression than the others, and both the current events and insight-oriented groups were significantly more internally oriented than the control group. The authors believe that this may be due in part to the buffering effects provided by the social support system that may be developed within the group setting.

Fifty adults with MS were studied by Braham, Houser, Cline, and Posner (1975) to assess their social needs (nonmedical support or action). Findings of the study indicated that the greatest number of needs were found in (1) subjects' and spouses' reactions to the illness, (2) the marital relationship, and (3) children's adjustment. Eighteen subjects said they adjusted without any outside help, or with the help of their families, and 34 spouses had needs that were met through their own adjustments or from within or outside the family.

McIvor, Riklan, and Reznikoff (1984) studied depression in a sample of 120 persons with MS and noted that the most significant correlation was between severity of depression and perceived social support from family and friends. The more depressed a subject was, the more likely he or she was to perceive little or no social support.

Hope, Social Support, and Adaptation to Multiple Sclerosis

Because no studies noted in the literature examined hope and adjustment to MS, and because there is a paucity of research related to social support and MS, a descriptive correlational study was done to determine if relationships existed between hope and adaptation to MS and between social support and adaptation to MS in a convenience sample of 30 adults (Hastings, 1989). Secondary purposes of the study were to ascertain if the select demographic variables of severity of disability, support group membership, and length of time since diagnosis were related to adaptation, hope, and social support. Pearson product moment correlation coefficients were calculated to see if relationships existed among the variables. An exploratory qualitative component was also used to determine patterns or themes that were descriptive of the process of adjustment to MS and to define the factors important to personal adjustment from the subjects' own perspectives. Data were collected by tape-recorded interviews that were transcribed verbatim. The data were analyzed using a content analysis, data-reduction approach.

Analysis of the data demonstrated significant negative relationships between adaptation and hope ($r = -.5151; p = .002$), and adaptation and social support ($r = -.4186; p = .011$). *Lower scores on the adaptation measure indicate more successful adaptation.* Those who have better adaptation have higher levels of hope and perceived social support. In addition, a significant positive relationship was found between hope and social support ($r = .6413; p = .000$). A significant negative relationship also existed between adjustment and support group membership ($r = -.4541; p = .006$). The more adaptation increased, the more likely it was that subjects would belong to a support group. Other correlations between adaptation, hope, and social support and the demographic variables were not significant.

Analysis of the qualitative data revealed that reactions to the diagnosis of MS ranged from relief to denial, and subjects felt such emotions as fear and sorrow. The work of adaptation was found to be difficult; however, most subjects came to either accept or adapt to the process. Adaptation was described as a continual, daily process that for some had beneficial outcomes but also involved having to pace oneself and make lifestyle modifications.

Four categories of coping resources emerged from the data: (1) social support resources, (2) religion or faith, (3) inner strengths such as self-determination and a positive attitude, and (4) knowledge about the disease. Support from family and friends was the most important means of assisting with the adaptation process for the sample (Hastings, 1989).

Implications for nursing practice emerged from the study findings. In light of the correlations between hope and adjustment, and social support and adjustment, it is felt that patients could benefit from a more thorough investigation of their hope states and social support resources as part of a routine nursing assessment. Findings from a hope assessment could be used as a basis from which hope-inspiring strategies could be generated. The social support assessment could pinpoint inadequacies or problems in the client's social support system for which appropriate nursing interventions could be instituted. Understanding the factors that are significant to an individual's illness adaptation will help nurses focus on personal strengths that will facilitate the adjustment process.

The last section of this chapter presents an in-depth case study that deals with adaptation to MS. Nursing assessment and interventions are based upon use of the Neuman Systems Model (Neuman, 1994).

SECTION 3: CASE STUDY USING THE NEUMAN SYSTEMS MODEL

Ann is a 40-year-old woman, married with two children, ages 10 and 14 years, who was given a diagnosis of MS 8 years ago. She was referred to a nurse-managed MS clinic at a large teaching hospital by her physician for evaluation of her inability to adapt to the illness-related disabilities, which included progressive upper and lower extremity weakness, intention tremor, and bladder dysfunction. She has also admitted having difficulty in maintaining a supportive marital relationship.

The clinic uses an interdisciplinary holistic framework, with a nurse practitioner as primary caregiver and manager as described by Winters, Jackson, Sims, and Magilvy (1989). They stated that the uniqueness of this multidisciplinary approach is that a client has one evaluation conducted concurrently by several professionals, who are then able to coordinate their efforts to construct a thorough plan of care. Other health-care professionals include a neurologist, physiatrist, physical therapist, psychologist, and occupational therapist.

Nursing care in the clinic is based on the Neuman Systems Model, a comprehensive systems-based conceptual framework which, according to the author, fits with the wholistic interrelationship of mind, body, and spirit of the client in a constantly changing environment and society (Neuman, 1994, p. 10). Based on the concepts of stress and the reactions to it, the model views the client as a composite of five interacting and interrelated variables: (1) physiological, (2) psychological, (3) sociocultural, (4) developmental, and (5) spiritual, ideally existing in harmony with internal and external environmental forces to which the system is subjected at any given point in time (Neuman, 1994). Environment, both internal and external, therefore, is a critical element of the model. Stressors, which comprise the environment, are either intrapersonal, interpersonal, or extrapersonal (Harris, Hermiz, Meininger, & Steinkeler, 1994). Health is viewed as optimal system stability or the best possible wellness state at a given time, whereas nursing's major concern is stability of the client system through accurate assessment of actual and potential effects of environmental stressors as well as assisting clients to achieve optimal levels of wellness. Nursing intervention is based on the point in time at which the stressor is suspected or identified. Intervention typology includes primary, secondary, or tertiary prevention (Neuman, 1994).

Nursing History

Ann came to the MS clinic for her first appointment with her husband, but he did not participate in the intake interview and waited in another room. The initial interview was done by the nurse practitioner, who used Neuman's (1994) assessment and intervention tool to ascertain the perceived patient stressors. The nurse practitioner noted that Ann, a heavy, very well-dressed woman, whose hair and makeup were poorly done, entered the room in a motorized wheelchair, and as they began to speak, she noted that the client had difficulty keeping eye contact with her. The client stated that her husband was a successful attorney and that she had never had to work, although she held a degree in elementary education. She described her two children as "what I live for. They give me a reason for waking up in the morning."

STRESSORS AS PERCEIVED BY THE CLIENT

The client stated that her health status was the major stressor in her life as it has been only within the last year that the disease has had such an impact on her life. Her lifestyle had completely changed. Until then she had been able to ambulate independently, with occasional wheelchair use for long distances. Because of progressive weakness in her legs, she has had to use a motorized wheelchair for the last year, and progressive upper extremity weakness and intention tremor have made performance of activities of daily living (ADLs) difficult. She stated, however, that she refuses to have anyone come in to help her with grooming, although she admits to the difficulties her attitude is causing. She must make frequent trips to the bathroom, and transferring has become difficult. Ann admitted to having frequent "accidents" because of her difficulty getting to the toilet.

She stated that her greatest joy in life was caring for her husband and children. Now she is forced to have domestic help for meal preparation and cleaning except for weekends when the family is home. "I've always prided myself on how well I cared for my family and how tidy my house was. Now I can hardly use a feather duster. My daughters are a tremendous help on the weekends. They clean and cook for the family. They've given up many activities to help me out. They want to help me bathe and wash my hair for me, but I can't let them see that their mother can't do this for herself, and I just can't give up everything. They would also see how fat their mother has gotten. I'm so ashamed of myself. I just look terrible." She stated that she was 5 feet 2 inches tall and weighed 165 pounds. She has had a significant weight gain within the last year since using the wheelchair. "I smell terrible, too, no matter how much I clean myself; the odor from the urine is overwhelming."

The nurse practitioner asked her if she had ever experienced any other significant life events and how she had handled them in the past. Ann stated that her diagnosis of MS was certainly significant but that previously, because she did not have the deficits she was now experiencing, she had been able to push problems out of her mind. "If there was nothing tangible, then it did not exist." She did, however, compare this time in her life to the lingering death of her mother with cancer when Ann was 25 years old. Although she stated that it was very difficult for her, her main coping strategy was her faith in the Lord and her daily readings from the bible. When asked if she still had strong religious beliefs, Ann stated that she felt the Lord had deserted her. "While I'm still a Christian, I do not want to go to church. He must be terribly angry with me to have let this happen." When asked what else she does to relieve stress, Ann stated that she watches television and eats candy. "I used to go out and work in the garden or call a good friend if something was bothering me. But, what else is there to do when you're in a wheelchair? I have no friends anymore. It's not that they don't want to be friends with me, I just can't do the things that they want to do. Besides, why should they be burdened with a cripple? At least when I eat, I can have something that I choose. Of course, it isn't doing much for my waistline, and watching TV is certainly not productive, but when you're sitting in a wheelchair, what does it matter?"

When asked what she anticipates for the future, Ann laughed. "You're seeing the future sitting before you. This is the future, only it will probably be worse. This situation is hopeless. When you have MS, there is no future."

The nurse practitioner then asked Ann what she was doing to help herself at this time. Ann stated, as she did previously, that caring for her own needs, as difficult as it may be, was the only thing she could do to help herself at this time. "I am not capable of doing anything else." When asked to state what else she felt she could be doing for herself, she said, "As I just told you, I am not capable of doing anything else."

When asked what she felt others could be doing for her, Ann replied, "As I said, my children do a lot for me and would do more if I let them. My husband, on the other hand, well, I'm surprised he even came here with me. He's too busy with his clients to do a thing for me. It's the children that help me get into bed and make sure I'm comfortable, not him. He hasn't touched me in a year, not that I can blame him. There's not much I can do in that realm anymore, and, besides, I look so awful now. I think he stays with me out of obligation and for the children's sake. Not that he does much with them, either. Before the MS got so bad, we did everything together as a family. He may be at home with us, but he's really not. Do you know what I mean?"

When the interview was over, the nurse practitioner made a second appointment with Ann so that they could discuss the interview and her other evaluations, which would be done this same day, and devise a plan of care. The nurse practitioner also asked that Ann's husband be present at the next session. Ann, however, felt that at this time it would not be a good idea to involve him.

STRESSORS AS PERCEIVED BY THE CAREGIVER

After Ann left, the nurse practitioner reviewed the interview data to evaluate her own perception of the client stressors. The nurse agreed with Ann's perception of her declining health status being the major stressor. Several other significant stressors flowed from the pivotal stressor. The client's deteriorating relationship with her husband was seen as significant. It appears that he is unable to adjust to the change in his wife's health status and avoids interactions with her as a way of coping with the situation. His avoidance sets up tensions within the household, and Ann must turn to her children for the support she wants and needs from her husband. His attitude in turn affects her adjustment to the illness.

Although Ann's continued pursuit of accomplishing her own self-care needs could be viewed as a strength, the nurse also viewed this as a source of stress because the energy used to complete her ADLs will lead to increased fatigue. The nurse noted a study by Hart (1978) that found that clients with MS when fatigued had an accentuation of disease symptoms and greater indications of emotional stress.

Self-esteem and body image were noted to be stressors. The nurse saw that Ann derived the majority of her self-esteem needs from caring for her family and home, and this was no longer possible. Ann mentioned no outside interests during the interview. Although the nurse felt that Ann saw her altered body image as due to her weight gain, the nurse also saw Ann's body image alterations in terms of her perception of being wheelchair bound and, perhaps, seeing herself only as an extension of the wheelchair. Her decreasing bladder function was also felt to have an effect on her body image perception. All the data pointed to very significant lifestyle changes for both Ann and her family.

According to the client, she was able to cope successfully with her mother's illness and eventual death because of her belief in God. However, she is now experiencing spiritual distress and is unable to use this once-effective coping mechanism. She apparently has no other means of effective coping, an area that, if Ann is willing, will need improvement.

The nurse felt that Ann was experiencing feelings of hopelessness and powerlessness due to her present situation. Ann's perception of the future is one that someone experiencing feelings of hopelessness would describe; that is, she does not have a future orientation, and what she does see is related to a worsening of the situation. Feelings of powerlessness were apparent in the client's statements regarding her inability to do anything but care for her own needs. She felt inadequate because she was unable to care for her home and family and did not give any suggestion of what else she could do. The nurse thought that the feelings of powerlessness and hopelessness were tied to Ann's level of self-esteem.

Finally, it was evident that Ann expected much more from her husband than he was either willing or able to give. In addition, their sexual relationship had completely deteriorated, although it was hard to determine from the client's comments how this situation had evolved. She intimated that she was unable to satisfy his needs in this area but also spoke of his lack of affection toward her.

Although Ann spoke of caregivers only in terms of family, the nurse felt that her perception of outside caregivers was important. Because Ann was not willing to accept outside help for her personal needs, the nurse felt that her refusal might be an issue of control. By allowing someone to help with her care, she would be giving up the only control she feels she has over the situation. This would increase her feelings of powerlessness.

SUMMARY OF IMPRESSIONS

After completing her evaluation of client stressors, the nurse wrote her summary of impressions.

INTRAPERSONAL FACTORS

Physical factors influencing the client situation that were noted by both the nurse and the client were the progressive MS symptomatology, which included progressive lower extremity weakness impeding mobility, progressive upper extremity weakness, intention tremor, and bladder dysfunction affecting achievement of ADLs. The nurse also saw the bladder dysfunction affecting body image and both the lower extremity weakness and bladder dysfunction potentially affecting skin integrity.

Psychosocial evaluation included the nurse's perception of the client's spiritual distress as evidenced by her feelings that God was angry with her. The nurse also felt that the client used ineffective coping mechanisms to deal with stress. The client was in partial agreement when she stated that her eating was affecting her weight.

Developmentally, tasks of this client's age group include: (1) acceptance of self and a stabilizing self-concept and body image, (2) establishment of an intimate bond with another, (3) establishment of and management of a home, (4) finding a congenial social group, (5) deciding whether or not to have a family, (6) formulating a meaningful philosophy of life, and (7) becoming established in a vocation or profession that makes one feel that he or she is making a contribution to society (Murray & Zentner, 1993). It was evident to the nurse that the patient was having difficulty achieving some of these developmental tasks.

1. Self-concept and body image were significant problems.
2. Maintaining an intimate spousal relationship was difficult.
3. Ability to maintain the family home was unachievable because of the client's physical and emotional condition.

4. A supportive social network was not maintained.
5. No vocation has been pursued posteducation, and the client has disclosed that at this point in time, she does not see herself as a productive member of society.
6. Client's philosophy of life is difficult to ascertain because everything seems rooted in the here and now; she sees no future.

As noted earlier, the client is suffering from spiritual distress, which, according to Burnard (1987), is the "result of total inability to invest life with meaning" (p. 377) and can be demotivating, painful, and the cause of anguish. The client's feelings of hopelessness and powerlessness may be related to her spiritual distress, as hope is predicated on a belief in God's control over a situation and support of an individual through the crisis. Meaning and purpose in life and in suffering can be found in one's relationship with God and having knowledge of this Supreme control. However, this relationship and knowledge cannot provide hope forever without the possibility of a meaningful and purposeful future as hope ultimately depends on the promise of eternal fellowship with the Lord (Shelly & Fish, 1988).

INTERPERSONAL FACTORS

Interpersonal factors related to the situation include the relationships the client has with her spouse and daughters. Spousal support has been shown to be a significant factor in adjustment to chronic illness. Strauss et al. (1984) noted that the most important work that a caring spouse does for the mate who is ill is "psychological" work, that is, those tasks which are basically uncomplicated, such as bolstering spirits to those that involve complex maneuvering (p. 103). Corbin and Strauss (1984, 1988) studied 63 couples managing chronic illness at home and found that those who collaborated in managing the illness felt that they had the internal and external resources to continue the work, no matter what may happen in the course of the illness, and that their relationships had grown even closer from having to work together. Klinger (1984) found that social support was the single most helpful factor in complying with the medical regimen, for 60 clients post–myocardial infarction, with spousal support being cited most often. Dimond (1979) found a positive relationship between spousal support and morale in a study of 36 patients undergoing hemodialysis, and Northouse (1988) found that adjustment to breast cancer was facilitated by higher levels of spousal support in a sample of 50 clients who had undergone mastectomy.

The difficulty of spousal adjustment as noted in the intake interview correlates with the findings of Braham et al. (1975), who found that of 47 subjects with MS and their families both the subject and the spouse had the most difficulty accepting the disease, and 32 couples had need for help with their marital relationships. Because of the specifics of the disease, perhaps the adjustment needs of MS patients and their spouses are different than those of other chronic illnesses.

The nurse noted, as did the client, that her children were her main source of support. In the study by Hastings (1989), children were found to be sources of help and encouragement for the client with MS. However, in a qualitative study of three mothers with MS and their daughters, Friedmann and Tubergen (1987) found that, although parenting patterns were distinct in each family, all mothers had high expectations of the daughter who was described as the "good" child (p. 47). All three daughters experienced either physical or emotional symptomatology, which suggests the presence of stress within the family. All three daughters were excellent students, which may be a reflection of the children's efforts to live up to their mothers' expectations. This study led the nurse to question further the dynamics of Ann's family.

EXTRAPERSONAL FACTORS

The extrapersonal factors related to Ann's situation and that influence both the intrapersonal and extrapersonal variables were the use of outside agencies and Ann's inability to sustain social relationships. It is evident that if a home health aide assisted with her personal care, less energy would be expended by the client, leaving her with more time and less fatigue so that perhaps outside interests might be more enticing. The family should also feel a sense of relief knowing that someone would be of assistance, and the daughters may not feel as obligated to help with personal needs. However, the nurse questioned if Ann was ready to give up this source of independence.

Friends have been shown to be significant sources of support. Hastings (1989) found that several persons with MS stated that friends, both those with MS and others, have helped in the adjustment process. McIvor et al. (1984) found that a significant correlation existed between severity of depression and perceived social support from family and friends in a sample of 120 persons with MS. According to these authors, the loss of emotionally significant persons, be it family or friends, apparently adds a further threat to the severe burden of loss of functional ability and knowledge of the presence of MS. This is apparently one or more loss Ann is sustaining in addition to the independence she seems to crave.

NURSING DIAGNOSES

Based on this assessment, the nurse practitioner decided that because symptomatology was already present, secondary prevention was

Table 12.3 ➤ **NURSING DIAGNOSES APPROPRIATE FOR ANN**

Nursing Diagnosis	Etiologies
1. Potential for total self-care deficit	Increased tremor of the upper extremities and weakness of the lower extremities
2. Alteration in urinary elimination	Altered nerve innervation (Kelly & Mahon, 1988)
3. Potential for alteration in skin integrity	Increased immobility and incontinence
4. Potential for injury	Increased lower extremity weakness and upper extremity tremor
5. Self-esteem, low: situational	Inability to accomplish usual homemaking and family tasks
6. Body image disturbance	(a) Substantial weight gain, (b) difficulty accepting wheelchair confinement, (c) bladder dysfunction
7. Spiritual distress	Perception of the Lord's desertion and anger
8. Ineffective individual coping	Inability to use past successful coping mechanisms
9. Diversional activity deficit and social isolation	Altered self-concept (seeing self as a cripple and burden)
10. Hopelessness	Inability to perceive any positive outcomes for the future
11. Sexual dysfunction	Altered nerve innervation (Kelly & Mahon, 1988) and dissatisfaction with the marital relationship
12. Powerlessness	Declining physical capabilities leading to the perception of the inability to have control over own life
13. Impaired adjustment	Increasing disability and perceived lack of spousal support
14. Possible ineffective family coping	Spouse's perceived inability to accept wife's declining health (The nurse was not able to speak with the husband, who would have been able to assist in validating the diagnosis.)

the appropriate level of intervention. Secondary prevention is aimed at providing treatment of symptoms so that optimal client stability or wellness and energy conservation are attained (Neuman, 1994). Table 12.3 lists the nursing diagnoses that were thought to be appropriate for Ann's situation.

MULTIDISCIPLINARY EVALUATION

When Ann returned for her second visit, she and the members of the interdisciplinary team discussed the results of their respective assessments. It was decided that Ann would come to the clinic twice weekly for physical therapy for upper and lower extremity strengthening exercises to facilitate ADL completion and transferring and to prevent lower extremity contractures, and to see the occupational therapist for help with the fitting and use of adaptive devices and techniques necessary for use because of the intention tremor. The neurologist felt that

Ann should see a urologist for urodynamic studies and measurement of postvoiding residual urine to define the type of bladder dysfunction and determine the appropriate therapy (Kritchevsky, 1988). The psychologist suggested that Ann and her husband begin counseling sessions as a means of helping to strengthen their marital and sexual relationships. At a later date, the children would be included in therapy sessions.

It was thought that it would be more appropriate to have physical and occupational therapy treat the self-care deficit and injury potential, and ineffective family coping would be best left to the psychologist. Physical and occupational therapy would also facilitate the avoidance of a disruption in skin integrity. Alteration in urinary elimination would be explored after Ann saw the urologist. Sexual dysfunction would be dealt with after the urology consult and after the psychologist was able to make an evaluation of the couple's progress in counseling. The nurse practitioner would coordinate all efforts by the team.

NURSING CARE PLAN

The nurse and Ann reviewed the nursing diagnoses and prioritized them in terms of immediate and long-term importance. Although all the diagnoses were believed to be significant, it was thought that by resolving hopelessness, spiritual distress, and powerlessness, work on the other diagnoses would be facilitated. The three nursing diagnoses are intricately intertwined with one another, as spiritual distress can promote both feelings of hopelessness and powerlessness. Figure 12.1 represents a diagrammed version of holistic nursing assessment and intervention for the client with MS. As noted in Neuman's model (Neuman, 1994), the client with MS is viewed from a systems perspective as an integrated whole being composed of interactive and interrelated components. One can appreciate the reciprocal nature of the assessment and intervention phases as both the client and nurse are integral and active participants in the entire process. In the assessment phase, both the client and nurse identify perceived stressors. After the stressors are identified, both parties collaborate on the actual plan of care.

The following nursing care plan was devised by the nurse, with full acceptance by the client.

HOPELESSNESS

Short-Term Goals

The client will be able to list factors promoting feelings of hopelessness.

The client will be able to name personal resources necessary to help inspire hope.

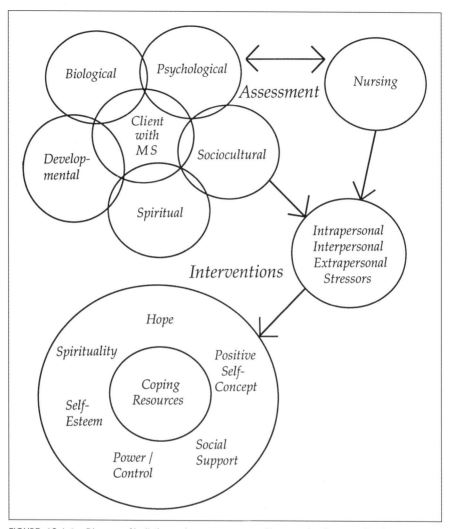

FIGURE 12.1 ➤ Diagram of holistic nursing assessment and intervention for care of a client with MS.

Long-Term Goal

The client will successfully integrate and use hope-inspiring strategies.

Interventions

1. Use a life-promoting framework so that the client is viewed as a potentially powerful and productive person with illness being only one facet of personality (Miller, 1985).

2. Help the client to explore those factors that contribute to feelings of hopelessness (Lederer, Marculescu, Mocnik, & Seaby, 1990).
3. Explore in depth the reasons why those factors are felt to promote hopelessness, and determine the factors that have given the client hope in the past.
4. Facilitate client's use of past successful hope-inspiring mechanisms.
5. Teach reality surveillance, the reconstructing of past events and assigning logic and reasoning to them, so that the client is able to avoid thinking about negative outcomes while looking for clues that affirm the maintenance of hope is possible (Miller, 1985).
6. Assess client for potential success of using relaxation techniques as a means of stress reduction and to facilitate coping so that other hope-inspiring strategies are reinforced.
7. Suggest the use of MS support group membership. Spiegelberg (1980) noted that MS support groups play an important role in allaying fears, helping members to use their strengths, and in helping to reach other clients.
8. Based upon the results of the psychological counseling sessions, potentially include the family relationships as a way of further inspiring hope. According to Miller (1985), one way to inspire hope is through emphasizing to the client that the presence and hopefulness of his or her sustaining relationships are important, because client's loved ones have the strongest influence on helping a client sustain hope.
9. Assist the client to set small, measurable goals so that a future orientation may be established.
10. Integrate interventions from both the spiritual distress and powerlessness nursing diagnoses.

SPIRITUAL DISTRESS

Short-Term Goal

The client will verbalize the reasons why chronic illness may precipitate distress of the human spirit.

Long-Term Goal

A renewed and more meaningful relationship with God will emerge.

Interventions

1. Perform a thorough spiritual assessment to determine past religious and spiritual practices.

2. Assist the client to examine the consequences of MS, which may arouse feelings of anger and of being abandoned by God.
3. Allow the client to express feelings of anger and abandonment.
4. Facilitate exploration of the client's past relationship with God and how it was successful in helping to manage stress-inducing situations.
5. Explain how a meaningful and purposeful relationship with God can help to maintain feelings of hope and control.
6. Establish the therapeutic use of self by employing listening, empathy, vulnerability, humility, and commitment (Shelly & Fish, 1988).
7. Facilitate the use of prayer and scripture as a means of comfort and support.
8. Integrate appropriate interventions from the hopelessness and powerlessness diagnoses.

POWERLESSNESS

Short-Term Goals

The client will identify those factors and situations that precipitate feelings of powerlessness.

The client will actively participate in decision making related to her plan of care.

Long-Term Goal

The client will begin to express feelings of control over her present situation and will identify actions that she feels are within her control.

Interventions

1. Collaborate with the other members of the multidisciplinary team to help encourage the client's participation in decision making regarding her plan of care and her own self-care needs, in addition to keeping her informed of her ongoing progress.
2. Encourage the client to express her feelings about her current illness situation, facilitating the view of illness as an experience, thereby promoting feelings of personal significance (Roberts, 1978).
3. Once the client is comfortable participating in decision making regarding her care, encourage her to participate in family-related decision making (also considering her progress in counseling).

4. Because maintenance of positive self-esteem has been determined to be an area of difficulty, and because positive self-esteem has been noted to be a power resource, use strategies to enhance self-esteem such as the promotion of positive self-statements and encouraging positive social experiences (tying into the problem of social isolation and diversional activity deficit).

5. Because powerlessness is a factor contributing to overeating, an identified client problem related to body image, help the client to further explore the reasons for overeating and begin to assist her to establish healthy eating habits.

6. Integrate the appropriate interventions related to the diagnoses of hopelessness and spiritual distress. The maintenance of hope and spiritual well-being facilitates an empowered state.

SUMMARY

MS and its potential for a downhill trajectory can promote a situation in which a person can feel vulnerable and experience a loss of control. Adjustment to a chronic illness such as MS is a dynamic, complex process influenced by a diverse number of variables, all needing further research. Despite the course that the illness may take, nurses can facilitate adjustment to chronic illness, and specifically MS, through the use of a holistic systems framework and assist the patient toward developing effective coping resources such as hope, spiritual well-being, and social support.

REFERENCES

Baldree, K. S., Murphy, S. P., & Powers, M. J. (1982). Stress identification and coping patterns in patients on hemodialysis. *Nursing Research, 31,* 107–112.

Braham, S., Houser, H. B., Cline, A., & Posner, M. (1975). Evaluation of the social needs of nonhospitalized chronically ill persons. *Journal of Chronic Diseases, 28,* 401–419.

Brandt, B. T. (1987). The relationship between hopelessness and selected variables in women receiving chemotherapy for breast cancer. *Oncology Nurses Forum, 14,* 35–39.

Brockopp, D. Y., Hayko, D., Davenport, W., & Winscott, C. (1989). Personal control and the needs for hope and information among adults diagnosed with cancer. *Cancer Nursing, 12,* 112–116.

Brooks, N. A., & Matson, R. R. (1982). Social-psychological adjustment to multiple sclerosis. *Social Science and Medicine, 16,* 2129–2135.

Burnard, P. (1987). Spiritual distress and the nursing response: Theoretical considerations and counselling skills. *Journal of Advanced Nursing, 12,* 377–382.

Cantanzaro, M. (1980). Nursing care of the person with MS. *American Journal of Nursing, 80,* 286–291.

Cohen, S., & Syme, S. L. (1985). Issues in the study and application of social support. In S. Cohen & S. L. Syme (Eds.), *Social support and health* (pp. 3–21). Orlando, FL: Academic Press.

Colliton, M. A. (1981). The spiritual dimension of nursing. In I. L. Beland & J. Y. Passos, *Clinical nursing. Pathophysiological and psychosocial approaches* (14th ed., pp. 492–501). New York: Macmillan.

Corbin, J. M., & Strauss, A. L. (1984). Collaboration: Couples working together to manage chronic illness. *Image: Journal of Nursing Scholarship, 16,* 109–115.

Corbin, J. M., & Strauss, A. L. (1988). *Unending work and care: Managing chronic illness at home.* San Francisco: Josey-Bass.

Craig, H. M., & Edwards, J. E. (1983). Adaptation in chronic illness: An eclectic model for nurses. *Journal of Advanced Nursing, 8,* 397–404.

Crawford, J. D., & McIvor, G. P. (1985). Group psychotherapy: Benefits in multiple sclerosis. *Archives of Physical Medicine and Rehabilitation, 66,* 810–813.

Davison, A. N. (1982). Multiple sclerosis: Recent advances in research. *Physiotherapy, 68,* 151–153.

Derogatis, L. R., & Lopez, M. C. (1983). *The psychosocial adjustment to illness scale. Administration, scoring, & procedures manual-I.* Baltimore: Clinical Psychometric Research.

Dimond, M. (1979). Social support and adaptation to chronic illness. The case of maintenance hemodialysis. *Research in Nursing and Health, 2,* 101–108.

Dimond, M. (1983). Social adaptation of the chronically ill. In D. Mechanic (Ed.), *Handbook of health care and the health professional* (pp. 636–654). New York: Free Press.

Feldman, D. J. (1974). Chronic disabling illness: A holistic view. *Journal of Chronic Diseases, 27,* 287–291.

Fischbach, F. (1995). *A manual of laboratory diagnostic tests* (5th ed.). Philadelphia: JB Lippincott.

Forsyth, G. L., Delaney, K. D., & Gresham, M. L. (1984). Vying for a winning position: Management style of the chronically ill. *Research in Nursing and Health, 7,* 181–188.

Franklin, G. M., & Burks, J. S. (1985). Diagnosis and medical management of multiple sclerosis. In F. P. Maloney, J. S. Burks, &. S. P. Ringel (Eds.), *Interdisciplinary rehabilitation of multiple sclerosis and neuromuscular disorders* (pp. 32–47). Philadelphia: JB Lippincott.

Friedmann, M. L., & Tubergen, P. (1987). Multiple sclerosis and the family. *Archives of Psychiatric Nursing, 1,* 47–54.

Gottlieb, N. H., & Green, L. W. (1984). Life events, social network, lifestyle, and health: An analysis of the 1979 National Survey on Personal Health Practices. *Health Education Quarterly, 11,* 91–105.

Gould, M. T. (1983). Nursing diagnoses concurrent with multiple sclerosis. *Journal of Neurosurgical Nursing, 15,* 339–345.

Gulick, E. E. (1984). Multiple sclerosis: The nurses' role using a self-care framework. *Journal of Community Health Nursing, 1,* 247–255.

Gulick, E. E. (1989). Model confirmation of the MS-related symptom checklist. *Nursing Research, 38,* 147–153.

Gurklis, J. A., & Menke, E. M. (1988). Identification of stressors and use of coping methods in chronic hemodialysis patients. *Nursing Research, 37,* 236–239, 248.

Harper, A. C., Harper, D. A., Chambers, L. W., Cino, P. M., & Singer, J. (1986). An epidemiological description of physical, social and psychological problems in multiple sclerosis. *Journal of Chronic Diseases, 39,* 305–310.

Harris, S. M., Hermiz, M. E., Meininger, M., & Steinkeler, S. E. (1994). Betty Neuman systems model. In A. Marriner-Tomey, *Nursing theorists and their work* (3rd ed., pp. 361–388). St. Louis: CV Mosby.

Hart, L. K. (1978). Fatigue in the patient with multiple sclerosis. *Research in Nursing and Health, 1,* 147–157.

Hastings, D. (1989). *Hope, social support, and adaptation to multiple sclerosis.* Unpublished master's thesis, Marquette University, Milwaukee.

Herth, K. A. (1989). The relationship between level of hope and level of coping response and other variables in patients with cancer. *Oncology Nurses Forum, 16,* 67–72.

Hibbard, J. H. (1985). Social ties and health status: An examination of moderating factors. *Health Education Quarterly, 12,* 23–34.

Holland, N. J., McDonnell, M., & Wiesel-Levison, P. (1981). Overview of multiple sclerosis and nursing care of the MS patient. *Journal of Neurosurgical Nursing, 13,* 28–33.

Holland. N. J., Wiesel-Levison, P., & Madonna, M. G. (1984). Community care of the patient with multiple sclerosis. *Rehabilitation Nursing, 9,* 18–20.

Hubbard, P., Muhlenkamp, A. F., & Brown, N. (1984). The relationship between social support and self-care practices. *Nursing Research, 33,* 266–270.

Hungelmann, J., Kenkel-Rossi, E., Klassen, L., & Stollenwerk, R. (1989). Development of the JAREL spiritual well-being scale. In R. M. Carroll-Johnson (Ed.), *Classification of nursing diagnoses. Proceedings of the eighth conference* (pp. 393–398). Philadelphia: JB Lippincott.

Kelly, B., & Mahon, S. M. (1988). Nursing care of the patient with multiple sclerosis. *Rehabilitation Nursing, 13,* 238–243.

Klinger, M. (1984). Compliance and the post-MI patient. *The Canadian Nurse, 80,* 32–36.

Korner, I. N. (1970). Hope as a method of coping. *Journal of Consulting and Clinical Psychology, 34,* 134–139.

Kritchevsky, M. (1988). Multiple sclerosis. In W. C. Wiederholt (Ed.), *Neurology for non-neurologists* (2nd ed., pp. 177–186). New York: Grune & Stratton.

Lange, S. P. (1978). Hope. In C. E. Carlson & B. Blackwell (Eds.), *Behavioral concepts & nursing interventions* (2nd ed., pp. 171–190). Philadelphia: JB Lippincott.

LaRocca, N., Kalb, R., & Kaplan, S. R. (1983). Psychological changes. In L. C. Scheinberg (Ed.), *Multiple sclerosis. A guide for patients and their families* (pp. 175–194). New York: Raven Press.

Lederer, J. R., Marculescu, G. L., Mocnik, B., & Seaby, N. (1990). *Care planning pocket guide. A nursing diagnosis approach* (3rd ed.). Redwood City, CA: Addison-Wesley Nursing.

Matson, R. R., & Brooks, N. A. (1977). Adjusting to multiple sclerosis: An exploratory study. *Social Science and Medicine, 11,* 245–250.

McIvor, G. P., Riklan, M., & Reznikoff, M. (1984). Depression in multiple sclerosis as a function of length and severity of illness, age, remissions, and perceived social support. *Journal of Clinical Psychology, 40,* 1028–1033.

Mechanic, D. (1977). Illness behavior, social adaptation, and the management of illness. A comparison of educational and medical models. *The Journal of Nervous and Mental Disease, 165,* 79–87.

Miller, J. F. (1985). Inspiring hope. *American Journal of Nursing, 85,* 22–25.

Miller, J. F. (1992). *Coping with chronic illness. Overcoming powerlessness* (2nd ed.). Philadelphia: FA Davis.

Morgante, L. A., Madonna, M. G., & Pokiluk, R. (1989). Research and treatment in multiple sclerosis: Implications for nursing practice. *Journal of Neuroscience Nursing, 21,* 285–289.

Murray, R. B., & Zentner, J. P. (1993). *Nursing assessment & health promotion through the life span* (5th ed.). Englewood Cliffs, NJ: Prentice-Hall.

Neuman, B. (1994). *The Neuman systems model* (3rd ed.). East Norwalk, CT: Appleton & Lange.

Northouse, L. L. (1988). Social support in patients' and husbands' adjustment to breast cancer. *Nursing Research, 37,* 91–95.

O'Brien, M. E. (1982a). Religious faith and adjustment to long-term hemodialysis. *Journal of Religion and Health, 21,* 68–79.

O'Brien, M. E. (1982b). The need for spiritual integrity. In H. Yura & M. B. Walsh (Eds.), *Human needs 2 and the nursing process* (pp. 85–113). Norwalk, CT: Appleton-Century-Crofts.

Pallett, P. J., & O'Brien, M. T. (1985). *Textbook of neurological nursing.* Boston: Little Brown.

Pollock, S. E. (1986). Human responses to chronic illness: Physiologic and psychosocial adaptation. *Nursing Research, 35,* 90–95.

Poser, C. M. (1983). The diagnosis. In L. C. Scheinberg (Ed.), *Multiple sclerosis. A guide for patients and their families* (pp. 17–33). New York: Raven Press.

Reed, P. G. (1987). Spirituality and well-being in terminally ill hospitalized adults. *Research in Nursing and Health, 10,* 335–344.

Rideout, E., & Montemuro, M. (1986). Hope, morale, and adaptation in patients with chronic heart failure. *Journal of Advanced Nursing, 6,* 157–169.

Roberts, S. (1978). *Behavioral concepts and nursing throughout the life span.* Englewood Cliffs, NJ: Prentice-Hall.

Ruffing-Rahal, M. A. (1984). The spiritual dimension of well-being. Implications for the elderly. *Home Healthcare Nurse, 2,* 12–16.

Scheinberg, L. (1983). Introduction. L. C. Scheinberg (Ed.), *Multiple sclerosis. A guide for patients and their families* (pp. 3–6). New York: Raven Press.

Scheinberg, L., & Geisser, B. S. (1983). Drug therapy. In L. C. Scheinberg (Ed.), *Multiple sclerosis. A guide for patients and their families* (pp. 45–55). New York: Raven Press.

Schneider, J. S. (1980). Hopelessness and helplessness. *Journal of Psychiatric Nursing and Mental Health Services, 18,* 12–20.

Schneitzer, L. (1978). Rehabilitation of patients with multiple sclerosis. *Archives of Physical Medicine and Rehabilitation, 59,* 430–436.

Shelly, J. A., & Fish, S. (1988). *Spiritual care. The nurse's role* (3rd ed.). Downers Grove, IL: InterVarsity Press.

Sims, C. (1987). Spiritual care as a part of holistic nursing. *Imprint, 34,* 63–65.

Slater, R. J., & Yearwood, A. (1980). MS. Facts, faith, and hope. *American Journal of Nursing, 80,* 276–281.

Sodestrom, K. E., & Martinson, I. M. (1987). Patients' spiritual coping strategies: A study of nurse and patient perspectives. *Oncology Nurses Forum, 14,* 41–46.

Soeken, K. L., & Carson, V. J. (1987). Responding to the spiritual needs of the chronically ill. *Nursing Clinics of North America, 22,* 603–611.

Spiegelberg, N. (1980). Support group improves quality of life. *Association of Rehabilitation Nurses, 5,* 9–11.

Stoner, M. J. H. (1982). Hope and cancer patients. (Doctoral dissertation, University of Colorado, 1983). *Dissertation Abstracts International, 44,* 115B.

Strauss, A. L., Corbin, J., Fagerhaugh, S., Glaser, B. G., Maines, D., Suczek, B., & Wiener, C. L. (1984). *Chronic illness and the quality of life* (2nd ed.). St. Louis: CV Mosby.

Stuart, E. M., Deckro, J. P., & Mandle, C. L. (1989). Spirituality in health and healing: A clinical program. *Holistic Nursing Practice, 3,* 35–46.

Surridge, D. (1969). An investigation into some psychiatric aspects of multiple sclerosis. *British Journal of Psychiatry, 115,* 749–764.

Sutherland, J. M. (1986). Multiple sclerosis—clinical. In P. A. Downie, (Ed.), *Cash's textbook of neurology for physiotherapists* (4th ed., pp. 383–397). Philadelphia: JB Lippincott.

Tan, S. Y. (1986). Psychosocial functioning of adult epileptic and MS patients and adult normal controls on the WPSI. *Journal of Clinical Psychology, 43,* 528–534.

Thompson, J. M., McFarland, G. K., Hirsch, J. E., Tucker, S. M., & Bowers, A. C. (1989). *Mosby's manual of clinical nursing* (2nd ed.). St. Louis: CV Mosby.

Tilden, V. P. (1986). New perspectives on social support. *Nurse Practitioner, 11,* 61–62.

Weiss, R. S. (1974). The provisions of social relationships. In Z. Rubin (Ed.), *Doing unto others* (pp. 17–26). Englewood Cliffs, NJ: Prentice-Hall.

Whitaker, J. N. (1983). What causes the disease? In L. C. Scheinberg (Ed.), *Multiple sclerosis. A guide for patients and their families* (pp. 7–16). New York: Raven Press.

Whitlock, F. A., & Siskind, M. M. (1980). Depression as a major symptom of multiple sclerosis. *Journal of Neurology, Neurosurgery, and Psychiatry, 43,* 861–865.

Whittington, L. (1983). Multiple sclerosis. Dealing with reality. *The Canadian Nurse, 79,* 34–38.

Wierenga, M. (1993). Alterations in motor function. In C. M. Porth (Ed.), *Pathophysiology. Concepts of altered health states* (5th ed., pp. 847–867). Philadelphia: JB Lippincott.

Winters, S., Jackson, P., Sims, K., & Magilvy, J. (1989). A nurse-managed multiple sclerosis clinic: Improved quality of life for persons with MS. *Rehabilitation Nursing, 14,* 13–16.

Zeldow, P. B., & Pavlou, M. (1984). Physical disability, life stress, and psychosocial adjustment to multiple sclerosis. *Journal of Nervous and Mental Disease, 172,* 80–84.

➤ 13

Coping with Chronic Lung Disease: Maintaining Quality of Life

➤ Anne M. McMahon

Adults with chronic lung disease experience a succession of distressing physical, psychological, and spiritual responses that challenge personal resources for coping. Progressive dyspnea and fatigue impair functioning in physical, emotional, and social dimensions of daily living. Human responses commonly experienced by adults with emphysema and chronic bronchitis and interventions designed to promote optimal coping are described in this chapter. Pathophysiological changes, challenges to quality of life, and a case study are reviewed. A model of quality of life for persons with chronic obstructive pulmonary disease (COPD) described in this chapter provides a framework for organizing research and nursing interventions.

Clients have identified the sense of mastery, or feeling of control, over the disease as an important aspect of quality of life in coping with impaired breathing (Guyatt, Townsend, Berman, & Pugsley, 1987). Nursing interventions during all phases of disease progression are directed at enhancing this sense of mastery.

PATHOPHYSIOLOGICAL CHANGES

Human responses to chronic lung disease are related to alterations in the structure and function of the airways and lungs (Carrieri & Janson-Bjerklie, 1993; Porth, 1993; West, 1991). Chronic bronchitis and emphysema cause irreversible changes that result in obstruction to the normal flow of air, hence the term *chronic obstructive pulmonary disease*. Persons who have one of these conditions often have both, partly because the causative factors of cigarette smoking and air pollution are common to both. Persons with these conditions often also have some degree of asthma, which causes episodes of airflow obstruction in response to irritating stimuli.

The pathophysiological changes that accompany chronic bronchitis have three main effects: hypertrophy of mucus glands in the large bronchi, hypertrophy of the bronchial smooth muscle surrounding the airways, and chronic inflammation and edema of the small airways. These changes obstruct airflow by narrowing the airways and by impairing the mucociliary system that normally clears foreign bodies from the airways. Persons with chronic bronchitis experience a chronic cough, productive of sputum that is purulent during acute exacerbations. In the later stages, ankle edema and fluid retention characteristic of right ventricular failure commonly appear.

The obstruction to airflow that accompanies emphysema has a different etiology. Pathophysiological changes cause the eventual destruction of alveolar walls, a process that destroys the capillary bed in which diffusion of respiratory gases occurs. This process weakens the supporting structure of the lungs and reduces the radial traction that maintains the patency of airways. Persons with this condition have "air trapping," a condition in which there is overinflation of the lungs and obstruction to airflow during expiration. Loss of the lung's normal elastic recoil causes bronchioles to collapse during exhalation, trapping air in the distal bronchioles and alveoli. Eventually the shape of the thorax becomes distorted and movement of the diaphragm during breathing is impaired.

Persons whose lung disease has an asthmatic component experience acute episodic obstructions to airflow, caused by spasms of the bronchial smooth muscle. Bronchospasm may be precipitated by irritating stimuli such as dusts, aerosols, or other allergens; exercise; exposure to cold air; or stressful psychological stimuli. Bronchoconstriction, which is responsive to treatment by bronchodilators, is labeled *reversible* airflow limitation. The airflow obstruction in asthma is compounded by edema of the bronchial walls and by thick, tenacious mucus produced by hypertrophied mucous glands.

Pulmonary function tests (PFTs) provide clinical measures of the airflow impairments caused by COPD. Clients achieve low values for measures of expiratory airflow such as forced expiratory volume in 1 second (FEV_1), the forceful, timed exhalation of vital capacity. High values for residual volume (RV) provide evidence of air trapping.

Arterial blood gases (ABGs) provide data on impaired diffusion of respiratory gases across the alveolar-capillary membrane and on the mismatching of ventilation and perfusion in the lung. Hypoxemia, hypercarbia, and respiratory acidosis are common patterns. Hypoxemia, with arterial Po_2 below 55 mm Hg, predisposes to the development of right-sided heart failure (Porth, 1993; West, 1991).

Comprehensive Assessment

A guide for nursing assessment of the person with a pulmonary disorder is summarized in Table 13.1. The assessment format is based on Gordon's (1994) 11 functional patterns.

The nursing diagnoses Ineffective Airway Clearance, Ineffective Breathing Patterns, and Impaired Gas Exchange summarize the principal alterations in pulmonary function that accompany COPD. Each diagnosis may have one or more causes for a given individual.

Ineffective airway clearance is defined as a state in which an individual is unable to clear secretions or obstructions from the respiratory tract to maintain airway patency. Causes may include airflow limitation, airway infection, the presence of an artificial airway, or other conditions that disturb the production or clearance of mucus. An effective cough requires the ability to collect a large volume of air in the chest and to exhale forcefully and rapidly. Persons with COPD have difficulty coughing to clear the airways effectively because of weakness of the respiratory muscles and the production of excessive, abnormally viscous mucus (DeVito, 1985; Kim & Larson, 1987).

Ineffective breathing patterns are defined as states in which the individual's inspiratory and/or expiratory pattern does not provide adequate ventilation. Causes may include airflow limitation, respiratory muscle fatigue, or decreased lung expansion. Aspects of normal breathing patterns that are altered may include respiratory rate, tidal volume, ratio of inspiratory time to expiratory time, and the coordinated motion of respiratory muscles. For COPD clients, the altered breathing pattern usually produces rapid shallow breathing, a pattern that increases the work of breathing by increasing ventilation of physiological deadspace. This pattern is inefficient and eventually ineffective in meeting ventilatory needs (Kim & Larson, 1987).

The diffusion of oxygen and carbon dioxide in the pulmonary capillaries is impaired by the loss of surface area in the lungs and by uneven distribution of air in the lungs. Hypoxemia results when blood flows past poorly aerated areas of lung tissue. Hypercarbia and acidosis result from impaired excretion of carbon dioxide. Clients with impaired

Table 13.1 ➤ **NURSING ASSESSMENT FOR CLIENTS WITH PULMONARY DISORDERS**

Activity-exercise pattern
  Dyspnea
    Self-report of experience
    Rating on visual analog scale (Gift, 1989)
    Frequency
    Precipitating factors
    Patterns from dyspnea log (Carrieri, 1989)
    Improvement or worsening (Mahler, Weinberg, Wells, & Feinstein, 1984)
  Cough
    Frequency
    Sputum: appearance, amount
    Precipitating factors
    Relieving factors
  Daily activities
    Functional independence in self-care activities
    Driving or alternative transportation
    Has handicapped parking permit
    Exercise patterns
    Access to fitness equipment
    Work: current, past
    Hobbies and recreation
    Other health problems that limit activity and mobility
    Former activities given up because of lung disease
Chest
  Inspection
    Anterior-posterior diameter
    Breathing pattern
      Rate
      Depth
      Inspiration:expiration ratio
      Coordination of abdomen and chest muscles
      Use of intercostal, neck, and shoulder muscles
  Percussion
    Hyperresonance
  Auscultation
    Breath sounds: diminished, bronchial
    Adventitious sounds: crackles, rhonchi, wheezes
Pulse: rate, rhythm
Neck vein distention
Color
  Skin
  Mucous membranes
  Nailbeds
Skin turgor
Edema
Posture and positioning
  Sitting
  Standing
Exercise tolerance
  Six-minute walk test (Guyatt et al., 1985; McGavin, Gupta, & McHardy, 1976)
  Rating of dyspnea: Borg Scale (Borg, 1982)
  Pulse oximetry: resting, walking
Data from medical assessment
  Pulmonary function testing
    Tidal volume
    Vital capacity

Table 13.1 ➤	**NURSING ASSESSMENT FOR CLIENTS WITH PULMONARY DISORDERS (Continued)**

Residual capacity
  Total lung capacity
  Forced expiratory volume in 1 second (FEV_1)
  Diffusing capacity for carbon monoxide (D_LCO)
  Arterial blood gases
    Oxygenation
    Acid-base balance
  Chest x-ray
Diagnosis
Medical management
Other health problems
Nutritional-metabolic pattern
  Appetite
  Diet
    Normal day's or week's intake: types and amounts
    Recent changes
    Diet log, if indicated
  Usual fluid intake
  Weight gains or losses within past year
  Dyspnea with meals
  Abdominal discomfort
  Drug and alcohol consumption
  Weight, height, ideal weight
  Appearance: Body build
  Oxygen saturation while eating, if indicated
Elimination pattern
  Bowel elimination patterns
  Bladder elimination patterns
    Stress incontinence
Sleep-rest pattern
  Usual sleep and rest patterns, including naps
  Number of pillows used
  Paroxysmal nocturnal dyspnea
  Feeling adequately rested
  Factors that prevent rest
  Factors that promote rest
  Sleep study data, if available
Cognitive-perceptual pattern
  Sensory deficits
  Memory: short-term, long-term
  Ability to concentrate
  Decision-making ability
  Education
  Self-care knowledge
Self-perception–self-concept pattern
  Feelings of anxiety, restlessness, being down or blue, powerlessness
  Sense of mastery in managing disease
  Activities that provide a sense of accomplishment, satisfaction, of "being me"
  Body image concerns:
    Sputum
    Shortness of breath
    Noisy respirations
    Presence of oxygen
    Appearance
  Motivation for rehabilitation
  Goals

Table 13.1 ➤	**NURSING ASSESSMENT FOR CLIENTS WITH PULMONARY DISORDERS (*Continued*)**

Coping-stress tolerance pattern
  Current sources of stress
  Factors that relieve stress
  Family support available
  Other resources for coping with stressors
  Communication
    Verbal
    Nonverbal
Role-relationship pattern
  Significant other(s)
  Positive aspects of relationship(s)
  Changes related to lung disease
  Other roles and relationships
    Family
    Work
    If retired, past work history
    Clubs, hobbies
  Concerns about roles and relationships
Sexuality-reproductive pattern
  Changes related to impaired breathing
  Satisfaction with present patterns
Health perception–health management pattern
  Past medical history, hospitalizations
  Current treatments
    Medications
    Oxygen
    Nebulizer
    Chest physiotherapy
    Respiratory muscle training (Kim, 1984)
Adherence to prescribed treatments
Risk factors
  Respiratory irritants: smoke, aerosols, sprays, dusts, allergens
    At home
    Away from home
  Response to environmental conditions
  Smoking history, if applicable
    Currently smoking?
    Attempts to quit
      Methods used
      Successes
  Preventive practices
    Immunizations for influenza, pneumococcus
    Use of air conditioner, humidifier, air cleaners
Value-belief pattern
  Spiritual resources
  Feelings of hope or hopelessness
  Religious affiliation and practices
  Sources of strength to transcend suffering

gas exchange may have tachycardia, weakness, fatigue, restlessness, and confusion (DeVito, 1985).

QUALITY OF LIFE AND CHRONIC OBSTRUCTIVE PULMONARY DISEASE

For persons with a chronic illness, quality of life is dependent upon changes related to illness phenomena, perceptions, functional capacity, and personal resources. *Illness phenomena* refers to individuals' subjective responses to the changes induced by disease. Disease comprises the structural and pathophysiological changes that can be evaluated using objective clinical measures, such as pulmonary function testing and ABGs. Illness phenomena encompass individuals' subjective experiences, such as dyspnea and fatigue, related to these changes. *Perceptions* refers to individuals' unique interpretations of their health status, functioning, well-being, and quality of life. *Functional capacity* refers to the ability to perform activities in the physical, emotional, and social aspects of daily living. *Personal resources* refers to physical, cognitive, emotional, social, and economic assets available to the individual (Dracup & Raffin, 1989; Gilson et al., 1975; Padilla et al., 1983; Wenger, Mattson, Furberg, & Elinson, 1984).

As a progressive disease affecting the vital supply of oxygen to muscle, brain, and other body cells, COPD affects all four aspects of life quality discussed. The broad range of responses experienced by clients is indicated by the nursing diagnoses associated with each of the four aspects (Table 13.2). Nursing interventions are directed at modifying clients' responses in each of the four areas.

Illness Phenomena in Chronic Obstructive Pulmonary Disease

DYSPNEA

Dyspnea is a prevalent response reported by persons with chronic lung disease. Sometimes used interchangeably with the term "breathlessness," dyspnea is a sensation of difficult or uncomfortable breathing, as perceived and interpreted by the individual. It occurs when the demand for ventilation, as perceived by the individual, is out of proportion to the ability to respond to that demand. For persons with COPD, the increased demand for ventilation is related to inefficient pulmonary gas exchange. The reduced ability to respond to ventilatory needs is caused by abnormal mechanics of the lung, diaphragm, and other respiratory muscles and by respiratory muscle fatigue (Carrieri, Janson-Bjerklie, & Jacobs, 1984; West, 1987).

Table 13.2 ➤ **DIMENSIONS OF LIFE QUALITY AND ASSOCIATED NURSING DIAGNOSES* FOR PERSONS WITH CHRONIC OBSTRUCTIVE PULMONARY DISEASE**

Illness phenomena
  Decreased cardiac output
  Constipation
  Fatigue
  Fluid volume deficit
  Fluid volume excess
  Potential for infection
  Potential for aspiration
  Ineffective airway clearance
  Ineffective breathing patterns
  Impaired gas exchange
  Alteration in oral mucous membrane
Perceptions
  Anxiety
  Altered comfort
  Ineffective denial
  Fear
  Grieving, actual and anticipatory
  Dysfunctional grieving
  Hopelessness
  Powerlessness
  Self-concept disturbance
  Body-image disturbance
  Self-esteem disturbance
Functional capacity
  Activity intolerance
  Impaired verbal communication
  Diversional activity deficit

Functional capacity (*continued*)
  Potential for disuse syndrome
    (end-stage)
  Altered health maintenance
  Impaired home maintenance
    management
  Potential for injury
  Impaired physical mobility
  Altered role performance
  Self-care deficit
  Altered sexuality patterns
  Impaired social interactions
  Social isolation
Personal resources
  Ineffective individual coping
  Ineffective family coping
  Compromised family coping
  Defensive coping
  Altered family processes
  Knowledge deficit
  Noncompliance
  Altered nutrition: less than body
    requirements
  Sleep pattern disturbance
  Spiritual distress
  Impaired swallowing
  Altered thought processes

*Nursing diagnosis labels based on Carpenito (1997).

Persons with emphysema typically describe their dyspnea as a constant, unrelenting pervasive body sensation of difficulty breathing or "difficulty getting the air out" (Carrier & Janson-Bjerklie, 1993). Persons with asthma more commonly refer to sensations of constriction and chest tightness in describing their experience of dyspnea (Janson-Bjerklie, Carrier, & Hudes, 1986). In recalling episodes of acute dyspnea, COPD clients have reported concomitant feelings of fear, helplessness, loss of vitality, preoccupation, and concern about having difficulty convincing others of the seriousness of their distress (DeVito, 1990).

In the early stages of COPD, clients experience dyspnea as a response to strenuous activity or intense emotions. As the disease progresses, dyspnea occurs with minimal activity in the absence of emotional arousal, and eventually dyspnea is present during rest. Changes in dyspnea over time can be assessed using tools such as the Baseline Dyspnea Index and the Transition Dyspnea Index, which quantify dyspnea in relation to the activities that provoke it and the effort expended (Mahler et al., 1984).

The severity of dyspnea reported by clients does not correlate directly with physiological measures, such as PFT results and ABG values. This observation supports the notion that dyspnea is a multidimensional phenomenon rather than a purely physiological one (Gift, Plaut, & Jacox, 1986; Hudson & Pierson, 1981).

Episodes of acute dyspnea are often accompanied by an intensely distressing sensation of panic (Janson-Bjerklie et al., 1986). Clients learn to prevent such dyspnea-panic episodes by avoiding the physical exertion and emotional experiences that precipitate them. This pattern of behavior leads to a progressively restricted lifestyle, in which the individual may eventually be unable to perform basic activities of daily living (ADLs), such as bathing, dressing, preparing meals, or even eating. Deconditioning of the cardiorespiratory system and the skeletal muscles then limits activity beyond the restrictions imposed by the pathophysiological changes (Glass, 1981).

Persons experiencing chronic dyspnea report using a variety of coping strategies. Problem-focused strategies include modifying grooming, eating, and other ADLs; modifying activities by planning ahead or using breathing stations; self-selected treatments, such as adjusting medications; and protective behaviors. Emotion-focused strategies include emotional distancing, adopting a positive attitude, social isolation, and tension-reduction strategies. Seeking social support is a mixed problem-emotion–focused strategy (Carrier & Janson-Bjerklie, 1986).

FATIGUE

Another response frequently experienced by persons with chronic lung disease is fatigue, a pervasive sense of energy depletion that affects many aspects of functioning and well-being. It is related to hypoxemia, dyspnea, altered sleep and rest patterns, and altered mood states. It is aggravated by the process of cardiovascular and skeletal muscle deconditioning that often accompanies the experience of chronic dyspnea. Clients report feeling low in energy, worn out, and sluggish. Fatigue is associated with reports of psychological distress (Guyatt et al., 1987; Janson-Bjerklie et al., 1986; Kinsman et al., 1983).

Fatigue and the accompanying management tasks present a challenge to clients' resources of time, energy, and money. For persons fortunate enough to have a dependable support system, the problem of energy depletion strains the resources of the members and necessitates ongoing trade-offs of one resource for another. It becomes increasingly necessary to use the energy of family members, other caregivers, and community agencies for household maintenance and for meeting basic needs (Fagerhaugh, 1973).

Perception: Sense of Mastery

Clients' perceptions of their illness and its impacts are important aspects of life quality. This emphasis on clients' subjective interpretations is consistent with the phenomenological view that individuals' perceptions of reality are more important than the reality itself (Dracup & Raffin, 1989).

A perception rated as important by persons with COPD is the sense of mastery over symptoms and functioning (Guyatt et al., 1987). The sense of mastery is threatened by dyspnea, fatigue, and altered mood states that accompany disease progression. Diminution of the sense of mastery can precipitate feelings of powerlessness and depression. There is evidence that persons who have a diminished sense of mastery use emergency services more than other COPD clients (Traver, 1988).

Empirical observations indicate that the sense of mastery is bolstered by effective medical management and by developing competence with skills such as controlled breathing patterns and energy-conservation techniques that help to avert or attenuate the experience of dyspnea. A primary goal of nursing care is to assist clients in maintaining or enhancing the sense of mastery by mobilizing their resources for coping. The sense of mastery is influenced by perceived changes in one's physical self (body image) and self-worth (self-esteem).

Altered Body Image

Physical changes that accompany disease progression may require coping with alterations in body image. As the anterior-posterior diameter of the chest increases and accessory muscles of breathing in the neck hypertrophy, clients note that shirts and blouses no longer fit properly and can no longer be buttoned at the neck.

Embarrassment related to symptoms and treatments can be a problem. Clients report feeling embarrassed by coughing and noisy breathing and by using medications or breathing treatments in public places (Guyatt et al., 1987). For clients receiving continuous oxygen by cannula, the presence of nasal prongs and tubing gives unspoken evidence of disability.

Diminished Self-Esteem

A number of threats to self-esteem accompany the progression of COPD. Clients may experience guilt about having smoked or being unable to quit smoking. The need to accept assistance with transportation, household chores, and, eventually, self-care activities threatens autonomy and may induce feelings of diminished self-worth. Inability to fulfill role expectations on the job, at home, and in social settings presents the need for the client to redefine his or her sense of identity and to find alternative sources of self-affirmation.

Functional Capacity

The progression of COPD is characterized by a steady deterioration in function, with episodic acute exacerbations that may require hospitalization. Because effective breathing is essential to physical, cognitive, psychological, and social functioning, persons with impaired breathing experience difficulties with functioning in many aspects of daily living. Typically, in the fifth and sixth decades of life, persons with COPD may have coexisting health problems, such as arthritis, heart disease, or sensory deficits, which compound functional limitations. Psychological responses such as depression or ineffective coping may further limit energy levels and vigor.

Human responses to chronic lung disease are a unique product of the pathophysiological changes caused by the disease and the personal resources of the individual. Pathophysiological processes produce typical patterns in clinical testing, as previously discussed. But these data alone are not predictive of the physical, emotional, cognitive, social, or occupational functioning of a given individual. Persons with identical abnormal pulmonary function and ABG results may differ greatly in their level of functioning and quality of life (Foxall, Ekberg, & Griffith, 1987; McSweeney, Grant, Heaton, Adams, & Timms, 1982; Prigatano, Wright, & Levin, 1984).

Functional capacity can be viewed as a quotient of the opposing effects of disease progression on the one hand and individuals' personal resources for coping on the other. The relationship of these factors is illustrated by the model in Figure 13.1, which is based on the concept of trajectory formulated by Strauss et al. (1984). Pathophysiological changes are associated with a trajectory or course of progressively declining functional capacity. This decline in functioning is characterized by fluctuations, which are related to acute exacerbations to the effects of atmospheric conditions on breathing and to physical and psychological factors. Individuals may have a level of actual functioning that is considerably below their potential functional capacity. Actual functioning is enhanced by personal resources for coping, including physical, cognitive, social, economic, and spiritual resources. Persons with optimal resources, including knowledge and motivation, are able to achieve a level of actual functioning that approaches or matches their potential functional capacity. According to this model, deficits in resources are correlated with impaired functioning, an observation supported by clinical studies (McDonald, Borson, Gayle, Deffebach, & Lakshminarayan, 1989; Moser, Bokinsky, Savage, Archibald, & Hansen, 1980). A goal of nursing care and of pulmonary rehabilitation is to assist clients in mo-

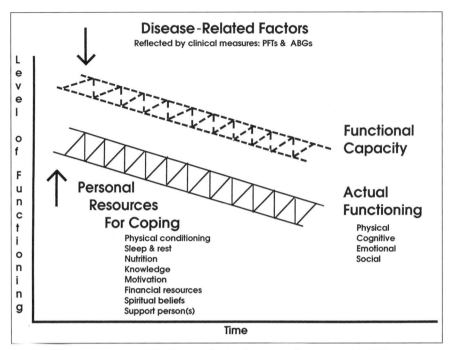

FIGURE 13.1 ➤ Proposed model of factors affecting functioning for persons with COPD.

bilizing their resources to maintain functioning at the maximal level allowed by disease progression. Assessment modalities and research findings related to each component of functioning are reviewed subsequently.

Assessment of Functional Capacity

Because of the pervasive effects of dyspnea and fatigue on functioning in all aspects of daily living, a comprehensive assessment of clients' functioning is essential. Standardized questionnaires such as the Sickness Impact Profile (SIP) (Bergner, Bobbitt, Carter, & Gilson, 1981), the Pulmonary Impact Profile Scale (PIPS) (Weaver & Narsavage, 1989), and the Chronic Respiratory Disease Questionnaire (CRQ) (Guyatt, Berman, Townsend, Pugsley, & Chambers, 1987) are useful adjuncts to the comprehensive initial nursing assessment in Table 13.1. These tools provide comprehensive data on clients' functioning in ADLs, including physical, emotional, and cognitive aspects. They can be readministered for subsequent evaluation of clients' responses to intervention programs or to disease progression. The PIPS and CRQ were designed specifically for the assessment of adults with chronic lung disease.

Several studies of large groups of clients have documented the broad range of functional impairment accompanying COPD. A study of quality of life for 985 persons with COPD with mild hypoxemia revealed moderate to severe impairment of function in most dimensions of daily living measured by the SIP, including ambulation, mobility, social interaction, communication, alertness behavior, emotional behavior, sleep and rest, home management, recreation and pastimes, and employment. Persons with COPD differed significantly from control subjects on all measures except the two dimensions of body care and movement, and eating (Prigatano et al., 1984). Also responding to the SIP, 203 persons with advanced COPD reported impaired life quality on all parameters assessed. Areas severely affected included home management, ambulation, mobility, sleep and rest, and recreation and pastimes. Eating and communication were moderately affected (McSweeney et al., 1982).

Noting the increasing incidence of COPD among women, Sexton and Munro (1988) investigated the life quality of 72 women with COPD. One-third of subjects with COPD reported shortness of breath and fatigue as their biggest problems. The ADLs most affected were physical activity and sleep. Fear of having a dyspneic attack while away from home restricted activity for many of the women. Because energy fluctuated widely from day to day, many reported difficulty in planning household and social activities.

Emotional Dysfunction

Persons with COPD have indicated that changes in emotional functioning are an important factor affecting their quality of life (Guyatt, Berman, Townsend, Pugsley, & Chambers, 1987). In coping with COPD, they encounter a succession of stressful experiences. Those mentioned in a support group discussion included being unable to do previously enjoyable activities, aging-related changes, family stresses, the effects of weather on breathing and energy levels, unrealistic family expectations, the distress of symptoms, financial concerns, and dietary changes. The anxious thoughts that accompany stressful experiences can precipitate rapid, shallow breathing. The result may be an escalating episode of anxiety, dyspnea, and panic, which is typically very difficult to interrupt. Episodes of acute anxiety are accompanied by other stress responses, such as poor appetite. Clients also report a more chronic state of anxiety, which is characterized by feeling worried, tense, restless, and fidgety (Gift et al., 1986; Janson-Bjerklie et al., 1986; Sexton & Munro, 1988).

Episodes of acute dyspnea are accompanied by both anxiety and depression (Gift & Cahill, 1989). Clinical observations and research data indicate high incidences of anxiety and depression among persons experiencing chronic dyspnea. Other responses reported by clients include episodes of anger, hostility, frustration, and responses indicating repression of feelings and cognitive impairments. Emotional dysfunction is attributed in part to an inadequate supply of oxygen to the limbic system and other areas of the brain that mediate emotional behavior (McSweeney et al., 1982).

Empirical observations support the theory that persons with COPD live in an "emotional straitjacket" (Dudley, Wermuth & Hague, 1973). According to this theory, emotional states are directly related to breathing. Active emotional states, such as anger and anxiety, increase metabolic demands for oxygen to levels that eventually exceed the limited oxygen supply available to persons with chronically impaired breathing. Conversely, inactive emotional states, such as depression, diminish breathing to the point at which ventilation is inadequate. In both cases, the subsequent distress causes clients to limit their expression of, and eventually even their experience of, these emotions. The result is learned patterns of emotional repression and social isolation.

Feelings of helplessness, hopelessness, and depression are commonly reported by persons with unremitting dyspnea. Reactive depression may occur in response to physical dysfunction, job loss, disruptions in family life, or thoughts about impending death. Depression has been attributed partly to fatigue, which depletes physical and psychic energy, and to a pattern of social isolation commonly adopted by persons experiencing chronic dyspnea. Indications that might signal depression in persons with COPD include insomnia, decreased appetite, social withdrawal, indecisiveness, a sense of failure or disappointment in oneself, sadness, difficulty in concentrating, dyspnea, suicidal ideation, lethargy, and feelings of helplessness or hopelessness (Janson-Bjerklie et al., 1986; Kinsman et al., 1983; Light, Merrill, Despars, Gordon, & Mutalipassi, 1985; McSweeney et al., 1982; Prigatano et al., 1984; Sandhu, 1986; Sexton & Munro, 1988).

Impaired Cognition

Problem solving, abstract thinking, and judgment are important resources for successful coping with life events. These intellectual skills can be impaired by the hypoxemia and respiratory acidosis that accompany advanced COPD. A study of 121 persons with advanced COPD revealed cognitive impairments in three-fourths of the subjects. The skills most frequently affected were abstracting ability, perceptual-motor integration (problem solving and other complex skills), simple motor skills, and attention. Skills involving language and memory remained generally intact (Grant, Heaton, McSweeney, Adams, & Timms, 1980). Long-term oxygen therapy for these clients resulted in small but definite improvements in cognitive function (Heaton, Grant, McSweeney,

Adams, & Petty, 1983). Clients in another study reported forgetfulness, confusion, and difficulty with concentrating, focusing attention, reasoning, and solving problems (Guyatt, Berman, Townsend, Pugsley, & Chambers, 1987).

Altered Role Functioning: Impacts on Client and Family

Spouse, employee, parent, club member, friend, neighbor, grandparent, community member—these roles and others change for individuals with COPD. Successful coping entails grieving for the losses that accompany changes and establishing new balances of personal and family resources (McSweeney et al., 1982; Sexton & Munro, 1985, 1988).

Clients and their support networks face the tasks of adapting to diminished energy reserves, mobilizing the resources of family members and community services, and finding a new equilibrium in response to the progressive nature of the disease. Optimal coping necessitates setting priorities, making decisions, and trading off one resource for another. For the client, this may mean allocating time for rest in order to maintain roles central to one's self-concept, coping with feelings of loss and social isolation, and learning energy-conserving techniques to use in maintaining selected roles and responsibilities. For the family, it may mean reallocating roles and responsibilities, spending money to pay for help with household chores, giving up some social and recreational activities, and finding new diversional activities.

As the roles of the ill member contract, the role of family members and others must correspondingly expand or help must be obtained from outside sources. The wives of 46 men with COPD reported taking on the roles of caretaker, decision maker, financial manager, and errand runner, while maintaining previous roles in the household (Sexton & Munro, 1985). Role synchrony is facilitated when the client, family, and others are realistic about the extent of disability (Barstow, 1974).

For caregiving spouses, COPD presents a number of challenges. The disease occurs at a time in life when the caregiving spouse may also be experiencing acute or chronic health problems. Wives of men with COPD reported personal health problems that included arthritis, hypertension, cataracts, and heart disease (Sexton & Munro, 1985). The tasks of caregiving can aggravate health problems or limit time and financial resources for managing health problems. During even a short-term illness or hospitalization, caregivers may find it difficult to find reliable assistance with household maintenance and caregiving roles.

Social isolation can become a problem for both client and spouse. Spouses must deal with the losses of social and recreational activities, especially when shared activities such as dancing, traveling, or bridge playing are affected. Successful coping involves exploring new pastimes that match the affected partner's energy and tolerance.

Driving is a role that can provide not only mobility, but self-esteem. When the client is the only driver in the household, mobility and social interaction for both client and spouse may be restricted. Transportation problems can restrict access of both persons to needed supplies and services including groceries, medications, banking, and health-care appointments. Limited access to social contacts can affect the well-being of both partners.

Some couples have reported positive responses to some of the effects of COPD. The changes that accompany the disease bring a slower pace of life and a sense of the tenuous nature of life, factors that have increased the closeness and interdependence in some marriages (Hanson, 1982). Of the married women studied by Sexton and Munro (1988), more than half indicated that their illness had increased their closeness with their husbands. Only one-tenth indicated that their disease had caused a distance from spouses.

Occupational Role

The stresses associated with a planned and timely retirement are well known. As a progressive disease occurring during the productive decades of middle adulthood, COPD often necessitates premature retirement because of disability. The individual may experience isolation from a network of significant social contacts and the loss of a role central to identity. These losses may be compounded by the economic impact of the job loss (Stollenwerk, 1985).

A positive correlation has been found between IQ and successful coping with the occupational changes consequent to COPD. This has been attributed to the fact that persons with higher IQ scores are more likely to have less physically strenuous jobs, which can be maintained further into the disease process (Daughton, Fix, Kass, Patil, & Bell, 1979). Persons with a higher IQ may have greater resources of time and money to facilitate their coping.

Women carrying out traditional roles in the household may have special problems in adapting to the limitations imposed by COPD. Because of the constant nature of household responsibilities, retirement is usually more difficult for these individuals. Women studied by Barstow (1974) continued to perform household chores despite functional impairments. They reported incorporating pauses for rest and seeking help with heavy chores.

Recreational Activities

While experiencing the progression of COPD, clients and families may note several changes in the time available for recreational activities. Early in the disease process, while maintaining occupational roles, clients may conserve energy by reducing recreational activities and hobbies. As function is further impaired, some persons who are required to retire early report having increased time for recreational activities, a change seen as a short-term positive side effect of the disease (Foxall et al., 1987).

As fatigue and dyspnea advance, minimally strenuous activities such as sewing or card-playing can become luxuries for the person with COPD. The loss of hobbies and pastimes curtails sources of recreation, identity, and socialization that make life pleasurable.

Social and recreational activities often involve exposure to second-hand smoke, which can precipitate dyspnea and coughing. Even in restaurants, public transportation, and public areas where smoking is restricted, small amounts of smoke can impair breathing in persons who are sensitive to inhaled irritants. For many clients with COPD and their families, this factor restricts social and recreational activities.

Sexual Dysfunction

Because of its physical and psychological effects, chronic lung disease may impair sexual and affectional expressions. A group of 128 subjects studied by Hanson (1982) rated this impact of the disease a highly important one. Correlational data indicate that worsening of lung disease is accompanied by worsening of sexual dysfunction (Fletcher & Martin, 1982). Both male and female clients have reported fear of becoming too tired or dyspneic during intercourse to continue (Dudley, Glaser, Jorgenson, & Logan, 1980). Other physical causes of sexual dysfunction include hypoxemia, inadequate cardiopulmonary reserve, coughing, wheezing, and effects of medications. Psychological responses including anxiety, depression, repression of emotions, social isolation, and diminished self-esteem also have detrimental effects on sexual function (Campbell, 1987; Timms, 1982).

Sexual dysfunction in one partner integrally affects affection, identity, and self-esteem for both. Of 46 wives of men with COPD, more than half reported that they no longer engaged in sexual intercourse. Some women identified this as a problem and others did not (Sexton & Munro, 1985).

Efforts to Adapt to Altered Functional Capacity

Individuals adapt to changing energy levels in ways that may or may not promote optimal functioning. Both denial of the disability and exaggeration of it can result in behaviors that compound the physiological deficits and restrict functioning unnecessarily. Denial is a common early response, in part because dyspnea is by nature a subjective experience that may not be accompanied by overt signs. Affected persons may engage in activities that tax their energy reserves beyond capacity and subject them to episodes of extreme fatigue, frustration, and feelings of anger or depression (Dudley et al., 1980). Early in the disease process, family members may also deny the illness and place undue expectations on the ill member (Sexton & Munro, 1988).

Exaggeration of activity intolerance can cause clients to restrict their functioning prematurely in the disease process. Family dynamics may be a contributing factor. A spouse experiencing guilt may be overly protective and solicitous and may unconsciously foster dependence. Such patterns can compound the loss of function associated with physical deconditioning. These patterns may contribute to emotional dysfunction and diminished self-esteem.

Clients interviewed in depth by Barstow (1974) reported a number of alterations used in managing ADLs. Most entailed "planning ahead to maximize economy of effort." Clients used the concept of simplification of activities, for example, eating only easily prepared foods, wearing slip-on shoes to avoid stooping and bending, and bathing less frequently. They applied the concept of pacing, for example, by bathing and dressing in stages with rest pauses.

In interviewing using a grounded theory approach, Fagerhaugh (1973) found that clients used similar adaptations in coping with breathlessness. They used the process of "routing" to set priorities and efficiently expend limited reserves of energy. They described complex systems of planning ahead for shopping and household chores, using "puffing stations" to unobtrusively recover from breathlessness in public places. They carefully monitored energy expenditure. Their lives were characterized by careful balancing of the resources of time, energy, and money to maintain equilibrium. One resource essential in this dynamic process was the use of "mobility assistants," family members and others who provided energy-conserving transportation and assistance.

For persons requiring continuous oxygen, portable oxygen systems bring mixed blessings for physical mobility and daily functioning. For some individuals, the oxygen systems are portable reservoirs of energy. Carts, shoulder straps, and backpacks enhance the systems' portability, allowing such activities as golfing, shopping, travel, and even swimming. Other persons paradoxically limit their activity after receiving oxygen systems. Some perceive the systems as cumbersome. Others see them as a symbolic burden and a sign of disability. Uninformed and insensitive comments by others who identify oxygen as a risk for explosion or fire can aggravate the social isolation.

Personal Resources

The physical, psychological, social, financial, and spiritual resources of clients and families determine the responses and options available as pathophysiological changes progress. Functioning and quality of life are integrally related to these resources.

NUTRITION

Optimal nutritional status is essential for effective breathing and for functioning of the immune system. Malnourishment puts individuals at risk for respiratory muscle fatigue and for infections affecting the lungs and other body systems. These problems can necessitate hospitalization and mechanical ventilation and may be life threatening (Openbrier & Covey, 1987).

Weight loss and malnutrition are commonly seen with advancing COPD. These responses are attributed to increasing metabolic demands and to decreasing ingestion of needed calories and nutrients. Metabolic requirements are elevated by the increased work of breathing associated with chronic airflow limitation. Smoking further increases metabolic rates (Braun et al., 1984).

Appetite and eating can be adversely affected by a number of factors, including fatigue, dyspnea, expectoration of sputum, and dry mouth. Taste and smell are blunted by malnutrition and by smoking. Gastric irritation is a common side effect of bronchodilating agents and steroids. Ineffective breathing patterns cause difficulty with simultaneously breathing and eating, resulting in meal-related dyspnea. Some clients experience oxygen desaturation during meals, attributed to ineffective diaphragmatic function associated with gastric fullness (Openbrier & Covey, 1987).

SLEEP AND REST

Sleep and rest promote coping by restoring physical and psychic energy. The physical and psychological responses that accompany COPD interrupt normal sleep and rest patterns.

Sleep disturbances and daytime somnolence compound the problem of fatigue for many persons with COPD. Problems reported by clients include difficulty with initiating and maintaining sleep, nightmares, and excessive daytime sleepiness (Kinsman et al., 1983; Klink & Quan, 1987; Sexton & Munro, 1988). Oxygen desaturation due to disordered breathing during sleep is one probable cause for sleep disturbances (Douglas & Flenley, 1990; Fulmer & Snyder, 1984). Sleep is also disrupted by orthopnea, coughing, and shortness of breath.

For couples, the sleep disturbances of one partner can have adverse effects for both. The client's nocturnal restlessness, coughing, and orthopnea make it necessary for the client and spouse to sleep in separate beds or even separate rooms (Sexton & Munro, 1985). A related challenge for couples is finding alternative expressions of closeness and affection.

SUPPORT PERSON

A vital resource in successful coping with chronic lung disease is the assistance of a competent and dependable person, usually a spouse or other family member. In the stages before the client requires direct assistance and care, the support person becomes a valuable source of energy for meeting daily needs for food, clothing, household mainte- nance, and illness management. This person often helps to attenuate fluctuations in mood, gives encouragement, fosters motivation, and pro- vides surveillance in observing daily changes in appearance, energy, and response to treatment. Specific functions performed by this person include helping with household chores, assisting with treatments, and discussing feelings and choices (Barstow, 1974; Fagerhaugh, 1973; Hanson, 1982; Sexton & Munro, 1988).

Deficits in or absence of a dependable support system will have a dramatic impact on quality of life as the disease progresses. Persons without reliable help in the home require earlier referral for home care and other resources, the availability of which often depends upon ability to pay. Nursing home placement, with the attendant changes and losses, becomes necessary earlier in the disease process for individuals lacking assistance from family and other caregivers.

FINANCIAL RESOURCES

Energy is a valuable commodity for persons with COPD. As per- sonal reserves of energy are depleted, financial resources can be used to purchase needed assistance with home maintenance, transportation, household chores, and care of personal needs.

The financial impact of COPD is an important concern for many clients and families. For those who must reduce work hours or retire prematurely, income may be unexpectedly diminished. Discretionary expenditures may be greatly altered as money is needed for medica- tions, oxygen, modifications of the home environment, help with home maintenance chores, and home care. Medications alone can become a major monthly expense. Clients often express frustration at the expense accompanying frequent changes in prescriptions.

Health insurance that covers home-care services can lengthen the time clients are able to remain at home. Persons lacking this re- source need to seek care in a long-term care facility earlier in the dis- ease process.

VALUES AND BELIEF SYSTEM

Persons with advancing COPD may find it difficult to sustain inner resources at the very time when they are experiencing threats to hope and spiritual well-being. Fatigue and episodes of coughing or labored breathing may preclude attendance at church services. Awareness of personal vulnerability and mortality may cause doubts about beliefs previously unquestioned, precipitating hopelessness, powerlessness, or spiritual distress. Awareness of the importance of breathing as a powerful symbol of life and health can intensify this distress.

NURSING INTERVENTIONS

A case study at the end of this chapter discusses the application of specific interventions in the case of a client coping with the progression of COPD. Interventions related to each of the four components of life quality are presented here.

A goal of nursing care is to identify, mobilize, and augment clients' and families' resources for coping with the changes related to illness phenomena, perceptions, and diminished functional capacity. Nursing care is often provided in the context of a pulmonary rehabilitation program, a holistic multidisciplinary program that might include a pulmonary nurse specialist, physician, respiratory therapist, physical therapist, occupational therapist, dietitian, social worker, vocational counselor, psychiatrist or psychologist, the individual with COPD, and a family member or caregiver. Other disciplines may be available for referral. In most such programs, roles are not mutually exclusive and team members work cooperatively to meet client needs. Members of each discipline reinforce client compliance with the interventions provided by other members of the rehabilitation team. A nurse often serves as coordinator for the pulmonary rehabilitation program (Borkgren, 1989; Hahn, 1988; Kirilloff, Carpenter, Kerby, Kigin, & Weimer, 1986). Participation in a pulmonary rehabilitation program results in positive outcomes such as improved functioning in ADLs, enhancement of self-concept, and decreased depression and anxiety (Emery, Leatherman, & MacIntyre, 1989; Kersten, 1989a, Moser et al., 1980; Shenkman, 1985).

Whenever possible, interventions should include both client and family. Even client-centered interventions, such as breathing exercises, are enhanced by the understanding and reinforcement of family members. Other interventions, such as postural drainage and chest percussion, may require assistance from a caregiver in the household.

Interventions Related to Illness Phenomena

BREATHING RETRAINING

Breathing retraining interventions can help clients to modify dyspnea and to increase functional capacity. Pursed-lip breathing—exhaling slowly through pursed lips—increases tidal volume, slows respiratory rate, and decreases the collapse of small airways by increasing intra-airway pressure. Diaphragmatic or abdominal breathing involves relaxing the abdominal muscles during inspiration and mildly tightening them during expiration to augment the diaphragm's upward movement. The result is to increase the use of the diaphragm during inspiration (Lareau & Larson, 1987). After clients master these breathing patterns, they can be taught to integrate them into exercises and ADLs. Such coordinated breathing involves inhaling during the resting phase of activities and exhaling during the exertion phase, for example, while placing groceries on shelves, dressing, cleaning, or getting into a car. Mastery of this skill can remarkably improve quality of life by increasing activity tolerance and daily functioning. Although these breathing patterns are widely used, their long-term efficacy has not been systematically studied (Carrieri et al., 1984).

BRONCHIAL HYGIENE

To enhance airway clearance, clients can be taught about exercise and adequate fluid intake. Supervised practice with coughing maneuvers can assist clients in clearing airways effectively without breathlessness and fatigue. Controlled coughing involves inhaling by sniffing, followed by pursed-lip exhalations to move secretions into large airways. The final exhalation is a staggered huffing effort, which keeps intrathoracic pressure low, preventing premature airway closure. Bronchial hygiene measures such as chest percussion and postural drainage may be necessary for persons unable to cough effectively (DeVito, 1985).

INSPIRATORY MUSCLE TRAINING

Inspiratory muscle training (IMT) involves a program of exercise for the diaphragm and other respiratory muscles, similar to training for skeletal muscles. Clients on such a program breathe for 15 to 30 minutes daily through a small hand-held device that increases inspiratory pressure loads (Larson, Kim, Sharp, & Larson, 1988). There is evidence that such a program may be useful in preventing respiratory fatigue and improving exercise tolerance, effects thought to be mediated by increased strength and endurance of the respiratory muscles (Kim, 1984).

OXYGEN THERAPY

For clients with impaired gas exchange, therapeutic use of low-flow supplemental oxygen may be necessary to maintain partial pressure of arterial oxygen (PaO_2) at about 60 mm Hg (Porth, 1993). The Nocturnal Oxygen Therapy Trials demonstrated the efficacy of continuous low-flow oxygen in prolonging life for persons with hypoxemia (Nocturnal

Oxygen Therapy Group, 1980). The goal of oxygen therapy is to maintain Pao_2 levels without suppressing the client's hypoxic drive to breathe. This requires careful monitoring of ABG measurements.

Clients receiving oxygen who are concerned about the appearance of conventional nasal cannulas may be candidates for transtracheal oxygen systems. These systems deliver oxygen directly into the trachea through a small flexible tube implanted surgically under local anesthesia. The tube provides an efficient method of supplying oxygen that can be hidden under clothing. Advantages include the cosmetic effects, cost savings because of reduced oxygen consumption, and improved mobility resulting from use of smaller portable reservoirs. Clients must be well informed about self-care of the catheter and must be carefully assessed for motivation to comply (Christopher et al., 1987; Lucas, Golish, Sleeper, & O'Ryan, 1988).

CARE DURING ACUTE EPISODES

In a qualitative study of hospitalized clients' experiences during episodes of acute dyspnea, 96 clients recalled nurse behaviors they perceived as helpful. These included directly communicating acknowledgment of clients' fear, demonstrating simple breathing techniques for clients to imitate, assisting with self-care activities, validating the severity of the dyspneic episode, and facilitating clients' concentrating on breathing (DeVito, 1990).

Interventions Related to Perceptions

SELF-MONITORING

Self-monitoring is an essential skill for successful coping with chronic lung disease. Self-monitoring interventions often precipitate spontaneous changes in individuals' behavior patterns (Ryan, 1989). By recognizing triggering events and early signals of dyspnea and anxiety, clients can learn to avert acute episodes. Recognition of the slight changes in sputum and breathing that herald a respiratory infection is a requisite skill in securing prompt treatment and avoiding hospitalization.

Even slight variations in air quality, temperature, and humidity can affect breathing for persons with COPD (Fagerhaugh, 1973). Becoming attuned to the sensations of breathing, breathing patterns, and the effects of changing weather conditions is a first step in learning to plan activities to maximize breathing and functioning.

A useful initial intervention in promoting a sense of mastery over symptoms is having the client keep a detailed log of daily activities and the accompanying sensations, symptoms, and weather conditions. This tool can help to identify patterns and precipitating factors that might otherwise go undetected. An adaptation of this idea is a dyspnea log, in which clients record the time, severity, and factors related to all episodes of dyspnea (Carrieri, 1989; Kersten, 1989b). In using such a log, one client discovered that she often experienced dyspnea episodes in the early afternoon, on days when she prepared and ate a large mid-day meal. By getting accustomed to smaller meals that are more easily prepared and digested, she was able to alter this pattern of dyspnea and achieve a sense of mastery.

Clients' experiences of dyspnea, fatigue, exertion, and anorexia can be rated on a visual analog scale. A common format is a vertical or horizontal line, usually 100 mm in length, with verbal descriptors such as "extreme difficulty breathing" and "no difficulty breathing" at either end (Fig. 13.2). The client is directed to make a mark indicating present, usual, or worst dyspnea. Measuring the interval marked on the scale provides an objective measure of this subjective experience; it can be used to compare episodes of dyspnea and to evaluate the effects of interventions. Because of their simplicity, such scales can be used by acutely dyspneic clients, including those in emergency rooms or on ventilators (Brown, 1988; Gift, 1987, 1989; Lush, Janson-Bjerklie, Carrier, & Lovejoy, 1988; Openbrier & Rogers, 1989).

In using the Modified Borg Scale, clients indicate their experience of dyspnea or other symptoms by using numbers from 0 to 10 to correspond to verbal descriptions (Fig. 13.3). This scale is useful for rating changes in dyspnea, exertion, or fatigue during exercise (Borg, 1982).

Biofeedback tools can be used to demonstrate the efficacy of interventions. Pulse oximetry monitors give immediate feedback on the effects of diaphragmatic breathing patterns on oxygen saturation (Tiep,

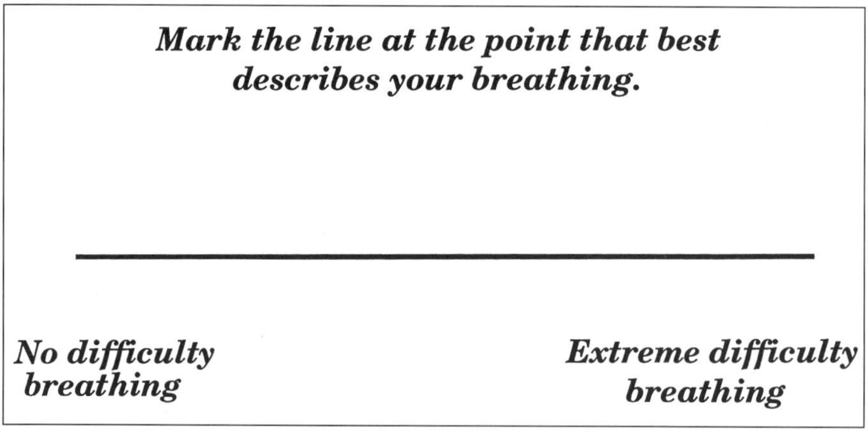

Mark the line at the point that best describes your breathing.

No difficulty breathing   *Extreme difficulty breathing*

FIGURE 13.2 ➤ Dyspnea visual analog scale.

Circle the number that best matches your shortness of breath.

0	*None at all*
0.5	*Very, very slight (just noticeable)*
1	*Very slight*
2	*Slight*
3	*Moderate*
4	*Somewhat severe*
5	*Severe*
6	
7	*Very severe*
8	
9	*Very, very severe (almost maximal)*
10	*Maximal*

FIGURE 13.3 ➤ Modified Borg scale. (Source: Borg, 1982.)

Burns, Kao, Madison, & Herrera, 1986). Clients are often surprised to learn that they can significantly increase saturation levels during an initial effort at controlled breathing. Pulse monitoring can be useful in observing the effects of relaxation techniques and exercise.

TEACHING

Clients can benefit from information about comfort measures. Temperature extremes affect oxygen demand and consumption. Maintaining humidity at about 40 percent, using an air conditioner or humidifier if necessary, and keeping room temperature at 68° to 72°F is optimal (Curigan & Gronkiewicz, 1988). Clients who experience a sense of suffocation with impaired breathing often find some relief with an electric fan blowing on the face.

Living with lung disease involves adapting to and using the tools of its medical treatment. Clients need to adjust treatment modalities to their lifestyles and to make decisions about using these treatments in response to self-assessments. Knowledge can promote a sense of mastery in using these resources. A teaching program for clients with COPD using principles of adult education has demonstrated short-term increases in knowledge and skills for coping (Perry, 1981). Areas in which clients may need information include medications and use of metered-dose inhalers, nebulizer devices, oxygen delivery systems, bronchial hygiene techniques, and use of IMT devices (Davido, 1981; Kersten, 1989b; Larson et al., 1988; Lindell & Mazzocco, 1990; Lucas et al., 1988; Openbrier, Fuoss, & Mall, 1988; Openbrier, Hoffman, & Wesmiller, 1988; Sexton, 1990). Clients who are candidates for transtracheal oxygen require carefully tailored assessment and teaching (Christopher et al., 1987; Heimlich & Carr, 1989).

Clients on continuous oxygen who are interested in traveling need specialized teaching and referral to medical equipment vendors (Sleeper, 1988; Traver, 1985). Information about cruises for persons with pulmonary disease may be appropriate for many clients, including those receiving continuous oxygen (Burns, 1987).

Interventions Related to Physical and Emotional Functioning

Exercise Program

A program of progressive exercise is a key component of pulmonary rehabilitation. Many clients with mild to moderate disease have restricted their activity in response to fear of dyspnea and are surprised to learn that they can comfortably exercise at more intense levels than before rehabilitation. Therapeutic exercise should be designed to promote the functional activities needed by the individual. Arm exercises, such as using an arm ergometer or arm lifts using dowels or weights, promote the upper body strength needed for self-care, household, and recreational activities. Walking and exercising on a stationary bicycle promote cardiopulmonary conditioning and are exercises suited to the lifestyles of most individuals. Using a treadmill and water exercises are other options (Hughes & Davison, 1983; O'Hara et al., 1987; Ries, Ellis, & Hawkins, 1988).

Regular exercise is correlated with significant improvements in function in daily activities, self-care, sense of well-being and mastery, and control over the fear of dyspnea. Although exercise conditioning is not associated with improvement in pulmonary function parameters or ABGs, its positive effects on exercise tolerance and daily functioning are associated with improved quality of life (Braun, Fregosi, & Reddan, 1982; Holden, Stelmach, Curtis, Beck, & Stoller, 1990; Stratton, 1989). Progressive exercise supervised directly by a health-care professional may have the effect of deconditioning clients to the fear of dyspnea, resulting in increasing tolerance of activity (Glass, 1981).

ENERGY-CONSERVATION TECHNIQUES

Persons who live with chronic lung disease devise ways of conserving vital energy by, for example, using carts for carrying groceries and laundry, planning rest stops during strenuous activities, wearing clothing that is easy to put on, and using energy-saving devices such as microwave ovens and remote-controlled television. Even very resourceful individuals can benefit from discussing principles of energy conservation and planning ways to apply them in meeting present and future needs. Calling ahead to stores, shopping centers, and office buildings can yield important information about accesses with few stairs, merchandise available, and locations of offices or items. Obtaining and using a handicapped parking permit decrease the amount of walking needed for completing errands. Getting into and out of cars can be eased by placing a large plastic bag on the seat to reduce the adherence of clothing and upholstery. Combing hair and applying makeup consume less energy and tax breathing less when elbows are supported on a table.

Promoting Emotional Functioning

RELAXATION TECHNIQUES

Anxiety can trigger dyspnea and tax cardiopulmonary function. To gain mastery over these distressing responses, many clients benefit from reflecting on their responses to stress and applying principles of behavior modification to respond in ways that place fewer demands on cardiopulmonary reserves. Relaxation training and meditation techniques can be effective tools in the relief of anxiety. Progressive muscle relaxation has been shown to be effective in helping clients to slow breathing rates. This technique can be taught in one session and reinforced with a tape recording, before following up with two or three weekly outpatient sessions (Renfroe, 1988). Such techniques can be supplemented by the use of biofeedback to control tension in respiratory and peripheral muscles (Sandhu, 1986).

CLIENT AND FAMILY COUNSELING

Resources are best used when the client, family, and others are realistic about the disease and its impact. Counseling skills can be used to assist both client and family to acknowledge the thoughts and feelings accompanying limitations and losses. For clients overwhelmed by losses, summarizing the coping resources they and their support network possess can provide needed affirmation.

Sudden, unexplained changes in behavior may be related to physical or psychological factors. Nurses can apply advanced skills in assessment and counseling to assist families to understand and cope with this source of frustration (McDonald, 1981). To interrupt patterns of blame and anger, clients and families can be taught to attribute the emotional effects of COPD to the disease process and not to one another (McSweeney et al., 1982). They can be guided to increase their exposure to experiences that are psychologically rewarding.

A multidisciplinary approach can be used for clients with impaired emotional functioning. Pulmonary clients with depression have shown positive responses to antidepressant medications, including improvements in functional ability and quality of life (McDonald et al., 1989). Nurses can play a key role in recognizing signs of depression, making referrals for medical treatment, and evaluating client responses. Clients with severe depression or potential for suicide should be referred to a mental health professional.

ASSERTIVENESS TRAINING

Clients who learn and apply principles and techniques of assertive communication exhibit enhanced physical and emotional functioning. Such skills can help clients take effective action to communicate their needs, conserve energy, avoid exposure to respiratory infections, and control episodes of dyspnea. Success with assertive communication can bolster self-esteem.

One client coined the phrase "I need to take 10" to briefly communicate to family and friends her needs for rest or relaxation. She used this technique, along with self-monitoring, to arrest episodes of dyspnea and anxiety before her symptoms became severe. Another client pleased with new-found skills in assertive communication, commented, "Sometimes the best medicine is saying 'No!'"

SEXUAL COUNSELING

For persons with COPD, planning ahead is an essential coping skill applicable to most activities, including sexual expression. A program of exercise conditioning can result in improved breathing and energy levels during sexual activity. Like other exercises requiring energy expenditure, sexual activity is optimized at times of the day when breathing is best, often late morning or early afternoon. In the early morning, coughing may be a problem because respiratory secretions accumulate during the night. Sexual activity can be planned to coincide with the peak action of medications. Breathing is enhanced when clients avoid a large meal or physical exertion before sexual activity. Shared pleasure is heightened when both partners are relaxed and approach encounters by pacing, going slowly, and adopting an attitude of playfulness (Hahn, 1989).

Inhaled bronchodilators can be taken before or during sexual activity. Clients receiving oxygen should maintain usual flow rates or increase flow by 1 liter (Cooper, 1986). Pursed-lip breathing and diaphragmatic breathing should be used to improve breathing. Positions that will minimize pressure on the chest, such as side-lying or sitting, may be necessary (Katzin, 1990).

Interventions Related to Personal Resources

PROMOTING OPTIMAL NUTRITION

Because malnourishment predisposes clients to impaired breathing and infections, dietary intake and nutritional status should be carefully assessed. Assessment should include factors in the social history that predispose to malnutrition: inadequate income, absence of a person with whom to eat, inadequate facilities, smoking, and impaired mobility and dexterity (Openbrier & Covey, 1987).

Measures to maximize oral intake include snacks and meals high in calories and nutrients, using hard candy or gum to stimulate salivation before meals, planning the largest meal when hunger is greatest, and cooking aromatic foods to stimulate appetite. Meal-related oxygen desaturation can be assessed with oximetry and treated with increased liter flows. Stabilizing the chest by resting elbows on the table can facilitate breathing. Relaxation techniques and a general exercise program can relieve anxiety and promote appetite. Medication and treatment schedules can be revised to minimize gastric irritation, dry mouth, or expectoration of sputum. Gas-forming foods that impair function of the diaphragm should be identified and avoided.

Diet supplements can be used to provide calories and nutrients. There is an abundance of products available that are tailored to meet individual needs. One product, formulated in response to concerns about carbon dioxide production after ingestion of carbohydrates, contains 28 percent carbohydrate and 55 percent fat (Openbrier & Covey, 1987).

ENHANCING SLEEP

Measures that provide some relief from sleep-disturbing orthopnea include elevating the head of the bed on blocks, procuring a hospital bed, or sleeping or napping in a reclining chair. Clients with severe orthopnea may sleep best at a table, with the arms and upper body supported on pillows. Clients often report that a fan blowing on the face minimizes the sense of suffocation that accompanies dyspnea. Keeping the temperature comfortably warm and controlling humidity minimize oxygen demands and promote comfort and rest. Previously used habits and bedtime rituals should be identified and encouraged. Nocturnal oxygen administration is indicated for persons with sleep-related hypoxemia (Douglas & Flenley, 1990).

SOCIAL SUPPORT

Because an effective support system is essential for optimal coping, nursing care encompasses assessment of the support system, mobilization of the resources of that system, and interventions directed at maintaining the well-being of the entire network. The nurse can help clients identify what type of support would be most helpful during a given phase of illness and which expressions of support are not perceived as helpful (Woods, Yates, & Primomo, 1989).

Support groups for both clients and those affected by their disease can be a source of affirmation, sharing, and problem-solving ideas. Groups may employ a variety of formats. Members of the rehabilitation team and other community experts can present educational programs on topics of interest. Examples are summarized in Table 13.3. With a competent group leader, discussions of experiences, resources, and prob-

Table 13.3 ➤ **TOPICS FOR EDUCATIONAL PROGRAMMING FOR PULMONARY SUPPORT GROUPS**

Topic	Resource
Using humor in coping	Nurse
Expressing love and sexuality	
Expressing anger constructively	
Decisions about life-support	
Coping with change and loss	
Coping with stress	
Energy conservation	Occupational therapist
At home	
Away from home	
Medications, effects, and side effects	Pharmacist, physician, nurse
Air quality	Meteorologist
Options for exercise	Physical therapist
Optimal nutrition	Dietitian
Nebulizers for aerosol therapy	Respiratory therapist
Home oxygen systems	
Traveling with oxygen	
Transtracheal oxygen	Nurse and respiratory therapist
Financial aspects	Social worker and nurse
Community resources	
Home-care options	
Long-term care options	
Family relationships	
Personal safety at home and away from home	Hospital security officer

Source: Adapted from White (1989).

lem-solving methods can be helpful. Structured group exercises can be used to point out the psychosocial aspects of COPD and suggestions for coping with them. Both clients and family members can benefit from informal communication with persons sharing similar experiences, in a group setting or during a refreshment break.

FINANCIAL RESOURCES

Lost earnings combined with illness-related expenditures can be a source of distress. A social worker can provide invaluable assistance in evaluating financial assets and providing information about programs of assistance for which clients qualify.

SPIRITUAL RESOURCES

Spiritual beliefs and practices can provide meaning and sustenance for clients confronting the changes and losses accompanying COPD. Nurturing this resource can avert or lessen the distress experienced by clients with COPD and their families.

Life review, with emphasis on achievements and accomplishments, can be a useful tool in providing a sense of purpose and order to clients' experiences (Stollenwerk, 1985). For persons experiencing spiritual distress, interventions include prayer and discussion of concerns. A referral for pastoral care may be indicated. Clients unable to attend church services may benefit from home visits by a pastor and church members.

CAREGIVER SUPPORT

Because the long-term assistance of one or more support persons is critical to successful coping, planning may be necessary to maintain the resources of these individuals. Age and the stresses of caregiving put the caregiver, usually a spouse, at risk for health problems. The nurse should plan with the spouse for personal health management. Interventions may include stress management and relaxation techniques, referral to a support group, or attention to personal health needs. Volunteers may be available for weekly visits or for assistance with shopping and home maintenance. For clients with advanced disease, respite care in the home or an inpatient facility can assist the caregiver during times of stress or illness (Sexton & Munro, 1985).

Planning for Long-term Care

As the progression of illness impairs function, client and family may need assistance in making arrangements for long-term care. Coping tasks include acquiring information, setting priorities, allocating financial resources, and confronting the feelings accompanying multiple changes. In making decisions about home care or admission to a long-term care facility, clients and family members can benefit from the expertise of a social worker in evaluating financial assets and insurance coverage. Care in the home, even with ample assistance from other professional caregivers, requires a competent and dependable primary caregiver (Heslop & Bagnall, 1988; White & Briggs, 1980).

Preparing for Death

Preparing for the eventuality of death involves other coping tasks for the client and family. These include dealing with feelings and the accompanying behaviors, such as repression of fears and withdrawal from spouse and family members. Clients may need help in anticipating possible episodes of acute respiratory insufficiency and discussing with the physician how aggressively these will be treated. The implications of intubation and mechanical ventilation can be discussed before an acute problem occurs. Hospice care, at home or in an inpatient facility, is a resource that can be suggested and explored before the disease is at end-stage. Living will and power-of-attorney documents can be used by clients to communicate their wishes to family members and caregivers. After death, bereavement visits can assist family members in accepting changes and the associated feelings and integrating these into their life experience.

➤➤➤ Case Study

RUTH P.

The experiences of Ruth P., summarized as follows, illustrate some of the changes in quality of life experienced by an individual coping with COPD and some of the interventions that can be used to enhance quality of life at successive stages of the disease.

> Ruth P., age 72 years, reminisces during a home visit. Her narrative is cut short by dyspnea, but her story unfolds in subsequent visits. In her early 60s, after over 40 years of smoking 20 to 30 cigarettes a day, Ruth became increasingly aware of her "smoker's cough" and occasional shortness of breath. Her doctor told her she had emphysema. For several years, the diagnosis had little impact on her life. Widowed, with three adult children, she maintained her large first-floor flat, made and sold quilts, entertained, and went out with friends.
>
> The changes began insidiously. In her late 60s, Ruth noticed increasing shortness of breath while walking to the grocery store. She became so fatigued while shopping that, on arriving home, she collapsed exhausted into a chair. After resting, she was able to put the groceries

on cupboard shelves. She experienced increasing dyspnea while climbing the stairs to her daughter's second-floor apartment. Eventually this became so uncomfortable that she went up only with great effort and felt fatigued for the rest of the day. She now required help with heavier household chores, such as scrubbing floors and carrying baskets of laundry up and down the basement stairs.

"By this time," Ruth said, "the term 'emphysema' had personal meaning for me." She took an oral theophylline preparation and digitalis as prescribed and saw the physician when her sputum increased or became yellow-tinged, signs that she knew indicated a respiratory infection. She had repeated visits to the emergency room for episodes of acute dyspnea and the panic that invariably accompanied them. She was hospitalized with increasing frequency for treatment with intravenous and aerosol bronchodilators and oxygen and medical management of heart failure.

At the urging of her physician, Ruth reluctantly accepted a referral to an outpatient pulmonary rehabilitation program. At her first appointment, she received an overview of the 12-week program. At this visit the nurse did an assessment and interview, focusing on Ruth's experience with her lung disease and its impact on her life. Ruth manifested compromised quality of life in all areas: illness phenomena, perceptions, functional capacity, and personal resources. Team members collaborated in identifying Ruth's current problems and her resources for coping with her lung disease (Tables 13.4 and 13.5). Based on her personal goals, needs, and resources, they identified objectives and developed a plan of care (Table 13.6). Over the next 3 months, Ruth had individualized weekly appointments with members of the rehabilitation team, for monitored walking, breathing exercises, and teaching and counseling.

When asked to identify her greatest problem in living with lung disease, Ruth immediately mentioned episodes of acute breathing difficulty, which she experienced with increasing frequency and acuity.

Table 13.4 ➤ **NURSING DIAGNOSES OF RUTH P.**

Ineffective breathing patterns related to airflow limitation
Anxiety related to episodes of dyspnea
Impaired mobility related to dyspnea, fatigue, and deconditioned state
Altered self-esteem related to reliance on family members
Altered health maintenance: neglect of other health needs (dental, podiatric) related to dyspnea and fatigue
Potential for noncompliance related to cost of medications and difficulty getting to pharmacy
Self-care deficit: bathing, cooking, laundry, related to dyspnea and deconditioned state
Knowledge deficit about self-assessment, medications, energy conservation, breathing exercises
Impaired health maintenance related to smoking

Table 13.5 ➤	ASSESSMENT OF RESOURCES FOR COPING WITH LUNG DISEASE FOR RUTH P.

Assets	Deficits
PERSONAL	
Sense of humor	Limited skills in assertive
Personal and family experience with illness	communications
Cognitive skills	Little knowledge of lung disease and
Trust in physician, medications	coping strategies
Age and life-experience: effects on	
expectations	
Low-energy hobbies	
SOCIAL	
Significant person: daughter	Concern about other daughter's
Son, daughter-in-law	impending divorce and finances
Sister in Arizona	
Other family members	
Network of friends	
Pet dog	
SPIRITUAL	
Faith	Difficulty attending church
Good relationship with pastor	
PHYSICAL	
Good appetite	Cardiorespiratory pathology
Prepares well-balanced meals	Deconditioned state
	Arthritis
	Obesity
	Smoking
	Hearing deficit
FINANCIAL	
Income supplemented by hobby (selling her	Gaps in insurance coverage
quilts)	Cost of medications
Financial resources for energy-saving	Expenses of maintaining large home
devices	
ENVIRONMENTAL	
No other smokers in home	Maintenance of large home
	Use of sprays and aerosols

While eating in a restaurant, a pleasure she savored, she would suddenly experience dyspnea and panic so acute that she would rush outside panting and pale, leaving her meal untouched, her companion deserted, and Ruth exhausted for the rest of the day. The sense of powerlessness evoked by these episodes was a distressing aspect of the illness. She admitted taking extra puffs of her metered-dose inhaler at these times but found that this offered limited relief. When told that pulmonary rehabilitation might provide help in gaining control over these episodes, Ruth was skeptical but willing to participate.

Table 13.6 ➤ **PLAN OF CARE FOR RUTH P.**

Personal goals identified by Ruth
1. To receive a medication or treatment to control panic attacks
2. To depend less on family members for household chores
3. To visit sister in Arizona, if possible
4. To remain in home for as long as possible

Objectives developed by Ruth and rehabilitation team. Ruth will:
1. Verbalize awareness of her resources for coping with effects of her lung disease
2. Demonstrate knowledge and skill in maintaining an effective equilibrium of physical and psychological resources including:
    Knowledge for coping with lung disease
    Management of dyspnea-panic episodes
    Health maintenance: optimal nutrition, rest, and exercise
    Self-care of personal needs
    Home management skills
    Effective self-administration of prescribed medications, including oxygen if needed
    Stress management
    Satisfying relationships
    Financial resources
3. Use resources for smoking cessation
4. Demonstrate improved exercise tolerance
5. Exhibit increased function in ADLs
6. Lose 20 lb
7. Consider plans and options for making a trip to Arizona to visit her sister
8. Report increased satisfaction with her quality of life

Interventions. Teaching and counseling related to:
1. Living with lung disease
    Awareness of energy, fatigue, and early sensations of dyspnea
    Recognizing and promptly reporting signs of infection
    Avoiding respiratory irritants
      In the home environment
      In public places
      Seasonal conditions
        Ozone, humidity in summer
        Cold weather in winter
2. Breathing retraining exercises
    Diaphragmatic breathing
    Pursed-lip breathing
    Coordinated breathing
    IMT as prescribed
3. Stress management
    Identification of stressors
    New responses to stress
    Assertive communication principles and skills
    Relaxation techniques
4. Smoking cessation
    Exploring personal motives to quit
    Referral
    Individualized program
5. Energy-conservation techniques
    Planning ahead
    Rest periods
    Work simplification
    Organizing supplies
    Positioning for efficiency
    Saying "no"

(Continued)

Table 13.6 ➤ **PLAN OF CARE FOR RUTH P. (Continued)**

6. Nutritional assessment and counseling
    Control of obesity
        Behavior modification
        Cognitive restructuring
    Prevention of muscle atrophy
    Control of CO_2 production
        Decreasing carbohydrates
        Increasing polyunsaturated fats
7. Exercise program
    Progressive exercise
        Walking
        Stationary cycling
        Arm exercises
    Application of coordinated breathing
    Self-monitoring, safety precautions

Ruth was taught controlled breathing patterns, designed to make more effective use of her diaphragm and other respiratory muscles. First she learned diaphragmatic breathing, relaxing her abdomen while inhaling and moderately tightening abdominal muscles while exhaling. In later visits, she learned and practiced pursed-lip breathing, exhaling slowly through lips tightened almost into a whistling position. The pulse oximeter was used as a biofeedback tool to give Ruth immediate visual evidence of the efficacy of her new breathing pattern. She was able to increase her oxygen saturation from 86 to 94 percent with a few minutes of pursed-lip breathing.

Next she learned coordinated breathing, integrating the controlled breathing patterns into movements and ADLs. The effort-expending portion of activities, she learned, should be done while exhaling slowly. She demonstrated her skill in applying this pattern while placing groceries on shelves, inhaling while resting and exhaling while lifting items to shelves. At the nurse's suggestion, she placed smiling-face stickers as visual cues in her home environment to remind her to use controlled breathing patterns while bathing, and dressing, preparing meals, changing bed linens, and performing other ADLs.

With some reluctance, Ruth participated in learning relaxation techniques, using tape-recorded exercises twice a day to progressively relax muscle groups and induce a state of mental quietude. Focusing attention on herself was a new experience for her, and she needed regular encouragement to continue with this. As she became attuned to the feeling of tension in her neck and shoulder muscles, she could see how this affected her breathing and how she could prevent episodes of dyspnea by arresting the developing tension.

Ruth's variable level of energy was a daily problem, which she felt powerless to control. She could not anticipate what her energy level would be on any given day or time of day. Her fluctuating energy level seemed to be affected by how well she had slept, the air quality, humidity, and her psychological state. When she pushed herself too hard, the ensuing exhaustion reinforced the need to take control of this aspect of her disease. A goal for this problem was for Ruth to balance rest and activity to prevent episodes of extreme fatigue and dyspnea. Interventions involved helping Ruth to learn new skills: sensitivity to her body's sense of energy or fatigue and the ability to identify factors that affected her energy level. She was helped to adopt new attitudes: accepting her fluctuations in energy and learning to consider all plans tentative. She was taught to apply skills in assertive communication in making her needs known to family and friends. Like her, they needed to learn that coping with lung disease may require last-minute changes in plans. Ruth learned to be flexible, changing plans when her energy level was unexpectedly low and, when necessary, canceling appointments or plans with friends.

During summer, when air quality in the city could deteriorate, Ruth learned to monitor meteorologists' reports of ozone levels, air quality, and humidity, available on radio and television news and on telephone recordings by the local weather service and the Department of Natural Resources. When ozone levels were high or the air-quality index was low, she avoided going out if possible. She learned to schedule appointments and do shopping early in the morning to avoid peak ozone levels, which usually occur in the afternoon. She found humidity oppressive and, on particularly bad days, sought refuge in her air-conditioned bedroom.

Smoking Cessation

During the first 6 years after diagnosis of her emphysema, Ruth had made 5 aborted attempts to quit smoking. She attended a group program with a friend, but her hearing deficit made it difficult to participate. On her own, she cut back to about 15 cigarettes a day but was unable to quit. "I truly enjoy those cigarettes!" she said with conviction. While attending the pulmonary rehabilitation program, she half-heartedly agreed to participate in individualized counseling by a graduate nursing student. Through this program, supplemented by exercises from the American Lung Association's (1986) booklet *Freedom from Smoking in 20 Days,* she was eventually successful in total smoking cessation. Especially helpful to her was her list of smoking substitutes: activities she enjoyed that did not involve smoking (Table 13.7). During this time, she became a connoisseur of teas and sugar-free candies; she immersed herself in her hobbies, making piles of quilts and afghans. She commented, "Sometimes I get so absorbed in my sewing that I don't think of smoking for several hours."

Table 13.7 ➤	**RUTH'S LIST OF THINGS I ENJOY THAT DO NOT INVOLVE SMOKING**
Sewing a square for quilting	Playing solitaire
Caring for my plants	Crocheting a section of an afghan
Eating a gooey dessert	Typing a letter
Working a jigsaw puzzle	Making popcorn
Combing the dog's coat	Playing cards with a friend
Taking a warm bath	Making holiday decorations
Drinking a cup of tea	

Ruth discussed her ambivalence about quitting smoking. "I surprised myself. I never believed I'd quit." She also saw this as a loss of one of her greatest pleasures, at a time when her life was becoming constricted by her disease. One of the nursing goals at this time was for Ruth to view her smoking cessation more as a successful achievement and less as a loss. Principles of client contracting (Steckel, 1982) were used to help her to reinforce nonsmoking. Weekly goals were set, with the main criterion that they be easily achievable. The first goal was for Ruth to make a list of 6 things she enjoyed that cost no more than $5. She readily agreed to this and returned the next week with her list (Table 13.8).

She learned to use these rewards to reinforce her nonsmoking behavior and to build her sense of self-esteem as a nonsmoker. She continued to find it especially difficult to avoid smoking during the first hour of the morning. She was instructed to build into her environment cues that stimulated behaviors other than smoking. For example, she set the table for breakfast before going to bed. Upon arising, she brushed her teeth and proceeded immediately to prepare breakfast, avoiding cues to her former habit of reading the newspaper in the living room with a cup of coffee and a cigarette. After getting through this first hour smoke-free, she was instructed to reinforce her behavior with a reward from her list. She grew to relish using these rewards to reinforce her nonsmoking behavior and reported satisfaction at her hard-won victory over smoking.

Table 13.8 ➤ **RUTH'S LIST OF THINGS I ENJOY THAT COST NO MORE THAN $5**	
Watching the *Today* show	Doing light gardening
Reading a biography from the library	Reading *People* magazine
Buying flowers	Sitting out in the yard
Calling my sister in Arizona	Watching the late movie
Staying in my robe and slippers all morning	Listening to music
Going out to lunch with my daughter	Having a neighbor over for coffee

Exercise Program

Ruth attempted to participate in the physical-conditioning aspect of the rehabilitation program. In favorable weather, she would begin a walking program, but had difficulty sustaining the effort. Inclement weather limited her walking, and she had no interest in the stationary bicycle that was recommended. "I've never been one to exercise much," she said, "and, to be honest, I have trouble believing it can help me now." Interventions were designed: a discussion and demonstration by a client who experienced markedly increased exercise tolerance after beginning a walking program, and a demonstration of the effects of exercise on Ruth's pulse rate.

Ruth agreed to participate in a program of arm exercises, designed to help her to prevent the limitation of arm function that often accompanies chronic lung disease. During clinic visits, she used the arm ergometer in supervised exercise sessions with the physical therapist. At home, she did exercises taught by the therapist, lifting a 36-inch wooden dowel overhead repetitively while using coordinated breathing. Ruth was motivated to comply with the arm exercise program because "My arms are stronger and that makes a difference in my life. I can see that it's easier to lift big pieces of fabric, bathe myself, comb my hair, and cook."

Energy Conservation

The aspect of the program that Ruth enjoyed most was learning the energy-conservation techniques taught by the occupational therapist. She learned ways to simplify daily activities that soon became habits, such as rolling laundry in a sheet and pushing it down the basement stairs, and placing clean laundry on hangers in the basement to be carried up later by visiting family members.

She completed the 12-week rehabilitation program, participating in the components with varying degrees of enthusiasm. The most salutary outcome for her was a marked increase in her daily activities. "The coordinated breathing has made all the difference for me," she reported in a postprogram evaluation. "I've learned to pace myself. Now I can do things that I hadn't done for the past year—vacuum my own carpet, put my groceries away without getting exhausted, enjoy time with my grandchildren again." She was exhilarated at the liberation of again being able to climb stairs, exhaling through pursed lips while climbing and pausing to inhale and rest on every third stair.

Group Support

Ruth began attending the monthly meetings of a support group for clients with chronic lung disease and their families and friends, coordinated by the nurse manager of the pulmonary rehabilitation program.

The format of meetings consisted of a brief practice of breathing exercises, an educational program on an aspect of living with lung disease, group discussion, and informal conversation and refreshments. Ruth and her daughter attended meetings when possible. It was a new experience for Ruth to see other people coping successfully with lung disease more advanced than hers. She was heartened to hear a man with portable oxygen discussing his golf score. She empathized with group members who discussed the hazards of using handicapped parking permits when one has an "invisible handicap." She cheered their stories of using assertive communication in responding to unfeeling comments by strangers in restaurants and shopping centers. She incorporated information from the educational sessions into her own self-care practices.

Relocation

Over the next 2 to 3 years, her lung disease became the central fact of Ruth's life. She experienced a series of changes and losses and came to rely heavily on her daughter's daily assistance.

As Ruth became unable to maintain her home, her daughters searched for a satisfactory housing unit for elderly people, completed the extensive application forms, sold much of her furniture, packed, moved, and set up the new household in a way that would conserve Ruth's now limited energy. The pulmonary rehabilitation nurse assisted with planning for energy conservation. She recommended investing in several new appliances—a microwave oven, a remote-control television, and an apartment-size air conditioner. A reclining chair was also suggested for rest periods with feet elevated. Ruth and her daughter were advised to set up "living stations," that is, chairs in two or three areas of the home where needed supplies would be within easy reach. Ruth's daughter set up a chair by the bathroom sink and placed all toiletry supplies within arm's reach. In the kitchen, she placed frequently used articles on countertops or in waist-level drawers, to minimize bending and reaching, which impair ventilation and consume energy. In the living room, the reclining chair was placed within easy reach of a floor lamp, magazine rack, and a table that held commonly used items: telephone, television remote control, writing supplies, crocheting and sewing supplies, nail file, and tissues. In the bedroom, the sewing machine was similarly equipped with all needed items within easy reach.

Ruth experienced fatigue and difficulty sleeping, which were attributed to nocturnal oxygen desaturation. This was documented using oximetry, and nocturnal oxygen was prescribed. The oxygen proved to be a mixed blessing, increasing Ruth's energy while presenting several new challenges.

When Ruth's associates in the building saw the "Oxygen in Use" sign on her apartment door, some of them expressed anxiety and began avoiding her. The nurse suggested having a question-and-answer session on oxygen presented for her friends, the building manager, and other interested tenants. Ruth sent invitations and was happily surprised when 12 people appeared at the appointed time. They listened attentively to the nurse's explanation of the system and raised questions about the combustibility of oxygen, the possibility of a cylinder exploding, and the belief that only terminally ill people are treated with oxygen. Several expressed relief in learning that oxygen is a safe treatment that poses no threat to people nearby. Their altered beliefs enabled Ruth to demonstrate that nothing essential had changed despite the oxygen cylinder and nasal cannula.

As Ruth's hypoxemia progressed, her pulmonologist prescribed continuous oxygen therapy. It now became necessary for Ruth to let the delivery person from the durable medical equipment (DME) company into her apartment every 3 to 4 days to replace empty cylinders. Ruth experienced this as an intrusion into her privacy and schedule. On delivery days, Ruth would be certain to be dressed by midmorning. Because of her hearing deficit, she worried that she would fail to hear the doorbell, especially when she was resting. She curtailed rest periods until the oxygen had been delivered. Walking to the door and carrying on a short conversation consumed precious energy. In discussing principles of energy conservation, Ruth admitted, "This is all too fatiguing." With her approval, the nurse arranged for Ruth's friend across the hall to have a key to her apartment and to let the delivery person in.

With Ruth now receiving continuous oxygen, the DME supplier suggested an oxygen concentrator as an option. At the nurse's next visit, Ruth raised questions about concentrators and expressed reluctance to make a change. The nurse explained the function of the concentrator, removing nitrogen and other gases from the air to provide a concentrated supply of oxygen. She pointed out the advantages for someone on continuous, low-flow oxygen: it would be less costly and require less frequent service, helping Ruth to conserve energy. About the size of an end table, with a wood grain finish, the concentrator would be more pleasant to look at. She also made Ruth aware of the differences from her present system. Because concentrators are powered by electricity, Ruth would still require an oxygen cylinder as a backup system in case of power failure. She could expect to become accustomed to the low-pitched mechanical humming sound of the concentrator after the first few days.

Upon trying the concentrator, Ruth realized that its smooth functioning allowed her to plan her daily rest periods without the previously bothersome interruptions. She expressed anxiety about the possibility of a power failure. "I'll just have to call the paramedics," she said, revealing anger at her sense of powerlessness. The nurse used demonstrations, with return demonstrations by Ruth, to teach her to disconnect her tubing from the concentrator and connect it to the cylinder in the closet, after turning the flow meter to 2 liters. Reliance on the oxygen delivery system induced in Ruth feelings of vulnerability, dependency, anger, and depression. During home visits, Ruth was encouraged to express these feelings. An effective strategy was providing Ruth with feedback and summaries of her successful coping behaviors, aimed at helping her to maintain her self-esteem and sense of autonomy despite increasing limitations. She learned to accept the oxygen and to successfully make the lifestyle adjustments associated with it.

At first, the oxygen therapy caused Ruth to restrict her mobility outside of her apartment building. The nurse taught Ruth's daughter to manage the portable cylinder and procured a wheelchair. Ruth enjoyed the freedom of short outings, for a meal at a restaurant and for appointments.

At the outset of her pulmonary rehabilitation program, Ruth had expressed a tentative wish to travel to Arizona to visit her sister. "I know it's probably too late," she had said, "but some days I think I could do it." With considerable support and coordination by the rehabilitation team, this dream became a reality for Ruth. She traveled by train, accompanied by her daughter. Liquid oxygen was supplied along the route and in Phoenix by vendors carefully orchestrated by the respiratory therapist. Upon her return, Ruth expressed gratitude for this opportunity. "The things I learned in the rehab program gave me the energy and confidence to make the trip," she said. Her sense of personal accomplishment was evident.

Declining Trajectory

For the next 10 months, Ruth enjoyed a high level of function in her daily activities. She then developed a fever and acute dyspnea, diagnosed as pneumonia. Hospitalized in the intensive-care unit, she received intravenous and aerosol bronchodilators and intravenous antibiotics. Blood gases were monitored frequently and a ventilator was on standby. When asked if she had fears, Ruth said to her nurse, "This is the closest I've ever come to dying. I'm afraid I'll suffocate. But I don't want to be put on any machines. And I don't want a tube in my throat." Aware of the physician's plans for intubation if necessary, the nurse consulted the clinical nurse specialist (CNS). The CNS asked Ruth about her impressions of intubation and mechanical ventilation, pointed out the need to support respiratory muscles during episodes of fatigue, and clarified Ruth's misconceptions. Ruth held firmly to her insistence on "no tubes or machines for breathing." The CNS communicated Ruth's wishes to the physician, who met with Ruth and her family and reluctantly agreed to comply with her wishes for no intubation. Ruth recovered from this episode and returned home.

Over the coming months, her quality of life declined precipitously as Ruth experienced greater energy deficits and constant dyspnea. She required the help of a home health aide for laundry, housecleaning, meal preparation, and bathing. In the shower she experienced acute feelings of suffocation, so a hand-held shower and shower chair were supplied. Most of her limited energy was now directed at easing her breathing. As dressing became exhausting, she wore only a nightgown and slippers. She spent much of her time sitting with her elbows propped on the kitchen table, a position that best eased her dyspnea. A fan blowing on her face provided some relief from the constant feeling of suffocation. As Ruth experienced impairment of her attention span and short-term memory, her reading was limited to short magazine articles. Television provided some diversion, but eating aggravated her shortness of breath. Because the effort of chewing impaired her breathing, she ate mainly soft foods, augmented with diet supplements. Within a 10-week period she lost 25 pounds, despite meal assistance. To ease orthopnea, the head of her bed was elevated on blocks and she used several pillows. Her sleep was fitful and she napped intermittently, night and day, in the reclining chair. Digitalis and diuretics had little effect on her pitting edema. Eventually a commode became necessary, because walking to the bathroom became too great an effort.

Nursing care during this time was directed at meeting Ruth's basic needs, supporting her and her family in adapting to the changes imposed by her disease, and planning for her future needs. At times Ruth and her family coped ineffectively with the losses, stresses, and demands of illness. Some family members began avoiding Ruth. The nurse interpreted their behaviors, reminding Ruth that they loved her but felt powerless to make her comfortable and feared losing her. She encouraged Ruth to discuss her feelings with them. Ruth's family sometimes expressed frustration at her irritability and forgetfulness. When they recognized these as signs of hypoxia, they were better able to accept her without blaming and to help in planning for her safety. When Ruth recognized her powerlessness to control her body and the changes brought by her now end-stage disease, she attempted to control family members through demanding and manipulative behaviors. The nurse supported family members in setting realistic limits. She helped Ruth and her family to express their feelings about loss and death. Ruth's daughter later said, "The turning point for me was when the nurse said our job is to care for Mom, not to get a cure for her. After that I could put my energy into trying to make her comfortable."

During this time, Ruth experienced times of spiritual distress, questioning the need for her suffering and expressing hopelessness about the prayers that had previously sustained her. The nurse contacted a nearby parish, and Ruth began receiving weekly visits from the priest. She appreciated the opportunity to receive communion, to pray with the priest, and to discuss concerns.

It became evident to Ruth and her family that her needs would soon exceed the resources available at home. Ruth feared being left alone, even for short periods. Her daughter was becoming exhausted from spending nights with her mother, working full time, and maintaining her own family and household. They acknowledged that a nursing home would be needed. After weighing the assets of available homes and prioritizing Ruth's needs—proximity to family and space for a small table where Ruth could sit with her arms supported and feet elevated with a fan blowing on her face—a home with these requisites was found.

Ruth's cardiopulmonary function continued to decline. Her breathing became increasingly labored, her skin became taut with edematous fluid, urine output lessened, and her awareness became obtunded. During her third night in the nursing home, Ruth died of acute heart failure caused by her lung disease.

Her daughter later reflected, "One difficult part of having a chronic illness is not knowing what is ahead, when an acute episode may occur in the middle of the night, when the end is coming. We thought Mom probably had weeks or months to live. If we had known her death was so near, we would have stayed with her for those 3 days at home. There was no way of knowing. Having a chronic disease gives you a chance to prepare and to lose a loved one in pieces, instead of all at once. At each stage, the nurses helped us to anticipate and plan for the problems of the next stage."

SUMMARY

Quality of life for persons with COPD is affected by illness phenomena, perceptions, functional capacity, and personal resources. Changes experienced by clients and families can be ameliorated by nursing strategies, provided within the framework of a rehabilitation team approach. Such strategies are associated with significant improvements in the four aspects of quality of life. Continued research is needed to evaluate the efficacy of specific interventions and to refine the selection of interventions for groups of clients having common characteristics.

REFERENCES

American Lung Association. (1986). *Freedom from smoking in twenty days.* New York: American Lung Association.

Barstow, R. E. (1974). Coping with emphysema. *Nursing Clinics of North America, 9,* 137–145.

Bergner, M., Bobbitt, R. A., Carter, W. B., & Gilson, B. S. (1981). The Sickness Impact Profile: Development and final revision of a health status measure. *Medical Care, 19,* 787–805.

Borg, G. A. V. (1982). Psychophysical bases of perceived exertion. *Medicine and Science in Sports and Exercise, 14,* 377–381.

Borkgren, M. W. (1989). Diversity in pulmonary rehabilitation: A geographic survey study. *Journal of Cardiopulmonary Rehabilitation, 9,* 63–71.

Braun, S. R., Fregosi, R. ,& Reddan, W. G. (1982). Exercise training in patients with COPD. *Postgraduate Medicine, 71,* 163–173.

Braun, S. R., Keim, N. L., Dixon, R. M., Clagnaz, P., Anderegg, A., & Shrago, E. S. (1984). The prevalence and determinants of nutritional changes in chronic obstructive pulmonary disease. *Chest, 86,* 558–563.

Brown, M. L. (1988). Measuring dyspnea. In M. Frank-Stromberg (Ed.), *Instruments for clinical nursing research* (pp. 369–378). Norwalk, CT: Appleton & Lange.

Burns, M. R. (1987). Cruising with COPD. *American Journal of Nursing, 87,* 479–482.

Campbell, M. L. (1987). Sexual dysfunction in the COPD patient. *Dimensions of Critical Care Nursing, 6,* 70–74.

Carpenito, L. J. (1997). *Nursing diagnosis: Application to clinical practice* (7th ed.). Philadelphia: JB Lippincott.

Carrieri, V. K. (1989). *Will the self-management/cognitive behavioral strategies used in the pain model decrease dyspnea?* Paper presented at the meeting of the American Thoracic Society, Cincinnati, OH.

Carrieri, V. K., & Janson-Bjerklie, S. (1986). Strategies patients use to manage the sensation of dyspnea. *Western Journal of Nursing Research, 8,* 284–301.

Carrieri, V. K., & Janson-Bjerklie, S. (1993). Dyspnea. In V. K. Carrieri, A. M. Lindsey, & C. M. West, *Pathophysiological phenomena in nursing: Human responses to illness* (2nd ed., pp. 191–218). Philadelphia: WB Saunders.

Carrieri, V. K., Janson-Bjerklie, S., & Jacobs, S. (1984). The sensation of dyspnea: A review. *Heart and Lung, 13,* 436–447.

Christopher, K. I., Spofford, B. T., Petrun, M. D., McCarty, D. C., Goodman, J. R., & Petty, T. L. (1987). A program for transtracheal oxygen delivery: Assessment of safety and efficacy. *Annals of Internal Medicine, 107,* 802–808.

Cooper, K. (1986). Sexual counseling of the patient with chronic lung disease. *Focus on Critical Care, 13,* 18–20.

Curgian, L. M., & Gronkiewicz, C. A. (1988). Enhancing sexual performance in COPD. *Nurse Practitioner, 13,* 34–35.

Daughton, D. M., Fix, A. J., Kass, I., Patil, K. D., & Bell, C. W. (1979). Physiological-intellectual components of rehabilitation success in patients with chronic obstructive pulmonary disease (COPD). *Journal of Chronic Diseases, 32,* 405–409.

Davido, J. (1981). Pulmonary rehabilitation. *Nursing Clinics of North America, 16,* 275–283.

DeVito, A. J. (1985). Rehabilitation of patients with chronic obstructive pulmonary disease. *Rehabilitation Nursing, 10,* 12–15.

DeVito, A. J. (1990). Dyspnea during hospitalization for acute phase of illness as recalled by patients with chronic obstructive pulmonary disease. *Heart and Lung, 19,* 186–191.

Douglas, N. J., & Flenley, D. C. (1990). Breathing during sleep in patients with obstructive lung disease. *American Review of Respiratory Disease, 141,* 1055–1070.

Dracup, K., & Raffin, T. (1989). Withholding and withdrawing mechanical ventilation: Assessing quality of life. *American Review of Respiratory Disease, 140,* S44–S46.

Dudley, D. L., Glaser, E. M., Jorgenson, B. N., & Logan, D. L. (1980). Psychosocial concomitants to rehabilitation in chronic obstructive pulmonary disease. *Chest, 77,* 413–420, 544–551, 677–684.

Dudley, D. L., Wermuth, C., & Hague, W. (1973). Psychosocial aspects of care in the chronic obstructive pulmonary disease patient. *Heart and Lung, 2,* 389–393.

Emery, C. F., Leatherman, N. E., & MacIntyre, N. R. (1989, November). *Psychological effects of a pulmonary rehabilitation program.* Paper presented at the meeting of the Gerontological Society of America, Minneapolis, MN.

Fagerhaugh, S. Y. (1973). Getting around with emphysema. *American Journal of Nursing, 73,* 94–99.

Fletcher, E. C., & Martin, R. J. (1982). Sexual dysfunction and erectile impotence in chronic obstructive pulmonary disease. *Chest, 81,* 413–421.

Foxall, M. J., Ekberg, J. Y., & Griffith, N. (1987). Comparative study of adjustment patterns of chronic obstructive pulmonary disease patients and peripheral vascular disease patients. *Heart and Lung, 16,* 354–363.

Fulmer, J. D., & Snyder, G. L. (1984). American College of Chest Physicians/National Heart, Lung, and Blood Institute national conference on oxygen therapy. *Heart and Lung, 13,* 550–562.

Gift, A. G. (1987). Dyspnea: A clinical perspective. *Scholarly Inquiry for Nursing Practice, 1,* 73–85.

Gift, A. G. (1989). Visual analogue scales: Measurement of subjective phenomena. *Nursing Research, 38,* 286–288.

Gift, A. G., & Cahill, C. A. (1989). Psychophysiological aspects of dyspnea in COPD. *American Review of Respiratory Disease, 139,* A245.

Gift, A. G., Plaut, S. M., & Jacox, A. (1986). Psychologic and physiologic factors related to dyspnea in subjects with chronic obstructive pulmonary disease. *Heart and Lung, 15,* 595–601.

Gilson, B. S., Gilson, J. S., Bergner, M., Bobbitt, R. A., Kressel, S., Pollard, W. E., & Vesselago, M. (1975). The Sickness Impact Profile: Development of an outcome measure of health care. *American Journal of Public Health, 65,* 1304–1310.

Glass, L. B. (1981). Exercise therapy for the patient with pulmonary dysfunction. *Topics in Clinical Nursing, 3,* 87–93.

Gordon, M. (1994). *Nursing diagnosis: Process and application* (3rd ed.). New York: McGraw-Hill.

Grant, I., Heaton, R. K., McSweeney, A. J., Adams, K. M., & Timms, R. M. (1980). Brain dysfunction in COPD. *Chest, 77S,* 308–309.

Guyatt, G. H., Berman, L. B., Townsend, M., Pugsley, S. O., & Chambers, L. W. (1987). A measure of quality of life for clinical trials in chronic lung disease. *Thorax, 42,* 773–778.

Guyatt, G. H., Thompson, P. J., Berman, L. B., Sullivan, M. J., Townsend, M., Jones, N. L., & Pugsley, S. O. (1985). How should we measure function in patients with chronic heart and lung disease? *Journal of Chronic Diseases, 38,* 517–524.

Guyatt, G. H., Townsend, M., Berman, L. B., & Pugsley, S. O. (1987). Quality of life in patients with chronic airflow limitation. *British Journal of Diseases of the Chest, 81,* 45–54.

Hahn, K. (1988). A nursing framework for multidisciplinary rehabilitation. *Rehabilitation Nursing, 11,* 6–10.

Hahn, K. (1989). Sexuality and COPD. *Rehabilitation Nursing, 14,* 191–195.

Hanson, E. I. (1982). Effect of chronic lung disease on life in general and on sexuality: Perceptions of adult patients. *Heart and Lung, 11,* 435–441.

Heaton, R. K., Grant, I., McSweeney, A. J., Adams, K. M., & Petty, T. L. (1983). Psychologic effects of continuous and nocturnal oxygen therapy in hypoxemic chronic obstructive pulmonary disease. *Archives of Internal Medicine, 143,* 1941–1947.

Heimlich, H., & Carr, G. (1989). The Micro-Trach: A seven-year experience with transtracheal oxygen therapy. *Chest, 95,* 1008–1012.

Heslop, A. P., & Bagnall, P. (1988). A study to evaluate the intervention of a nurse visiting patients with disabling chest disease in the community. *Journal of Advanced Nursing, 13,* 71–77.

Holden, D. A., Stelmach, K. D., Curtis, P. S., Beck, G. J., & Stoller, J. K. (1990). The impact of a rehabilitation program on functional status of patients with chronic lung disease. *Respiratory Care, 35,* 332–341.

Hudson, L. D., & Pierson, D. J. (1981). Comprehensive respiratory care for patients with chronic obstructive pulmonary disease. *Medical Clinics of North America, 65,* 629–645.

Hughes, R. L., & Davison, R. (1983). Limitations of exercise reconditioning in COLD. *Chest, 83,* 241–249.

Janson-Bjerklie, S., Carrieri, V. K., & Hudes, M. (1986). The sensations of pulmonary dyspnea. *Nursing Research, 35,* 154–159.

Katzin, L. (1990). Chronic illness and sexuality. *American Journal of Nursing, 90,* 55–59.

Kersten, L. (1989a). Changes in self concept during a pulmonary rehabilitation program. *American Review of Respiratory Disease, 139,* A194.

Kersten, L. (1989b). *Comprehensive respiratory nursing: A decision making approach.* Philadelphia: WB Saunders.

Kim, M. (1984). Respiratory muscle training: Implications for patient care. *Heart and Lung, 13,* 333–339.

Kim, M., & Larson, J. L. (1987). Ineffective airway clearance and ineffective breathing patterns: Theoretical and research base for nursing diagnosis. *Nursing Clinics of North America, 22,* 125–134.

Kinsman, R. A., Yaroush, R. A., Fernandez , E., Dirks, J. F., Schocket, M., & Fukuhara, J. (1983). Symptoms and experiences in chronic bronchitis and emphysema. *Chest, 83,* 755–761.

Kirilloff, L. H., Carpenter, V., Kerby, G. R., Kigin, C., & Weimer, M. P. (1986). Skills of the health team involved in out-of-hospital care for patients with COPD. *American Review of Respiratory Disease, 133,* 948–949.

Klink, M., & Quan, S. E. (1987). Prevalence of reported sleep disturbances in a general adult population and their relationship to obstructive airways diseases. *Chest, 91,* 540–546.

Lareau, S., & Larson, J. L. (1987). Ineffective breathing pattern related to airflow limitation. *Nursing Clinics of North America, 22,* 179–191.

Larson, J. L., Kim, M. J., Sharp, J. T., & Larson, D. A. (1988). Inspiratory muscle training with a pressure threshold breathing device in patients with chronic obstructive pulmonary disease. *American Review of Respiratory Disease, 138,* 689–696.

Light, R. W., Merrill, E. J., Despars, J. A., Gordon, G. H., & Mutalipassi, L. R. (1985). Prevalence of depression and anxiety in patients with COPD: Relationship to functional capacity. *Chest, 87,* 35–38.

Lindell, K. O., & Mazzocco, M. C. (1990). Breaking bronchospasm's grip with MDIs. *American Journal of Nursing, 90,* 34–39.

Lucas, J., Golish, J. A., Sleeper, G., & O'Ryan, J. A. (1988). *Home respiratory care.* Norwalk, CT: Appleton & Lange.

Lush, M. T., Janson-Bjerklie, S., Carrieri, V. K., & Lovejoy, N. (1988). Dyspnea in the ventilator-assisted patient. *Heart and Lung, 17,* 528–535.

Mahler, D. A., Weinberg, D. H., Wells, C. K., & Feinstein, A. R. (1984). *Chest, 85,* 751–758.

McDonald, G. (1981). A home care program for patients with chronic lung disease. *Nursing Clinics of North America, 16,* 259–273.

McDonald, G., Borson, S., Gayle, T., Deffebach, M., & Lakshminarayan, S. (1989). Nortriptyline effectively treats depression in COPD. *American Review of Respiratory Disease, 139,* A11.

McGavin, C. R., Gupta, S. P., & McHardy, G. J. R. (1976). Twelve-minute walking test for assessing disability in chronic bronchitis. *British Medical Journal, 1,* 822–823.

McSweeney, A. J., Grant, I., Heaton, R. K., Adams, K. M., & Timms, R. M. (1982). Life quality of patients with chronic obstructive pulmonary disease. *Archives of Internal Medicine, 142,* 473–478.

Moser, K. M., Bokinsky, G. E., Savage, R. T., Archibald, C. J., & Hansen, P. R. (1980). Results of a comprehensive rehabilitation program. *Archives of Internal Medicine, 140,* 1596–1601.

Nocturnal Oxygen Therapy Group. (1980). Continuous or nocturnal oxygen therapy in hypoxemic chronic obstructive lung disease. *Annals of Internal Medicine, 93,* 391–398.

O'Hara, W. J., Lasachuk, K. E., Matheson, P. C., Renahan, M. C., Schlotter, D. G., & Lilker, E. S. (1987). Weight training benefits in chronic obstructive pulmonary disease: A controlled crossover study. *Respiratory Care, 32,* 660–667.

Openbrier, D. R., & Covey, M. (1987). Ineffective breathing pattern related to malnutrition. *Nursing Clinics of North America, 22,* 225–247.

Openbrier, D. R., Fuoss, C., & Mall, C. C. (1988). What patients on home oxygen therapy want to know. *American Journal of Nursing, 88,* 198–201.

Openbrier, D. R., Hoffman, L. A., & Wesmiller, S. W. (1988). Home oxygen therapy: Evaluation and prescription. *American Journal of Nursing, 88,* 192–197.

Openbrier, D. R., & Rogers, R. M. (1989). Validity and reliability of visual analog scales (VAS) used to measure symptoms in patients with COPD. *American Review of Respiratory Disease, 139,* A244.

O'Ryan, J. A., & Burns, D. G. (1991). *Pulmonary rehabilitation: From hospital to home* (2nd ed.). St. Louis: CV Mosby.

Padilla, G. V., Presant, C., Grant, M. M., Metter, G., Lipsett, J., & Heide, F. (1983). Quality of life index for patients with cancer. *Research in Nursing and Health, 6,* 117–126.

Perry, J. A. (1981). Effectiveness of teaching in the rehabilitation of patients with chronic bronchitis and emphysema. *Nursing Research, 30,* 219–222.

Porth, C. M. (1993). *Pathophysiology: Concepts of altered health states* (5th ed.). Philadelphia: JB Lippincott.

Prigatano, G. P., Wright, E. C., & Levin, D. (1984). Quality of life and its predictors in patients with mild hypoxemia and chronic obstructive pulmonary disease. *Archives of Internal Medicine, 144,* 1613–1619.

Renfroe, K. (1988). Effect of progressive relaxation on dyspnea and state anxiety in patients with chronic obstructive pulmonary disease. *Heart and Lung, 17,* 408–413.

Ries, A. L., Ellis, B., & Hawkins, R. W. (1988). Upper extremity exercise training in chronic obstructive pulmonary disease. *Chest, 93,* 688–692.

Ryan, P. (1989). Noncompliance. In J. M. Thompson, G. K. McFarland, J. E. Hirsch, S. M. Tucker, & A. C. Bowers (Eds.), *Clinical Nursing* (pp. 1612–1615). St. Louis: CV Mosby.

Sandhu, H. S. (1986). Psychosocial issues in chronic obstructive pulmonary disease. *Clinics in Chest Medicine, 7,* 629–642.

Sexton, D. L. (1990). *Nursing care of the respiratory patient.* Norwalk, CT: Appleton & Lange.

Sexton, D. L., & Munro, B. H. (1985). Impact of a husband's chronic illness (COPD) on the spouse's life. *Research in Nursing and Health, 8,* 83–90.

Sexton, D. L., & Munro, B. H. (1988). Living with a chronic illness: The experience of women with chronic obstructive pulmonary disease (COPD). *Western Journal of Nursing Research, 10,* 26–44.

Shenkman, B. (1985). Factors contributing to attrition rates in a pulmonary rehabilitation program. *Heart and Lung, 14,* 53–58.

Sleeper, G. (1988). Traveling with oxygen. In J. Lucas, J. A. Golish, G. Sleeper, & J. A. O'Ryan (Eds.), *Home respiratory care* (pp. 95–108). Norwalk, CT: Appleton & Lange.

Steckel, S. (1982). *Patient contracting.* New York: Appleton-Century-Crofts.

Stollenwerk, R. (1985). An emphysema client: Self care. *Home Healthcare Nurse, 3,* 36–40.

Stratton, B. F. (1989). Pulmonary rehabilitation: For the breath of your life. *Journal of Cardiopulmonary Rehabilitation, 9,* 80–86.

Strauss, A., Corbin, J., Fagerhaugh, S., Glaser, B., Maines, D., Suczek, B., & Weiner, C. (1984). *Chronic illness and the quality of life.* St. Louis: CV Mosby.

Tiep, B. L., Burns, M., Kao, D., Madison, R., & Herrera, J. (1986). Pursed lips breathing training using ear oximetry. *Chest, 90,* 218–221.

Timms, R. M. (1982). Sexual dysfunction and chronic obstructive pulmonary disease. *Chest, 81,* 398–399.

Traver, G. A. (1985). *Information for home respiratory therapy patients: Traveling with oxygen.* Deerfield, IL: Travenol Laboratories.

Traver, G. A. (1988). Measures of symptoms and life quality to predict emergent use of institutional health care resources in chronic obstructive airways disease. *Heart and Lung, 17,* 689–697.

Weaver, T., & Narsavage, G. (1989). Reliability and validity of the Pulmonary Impact Profile Scale. *American Review of Respiratory Disease, 139,* A244.

Wenger, N. K., Mattson, M. E., Furberg, C. D., & Elinson, J. (1984). Assessment of quality of life in clinical trials of cardiovascular therapies. *American Journal of Cardiology, 54,* 908–913.

West, J. B. (1991). *Pulmonary pathophysiology: The essentials* (4th ed.). Baltimore: Williams & Wilkins.

White, H. A., & Briggs, A. M. (1980). Home care of persons with respiratory problems: Optimization of breathing and life potential. *Topics in Clinical Nursing, 2,* 69–77.

White, P. (1989, October). *Pulmonary support groups.* Paper presented at the meeting of the Nursing Assembly of the American Lung Association, Milwaukee, Wisconsin.

Woods, N. F., Yates, B. C., & Primomo, J. (1989). Supporting families during chronic illness. *Image, 21,* 46–50.

14

Empowering Persons Affected by Acquired Immunodeficiency Syndrome*

➤ JoAnne Bennett

Acquired immunodeficiency syndrome (AIDS) is a late-twentieth-century hallmark of both the advances and limitations of biopsychosocial sciences. It is a pandemic infection that can debilitate and threaten life in both young and old. Its epidemiology reflects the breadth and pace of late-twentieth-century social mobility, both globally and regionally. Unlike the acute infectious diseases that challenged society at the end of the nineteenth century (but like many noninfectious chronic diseases that became prevalent in the late-twentieth-century, postantibiotic era), the natural history of AIDS is slow and relatively silent. The uncertainties of dealing with a chronic illness are a constant for persons with AIDS (PWAs).[1]

Since the AIDS virus, human immunodeficiency virus type 1 (HIV-1),[2] was first identified in 1983, symptomatic disease has been recognized as the tip of an iceberg that includes a broad spectrum of illnesses

---

*Because of the detail and length of this chapter, an outline is included in Appendix A as a guide for the reader.

as well as asymptomatic organ dysfunction. A nonlinear progression of symptoms masks continuously progressing pathology. Like so many chronic diseases, HIV disease progresses silently and symptoms do not occur until the disease is considerably advanced. There is considerable individual variation in the length of the asymptomatic period, and although symptoms often occur before immunodeficiency is severe, there may be no symptoms even when severe pathology is present. Diverse manifestations that are discomforting or debilitating, but not life threatening, can be intermittent or persistent.

Although popular media previously promulgated a hopeless perspective for persons with AIDS, today's media report declining mortality, longer survival, more effective treatments, and even the possibility of an eventual cure. For those with advanced disease, particularly those who have tried many regimens through the course of their illness, each new treatment presents a gamble, not a promise. Treatments may cause uncomfortable side effects and possible cumulative and irreversible damage to nerves, liver, pancreas, kidneys, and/or bone marrow. Improvement may mean months of improved laboratory test results rather than longer survival or improved health.

In this disease, chronicity means not merely a long-term incurable illness, but rather unending, cumulative, and potentially or seemingly uncontrollable demands that the individual must integrate into daily life, along with uncertainty about the short- and long-term implications of the illness. "Impaired functioning is experienced in multiple body-mind and spirit systems" (Miller, 1992, p. 4).

Nurses may encounter PWAs in any health-care or community setting, whether its purpose is HIV-specific care, general health care, a clinical specialty unrelated to HIV (e.g., family counseling center, addictions treatment program, home care, college or university health service unit, family planning or obstetric center, nutrition or holistic care center, employee health service, mental health practice, long-term care), or in a setting not specific for health-care delivery (e.g., a homeless shelter, a church's meal program, a school or day-care center, a worksite employee assistance program, or a senior citizen's center). AIDS care can encompass counseling the worried well whose actual HIV risk may be negligible, or very great, as in pre-HIV-antibody test counseling. Nurses are involved in posttest counseling for positive and negative results, bereavement counseling, and supportive care to a PWA's family, friends, and larger social network. Some families have (or are grieving for) one or more infected adult members, sometimes along with one or more infected children. The nurse may also work with groups, such as a support group, a work group of volunteer caregivers, or a bereavement group.

Simultaneous regimens for palliative care and aggressive treatment are frequently needed in providing care to the PWA. Severe symptoms do not necessarily herald terminal disease. Surviving an acute opportunistic illness (OI) episode or starting a newly available treatment often brings remarkable reversal in disability and even prognosis. Prophylactic regimens remain important even in very late-stage disease.

The implications and impact of issues related to the disease's chronicity vary for an individual at different times. However, many concerns recur throughout the illness, such as choosing health-care providers, locating and accessing services, maintaining or obtaining insurance coverage, starting or changing treatments, stopping or returning to a job, disclosing health status to others, planning for financial growth and conserving resources, reconciling with significant others, appraising the personal implications of research findings, weighing the health-promoting potential and lifestyle implications of using newly available drugs, considering the end of life, preparing for potential dependency and/or incompetence by drafting a will and advance directives for health care, designating a health-care proxy and power of attorney, and planning for future guardianship of children who are minors as needed.

THE HUMAN IMMUNODEFICIENCY VIRUS/ACQUIRED IMMUNODEFICIENCY SYNDROME CHALLENGE

Distinguishing between AIDS and the rest of the HIV disease spectrum is rather artificial and can be misleading. HIV disease is a continuum of immunodeficiency, and an absence of symptoms does not indicate viral dormancy or latent disease. Immune dysfunction begins early in the disease—within a couple of weeks after the onset of infection. Manifestations vary, but all represent the ineluctable progression of underlying immunodeficiency and its sequelae.[3] In other words, the distinction between AIDS and earlier HIV disease is quantitative, not qualitative. AIDS is not a separate "stage" of pathology per se. Rather, a distinct case definition is maintained for epidemiological surveillance that is *not intended for clinical purposes*. By restricting surveillance definition for AIDS to manifestations that indicate the same degree of cellular immunodeficiency associated with the two diseases first identified as AIDS—*Pneumocystis carinii* pneumonia (PCP) and Kaposi's sarcoma (KS)[4]—epidemiologists have uniform criteria in defining the presence of AIDS. The clinical perspective, however, must be broader.

The Disease Course

Human immunodeficiency virus involves multiple pathogenic mechanisms. When it first enters the body, HIV rapidly infects a large number of CD4 T cells[5] and then continues to replicate rapidly (10 billion new virions per day), seeding various organs, particularly the lymphoid organs (lymph nodes, spleen, tonsils, and adenoids) (Pantaleo et al.,

1997). The immune system fights back by producing CD8 T lymphocytes (killer T cells) and B-cell-produced antibodies that directly attack HIV in the bloodstream, and CD8 cells that destroy HIV-infected cells. Local infection of nonlymphoid tissues, such as the central nervous system, is sustained and propagated by monocytic cells, which serve as reservoirs that hide accumulating virus from the immune cells.

The result is a flu or mononucleosis-like febrile illness (lymphadenopathy, malaise, anorexia, gastrointestinal [GI] symptoms, pharyngitis, esophagitis, aphthous ulcers, skin eruptions, myalgia, and arthralgia, with marked lymphopenia frequently followed by relative lymphocytosis [signs that the immune system has been activated]) 2 to 6 weeks after initial infection. The severity and duration of this primary illness vary. The affected person typically does not associate it with an HIV exposure and often does not even seek medical intervention. Thus, because the symptoms do not seem very different from those of other seasonal viral syndromes, the HIV infection remains undiagnosed.

The symptoms subside within 2 to 3 weeks (but may persist for 2 to 3 months); however, the virus is not eliminated. Indeed, viremia is remarkably high even in asymptomatic HIV-infected individuals. The continued viral replication in the lymph nodes causes progressive, ultimately irreversible damage. Paradoxically, the body's immune response to the persistent HIV infection creates favorable conditions for disease progression. The persistent infection induces cytokines to activate the immune cells in which the virus replicates. The virus replicates more rapidly in activated cells. The immune response effectively limits the viral replication *rate* until viral destructive capacity eventually exceeds the immune cells' replicative capacity. Then plasma viremia rises and immunodeficiency worsens.[7] The co-occurrence of rising viremia and falling CD4 lymphocytes thus signifies that the immune system can no longer maintain equilibrium against the virus. (CD4-cell counts greater than $500/mm^3$ are associated with viral loads of fewer than 10,000 HIV copies/mm^3).

The life-threatening opportunistic diseases that are the criteria for Centers for Disease Control and Prevention (CDC)-defined[4] AIDS typically manifest when the CD4-cell count drops to $200/mm^3$ or fewer. Immunodeficiency continues to worsen as the number of CD4 cells declines further and the CD8-cell count also drops dramatically. Extensive fibrosis of lymphoid tissue essentially eliminates trapping of viruses and other organisms, so circulating virus levels rise and eventually match those found in lymph nodes.[6] As immune controls continue to deteriorate, the virus replicates at a faster rate, boosting viremia ever higher.

Symptoms

Human immunodeficiency virus disease is a multisystemic disease, the chief sequelae of which are infectious and neoplastic opportunism secondary to immunodeficiency, autoimmune phenomena, and metabolic derangements. HIV itself directly affects the GI, cardiac, reproductive, endocrine, dermatologic, neuromuscular, and renal systems, each of which may also manifest one or more OIs or malignancies. Hence there is a wide range of possible symptoms. Chronic or intermittent symptoms can range from mild discomfort to severe disability, even in a person who has not experienced an AIDs-defining OI. The nonspecific symptoms of an activated immune system (such as fever, headache, myalgia, arthralgia, chills, night sweats, anorexia, and fatigue) may also be incapacitating.

The sequence and timing of symptom occurrence are quite variable. Some symptoms may be short term, others persistent or recurring. OIs may be missed if a person's risk is not accurately assessed. In addition, an atypical early presentation of an OI may not be recognized as HIV related. For example, HIV encephalopathy—known as AIDS dementia complex (ADC)—can precede symptoms of immunologic dysfunction, although clinically evident neurological dysfunction typically occurs later in the disease. Linear progression of symptoms is not typical.

The earliest symptoms of AIDS include lymphadenopathy (a sign of a functional immune response), dermatologic abnormalities (including seborrhea, psoriasis, perifolliculitis, pruritus, itchy red bumps on trunk and extremities), and oral lesions (such as aphthous ulcerations and hairy leukoplakia). When the number of CD4 cells drops below $500/mm^3$, skin and oral lesions become more common or worsen. Failing immunity is manifested by OIs, neoplasms, and/or severe and persistent constitutional signs and symptoms, including unexplained weight loss, intermittent fatigue, muscle aches and joint pain, headaches, and fevers, often with chills and/or profuse sweating. Recurrent episodes of diarrhea, shingles, thrush, vaginal candidiasis, bacterial sinusitis, and bronchitis are also typical. Persistent generalized lymphadenopathy (PGL) (defined as the involvement of two or three extrainguinal node-bearing areas that persists 3 months or longer) may or may not be evident. The subsiding of PGL is generally considered a late sign that heralds imminent marked immune deterioration.

The co-occurence of OIs makes definitive diagnosis difficult, particularly when symptoms overlap. With more advanced disease, comorbidity is more common and adverse drug effects occur more frequently and are often more severe. Drug tolerance can change with each addition to an individual's drug regimen and also with changes in one's health status. Also, the person with more advanced disease may be less able to tolerate discomforting or energy-draining side effects of treatment. As the disease progresses, the number of drugs prescribed is likely to be greater, further increasing the chance of both dangerous and unpleasant interactions. Drug-nutrient interactions also occur. Other adverse effects or interactions may be related to inadvertent misadministration of medications, especially when multiple providers are involved.

DIARRHEA

Sporadic or persistent diarrhea (defined by stool weight, frequency, or consistency) afflicts almost all PWAs at some point in the disease course. The incidence increases with advancing disease, symptomatic of opportunistic pathogens. When diarrhea persists for a month or longer, it is considered chronic. The most frequent cause is parasitic GI infections, but cytomegalovirus (CMV) colitis may be implicated in almost half of chronic diarrhea cases. Mycobacterial enteritis, resulting in fever and wasting, is another cause of diarrhea. Acute diarrhea with abdominal pains, sometimes with bloody stools, occurs with bacterial GI infections, including those with *Salmonella, Shigella, Campylobacter,* and *Clostridium difficile.* Nausea and vomiting suggest that the upper GI tract is also involved, whereas cramping, gas, increased bowel sounds (borborygmi), watery stool, and diarrhea with fasting indicate small-bowel disease. When the distal colon is involved, frequent small-volume stools are accompanied by urgency, followed by a sense of incomplete evacuation; lower abdominal pain and rectal bleeding may also occur.

The CD4-cell count directs the approach to differential diagnosis. When multiple stool tests are negative, sigmoidoscopy is used. When no specific cause for chronic diarrhea is found, the diagnosis of AIDS enteropathy is made. Enteropathic malabsorption may be caused by low-grade bacterial overgrowth or rare pathogens, including unusual viruses. Functional and morphologic abnormalities directly caused by HIV, including atrophy, increased mucosal permeability, and chronic inflammation, have also been implicated. Chronic unexplained diarrhea can be intractable, although it sometimes subsides spontaneously even after months of unsuccessful treatment. The diarrhea-associated opportunistic diseases that occur when CD4-cell counts drop to 100/mm³ or below are associated with a poor prognosis, particularly when there is weight loss and wasting.

Intervention

Treatment of chronic diarrhea includes bulking and antimotility agents along with antimicrobials. Diet manipulation is often helpful. Consultation with a nutritionist is important both to help determine the role of diet in the etiology and treatment of the diarrhea and, most important, to prevent wasting. Hydration, electrolyte balance, skin integrity, and psychological morbidity are also vital components of treatment.

HUMAN IMMUNODEFICIENCY VIRUS WASTING

Wasting or involuntary weight loss indicates disease progression, regardless of the degree of immunodeficiency. Women may be at greater risk because of low testosterone levels or other hormonal differences and also because of delayed access to health care. Malabsorption and/or diarrhea may be caused by one or more of many types of infections (parasites, viruses, bacteria), including HIV itself (AIDS enteropathy), or neoplasms. Weight loss may also reflect inadequate intake. Poor appetite, dysphagia, painful mouth ulcers, taste disturbances, fatigue, malaise, dyspnea, reduced finances, depression, and social isolation or withdrawal may alter a person's eating pattern, resulting in reduced intake while metabolic requirements are rising in response to (identified or unidentified) infection(s) or neoplasm(s). Some drugs may cause a person to feel bloated. Some PWAs, intending to promote their health and/or boost their immunity, restrict their diet to foods or eating patterns that are counterproductive, and this results in undernutrition. Weight loss despite good intake and the absence of diarrhea may reflect altered metabolism or malabsorption that is attributable to HIV-related atrophy of intestinal villi.

Weight loss per se is not the primary issue, but rather the loss of lean muscle mass that accompanies weight loss. Protein-calorie malnutrition concomitant with the weight loss (or accompanying weight gain in the absence of lean muscle development) furthers immunodeficiency. The greater the loss in lean body-cell mass, the higher the mortality. Thus, although overall dietary intake is important, the goal is not just an issue of calories and maintaining weight or fat. Changes in body composition and inadequate micronutrient intake can alter pharmacokinetics and thus affect drug efficacy and toxicity.

Undernutrition, in turn, can affect degree of energy and fatigue, mood, coping, one's capacity to manage activities of daily living (ADLs) and self-care, and the body's response to infectious diseases. Nutritional deficits can be easily overlooked. People who have previously been overweight may not perceive weight loss as undesirable. Others may attribute muscle loss to reduced activity or changes in exercise patterns, particularly if it is not accompanied by weight loss per se. Similarly, weight maintenance, even gain, may mask wasting if lean muscle mass is not replenished.

Intervention

Early attention to preventing the start of the wasting process is vital, because once started, it is difficult to reverse. Treating an underlying GI infection or eliminating an offending therapy can reverse some anorexia and diarrhea (Casey, 1997). Diet manipulation may also be effective in diarrheal management. When pathogens do not respond to treatment, antidiarrheal agents and hydration are key to weight control. Short-term peripheral parenteral nutrition may also be necessary. Cryptosporidiosis and Microsporida infections are particularly difficult to treat. Supplements and other strategies to increase nutrient intake are useful, but their potential efficacy is predicated on reversing underlying anorexia. Steroids, cyprohepatidine, hydrazine sulfate, dronabinol, thalidomide, and megesterol acetate are being evaluated for safety and/or efficacy in improving PWAs' appetite and weight maintenance (Cooper & Horn, 1997). Early indications are that their efficacy may be short-lived. Improved appetite is not always accompanied by weight gain. The social component of appetite must not be overlooked. Congregate meal programs can be organized not only to provide nutritious meals with food choices, but also to emphasize hospitality, social interaction, and camaraderie. While extending the PWA's food dollar, such programs can provide a venue for other support services, including nutrition consultation and other health teaching. Delivery of meals to the homebound can also provide an opportunity for social visiting.

Reviewing diet history and intake patterns is an important component of establishing the baseline for ongoing monitoring of nutritional status, which should include deliberate as well as incidental changes in intake and meal patterns. Physical assessment should include skin condition and inspection of oral mucosa in addition to weight and musculoskeletal physique. The diet diary is useful not only for assessing intake, but also as a teaching tool. It often starkly illustrates the (quantitative and qualitative) difference between actual and perceived intake and eating patterns and thus can help both the PWA and clinician recognize nutritional risk. Nutrition teaching must start early in the disease course, with the recognition that changing nutritional behavior is likely to take time and practice. The transtheoretical model of behavior change (Prochaska & DiClemente, 1984, Prochaska & Norcross, 1992) is a useful guide for planning effective teaching, reinforcement, and coaching. Simply providing information and explaining the purpose and importance of "dos and don'ts" are not adequate. Not only is repetition over time necessary, but separate appointments, with or without a dietitian, can provide the needed reinforcement and continued assessment of nutritional learning needs. Including family and household members in these sessions can help mobilize social support for the PWA and provide necessary teaching for others involved in meal preparation.

Teaching needs to address basic nutrition principles (nutrient requirements and the role of vitamin and mineral supplements, the five basic food groups with recommended amounts, food preparation, and the concept of whole foods and the value and limitations of supplement formulations), how to read nutrition information on packaged-food labels, and precautions against infection in food storage and preparation, including implications for shopping and eating out. Also to be included in teaching plans are nutrition-related management of nausea, vomiting, diarrhea, fever, fatigue, food intolerance, and early satiety as well as dealing with anorexia, xerostomia, stomatitis, and dysphagia. Supplements, such as Ensure, are not intended to replace regular meals. Eliminate consumption of low-nutrient-value foods that may be filling or promote bloating and explain how they can compromise nutritional adequacy.

Potential confusion or contradictions may be inherent in our instructions. For example, drug regimens that require an empty stomach may be counter to recommendations for frequent snacking to enhance intake. Prepare a specific schedule with the individual PWA that "fits" the PWA's sleep-wake-activity schedule. Evaluate this plan in terms of congruence with other household members' schedules. Review its 7-day-a-week applicability and design alternate plans, as needed, for certain days with variant schedules. Hands-on teaching in kitchen settings may enhance learning and assist people to learn how to integrate nutrition teaching, energy conservation, and work simplification into safe food preparation (Casey, 1997; Lehman, Muurahainen, Guenter, & Canteruci, 1996; Liss, Chan, McKinley, Ilaria, & Jacobs, 1996).

FATIGUE

Fatigue is multidimensional with biological, cognitive, affective, sensory, and sociobehavioral causes and manifestations. Fatigue is more prevalent in advanced disease. A detailed history is key to identifying sources of an individual's fatigue and understanding its impact. A fatigued person may feel weak, have motor difficulty, lack concentration, feel anxious or restless, be unable to sleep, and withdraw from social life. It is important to distinguish fatigue from depression.

Fatigue may be related to disease, to treatment, or both. Anemia, cachexia, high cytokines, hypogonadism, respiratory incapacity, anxiety, depressed mood, overexertion, sleep-wake disturbances, or other reasons for inadequate rest may underlie fatigue. Of course, an individual's fatigue may have overlapping causes. Sleep and rest can be disrupted by any number of symptoms, which also drain energy during waking hours. The work of illness-care routines clearly taxes energy reserves. Nokes and Kendrew (1996) pointed out that any illness that causes significant pain or discomfort or that is associated with metabolic disturbances can have a negative impact on both the quality and quantity of sleep. Neurological effects of disease or drug treatment may affect sleep quality. Sleeping pills do not adequately relieve disturbed sleep.

Intervention

Client teaching should include planning and organizing activities to conserve energy, setting priorities and choosing those activities that are most fulfilling, planning rest, and identifying energy-draining and energy-replenishing activities. Attention to nutrition is important in order to avoid a cycle of not eating because of being tired or skipping meals because of napping. Likewise, the raised endorphin level produced during exercise enhances feelings of energy and well-being. Pharmacological interventions being studied for possible benefits include psychostimulants, antidepressants, corticosteroids, and thalidomide, which lowers cytokine activity.

ENCEPHALOPATHY AND NEUROMUSCULAR SYNDROMES

AIDS dementia complex (ADC) is characterized by decreased concentration, slowed thought, loss of interest in activities, forgetfulness, poor judgment, and slowed motor movements. Routine activities may require concentrated effort. Mood and behavior change may be noted by others. Similar symptoms may be caused by focal lesions of OIs or lymphomas originating in or spreading to brain tissue or to the meninges.

Neuromuscular disorders may be the presenting symptom of HIV disease, but they are commonly masked by coexistent CNS problems such as dementia, focal brain lesions, or myelopathy (Simpson & Tagliati, 1997). In later disease, the insidious progression of peripheral neuropathy or myopathy may be missed by focusing on OIs or presuming that they are neuromuscular effects of antiretroviral or other drug regimens.

Myopathy may occur at any time in the course of HIV disease and is not associated with any particular stage of immunosuppression. The typical manifestation is slowly progressive muscle weakness, evident when climbing stairs or getting up from sitting in a chair. Myalgia, a nonspecific symptom in HIV infection, is present in less than half of those with myopathy. A definitive diagnosis is made by electromyogram and biopsy examination when limb weakness is accompanied by creatine kinase elevation. Myopathy-associated wasting (in the absence of malnutrition or other systemic causes) may improve with prednisone therapy. Because zidovudine-induced myopathy is clinically indistinguishable from HIV-induced myopathy, the initial treatment is always to stop zidovudine (ZDV) therapy. Not all patients experience improvement after ZDV withdrawal, but some who improve can resume taking ZDV without recurrence of the myopathy.

Different forms of peripheral neuropathy occur with greater frequency at particular disease stages. Acute and chronic inflammatory demyelinating neuropathy (IDN) occurs infrequently, typically when CD4-cell counts are high and the person is otherwise asymptomatic; the prevalence of distal symmetrical polyneuropathy (DSP) increases with immunosuppression. CMV, which manifests in advanced AIDS, may present as progressive polyradiculopathy (PR). With IDN, there is severe motor impairment and ataxia and absent or mild sensory symptoms. The acute form is marked by rapidly progressive weakness in two or more limbs and sometimes the face, along with generalized areflexia. When drug toxicity, nutritional, and metabolic etiologies have been ruled out, symptomatic treatment can include analgesics, tricyclic antidepressants, and anticonvulsants. Ganciclovir therapy is tried if muscle biopsy shows evidence of CMV disease. Otherwise immunomodulation with steroids, intravenous immunoglobulin, and plasmapheresis may be tried. None of these strategies have yet been evaluated in controlled clinical trials, however.

SENSORY-PERCEPTUAL ALTERATIONS

Visual disturbances caused by CMV retinitis occur late in the disease, when CD4 counts fall below 50 to 100/mm^3. Blindness will occur unless the infection is treated promptly. The vision loss, which is progressive and irreversible, can be limited by timely intervention.

Toxoplasma gondii and varicella-zoster virus (VZV) can also affect the eye, and KS can affect the eyelids and/or conjunctivae. Keratitis, uveitis, and blepharitis also occur.

PAIN, DEPRESSION, AND SUICIDAL VULNERABILITY

The prevalence of pain in PWAs is significant and includes peripheral neuropathy, headache, sore throat and dysphagia, abdominal pain and cramping, arthralgias and myalgias, headache, and skin conditions, including severe pruritus and the effects of advanced KS. Because pain syndromes respond best to specific interventions, a comprehensive assessment to define the pain syndrome and untangle its physical and psychological components is essential. Pain can be overlooked in the person who is confused, delirious, or demented and is often dismissed or undertreated in PWAs with a history of addiction. Effective pain relief depends on appropriately using pharmacological, psychosocial, and cognitive-behavioral interventions. Neuropathic pain responds well to antidepressants, anxiolytics, or anticonvulsants. Steroids are useful for the headaches of toxoplasmosis. Psychostimulants help reduce the sedative effects of narcotics while augmenting analgesia.

Disease-related depression is marked by persistent feelings of sadness, panic, worthlessness, and yearning for lost normalcy and certainty of one's personal world that are accompanied by increasing dysfunction, inability to anticipate pleasure, and suicidal preoccupation. Drug-induced depression is associated with a number of agents commonly used in HIV disease, including ZDV, interferon, sulfonamides, acyclovir, ethambutol, anticonvulsants, dapsone, isoniazid, nonsteroidal anti-inflammatory drugs (NSAIDs), neuroleptics, benzodiazepines, and ganciclovir (McEnany, Hughes, & Lee, 1996). Hence, pharmacological treatment of depression in a person with HIV is complex and requires careful monitoring of side effects. This should not preclude drug intervention; rather, it underscores the need for careful evaluation of selective polypharmacy. Individual and group psychotherapy targeted at depressive symptoms, as well as cognitive-behavioral interventions and other modalities to enhance coping and enrich social supports, is integral.

EMPOWERED OR OVERWHELMED?

Morse (1997) contended that nursing's mission is to help those whose self-integrity is threatened by disruptions in health. This mission is accomplished by nursing's focus on the experiential aspects of illness. Barrett's (1983, 1990) definition of power is appropriate for addressing the challenge that AIDS poses to the individual, family, and community. Barrett emphasized that power was the capacity for action, energy, and accomplishment and not control over means and others. Power encompasses an "affective feeling of strength, a volitional and cognitive recognition of choices, and behavioral activities" (Barrett, 1983, p. 6). It is a *knowing participation in change* with four interrelated dimensions: awareness, choice, freedom to act intentionally, and involvement in the process of change.

Power is not a tool; instead, it is recognized as integral to everyone's daily activities, existence, and growth. Rather than control, it is self-transformation and transformation of relationships with others. Power may be noted in information seeking, recognizing opportunities for self-improvement, initiative taking, and involvement with others. Nurses can coach clients and their families to recognize potentialities and tap sources of power, to acknowledge the options that are available, and to sort through multiple illness demands to set goals and plan for future potentialities.

Implications for Acquired Immunodeficiency Syndrome Care

For nurses and other health-care professionals, this paradigm of power and empowerment requires a renewed commitment to learn and to use the knowledge we acquire and to clarify our values and goals and the bases for them. We also must explore how others form their preferences and make their choices. Sharing ambiguities and uncertainties with PWAs and those who care for and about them may result in empowerment. Helping PWAs become competent in self-care and symptom management empowers them.

PARTNERSHIP

Empowerment includes the PWA's identifying potentials and setting goals collaboratively with professionals and informal caregivers. Few choices can be made in isolation by the client *or* clinician. Partnership and reciprocity may be essential for all sources of power. In other words, one person does not empower another. Rather, to "advocate for [PWAs] who have limited power to deal with a devastating disease, an inadequate health care delivery system, and a society that blames them for their illness" (Adinolfi, 1996, p. 220), we must engage in partnership with them at all levels of decision making. Determining needs and engaging in policy making about community-wide programs are needed.

The nature of the partnership that evolves varies with the individuals involved. The nurse recognizes not only the PWA's individuality or uniqueness, but also his or her personhood. In turn, the client recognizes the nurse's individuality and personhood as well as professionalism. As clients' needs and capacities vary along with nurses' abilities, so too will the quality and productivity of the partnerships that evolve. Mutuality is demonstrated when each shares his or her own intentions and goals and explicates the purpose and rationale that underlie them, while accepting the other's preferences, beliefs, and values. It is a reciprocal process of collaborative consciousness-raising. Acceptance conveys respect for the other and appreciation of the other's goals and prerogatives. It does not presuppose changing one's own view or adopting the other's goals as one's own. Nevertheless, both partners can expect to grow. The nurse's advice and suggestions must be offered tentatively, anticipating mutual evaluation of whether and how well it meets an individual's or family's needs in a particular circumstance.

CHAMPIONING SELF-HELP

Zerwekh (1991) identified four strategies that nurses can use to promote self-help and autonomous choice: "(1) *believing in* the clients' ability to make choices and helping the clients believe in themselves, (2) *listening* to what the clients want and starting there, (3) *expanding* families' vision of options, and (4) *feeding back* reality to help them see the patterns of their lives and the implications of unhealthy choices" (p. 213). She underscored the importance of timing. A nurse's encouragement for behavior change must match the individual's readiness. The nurse may need a one-step-at-a-time approach, *backing off* and not pressuring, *getting through the door* by behaving like a respectful guest and meeting clients at their level. The "do-not-take-over" caveat is especially relevant for introducing and encouraging health-protective lifestyle changes, help seeking, and discussion of diagnosis or worsening symptoms with significant others, as well as for presenting medical regimens that the PWA may be reluctant to pursue. One must be attentive to withdrawal clues such as lack of eye contact, missed appointments (or patterns thereof), or evasive or contradictory responses. The appropriate nursing response may be to postpone discussions, to make supplementary appointments, to be present and less directive. The PWA's receptiveness may seem to counter the goal of providing timely anticipatory guidance for the challenges, needs, and crises that may evolve.

ASSESSMENT

The nursing assessment of the PWA proceeds as a head-to-toe review of systems and functional health patterns according to the clinician's standard practice, which varies somewhat depending on setting, theoretical framework, and acuteness of the client's presenting complaint or purpose for hospitalization (nurse's or client's) visit. If the nursing goal is to facilitate and enhance the PWA's self-determination and effective health-promoting responses to illness demands, then the assessment must emphasize the person's competence to plan and implement action to seek information, help, and care; the efforts that he or she has taken; and his or her interpretation of responses to those efforts.

A more conversational approach, rather than a structured interview, can facilitate empathetic exchange between nurse and client while gathering data. Because many PWAs have repeatedly provided information, often quite personal, to other providers as part of "intake" procedures at diverse agencies (either to assess health-care needs or to access services, or to apply for entitlements such as insurance or disability benefits), it can be a challenge to personalize what can easily be perceived as a perfunctory routine using a scripted checklist. To keep the dialogue from seeming like an interrogation, beware of needlessly asking for information that can be accessed readily from the client record. Instead, go over information with the client to verify its accuracy or inquire about changes or subtle nuances. For example, probing, "Could you tell me more about that?" or "I'm not sure I understand what you mean by that" gives the person an opportunity to confirm, modify, or correct your impressions. Using "open-ended questions, rather than questions that can be answered with a simple yes or no, allows the patient to talk freely about personally relevant issues" (Adinolfi, 1996, p. 226).

A comprehensive baseline assessment is difficult, if not impossible, to achieve at first encounter. Continuing assessment involves ongoing conversation that parallels physical observations and direct inquiry with structured interviews. Client self-disclosure and candor about needs, values, goals, and concerns are thus the product of an ongoing relationship that is built with deliberate effort. Perception of the nurse's candor and honesty influences what information the PWA shares, what question he or she asks, how he or she evaluates the nurse's advice, and whether he or she decides to follow it. Trust is the foundation of a helping relationship, although as Zerwekh (1991) noted, it can sometimes be a difficult proposition when even family or friends may not be trusted by the PWA (p. 214). Moreover, many PWAs have a (firsthand or second-hand) history of negative experiences with the health-care delivery system and/or clinicians that have nourished their distrust and skepticism.

A nonjudgmental, empathetic interview style is important, though not sufficient to ensure success. There is no magic formula for conveying caring or achieving connectedness and trust. The nurse's intentionality, sincerity, patience, and acceptance of the relationship's limitations provide an initial glue with which one can attach expressions of interest, concern, and suggestions for what steps to take in the future. The more the PWA is permitted to talk, the better one can understand the situation and the more helpful suggestions can be. "Long-term involvement affords the opportunity to elaborate the therapeutic relationship in a unique way and to recognize that it is a partnership in which both learn and grow" (Bennett, 1988, p. 739).

Providing reassuring presence is unquestionably a core component of the nurse-PWA relationship. Even in short-term inpatient situations, there needs to be a moment for the nurse and client to connect without the requirement of accomplishing a task. Use of communication techniques that are helpful includes discussion of issues other than physical symptoms, an unrushed conversation about something that seems inconsequential, an exchange of personal history that allows a personality separate from one's illness (perhaps even separate from one's adulthood) to be recognized, or the sharing of a commonality that acknowledges the uniqueness of both. An attempt to understand the special uniqueness of this particular individual is important.

History

To put current observations in context of the illness trajectory, the history of currently observed and/or reported signs, symptoms, and daily functioning needs to be addressed. Changes can reflect new, persistent, or recurrent problems. How have medical and other interventions affected symptoms? To what extent has illness, its treatment, or being newly diagnosed with HIV disease disrupted the person's personal goals and ongoing life patterns, including daily activities and relating to others? Knowing what feelings are associated with AIDS in general can help provide context for the person's feelings about, and perceptions of, the current situation as well as for his or her expectations in the near and distant future.

Perceptions and expectations will be influenced by the PWA's past experience, including previous personal crises and illness experiences as well as having known others with AIDS. The latter is an important point of reference:

- How many people?
- What was the nature of the relationship?
- In what way(s) and at what stage of disease did one participate in or observe the other's illness experience?
- How much time was involved and what was the geographic proximity?

It is not unusual for a person to have known many people in his or her social network—or even in the immediate or extended family, including spouse and/or siblings—who have experienced the disease, including many who have already died from HIV-related illness. Spouse, siblings, or friends may currently be experiencing similar or different stages of illness. Some people can describe having lost a whole network, only to have rebuilt a social life in which still more people, perhaps even the majority of one's acquaintances, are also affected. Others who are working in the field of AIDS social services or health care may find the disease inescapable and include former and current coworkers among friends and acquaintances with the illness. Still, many people have had no firsthand experience, and their perceptions and expectations are thus partly shaped by media portrayals.

Self-Care Resources, Skills, and Strategies

Regardless of prior experience or preparation, reaction to receiving an HIV diagnosis is a singular experience, and one cannot anticipate the actual feelings of anxiety, fear, anger, guilt, social isolation, and grief or the changes in body image and social roles that accompany confronting a life-threatening process and potential debilitation. Exploring the PWA's experience with other illnesses and/or personal or family crises contributes to the baseline assessment of the person's reaction to, and management of, AIDS-related experiences. It provides a foundation for assessing the person's repertoire of coping skills and strategies, which is key to setting realistic goals and developing and improving supportive resources. The nurse should consider:

- How the PWA spends his or her time and what interests and motivates him or her. What difficulties are experienced managing time and coordinating illness-related activities, such as drug and nutrition regimens, obtaining supplies and resources, making and keeping appoint-

ments for health care, counseling, and/or social or supportive services?

- People, things, activities, and organizations that have
  had significance in the person's life.
- The nature of relationships with close friends and family
  members. What do they do together? What kinds of
  thoughts and feelings do they discuss? To what extent do
  they share feelings about the illness and its prognosis?
  How reciprocal is this exchange?
- Significant reminiscing and opportunities for sharing
  reminiscences with significant others.
- Ways in which the PWA's family typically deals with routine health maintenance and minor illnesses as well as
  ways in which they have handled previous crises. To
  what communities does the PWA feel connected—and in
  what ways?
- The extent to which family members, friends, neighbors,
  and coworkers are aware of the HIV diagnosis and actual
  health status (i.e., specific symptoms, recent changes in
  condition, medical regimens).
- How AIDS in general and the PWA's illness in particular have affected the lives and activities of significant
  others, including the PWA's ongoing interactions with
  them.
- Sexual relationships and satisfaction (the PWA's own
  and that of spouse, lover, or other significant partner[s]).
  How do they deal with changes necessitated by the infection or related symptoms?
- Adherence to prescribed prophylactic or maintenance
  therapies as well as antiviral regimens and other therapies. Evaluate these data in tandem with laboratory test
  results.
- The use and sources of nonprescribed treatments.
- Risk factors for repeated HIV exposure as well as for OI
  occurrence. Ask about recent sexual activity (specifying
  what activities and the precautions taken to avoid sexually transmitted disease), drug use and related behavior
  (including infection control precautions), travel, dietary
  patterns and alterations (including meal preparation
  routines, whether one eats at home or restaurants, food
  restrictions or preferences, and appetite and taste
  changes—and their relationship to drug therapies), adequacy of cooking and food storage facilities, pets (in the
  PWA's own home or wherever he or she may visit).

- Living arrangements, including the PWA's relationship to other household members and whether the situation is permanent or temporary, whose home it actually is, and adequacy of home maintenance.
- The extent of participation in various self-help and/or social support programs.
- The type of supportive resources available—how much and when—to the PWA *and* to those on whom he or she relies for help and/or companionship.
- The PWA's self-assessment of coping skills and the type, quantity, and quality of existing social support systems. What plans, if any, have been made for either the short- or long-term future? Has the PWA considered and/or prepared advance directive regarding health care and life support? With whom and to what extent have all concerned discussed these plans (health-care providers, family members, the health-care proxy)? How have these significant others responded to the PWA's plans? What conflicts exist, if any? How well does the PWA seem to understand the range of implications and applications of the stated plans, and does he or she recognize the prerogative to revise them? Do all concerned understand the terminology used—and the PWA's purpose and reasons?
- Responsibilities for dependent others and how well they are currently managed. Are changes anticipated? Have plans been made in case of hospitalization, prolonged disability, death, or for short- and long-term respite for the PWA, as needed, to meet one's own health-care or illness management needs? What about permanency planning for rearing children who are minors?

Social Support

Opportunities to meet and work with family members or others in the social network vary among diverse institutional and community settings. In any case, it is useful to attempt to learn not only the type and extent of support they can and do provide for the PWA, but also how the PWA's illness has affected *their* lives and how *they* are coping with its impact. How do they manage the tasks they are performing on the PWA's behalf? Do they feel competent and effective? What is their source of support? What do they expect the future to bring to the relationship, and how prepared do they feel for anticipated responsibilities? What other responsibilities do they have? Regardless of whether one can discuss these concerns with family members directly, it is worth exploring not only the PWA's perception of their involvement, but also the

PWA's assessment of their coping capacity and the illness's impact on them, regardless of how limited or extensive their involvement has been.

INFORMATION FOR SELF-CARE AND ILLNESS MANAGEMENT

Well-informed clients tend to experience less anxiety, to cope better with illness demands, and to adhere more successfully to self-care and medical regimens. However, a person's glib use of medical jargon and talk about laboratory data, viral load, immune status, and available drugs are not evidence that a person understands the terms or the implications or applications of information. It is important to "take time to review information the person has received from others, helping to sort what is applicable to his/her specific situation. Then continue to evaluate how well he or she pieces it together and uses it. Do not assume that a person is connected to information resources even if he or she seems to be" (Bennett, 1988, p. 739). Find out not only where and from whom the PWA obtains information, but also the focus of the information gathering and the schema that is used to organize information. The latter provides a frame of reference for the clinicians to understand how their explanations and instructions have been and will be processed.

There are many opportunities for inconsistency in clinicians' explanations and instructions to PWAs. PWAs may see many providers even within the same clinic. Explanations provided in one context can seem to contradict those in another; an analogy useful for one purpose may be confusing if the PWA remembers it when considering instructions received in another circumstance.

PLANNING AND MANAGING FINANCES

Financial status, including medical and disability insurance concerns, is not a nursing focus per se, but because the PWA's continued ability to seek care will often depend on such entitlements, it is imperative that someone (social worker, case manager, or financial counselor or advocate) indeed addresses these concerns. Financial counseling and perhaps advocacy may be necessary to calculate how an individual's work (including veteran status) and insurance history may affect entitlements, particularly as new criteria evolve under managed-care systems. Because disruptions in insurance can delay or even permanently threaten access to needed resources and interventions, instruction about the critical importance of not allowing insurance coverage to lapse must be addressed early in the illness trajectory. Coverage that has lapsed typically cannot be reinstated under similar conditions. Options must be explored in advance, for example, before a person stops working or changes jobs or employment status. In some states (e.g., New York), Medicaid may pay private insurance premiums for Medicaid-eligible PWAs in lieu of assuming medical costs. However, this option usually is not available once the original insurance coverage has expired.

Funding streams seem to be in a perennial state of flux, so it is important that a PWA and his or her caregivers and health-care providers have access to accurate, current information about the implications of changing insurance providers or plans. Specific areas that might be affected include choice of freedom to change health-care delivery site(s) and provider(s); coverage of various types of services, laboratory tests, and drugs, including "caps" on type and frequency; and range of available consultation services, particularly mental health, hospice, and home care. Continuity of care without disrupting established relationships with providers or caregivers cannot be assumed. It is important that these concerns be raised and confirmed before irrevocable actions are taken. These concerns also pertain to clients with Medicare and Medicaid, because their managed-care contracts are not uniform and may continue to change.

Federally funded, state AIDS drug assistance programs (ADAPs), designed to pay for selected drugs and other items (such as nutrition supplements and selected laboratory tests and medical equipment) not included in the insurance coverage of symptomatic individuals not eligible for Medicaid, continue to evolve and in some states devolve or shrink as managed-care contracts take effect. Not only do programs vary across states, but the programs' very continuation depends on annual reappropriation by Congress. Moreover, as demand increases (because of more people seeking treatment as disease incidence climbs and survival extends and because of the availability of more treatments that are started sooner and continued longer) and costs rise, ADAP coverage is necessarily constrained unless appropriations are increased. Hence, what is covered at any given time often may not match the recommended approach to treatment. For example, the program has not yet caught up with current recommendations of early, presymptomatic antiviral intervention. Many states' programs do not pay for three-drug antiviral regimens (the annual cost of a single agent may be between $12,000 and $14,000). In short, the gaps that the program was originally intended to fill often are not filled. Current constraints of local programs must, therefore, be considered when making treatment decisions.

The transition to untimely retirement from the workforce may be necessitated less by disability than by the cost of medical care, particularly drug treatment. The combination of earlier (i.e., longer) anti-HIV treatment and longer symptom-free life is likely to make this issue a growing concern in the coming years.

Stigma

The stigmatizing nature of illness, particularly serious, debilitating, or life-threatening illness, is well documented. The epidemiological profile of AIDS has augmented its stigma because the populations most affected were already targets of prejudice (Bennett, 1995; Herek & Glunt, 1988; Nelkin & Gilman, 1988). Fear of stigma and rejection places a heavy burden on newly diagnosed PWAs and indeed may deter them from seeking screening and/or help. Discrimination in housing, employment, insurance, and even health care has been a problem throughout the epidemic (Presidential Commission, 1988). Its impact on individuals' quality of life and life satisfaction has been quantified (Heckman, Somlai, Sikkema, Kelly, & Franzoi, 1997). Asking clients about their personal experiences invites them to ventilate their feelings and provides an opportunity to make more useful referrals as well as to direct them to appropriate ombudsmen for practical and, if indicated, legal resolution. The knowledge also enables clinicians to recognize patterns of discrimination so that broader advocacy and agency-level interventions beyond an individual's needs can be planned.

Like others with chronic, life-threatening illnesses, the PWA struggles with the effect of diagnosis, illness, and treatment on one's identity, roles, relationships, and daily activities and functioning. "Chronic illness can require that whole areas of living be reshaped or abandoned" (Catanzaro, 1990). A person who is hospitalized with an acute AIDS-defining illness has different immediate needs and is likely to differ in how he or she anticipates the future from a person who has recently been found to be HIV-antibody-positive with a low viral load and high CD4-cell count or who has recovered from multiple bouts of several OIs over several years. Timing is also relevant in terms of the person's stage in life and family development, including both family of origin and current (and perhaps intermediate) kin networks, whether biological, legal, or otherwise.

Although some PWAs put their lives on hold while they figure things out, others are determined not to let the disease intrude on their activities and relationships. They may attempt to compartmentalize activities and relationships. This approach may or may not reflect denial, which can be functional or problematic. Denial is a useful defense mechanism for relieving disruptive anxiety, maintaining hope, and relieving intrapsychic discomfort in the face of threatening situations. The perception of being in control can facilitate coping. Hence, denial that does not prevent productive behavior should not be assessed as inappropriate.

Both illness-related symptoms and therapeutic regimens may change repeatedly and thus require continuing adaptation and learning. Lifestyle adaptations, whether permanent or temporary, are often symptom driven rather than a reflection of considered decision making and future planning. Many encompass changes in self-concept, roles, and relationships and may reflect losses of health, strength, energy, independence, physical self (weight, muscles, hair, skin integrity, strength), specific functions (vision, cognition, libido, gait stability, balance, athleticism), goals, and future plans. Some of these losses are partially reversible. Some, such as lost income, can further complicate efforts to adapt and often limit the availability of supportive resources at different times during the illness. The expense of illness may limit one's financial options, even if the person maintains a job and does not have to take time off for illness-related concerns. In some cases, it can force a person to retire to become eligible for medical or disability benefits by reducing either financial resources or job-related activity.

Age and social situation also affect both the problems experienced and the person's ability to cope with them. For example, a person in his or her 50s regards "retiring" from work differently from a person in his or her 20s or 30s. He or she is also likely to have different options for eligibility for disability income and related entitlements (as well as the amount of such income), depending on work history.

Similarly, there are different considerations when a person lives alone in comparison to someone who lives with a spouse or partner who shares one's circumstances and with whom there is reciprocal caring and commitment. Likewise, a person with dependent family members has additional constraints and also must address issues related to the continuing care of those dependents. For example, a parent will need to make custodial and guardianship arrangements for children who are minors in case of incapacity or death. Although such "permanency planning" for dependent others requires legal consultation, the issues involved encompass more than legal questions. Considerations vary with the number and ages of children involved; their (and the PWA's) relationships to adults who are available and interested in caring for them; and the would-be caregivers' age, health status, and ability to provide for the children. Often, grandparents or others assume the responsibility by default for children, with few support systems in place.

The nurse needs to establish and build trust where there may have been none, to provide reassurance about possibilities of therapies, to provide consistency in the relationship, and to help the person plan "one day at a time." Regular medical care and social networks that support self-care need to be maintained. Acceptance of the person wherever he or she is; encouragement of personal growth (employment, volunteer work, job training, and other education); and "being there" are nursing challenges.

SUPPORTIVE CARE

The nurse quickly realizes that the physical care, as taxing and complicated as it becomes because of the vast symptomatology of AIDS, is only part of the nursing responsibility. Emotional, psychosocial, and spiritual challenges exist as well. With the diagnosis of AIDS, the physical and metaphysical come together. Along with these physical realities are the agonizing metaphysical questions for the client and the caregiver. "Why me?" "Am I being punished?" "Did God make a mistake when he created me?" "Am I to blame for my illness?" "What is the meaning and purpose of my life?" These questions form an important component of the care of AIDS clients (Murphy, Bass, Donovan, & Selman, 1988, p. 153).

Specific symptoms bring discomforts of varying intensity, as well as anxiety over advancing disease, fear of extreme suffering, and worry about adequacy of resources for managing continued illness. Suffering is linked to the impact of all symptoms, including psychosocial disease and spiritual distress.

Many PWAs, having known others with the disease, associate particular symptoms with specific negative outcomes. Their very occurrence, regardless of how easily or quickly relief follows, can have meaning for the individual (and his or her social network) even if their actual clinical implications are negligible or difficult to assess. Symptoms thus serve, often inaccurately, as benchmarks of disease severity and the imminence of more severe symptoms or progressive disability, as well as self-assessment that one has failed at "positive thinking and doing the right things."

Because uncertainty causes distress, explaining a symptom's cause, when possible, along with the rationale for suggested interventions, can be helpful. Teach the person to keep track of the timing of symptoms and associated activities, including eating and medicine taking. Being able to identify a pattern not only facilitates effective intervention, but also provides a sense of control if predictability regarding symptoms' occurrence is discovered.

Besides uncertainty about the disease and the meaning of symptoms in terms of health, their unpredictable (yet frequent) exacerbations make even the short term unpredictable and thus frustrate day-to-day planning. Can a weekend camping trip be planned? Should a dinner engagement be cancelled or will the diarrhea abate? Will coughing make attending a concert an agonizing event? Will the energy required to make preparations leave one too tired to enjoy others' company? Practical advice about symptom management must address organizing daily activities around the pattern of symptom occurrence and treatment regimens, as well as having alternative plans rather than avoiding planning altogether. No one system will meet everyone's needs, nor is an approach likely to remain suitable for an individual throughout the course of the illness. Continued trial and error can be frustrating for nurse as well as client when the nurse's repertoire of suggestions, often built on other clients' experiences and creative strategies for managing the demands of illness and symptom-imposed limitations, is depleted before a problem abates.

MEDICAL INTERVENTIONS

Medical treatment goals are to halt or eliminate viral activity (treatment and cure), to delay or slow disease progression (secondary prevention), to prevent the opportunistic sequelae of immunocompromise (tertiary prevention), to initiate timely treatment when these secondary diseases do occur (cure, reduce morbidity, mortality, and residual damage), to relieve symptoms (palliation), and to restore damaged organ function (rehabilitation). Treatment efficacy is ultimately measured by survival time post-HIV infection and post-AIDS, the absence of OI occurrence (including both time before first occurrence and subsequent disease-free periods between OIs), symptom relief, quality of life, and ability to perform and enjoy one's social roles and ADLs.

Laboratory tests to measure viral load and lymphocyte counts indicate ongoing pathophysiology, disease progress, and prognoses. Hence, they are intermediate measures (or surrogate markers) of an antiviral agent's efficacy in halting the virus and thus preventing or slowing immune damage. In other words, both viral load and immune function reflect the efficacy of *secondary prevention*. With fewer viruses, there is less damage; the longer it takes for immune damage to evolve and accumulate, the more effective the treatment. The efficacy of *tertiary prevention* is measured, in turn, by the absence of OIs *despite declining immunity:* The lower the CD4-cell count when an OI occurs, the more effective its prophylaxis has been.

Although advances in antiviral therapy have captured more recent headlines, the greatest progress in extending disease-free survival in the last decade and a half was in the prevention and treatment of OIs. By contrast, efforts to restore the damaged immune system, though promising, have not yet been productive. In fact, improved immune function is not always apparent when CD4-cell counts rise as viral load drops after antiviral therapy. In other words, HIV damage to the immune system is not merely a quantitative cellular loss, but also a qualitative functional loss that researchers have not yet fully described. Averting this loss, which might be irreversible, is one rationale in the argument for early treatment of asymptomatic infection even when CD4-cell levels are high.

Antiretroviral Options

Because the rate of disease progression reflects an individual's viral burden, and immunodeficiency worsens as viral burden rises, an infected person's immunity will progressively deteriorate unless HIV replication is effectively inhibited. Although the researcher's aims have always been to learn how to cure HIV infection, until the mid to late 1990s, almost all anti-HIV treatment was essentially aimed at tertiary prevention. That is, except for attempts at postexposure prophylaxis, available antivirals (or more accurately, antiretrovirals[8]) were used to treat disease after immune damage was evident (when CD4 cells had fallen to 500/mm^3 or fewer). Since 1996, the antiviral efficacy (viral kill power) shown by three- and four-drug regimens combining two or three types of antivirals, including a protease inhibitor (PI), has given some biomedical researchers confidence to suggest that viral elimination may be possible, at least with early treatment.

Three *types* of antiviral agents are being used against HIV infection today: nucleoside reverse-transcriptase inhibitors (NRTIs), non-nucleoside RT inhibitors (NNRTIs), and protease inhibitors (PIs) (Table 14.1). Because reverse transcriptase inhibitors (RTIs) and PIs act at different points in the HIV life cycle (Fig. 14.1), their combined use provides two targets for attacking the virus. Moreover, because PIs, NNRTIs, and NRTIs have different side effect profiles, they can usually be combined for antiviral synergy without risk of overlapping or augmenting adverse effects. Antivirals aimed at other targets on the virus (Fig. 14.1) have not yet shown clinical efficacy. In addition, drugs with diverse cell or tissue tropisms are also needed, but this efficacy has not yet been demonstrated by available drugs. Efficacy of new drugs and also combination regimens can differ between treatment-naive individuals and those who have previously taken antiretrovirals because of cross-resistance patterns.

The caveat tempering clinical excitement that a cure (an antiretroviral regimen that could eliminate the infection and thus the disease) is finally at hand comes from knowing that we have had only a few years of experience with either PIs or today's combination regimens. Questions about long-term efficacy and cumulative adverse effects remain to be answered. Moreover, regardless of whether the virus can be eliminated if a person starts treatment soon after infection, for tens of thousands of people treatment will be initiated only after several years of infection. Until drugs capable of eliminating virus sequestered in tissue are available, such individuals will need to continue treatment for years, perhaps decades.

PRINCIPLES GUIDING ANTIRETROVIRAL THERAPY

The goal of antiviral therapy is to suppress viral replication as much as possible, as soon as possible, and for as long as possible. Suppression is

Table 14.1 ➤ **ANTIRETROVIRAL AGENTS USED TO TREAT HUMAN IMMUNODEFICIENCY VIRUS**

Class of Drug	Generic Name	Brand Name	Instructions
Reverse transcriptase inhibitor Nucleoside analogs	Didanosine (ddI)	Videx	Take on empty stomach.
	Lamivudine also known as 3TC	Epivir	Take at least 1 h apart from ddI or antacids.
	Stavudine also known as d4T	Zerit	
	Zalcitabine also known as dideoxycytidine (ddC)	Hivid	
	Zidovudine (ZDV) also known as azidothymidine (AZT)	Retrovir	
Nonnucleoside analogs	Delavirdine mesylate	Rescriptor	
	Nevirapine	Viramune	
Protease inhibitors	Indinavir	Crixivan	Take 1 h before or 2 h after eating.
	Nelfinavir mesylate	Viracept	Take with meal or light snack.
	Ritonavir	Norvir	Refrigerate. Take with meals.
	Saquinavir mesylate	Invirase	

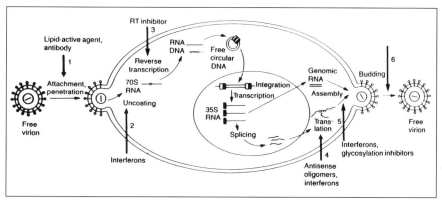

FIGURE 14.1 ➤ The HIV life cycle (left to right) entering, replicating within, and leaving the human host cell. After (1) binding to the cell membrane, HIV fuses with the cell surface and enters the cell (cytoplasm), where it is (2) uncoated (i.e., the viral envelope is opened) so that RNA can be transcribed into DNA. (3) Reverse transcriptase (RT) catalyzes initiation of the transcription process. Proviral DNA is integrated into the host cell chromosome (in the nucleus), where it remains until activated. (4) The viral DNA is transcribed into RNA when the infected cell is activated, then exits from the nucleus. (5) Additional proteins are synthesized and assembled into mature virions, which are released into the circulation by (6) budding from the host cell membrane. The process results in cell lysis (death). (With permission from Sha, B. E. (1992). The art of antiretroviral treatment: AZT, ddI, and ddC. This figure was reprinted from *The AIDS Reader* (1992; 2:153–160), Copyright © 1992, SCP Communications, Inc.)

necessary to avert or at least to delay outgrowth of virus resistant to the drugs being used. *Measuring viral load thus gauges a regimen's efficacy.* The time it takes to reduce viremia to undetectable levels will depend on how high the viral load is when treatment starts. A threefold (0.5 log) drop indicates an antiviral effect. A 10-fold (or 1 log) drop in HIV RNA is expected within 4 weeks of starting treatment, and detectable viremia (200 to 500 copies/mm^3) should be eliminated within 4 to 6 months.

The clinical benefit of incomplete suppression will depend on the extent of suppression achieved. Hence, when suppression is not fully achieved, no alternative viremic level is specifically targeted, but the lower the better.

The key to whether intervention with antiretroviral combinations could stem immune damage indefinitely, or even totally eliminate the virus, is likely to be not only an antiviral regimen's potency, but also how early in the disease process (i.e., how soon after infection) treatment starts. "The greatest and most durable beneficial impact on an individual's health is likely if treatment starts before either immunologic or virologic parameters evidence disease progression" (OAR, 1997). Hence, optimal timing would be before the infection involves tissue, essentially immediately after exposure, before the onset of primary illness, or as soon thereafter as possible. There is no theoretical cutoff for starting treatment (i.e., no CD4-cell level above which, nor viral load below which, one should hold off therapy) because there is no known threshold of viral replication below which disease does not progress. In other words, neither CD4-cell count, symptoms, nor viral load provides a yardstick for guiding treatment initiation. Although antiviral therapy is most beneficial the earlier it is begun, even if treatment is initiated when immunodeficiency is severe, a beneficial effect on survival can occur.

The next question is whether therapy could eventually be discontinued. Current viral load assays measure only virus in the peripheral circulation, not virus sequestered in lymph nodes, brain, and other tissue. Moreover, with current technology, *undetectable viremia does not mean absolutely zero circulating virus.* So mathematical models of both T-cell and virus replication are being used to estimate how long antiviral treatment should continue in the absence of detectable viremia. Some researchers have suggested that intermittent remissions may be achieved and sequential, periodic treatment could then be used to suppress subsequent viremia that might arise from activated sequestrations.

Drug resistance may occur after clinicians begin and stop the drug but also after individuals elect to discontinue a prescribed treatment or do not adhere to a prescribed regimen (e.g., skipping or reducing dosage). *Resistance has implications not only for the individual's prognosis, but also for public health.* The transmission of drug-resistant virus eliminates the promise of effective treatment by these new drugs.

Monotherapy is no longer recommended at any disease stage. No available agent can provide even short-term effective monotherapy, nor does any two-drug combination of available drugs produce significant, durable suppression.[8] The current recommendation (OAR, 1997) is to begin with a three-drug combination of two NRTIs and a PI, pending results of ongoing research with combinations that include NNRTIs or two-PI regimens.

Treatment initiation should not be staged. That is, a person should start taking all drugs in a combination regimen simultaneously. In the past, sequential addition of drugs to a multidrug regimen was often used to differentiate the potential sources of side effects and to allow clients to adapt to them, particularly those that tend to subside after a few weeks of therapy. This strategy is counterproductive, however, because even short-term monotherapy delays complete suppression and thus allows the accumulation of mutations that may contribute to multidrug resistance. The accumulation can be rapid, considering that an HIV-infected person can produce 10 billion new virions every day.

From a pharmacokinetic perspective, *the right combination for an individual depends on the person's previous anti-HIV therapy.* The key is not the number of drugs in a combination, but the total combined potency and the resistance patterns of the drugs being combined. The more potent the drugs and the less likely they are to be resistant, the fewer are needed. In other words, the impact of implementing treatment as currently recommended with combinations of available drugs will depend not only on the timing of treatment initiation vis-à-vis the extent of disease, but also on which drugs a person has previously taken and how (i.e., the duration of the treatments, the dosing that was used, whether treatment was interrupted). The goal is to select drugs that do not have resistance to similar viral mutation patterns as drugs the individual previously used. Toxic or intolerable side effects may further limit options.

The practical decision about *when to start anti-HIV treatment and what that treatment should be* must anticipate both potential benefit and the risks of incomplete suppression for a particular individual and take into account the potential toxicities as well as the individual's quality of life and commitment and ability to adhere to a chosen regimen. The risk of disease progression, and thus the urgency for antiviral intervention, is most immediate when CD4-cell counts at any level drop progressively (i.e., when the CD4-cell count is not stable), when they fall to 500/mm^3 or fewer, and when viremia of any level rises. If treatment is deferred because the CD4-cell count is high and/or the viral load is low and stable (<5000 copies/mm^3), viral load should be monitored every 3 to 6 months, or perhaps more often if clinical status suggests change. The risk of progression and death grows steadily with increasing viral load. At plasma levels above 10,000 copies/mm^3, the median time to death of people with 500 or more CD4 cells/mm^3 is 6.8 years. Treatment is urged when viral load is 30,000 copies/mm^3 or greater, no matter how high the CD4-cell count is.

There is no advantage to starting treatment without a client's full acceptance of the goal and strategy. Indeed, it is better to delay treatment until the client has been adequately counseled, understands the rationale for treatments, recognizes the implications of starting or not starting treatment on current and future health status and daily activities. The necessity to adhere fully to the regimen (particularly regimens that include a PI), without change or interruption, needs emphasis. Client resolve to follow a specific treatment course must be obtained. One of the most difficult challenges is not only to accept an unrelenting decision by a PWA to forgo or delay treatment or to reject the primary provider's (physician or nurse practitioner) recommendations, but to continue a supportive, nonjudgmental relationship.

When a PWA elects to begin antiviral treatment, continuing active collaboration between clinician(s) and client in decision making remains critical. Underdosing or intermittent adherence essentially guarantees drug resistance.

Deciding to change a regimen is another critical determination that can have long-term implications. Because future treatment options may be further limited by changing therapies prematurely, *failure to achieve complete suppression is not a universal criterion to abandon a regimen.* Incomplete suppression may be a result of persistent reservoirs of infection within chronically infected macrophages or incomplete drug penetration into tissue. Changing treatment is recommended when virus is detected after being suppressed to undetectable levels or when the level of incompletely suppressed virus begins to rise. These events or trends indicate emergent resistance. Clinical deterioration and persistent decline in CD4 T cells or a return to pretreatment level or percentage are also indications that a regimen is not working.

Viral load should drop threefold within a month of starting treatment. A subsequent rise to within 0.3 to 0.5 log of pretreatment levels usually reflects lack of efficacy. Because any single test result of viral load may be spurious, decisions to change treatment should be based on repeated measurements made at least 2 to 4 weeks apart. Serial measurement by the same assay method are likely to reflect true changes rather than measurement error. A single test result, however, may reflect viremic boosting when CD4 cells have been activated by another infection or an immunization. Of course, it is also important to ascertain whether a viral breakthrough (rise in viral load despite antiviral therapy) is caused by nonadherence or partial adherence to the regimen, an altered drug metabolism resulting from interactions with other drugs, or reduced drug absorption. Lack of improvement in CD4-cell count with clinical deterioration also suggests considering a regimen change.

The AIDS community has learned to anticipate reversals when new treatments are heralded as "promising" in either the popular or scientific media. Indeed, AIDS care takes place in an environment where the mingling of skepticism and hope yields both willingness to try unproven therapies and reluctance to accept authoritative claims about demonstrable efficacy. *Errors in perception and practice include* recommending lower antiviral dosages than necessary; viewing early disease treatment as not being useful; believing that drug efficacy declines after several months; denying different drug efficacy across ethnic groups; believing in the acceptability of taking a drug vacation to relieve stress, side effects, or even to promote its effectiveness; viewing occasional skipped doses as harmless; viewing treatments as being just as harmful to the immune system as to the virus, such as ZDV's toxicity being more damaging than the virus or any other treatment; and viewing drugs as poison that can only harm. Truth and mythology are inextricably intertwined. In addition, there is considerable mistrust of the medical establishment throughout many communities most affected by AIDS.

Hence, many PWAs remain determined not to use antivirals against HIV itself (although they may accept prophylactic therapy against OIs), regardless of physicians' (or other health-care providers') advice. Others hold fast to the view that antiviral intervention, with its potential deleterious effects, is a last resort to be avoided until natural resistance is exhausted. Some clinicians, concerned about the implications for resistance, may determine not to recommend early treatment to persons they deem likely not to adhere. In other cases, a PWA may strive to remain antiretroviral-naive in order not to exhaust his or her susceptibility to potentially more potent agents in the pharmaceutical "pipeline."

AIDS survival differs significantly according to whether medical care is provided by a physician experienced with AIDS (Kitahata et al., 1996). One home-care agency's study of 174 clients with HIV receiving antiretrovirals found that physicians had prescribed inappropriately for 40 percent of those on PI regimens (Ungvarski & Rottner, 1997).

With respect to *adherence,* practical dosing regimens and tolerable side effects are imperative if a drug is to be useful. Regimen complexity is a key determinant of adherence or nonadherence. AIDS regimens are often complex and are becoming more complex. Current treatment regimens involve multiple agents with more specific dosing requirements, including timing in relation to food and other drug intake. The range and severity of adverse effects of available antiretrovirals vary from headache, nausea, insomnia, and fatigue to bone marrow suppression and pancreatitis (Williams, 1997) (Table 14.2). In addition, the PIs have substantial interactions with many other agents, an important concern for the majority of PWAs even before the disease is well advanced. Research efforts to ease medicine taking and make regimens more user friendly must be a high priority. This research must include efforts to produce formulations that reduce both the number of pills a person must take and the dosing frequency, for example, for combination (multidrug) agents.

Directly observed therapy (DOT) has been the key to increased adherence in methadone-maintenance treatment for narcotic addiction and for tuberculosis treatment. Incentives such as meal coupons for fast-food chains, reimbursement for transportation, and stepwise bonuses for completion of each month of treatment can be used. Given the number of required daily dosings of current antiretroviral regimens for PWA, DOT as it has been implemented for TB control is not a viable option for large numbers of people. Creative ways to integrate medicine taking into PWAs' activities outside the clinic are needed, not only to help them to accomplish their individual goals, but from a proactive population-focused perspective, to stem a potential epidemic of drug-resistant HIV. Ways for this population to use diverse nonclinical as well as community-based venues need to be considered. Barriers to adherence vary from individual to individual. Stability of housing and quality of residential environment must be part of the equation when assessing adherence risk. Poor adherence should not be caused by clients' confusion (related to anxiety, stress, fatigue, physical distress, or being overwhelmed by information), misunderstanding of instructions regarding medicine taking (which can frequently result from inadequate instruc-

Table 14.2 ➤ **SIDE EFFECTS OF DRUGS COMMONLY USED IN HUMAN IMMUNODEFICIENCY DISEASE**

	AZT	ddl	ddC	d4T	3TC	SQV	RTV	IDV	NFV
Abdominal pain	+++	++	++	+++	++	+	++	++	+
Altered taste	++	+++	+	*NR*	*NR*	+	+++	+	*NR*
Anorexia Reduced appetite	+++	+	+	++	++	*NR*	++	+	+
Arthralgia Joint pain	+++	+	+	+++	++	+	+	+	+
Chills	+++	++	+	+++	++	+	+	+	*NR*
Constipation	+	+	+	++	*NR*	+	+	+	*NR*
Depression	+	+	+	++	++	+	+	+	+
Diarrhea	+++	+++	++	+++	+++	+	+++	+	+++
Dizziness	++	+	+	++	++	+	++	+	+
Fatigue	++	++	+++	++	+++	++	+++	++	+
Fevers	+++	++	+++	++	++	+	+	+	+
Headache	+++	++	+++	+++	+++	+	++	++	+
Insomnia	++	+	+	+++	++	+	+	+	+
Malaise	+++	+	+	+++	+++	*NR*	+	+	+
Myalgia Muscle pain	+++	++	++	+++	++	+	++	+	+
Nausea	+++	++	++	+++	+++	+	+++	+++	++
Nephrolithiasis Kidney stones	*NR*	*NR*	*NR*	*NR*	*NR*	*NR*	*NR*	+	*NR*
Neurological symptoms	+	+	++	+++	+	+	++	+	+
Neuropathy	+	+++	+++	+++	++	+	+	+	*NR*
Pancreatitis	*NR*	++	+	+	++ children	+	+	*NR*	+
Paresthesia Numbness, prickling, tingling	+	*NR*	*NR*	*NR*	*NR*	+	++	+	+
Rash	+++	++	++	+++	++	+	+	*NR*	+
Seizures	*NR*	+	+	*NR*	*NR*	*NR*	*NR*	*NR*	+
Vomiting	++	++	++	+++	++	+	+++	++	+

Source: San Francisco Project Inform, 1965 Market Street, Suite 220, San Francisco, CA 94103, August 1997. From Project Inform, for more information contact the Project Inform National HIV/AIDS Treatment Hotline, 800-822-7422.

AP = *aerosol pentamidine;* **AZI** = *azithromycin;* **CDV** = *cidofovir;* **CLA** = *clarithromycin;* **DLV** = *delavirdine;* **FLU** = *fluconazole;* **FOS** = *foscarnet;* **GCV(iv)** = *intravenous ganciclovir;* **IDV** = *indinavir;* **NFV** = *nelfinavir;* **NR** = *not reported;* **NVP** = *nevirapine;* **RBT** = *rifabutin;* **RTV** = *ritonavir;* **SQV** = *saquinavir;* **TS** = *Bactrim / Septra.*

tion or poor communication by providers), or misinformation from others. Everyone involved must interpret the instructions consistently. For example, "three times a day" does not specify dosage times.

Suggest that the client use a written record to check off when each dose is taken, and emphasize consistency about when to mark it (i.e., always mark it immediately after taking the medicine, not retrospectively or after pouring the medicine). Do not overlook atypical routines, such as weekends and out-of-town travel. Being available and welcoming

NVP	DLV	AZI	CLA	RBT	TS	AP	GCV (iv)	FOS	CDV	FLU
+	+	+	++	+	+++	+	+++	++	+++	++
NR	+	NR	++	+	NR	+++	+	+	+	+
NR	+	NR	NR	+	+	+++	+++	++	+++	NR
NR	+	NR	NR	+	+	+	NR	NR	+	NR
NR	+	NR	NR	NR	+	+++	++	++	+++	NR
NR	+	NR	NR	NR	+++	NR	+	+	+	NR
NR	+	NR	NR	NR	NR	+	+	++	+	NR
+	+	++	++	+	++	+	+++	+++	+++	+
NR	+	+	NR	NR	+++	+++	+	++	+	NR
NR	++	+	NR	+	++	+++	+	++	+++	NR
++	+	NR	NR	+	+++	+++	+++	+++	+++	NR
++	++	+	++	+	+++	+	+	+++	+++	++
NR	+	NR	NR	+	++	+	+	+	+	NR
NR	+	NR	NR	NR	+	+	+	++	+	NR
+	+	NR	NR	+	+	+	+	+	+	NR
++	++	+	+++	++	+++	+++	+++	+++	+++	+
NR	NR	NR	NR	NR	NR	NR	NR	NR	NR	NR
+	+	+	NR	+	+	+	++	++	+	+
NR	+	NR	NR	NR	+	NR	++	++	+	NR
NR	+	NR	NR	NR	+	+	+	+	NR	NR
+	+	NR	NR	NR	NR	NR	++	++	+	NR
+++	++	+	++	++	+++	+	++	++	+++	+
NR	NR	NR	NR	NR	NR	+	+	++	NR	+
NR	+	+	++	+	+++	+++	++	++	+++	+

phone calls to clarify concerns or answer questions between appointments can be reassuring and improve follow-up when problems or new circumstances arise, such as a skipped dose, compromised storage, changes in prescriptions from other providers, or the receipt of contradictory information from a friend. On-line communication via computer network links may facilitate communication between some PWAs and clinicians, but it may not be equally attractive or available to all.

Preventing and Treating Opportunistic Illness

Although the potent antiviral regimens of the late 1990s have brought more successful secondary prevention along with the hope that a cure may be on the horizon, the continually extended survival witnessed throughout the epidemic has been largely the result of improved management of OIs by prevention and treatment, earlier diagnosis (recognizing more subtle, earlier signs and symptoms), more effective use of available interventions (better dosing, longer treatment, combining and sequencing drugs); chemoprophylaxis against specific organisms, and new pharmaceutical agents to treat formerly untreatable infections and replace poorly tolerated drugs. A somewhat more difficult battle against neoplastic opportunism may emerge as mortality from infections is curbed and people live with immunodeficiency for longer periods, thus allowing neoplasms to develop. Meanwhile, the changing epidemiological profile of OIs suggests that new preventive strategies are needed for some diseases and that much broader efforts must be made to provide prophylaxis to all who need it (USPHA/IDSA Working Group, 1997).

Recommendations jointly published by the Centers for Disease Control and Prevention (CDC), the National Institutes of Health (NIH), and the Infectious Diseases Society of America (IDSA) in 1995 addressed 17 infections and were recently updated (USPHA/IDSA Working Group, 1995, 1997).[9] The guidelines differentiate regimens to prevent first episodes from those aimed at preventing recurrent disease. The efficacy of some recommendations reflect drug applications and dosing not approved by the Food and Drug Administration because they are based on clinicians' experience rather than empirical data. For these regimens, the guideline recommends discussing pros and cons with clients. The guidelines indicate that primary prevention for some diseases involves behavioral precautions to avoid exposure and recognize that inadequate or ineffective counseling may limit this recommendation's utility.

For ubiquitous opportunistic organisms (i.e., organisms that most people harbor without associated disease occurrence), such as PCP and *Mycobacterium avium* complex (MAC), chemoprophylaxis is universally implemented at specific levels of immunodeficiency (i.e., when the CD4-cell count falls to the level at which disease from the particular organism is predictable). For less ubiquitous organisms, such as *Mycobacterium tuberculosis* and *T. gondii,* screening to identify exposure or infection history is an additional criterion for prescribing prophylaxis at an appropriate level of immunity. However, debates continue about just how universal chemoprophylaxis should be, even for ubiquitous organisms. A risk-benefit assessment is needed to include how survival will be affected, current and expected quality of life, potential severity of illness occurrences, and the cost of using prophylaxis or not. Those with more advanced disease, who are already burdened by multiple symptoms and multidrug regimens, need more aggressive prophylaxis. Certainly for individuals who eschew or cannot tolerate antiretrovirals, as well as for those whose nonadherence limits the use of antivirals, tertiary prevention becomes the paramount focus. For PCP, once the major killer of PWAs, the answer has been clear.[10] Neither routine prophylaxis nor suppressive treatment to prevent recurrent disease is recommended for candidiasis or herpes simplex infections because effective therapy for acute disease is available, mortality is low, drug resistance is likely to develop, drug interactions are possible, and long-term prophylaxis is costly ($2000 to $5000 per year). The annual costs of the preventive regimens for PCP, toxoplasmosis, and tuberculosis (TB) are more reasonable.

CLIENT TEACHING

Client teaching for primary prevention of *Toxoplasma* infection is essential for all HIV-infected persons, but especially for those who lack immunoglobulin G (IgG) antibody to *Toxoplasma;* that is, for those who have not had prior exposure. Advise people not to eat raw or under-cooked meat or unwashed fruit or vegetables; to wash hands carefully after contact with soil (for example, when gardening); to peel and wash raw fruits and vegetables before eating; to keep cats inside and feed them only canned or dried commercial food or well-cooked table food; to wear gloves when handling litter boxes and to wash hands afterwards. See Table 14.3 for a general food safety guide.

Although careful pet care is important, parting with cats or having them tested for toxoplasmosis is not necessary. Water safety may be a concern in some communities. Teaching should include information about the relative benefits of filtered, boiled, and/or bottled water in specific circumstances. National hotline resources are listed in Appendix B.

Counseling regarding fertility control must include discussion about the relative risks involved for both mother and fetus. The risks vary according to the mother's disease stage (i.e., viral load, degree of immunodeficiency, overall health status, and antiretroviral regimen). Of course, fertility control concerns extend beyond the risks of pregnancy and perinatal transmission. The long-term impact of childbearing and childrearing needs to be considered. Breastfeeding is discouraged because HIV can be transmitted from mother to infant in breast milk.

HIV-positive men and women need to be concerned about reinfection, infection with other sexually transmitted diseases, and blood borne infections whose treatment may complicate or be complicated by their HIV disease. Reinfection may disrupt the precarious equilibrium between one's immune system and the virus challenge. One may experience a short, but devastating, boost in viral load, acquire more rapidly replicating or drug-resistant virus, or promote viral replication by activating one's immune system in response to new infection. Thus safe-sex

Table 14.3 ➤ **CHECKLIST FOR FOOD SAFETY***

Wash hands before beginning food preparations and again after each time you handle raw food. Also wash hands before serving food and/or before eating.

Keep refrigerator and other food storage areas clean. Check for mold.

Use food before expiration date. Discard bulging, leaking, or cracked cans.

Use a thermometer to check refrigerator temperature. It should be between 33°F and 40°F, and freezer temperature should be less than 5°F.

Thaw frozen meat in refrigerator or microwave, not at room temperature.

Keep cooking appliances (food processors, blenders, and juicers; can openers, ovens, and broilers, etc.) clean and free of food particles.

Clean countertops and cutting boards immediately before use. Sanitize with chlorine bleach solution (1 qt water:1 teaspoon bleach) periodically.

Wash fresh foods, even those that will be peeled, thoroughly under running water before preparing.

Use plastic or ceramic cutting boards, not wood. Clean with bleach solution (1:10) routinely (e.g., weekly).

Designate a specific cutting board for raw meat, poultry, and fish. Do not use this cutting board for cooked meats or for foods that will be eaten raw (e.g., fruit, vegetables, nuts, bread). Wash immediately after use.

Use a meat thermometer.

Do not allow cooked foods to stand before eating.

Keep hot foods hot and cold foods cold. Refrigerate or freeze leftovers within 2 h. If leftovers are not frozen, discard within 3–5 days.

Discard dirty sponges. (Sponges are more likely to harbor bacteria, so dishcloths are preferable.)

Launder dishclothes and dish towels regularly.

Use separate towels for hands and dishes/cookware.

*It is safe for PWAs to use the same cooking and eating utensils as other household members, and vice versa. Commercial cleaning preparations, such as directed, are adequate.

and needle-use precautions are important concerns for PWAs as well as for the uninfected.

ROUTINE IMMUNIZATIONS

Pneumococcal vaccine should be given soon after HIV diagnosis to anyone who has not received the vaccine within the previous 5 years, and revaccination every 5 years should be considered because the duration of efficacy is not known. More frequent immunizations are not recommended. Early vaccination is emphasized because there is probably a lesser humoral response in people with severe immunodeficiency. Pneumococcal vaccination administration during pregnancy may be deferred until antiretroviral treatment has begun to reduce the chance that HIV might be transmitted to the fetus as a result of a transiently boosted viremia after the immunization.

PWAs who do not carry antibody to hepatitis B virus (HBV) should receive a three-dose course of either Engerix B or Recombivax HB vaccine. *Haemophilus influenzae* type B is not generally recommended for adults because disease incidence is low. Varicella zoster immune globulin (VZIg) should be given to PWAs, including pregnant women, within

96 hours after exposure to chickenpox or shingles when one has no detectable VZV antibody or no history of chickenpox or shingles.

Despite concern raised in the early 1990s that flu vaccination might temporarily enhance HIV replication, there is now a consensus that it is safe (Fowke et al., 1997). In fact, some clinicians have suggested a second dosing after 6 to 8 weeks to ensure efficacy for the duration of flu season in case immunodeficiency shortened the vaccine-induced immunity. This booster is not a standard recommendation, however. Flu has never appeared to be a major problem among PWAs (albeit perhaps because no major flu epidemic has occurred during the AIDS era). In any case, it is reasonable to expect that people who work or live with people experiencing HIV-related or other immunodeficiency, including hospital and social service agency workers, should follow CDC recommendations to be immunized against flu each year.

SCREENING

Initial assessment soon after HIV diagnosis includes travel and residential history, previous GI and sexually transmitted diseases, and screening to detect latent infection with *T. gondii, M. tuberculosis,* CMV, HBV antigen. Screening for IgG antibody to *T. gondii* should be repeated when CD4-cell counts drop to 100/mm^3 or fewer. Repeated tuberculosis skin testing (TST) with the Mantoux method on a yearly basis is indicated only for HIV-positive individuals in populations with high risk of exposure to active TB and for those who have a known contact with an active case.

Because people with immunodeficiency may be less responsive to the tuberculin antigen, a 5-mm induration is used as the criterion for a positive result (instead of the 10-mm criterion that is generally used). People with positive TSTs should have a chest x-ray and physical examination to rule out active TB. Although anergy may cause a false-negative result in people with advanced immunodeficiency, anergy testing is recommended only for PWAs with a high risk for TB exposure. When anergy is present, TB should be considered when pulmonary symptoms are suggestive even if the TST is negative.

Because multifocal genital neoplasia is prevalent in women with HIV disease, Pap smears for the detection of cervical disease should be performed every 6 months. Colposcopy to obtain histological samples may be indicated.

SECONDARY CHEMOPROPHYLAXIS

PNEUMOCYSTIS CARINII PNEUMONIA

Systemic treatment (daily trimethoprim-sulfamethoxazole [TMP-SMX]) is indicated for all HIV-infected adults and adolescents with 200

CD4 T cells/mm³ or fewer or who experience oropharyngeal candidiasis or an unexplained fever above 100°F that lasts for 2 weeks or longer. Of course, it is not necessary to wait until the CD4-cell count actually reaches 200. If the count has been dropping, it is appropriate to start prophylaxis as the count approaches 200/mm³ (i.e., if the count falls to 250/mm³ or so). Pregnancy is not a contraindication. In fact, a pregnant woman requires daily double-strength dosing of TMP-SMX because her expanded plasma volume reduces drug concentration.

Unfortunately, PCP is still the most frequent first AIDS-defining illness diagnosed. This is sad evidence that availability of treatment does not ensure access. PCP prevention needs to be advertised in diverse public venues (e.g., buses, kiosks, newspapers). Clearly, such messages must be paired with those that promote self-appraisal of HIV risk and screening (HIV-antibody testing) so that infection can be identified sooner rather than later.

Breakthrough occurrences despite prophylaxis usually result with lower levels of immunity. Breakthrough cases may be milder and more easily treated, with quicker recovery and less residual damage. The same regimen is continued after a PCP episode to prevent recurrence. Desensitization may permit the person who has previously not tolerated TMP-SMX to use this first-line strategy.

M. TUBERCULOSIS

Twelve months of preventive isoniazid (INH) therapy is indicated for PWAs with a positive TST who have not previously completed TB treatment or prophylaxis, including pregnant women. Alternative antimyocobacterial agents may be indicated, depending on the risk of INH resistance. Chemoprophylaxis should be started in PWAs who are close contacts of persons with active TB (household members, coworkers, people living in a residential facility or attending a day-care program), regardless of skin test results or prior course of prophylaxis. If they remain negative after 3 months, discontinuation of the chemoprophylaxis may be considered. Pyridoxine must be included in INH regimens to prevent peripheral neuropathy. HIV infection is a contraindication for bacille Calmette-Guérin vaccine because it can cause disseminated disease in an immunodeficient person.

TOXOPLASMOSIS

Prophylaxis against toxoplasmic encephalitis (TE) is indicated for PWAs with 100 CD4-cell counts of 100/mm³ or fewer and is adequately provided by the TMP-SMX regimen used for PCP prophylaxis. People who cannot tolerate sulfa agents should take dapsone plus pyrimethamine. Other alternative anti-PCP regimens are not adequate protection against TE, however.

After a TE episode, the recommended suppressive therapy is a regimen of pyrimethamine plus sulfadiazine and leucovorin. Clindamycin is substituted for people who cannot tolerate sulfadiazine.

MICROBACTERIUM AVIUM COMPLEX

When CD4 cells drop to $50/mm^3$, macrolide (azithromycin or clarithromycin) monotherapy should be started if disseminated MAC disease is not present. Clients who have had disseminated MAC require combination therapy with at least one additional drug besides the macrolide, such as ethambutol or rifabutin. Prophylaxis may be withheld during the first trimester of pregnancy and clarithromycin should be used with caution.

FUNGAL DISEASES

Concerns about cost and resistance contraindicate routine prophylaxis against fungal diseases. When repeated recurrences affect a person's quality of life or a person has experienced more than one fungal disease (e.g., candidiasis, cryptococcosis, histoplasmosis), the cost may be warranted, especially for people with CD4-cell counts of $50/mm^3$ or fewer. An azole, such as fluconazole or itraconazole, may be prescribed in such cases.

HERPES VIRUSES

Ganciclovir may be given to PWAs with CD4 counts under $50/mm^3$ to prevent CMV, although its limited efficacy and the side effects of neutropenia and anemia are arguments against its use. Acyclovir and valacyclovir are not recommended. Once CMV has occurred, chronic suppressive therapy is required with ganciclovir, cidofovir, foscarnet, or combination regimens. Prophylaxis for herpes simplex virus is not recommended, except that daily suppressive acyclovir therapy may be used when recurrences are frequent or severe.

OTHER BACTERIAL INFECTIONS

Long-term therapy is required to prevent recurrence once a PWA has experienced *Salmonella* septicemia. Ciprofloxacin or another fluoroquinolone is used.

Nonallopathic Therapies

The small but growing armamentarium of effective pharmaceutical agents for fighting HIV and boosting immunity provides only one alternative in a wide range of options available for fending off disease, strengthening constitutional resistance, relieving symptoms, and generally enhancing health. Herbs, homeopathic and folk remedies, reflexology, reiki, aromatherapy, special diets and/or dietary supplements, and so forth may be used in conjunction with or as alternatives to allopathic regimens. PWAs (along with their caregivers, including physicians, nurses, and other licensed health-care providers) have found that a wide range of interventions that are not part of Western allopathic medical tradition can be useful for symptom relief and health promotion. These include acupuncture, yoga, guided imagery, chiropractic, relaxation therapies, humor, massage, and other touch therapies (Sowell et al., 1997). Some have been proposed as boosting the immune system.

Unfortunately, there is a lack of hard data describing the positive and negative effects of almost all nonallopathic options. Meanwhile, both misinformation and misinterpretation of available data can be widely disseminated.[11] Compelling personal testimonials as well as commercial advertisements fill an ever-growing consumer-generated literature in the PWA community. This plethora of information is not easily evaluated and can be overwhelming. It is known that some compounds may be harmful, even life-threatening, particularly if taken in large quantities. Some may interact adversely with drugs or interfere with nutrition. Others, though harmless, may simply be ineffective for their intended purpose and unnecessarily dilute a PWA's financial resources.

Like others with chronic and/or life-threatening disease, particularly diseases for which a cure is not readily available and adequate symptomatic relief is elusive, PWAs are not only susceptible to misinformation, but also easy prey for quacks, who not only promote questionable remedies, including some known to be useless, but sometimes also vigorously attempt to dissuade the use of physician-recommended antivirals and/or antibiotics. Some proponents of unconventional therapies are well intentioned and may ardently believe their recommendations. However, by not distinguishing beliefs from knowledge, they rarely acknowledge how little may be known about the remedies they espouse, even though their arguments may rely on pointing out the limitations of biomedical research about allopathic pharmaceutical agents.

Exploring the person's goals may be more relevant than elaborating the pros and cons of specific modalities. Often, adoption of alternatives to physician-recommended approaches reflects a desire to have and exercise options independently and to take control of one's health (Sowell et al., 1997, p. 25).

As newly available treatments alter the disease course, the health and medical care needs of those affected are continuously shifting. The challenge to nurses is to ensure that the *person* is not labeled by the diagnosis, to identify the response patterns that enhance each individual's potential to grow through the illness experience, and to assist in repatterning both individual and community responses that can be dispiriting. Competent, compassionate care must be bolstered by a raised consciousness about the need to address the diverse societal and community factors that continue to shape the epidemic and the caregiving environment. Client and family teaching must be coupled with raising the consciousness of others—such as hospital and managed-care administrators, government policy makers, community leaders, educators, and indeed the general public—about needed standards and the kinds of interventions and approaches to care delivery that could improve PWAs' quality of life. We must augment our compassion and clinical competence with an activist stance, within and outside our own workplaces, to ensure that those in need obtain effective, timely care. More important, nurses can support PWAs to reconstruct their lives, becoming skilled in self-care to manage the ups and downs of AIDS as a chronic illness while anticipating a future and maintaining hope.

The following case study illustrates one person's efforts to deal with the initial phases of diagnosis and treatment of AIDS.

➤➤➤ CASE STUDY

FRANK

Frank was a 42-year-old manager in an office supply store when he learned he was HIV-positive 3 years ago. He took the antibody screening test at a Department of Health anonymous test site because he had unprotected sex with 4 partners before beginning to use condoms consistently 6 years previously. He felt that he was well informed about AIDS and told the posttest counselor that he "knew what to do." When he got back to his office, he called a friend, George, and arranged to meet him after work. George was not prepared for Frank's news, although it was not the first time he had had such a conversation with or about a friend.

Frank and George had known each other for almost 15 years, and in that time had lost several mutual friends to AIDS. Frank said he did not want to tell any one else just yet because he did not have to talk about it. "I want to be able to keep some things normal," he said. "I have so much to think about." George assured him that friends would be understanding, but agreed that there was no rush to tell anyone. "It's your business; no one else needs to know anything you don't want them to know," he told him. Frank did plan to call his brother, who lived about

200 miles away, but not until after he had a medical examination and would have more information. Frank told George he wanted to "interview" a few physicians. "After all," he said, "I expect it to be a long relationship!" Frank had clear ideas about being a proactive client who would be in charge of his own care. George suggested that Frank go to the nearby AIDS service organization (ASO) to obtain information and offered to go with him. Weeks later, Frank would recall hearing himself refer to "my diagnosis" and thinking, "I will never be without this HIV. It is not erasable; things will never be the same. I have crossed an imaginary line. HIV is now my present *and* my future." In fact, such thoughts would intrude on him throughout the days ahead, distracting him not only at work but also when socializing with friends.

Care Seeking

Frank got the names of several physicians by calling the ASO hotline, and George suggested a physician who had taken care of another friend. Frank was not prepared, however, to discover that one physician on his list of five was not taking any new clients or that two others did not have available appointment times for the next 3 weeks. He was also surprised to learn that physicians were affiliated with specific hospitals, and disappointed that three of the five physicians he called were not affiliated with either of two hospitals he would prefer to use. An even bigger shock was to learn that they all expected him to pay with cash or check at the time of an initial appointment and that they would charge him "just to talk" even if there was no complete physical examination. He made two appointments, but eventually cancelled the second because he felt comfortable with the first physician.

Dr. C seemed to anticipate most of the topics Frank wanted to discuss, and he raised quite a few more. Frank felt confident, but also overwhelmed and somewhat unnerved; somehow he did not quite feel as though he was "taking charge" the way he had wanted to, the way he thought he was supposed to. In a way, it was a relief not to feel so responsible, but he also felt insecure about trusting his health to someone else.

The issue of trust in doctors and the health-care system would remain a topic for recurring debate among Frank and his friends, including new acquaintances that he met as a result of his illness. Every magazine and newsletter he would pick up seemed to say to be wary of doctors, that they definitely do *not* know best. He would listen to others spout medical jargon and knowingly assert conclusions about different therapies and wonder how they could be so sure when the more he read, the less sure he felt. He wanted to know that there was a right way and a wrong way, and the only persons who supported this view were those who insisted that listening to doctors and drug companies was the

wrong way. No one could say what the one right way might be, except those who advocated avoiding everything "unnatural" or synthetic, a view that Frank did not hold. He envied those who could be so sure as well as those who could be, or seemed to be, nonchalant. Having the prerogative to make decisions about his care did not make him feel in control. Eventually Frank decided that feeling he could trust his physician was actually a source of control. He wanted to understand what was going on and what the physician was thinking. But he also wanted to rely on the physician—not his own judgment or friends' opinions—to determine what options were available.

At that first medical appointment, Frank also learned that his 80 percent insurance coverage would leave a hefty bill for him to pay out of pocket. Drug therapies were not covered at all. The nurse case manager recommended that he talk to a financial advocate at the ASO to determine what entitlements to benefits he might have. Frank doubted that he had any benefits from his 3-year stint in the merchant marine after high school, but it was worth checking. Because his medical insurance did not cover drugs, he was given an application for state aid so that selected HIV-related therapies would be paid for by the state.

The news was not so good when he returned for his follow-up medical appointment 2 weeks later. His CD4-cell count was $300/mm^3$, and he had a viral load of 56,000 copies/mm^3. Dr. C told him that the virus had already significantly weakened his immune system. He also had a low platelet count ($54,000/mm^3$), which he learned was a common symptom. Given his high viral load and declining T-cell count, he needed to start taking several antiviral medicines sooner rather than later, preferably without delay. "These are powerful treatments," Dr. C explained, "and we should see results right away. But once you start taking them, you'll have to keep taking them indefinitely; otherwise they will lose their power and the virus will become resistant." The word resistant alarmed Frank. He asked if resistance was inevitable if he started treatment so early. Dr. C's response stunned him: "With your T-cell count and high viral load, we cannot think of this as early treatment. You have very active disease and we have to suppress it or you'll have serious symptoms soon."

Frank did not want to tell his boss about his illness, but he felt he needed to take time off from work to sort things out and "take care of business." There was no time during the day to make all the calls he needed to gather information and make appointments. Accustomed as he was to working 11-hour days and bringing work home on weekends, the extra-long lunch hours he had been taking in recent weeks meant that work was piling up. He felt distracted and was not returning calls to clients. Of course, the down side of taking time off was that he would be forfeiting commission income and spending vacation time that might be better saved for future use.

The next morning he overslept and called his boss to tell him there was a family emergency. He went into the office in the afternoon and arranged to take the next week off from work. He was vague about the nature of the emergency, and his boss and coworkers did not ask for details. For the remainder of the week, he immersed himself in catching up so that he could clear out his inbox before taking off. Just knowing that he had a plan, even if it was just a plan to get down to planning, seemed to help clear his head, and he postponed thinking about lab tests and drug therapies.

"Getting It Together"

"People talk about the shock of finding out you're positive and the immediate aftermath. For me, however, 'the week that was' actually came a month later. When I took that week off work, I was suddenly a full-time PWA. You could even say 'patient' if that word were politically correct." Frank laughed as he recounted these events, then stopped. "I wasn't laughing that week; there was nothing to laugh about. There was always one more problem for every one that I solved, and nothing was simple. Everything was 'hurry up and wait.' For every possibility, there seemed to be a catch-22. It was a damn run-around. Everyone talked like they wanted to be helpful, but no one wanted to help me do what I wanted or the way I wanted. It seemed like the CBOs [community-based organizations] were just as bureaucratic as government agencies and the whole health-care system. It was like a full-time job making and keeping appointments, jumping through hoops, going through these long 'intake' interviews, and listening to their advice. In a way, I wasn't being realistic; I can say that now. But back then, I was just totally frustrated and felt I was seeing my life fall apart even while I was perfectly healthy."

He had gone to the ASO the first thing Monday morning, only to find that it did not open until 10 o'clock. (Most clients found late hours more convenient, as Frank would in the coming months, particularly the evening hours that would go as late as 8:30 PM.) He waited an hour and a half, only to find that he needed to have an appointment for an intake interview, which could be scheduled only 2 days a week and generally 1 or 2 weeks in advance. It was a lost day as far as he was concerned, but he did pick up flyers, program announcements, and newsletters. Studying them when he returned home, he decided to call the hotline.

He learned that he could obtain several services without having completed the intake process, including the financial advocacy clinic and a weekly drop-in support group for the newly diagnosed. He was hesitant about the prospect of participating in a group. It did not seem to fit his style, and besides, what was the point of "joining" other PWAs? His goal was to normalize his life, not to build a new social life with AIDS at its core. The hotline counselor stayed on the phone with him for

almost 50 minutes and helped him articulate these and other feelings and also to identify his immediate goal: personalized information gathering. The group sessions seemed designed to accomplish just that, but Frank was not quite ready. He convinced himself to try it by telling himself that if he was not getting the answers he wanted, he could just leave.

Three others attended that first 2-hour session, including a man who had been given his diagnosis 2 years earlier. The topic of discussion was right on the top of Frank's agenda: "questions to ask your doctor." No one seemed rushed, and when the semi-formal discussion ended, the nurse stayed to answer additional questions. Frank asked about experimental treatment possibilities, and she explained the way clinical trials were organized, including the randomization process and its implications. There were also eligibility criteria to consider. Clinical conditions and lab test results could exclude him from some trials; so could treatment history. The nurse also explained how different treatment decisions could have long-term implications.

Later that week, Frank was able to complete an intake interview, which culminated in an appointment with a financial advocate. He signed a release that would allow agency staff members to talk to his physician. The interviewer also gave Frank a referral for legal planning for property and future care and suggested that Frank consider the agency's buddy program, particularly if he did not want to participate in a support group.

The financial advocate gave him a list of things he would have to research—a review of his work history, insurance policies, income tax forms from the previous 2 years, bank accounts, and retirement and death benefits that he had accrued (including pensions, annuities, and life insurance). The advocate emphasized the instruction not to do anything to jeopardize on-time payment of medical insurance premiums.

A Way of Life: Pills, Pills, and More Pills

When Frank returned to see his physician, they discussed treatment options again, including a calendar for monitoring treatment effects and gauging efficacy. He would have blood specimens drawn that day and then again in 2 weeks and 2 weeks after that. Then he could anticipate monthly monitoring for the next 6 months, and perhaps less frequently after that. Frank said he wanted to fight the virus aggressively and asked about possibilities to take part in clinical trials. Dr. C advised against the minimum month-long delay that start-up and enrollment in a trial would take. When Frank expressed his disappointment and said that he felt he was being given no choices, Dr. C explained that being in a trial at this time would limit possibilities. "If we didn't have something available that we knew would likely suppress your virus in the next few weeks, then I'd say let's try something unknown. But right now I suggest that we work with what we know—and if the trials suggest we add to that, then we can add to that. The trials being run now are comparing different combinations and dosages. We can use their results as quickly as they're known."

The argument was sufficiently convincing for Frank, but he still felt more than ever as though he had little control over anything that mattered to his health. The nurse tried to put a different spin on it: "What *is* in your control is sticking to the prescription, and that will be an achievement you can be proud of because it won't be easy," she told him. "Compliance doesn't just happen; you have to make it happen." After reviewing the prescriptions with him, she asked him about his daily and weekly routines and then pressed for details about exceptions. "We can work these medicines into your existing schedule or plan a schedule around the prescription. Which approach do you think will work in the long run?" After an hour's discussion, they had worked out a tentative plan, and she had learned more about Frank's life past and present than many of his friends put together, certainly more than he had ever imagined telling any stranger—nitty-gritty, concrete things, and also feelings about friendships, his relationship with his brother, his parents, and grandparents. As if that were not enough, he agreed to keep a diet diary for 4 consecutive days, including a weekend day. They made a follow-up appointment, and the nurse gave him a number to call her directly and urged him to use it if anything came up, especially questions about the medicines. "You'll think of something as soon as you leave or on the weekend. Whenever, just call and, if I'm not here, leave a message on the voicemail and I'll call you back. Don't worry, I won't say I'm a nurse or that I'm calling from a doctor's office." He was glad that she said that because it probably would not have occurred to him until he was faced with leaving a message for her to call him back, and then he would definitely have hesitated to leave his work number.

The four-drug regimen seemed to work, although his T cells dropped further before climbing back up to the 500 to 600/mm^3 range 2 months later, where they have remained ever since. Dr. C recommended that he continue the PCP prophylaxis that he had started to take when the T cells had dropped. He experienced no symptoms that could definitely be attributed to the medicines, although his frequently overwhelming fatigue was probably caused, at least in part, by drug-related anemia. He did not have the energy to jog in the morning as had been his custom, and he was not pleased with the paunch he developed despite continuing to work out at the gym three or four times a week.

Telling and Retelling

Frank usually talked to his brother by phone every 2 or 3 weeks. The first couple of times he talked to him after getting his positive antibody-

test result, it was not so difficult to avoid mentioning it. He just put himself on automatic and followed a standard script that reviewed his niece's activities, World Series results, and so forth. It became harder as he became more and more preoccupied with the stresses of finding a physician, getting other lab tests done, and starting treatment. His brother caught his inattention several times in the conversation, but Frank was able to beg off answering by saying he was going through a particularly busy period at work and had a lot on his mind. He decided that he wanted to tell him in person, and would wait until he saw him at Thanksgiving. He had to hold back tears as his father said grace before carving the turkey and included "being thankful that we all have our health." The next day, he went jogging with his brother before breakfast. He made a good show of keeping up with him, then slowed, and admitted feeling winded. He took his brother's teasing, and then said, "Well, it will be good news if I am going to get old. I may have some bad news, though." His brother's eyes grew wide with disbelief as Frank recounted the last 2 months' events. He reached for Frank's shoulder, "How long have you known? I should have guessed." "No," Frank said, "How could you have known? I didn't know."

Frank waited until shortly after the Christmas holidays to tell his parents. "That was the hardest thing I ever had to do," he would later tell George. "I could just see the worry and heartbreak in their eyes." After that, he took a rather nonchalant approach about disclosing illness information to others. Basically, he was a rather private person, and he did not see the need to discuss his life situation with those who were not involved. So he did not make formal announcements. On the other hand, he made no effort to hide evident accoutrements of his illness regimen: He casually took his pills in front of friends and occasionally commented on his declining viral load. Friends were taken aback at first, thinking that somehow they had either missed a cue or had inadvertently invaded a private moment. However, they were usually also grateful for the opportunity to digest the information, and sometimes even to discuss it with each other, before having to say something directly to Frank. It didn't change the situation, but initial communications about it could have been less awkward. Frank felt he was avoiding putting others—as well as himself—on the spot. It also helped him maintain a zone of privacy if he did not have to elaborate or "play" the client. The initial assessment of Frank is summarized in Table 14.4.

Continuing Challenges

Like many of his friends, gay and straight, Frank had for some years been on the periphery of activism in the AIDS community. He had participated in the annual AIDS Walk and written checks for other fundraising events that supported the ASO, a hospice for PWAs, and the community-based initiative for clinical AIDS research. He had occasionally

Table 14.4 ➤ **INITIAL NURSING ASSESSMENT OF FRANK**

The nurse identified Frank as a vigilant focuser and sensitizer (Miller, 1992, p. 23) who sought concrete assistance with self-monitoring and moderately detailed explanations for recommendations.

Diagnosis	Related to
Potential for ineffective coping	Feeling overwhelmed
	Unfamiliarity with requirements of health-care and social service systems
	Inexperience with care-seeking role
	Inexperience in dealing with bureaucratic agencies
Knowledge deficits about: available resources, how to access them, including eligibility requirements; treatments and illness-care regimens	Inexperience with dependence and help seeking
	Limited, superficial experience with AIDS-related problems of acquaintances
	Misinformation provided by friends as well as uninformed, but opinionated, acquaintances
	Outdated information continuing to circulate in PWA community
	Enormous quantity of information that is continually changing
Fear of illness progression and death concerns	Knowing the implications of viral load and T-cell count
	Having seen others' illness trajectory
Decisional conflicts about treatment choices	Unanticipated limited options and concern about toxicity and long-term effects
Risk (minimal) of poor adherence to treatment regimen	Lack of energy, complicated schedule and potential delay in adjusting thereto
	Possible forgetfulness, especially when normal schedule or routines are changed
Fatigue	Undetermined etiology (possibly secondary to immunodeficiency, metabolic demands of illness, and/or drug effects)
	Anemia
	Ongoing or intermittent anxiety or depression
Risk for inadequate nutrition	Increased needs secondary to illness
	Irregular schedule and meals now potentially further compromised by medicine schedule and finances (curtailing eating out and not accustomed to preparing meals)
Potential for social isolation	Not wanting to discuss illness with friends, coworkers, and social acquaintances
	Preoccupation with immediate demands of illness
	Friends' perception that they may be intruding or that Frank does not want them involved
	Close friends (such as George) feeling overwhelmed or disagreeing with Frank's illness-related decisions

Table 14.4 ➤ **INITIAL NURSING ASSESSMENT OF FRANK (Continued)**	
Strengths	**Problems/Potential Deficits**
Financial status and moderately flexible job schedule	Insurance coverage not adequate to cover regular, ongoing health-care expenses
Strong family ties	Lives alone; family not immediately
Reliable friends	available (located at moderate geographic
Actively seeks help	distance)
Able to identify sources for help	Advanced disease with evident decline in
Ability to verbalize frustration and identify preferences	immunity
Eager to follow medical advice	Frequent fatigue
Openness to new ideas	

attended community information forums about AIDS and felt that he was better informed than a lot of people, perhaps even the majority of gay men. In the years since his diagnosis, he had learned a lot more but he still did not consider himself an activist. Nevertheless, he was actively involved. AIDS was not his whole life, but he took part in various Body Positive (health club group) activities and attended a support group twice a month.

At times it would be hard to believe that there was an active disease inside him ready to take over if he let his guard down. It was hard to believe that his colorful handful of pills was a lifeline. Actually, he did not want to believe it. He wanted to believe the pills were just a crutch and that it was his own positive thinking that kept him well. Occasionally, his positive thinking was challenged. Eighteen months after his diagnosis, he experienced 6 months of transient, but frequently recurring, diarrhea that was complicated by a painful anal fissure. He would sometimes have severe cramping. The nurse instructed him regarding avoiding lactose and so forth. Despite referral to a gastroenterologist who specialized in HIV disease and put him through repeated extensive tests, no specific cause could be identified. He was exhausted. Treatments brought no relief. He even visited a homeopathic therapist. Finally, the diarrhea subsided as suddenly and inexplicably as it had started, leaving him a little apprehensive about whether and when it might occur again.

He noted dry, flaking, itchy patches of skin on his trunk, forearms, and sometimes his face. From time to time, the itch was so painful that topical analgesia was necessary. He went to a homeopathic therapist for these episodes. Worried that the skin eruptions were a sign that his immune system was failing or that the medicines were becoming toxic, he began practicing daily meditation to relax, and he inquired about the use of imagery to support healing and immunity. These modalities were taught at the ASO, and he signed up for several workshops as well as a consultation visit with the practitioner who taught the sessions.

After experiencing 4 bouts of extensive esophageal candidiasis within a 14-month period, he began a maintenance schedule of fluconazole (Diflucan). Recently he enrolled in a clinical trial that is evaluating interventions to alleviate fatigue, but he does not yet know to which group he will be assigned (exercise only, drug only, drug and exercise combination, no treatment).

The biggest disappointment came when, after 30 months of treatment, a routine viral load test showed that the virus was increasing. When a repeated test confirmed the finding, he had to change his drug regimen. He felt that he was starting all over—facing only unknowns. What would the right combination be? Would he have adverse effects from the new drugs? Would they work? His physician pointed out that in many ways, he was better off than during his first go-round. Although his viral load had begun to rise, it was still much lower than it had been when his illness was first diagnosed, and his T cells had not dropped. Nevertheless, Frank felt newly vulnerable.

A frequent topic of conversation at support group meetings was forming and maintaining intimate relationships. Frank was not eager to date when he was first diagnosed, largely because he was preoccupied with other concerns. Nevertheless, he could not help thinking about and dreading that the reality of his disease could get in the way of even meeting someone on a truly personal level, let alone getting more involved. After a while, as life became more settled, he would date occasionally and the issue of whether and when to disclose the fact of his diagnosis always loomed large. He would ruminate on whether a premature disclosure would derail a promising relationship. Frank's later diagnoses are shown in Table 14.5.

Thinking about Retiring

Finances became an issue rather quickly after Frank's diagnosis, and it was not altogether expected. Frank had a relatively good job and led a comfortable but nonextravagant life. The problem was that his major medical insurance plan did not cover his extraordinary outpatient expenses. The state aid covered most, but not all, of his medicines. He was spending about $1400 a month, sometimes more, on doctor and pharmacy bills, plus he contributed $900 a year to his medical insurance payments. He was not in a position to switch medical plans unless he continued his old coverage for a year while paying the new premiums (i.e., until the new insurer would no longer disqualify his HIV-related expenses as a preexisting condition). But that would add at least another $3000 to the year's health-care bill. He also wanted to make sure that he would be able to stay with Dr. C, which meant carefully selecting a plan that included Dr. C in its provider network. Frank decided not to change. The case manager suggested that he talk to Dr. C so that they could be

Table 14.5 ➤ **LATER DIAGNOSES OF FRANK**

Diagnosis	Related to
Fear of illness progression and death concerns	Occurrence(s) of diverse symptoms and opportunistic illnesses
	Persistent, difficult-to-treat symptoms for which physicians cannot provide exact diagnoses or explanations
	Increased abdominal girth
Altered self-concept associated with altered body image	Fatigue; reduced exercise tolerance
	Abnormal lab tests
Altered skin integrity manifested by rash, discomfort, reddening, and dryness	Unknown specific etiology
Risk for infection evidenced by recurrent candidiasis	Immunodeficiency secondary to HIV disease

sure to avoid unnecessary lab tests. For example, she would be sure to get copies of test results from the fatigue study so that Frank would not be undergoing and paying for duplicate tests.

From time to time, Frank thought about retiring. He knew other people who had quit work, and Medicaid had assumed their medical insurance payments. On one hand, he could not afford not to work; on the other, he almost could not afford to work. He would have almost as much income from disability insurance and social security if he stopped working as he now had left after his medical costs. He tried to tell himself that he should at least wait until he turned 50, but then he would wonder if he could count on enjoying another 4 years of health. He had been fortunate so far, but should he wait til he got sick and debilitated before taking time to relax and enjoy himself?

Of course, not working was not just an economic issue. Would he be able to fill his time? Now he seemed to never to have enough time, but he did not want to be bored or too poor to enjoy his freedom. His case manager suggested he talk to both a financial planner and a vocational counselor, as well as to his financial advocate. He might be able to continue working in a different capacity, for example, as a consultant with a different time arrangement. That way, he could not only maximize his income, but he could also be productive in an activity that he enjoyed. Or he might be able to afford to do volunteer work. His nurse discussed all of this with him and referred him to the financial planner. A financial planner could help him evaluate his assets and project his long-term and short-term needs for a variety of work-stopping and survival scenarios. The financial advocate would know what impact different decisions might have on his benefits.

The real question, Frank admits, centered on not being able, and to some extent, not wanting to be able to define the future. Would it be measured in years or decades? Frank says, "It wouldn't be so hard to make a 5-year plan or a 10-year plan, or even a 2-year plan if that is the case. But not knowing what you are planning for makes any decision seem reckless, especially because I know I want it to be more than 10, even more than 20. But is that realistic? Should I be trying to stick money into a retirement account or annuity that I won't touch for another 15 years?" He also acknowledges that rather than focusing on a survival trajectory, he would really like to be thinking in terms of a midlife career switch and is considering seeing a vocational counselor. Frank's nurse is "with him" as he faces uncertainty. Their relationship alleviates any sense of abandonment during crises and times of difficult decisions. Frank knows that he can count on her.

SUMMARY

Informational needs vary among PWAs. Their unique concerns, capacities, phase of adjustment, and preferences influence nurses' provision of information. The nursing interventions can enlarge an individual's focus, enable alternate perspectives, promote recognition of strengths, and provide safe space for voicing new ideas. Nurses can organize community resources, help clients prioritize needs, and monitor when varied resources need to be tapped. Nurses can help with problem solving and also offer anticipatory guidance about real and potential concerns that an individual has not yet considered. The nurse can help clients review their life course, engage in positive reminiscence, and find sources of hope. Transcendence of physical and emotional suffering should be an outcome of nursing intervention.

NOTES

[1]The acronym PWA is applied in this chapter to anyone with HIV disease, regardless of disease severity or manifestation, and is not reserved for those who meet the Centers for Disease Control and Prevention (CDC) surveillance criteria. Of course, people *affected* by AIDS include not only infected individuals, but families, friends, neighbors, coworkers, informal helpers and caregivers, health and social service providers, and others throughout the community. In truth, we are all affected by AIDS.

[2]Another virus, human immunodeficiency virus type 2 (HIV-2), also causes immunodeficiency. However, it appears to be less virulent—that is, the disease associated with it is less severe. Its epidemiology is different. There are fewer cases and it has not spread worldwide. Its pathology and pathogenesis have not been studied as extensively as those of HIV-1, and scientists do not know whether most HIV-2-infected persons will develop life-threatening AIDS (Kanki, 1997).

[3]An analogy has been made between HIV disease and a train going along a track that ends at a precipice (Coffin, 1996). There is no question about where the train is headed. The questions are how quickly it is moving toward the end of the track and whether it can be stopped before it gets there. Health care aims to prevent the train from starting in the first place (primary prevention of exposure to HIV) and then intervenes to slow the train (secondary prevention) or, better, to stop it (cure). The PWAs CD4-cell count is analogous to the distance to the precipice; the viral load is the train's speed.

[4]Twenty-six diseases are recognized as indicators of AIDS in adults in the United States and western Europe: esophageal, bronchial, tracheal, or pulmonary candidiasis; invasive cervical cancer; disseminated or extrapulmonary coccidioidomycosis; extrapulmonary cryptococcosis; chronic (>1 month) intestinal cryptosporidiosis; cytomegalovirus (CMV) disease other than those of the liver, spleen, or nodes; CMV retinitis with vision loss; HIV encephalopathy (AIDS dementia complex); herpes simplex bronchitis, pneumonitis, esophagitis, or chronic (>1 month) ulcer(s); disseminated or extrapulmonary histoplasmosis; chronic (>1 month) intestinal isosporiasis; KS; Burkitt's, immunoblastic, or primary brain lymphoma; disseminated or extrapulmonary *Mycobacterium avium* complex or *Mycobacterium kansasii;* pulmonary or extrapulmonary *Mycobacterium tuberculosis;* PCP; recurrent pneumonia; progressive multifocal leukoencephalopathy (PML); recurrent *Salmonella* septicemia; toxoplasmosis of brain; wasting syndrome (defined as involuntary weight loss of 10% or more of body weight for which there is no explanation other than HIV disease). To ensure that current counts represent essentially the same degree of immunodeficiency as the earlier surveillance case definitions (1982, 1985, 1986, 1987), a CD4-cell count $200/mm^3$ or fewer or less than 14% of total lymphocytes is also a criterion even in the absence of weight loss, neurological symptoms, or any OI (CDC, 1992). The CD4-cell count criteria recognize that absence of opportunistic disease in the presence of severe immunodeficiency is likely the result of chemoprophylaxis, as discussed on pages 400–406.

Children's immature immune systems make them susceptible to different diseases, so different criteria are used to define AIDS in children younger than 13 years (CDC, 1994): two bacterial infections within 2 years; candidiasis (thrush) persisting for 2 months or longer; cryptococcosis; cryptosporidiosis; CMV encephalopathy after 1 month of age; chronic (>1 month) herpes simplex ulcer(s); histoplasmosis; KS; lymph interstitial pneumonia (LIP); lymphoma; *Mycobacterium avium intracellulare;* disseminated tuberculosis; PCP; PML; toxoplasmosis; and failure to thrive. CD4-cell counts and percentages are incorporated into the definition according to age. The pediatric definition further classifies clinical findings as mildly, moderately, or severely symptomatic without indicating pathological stages.

The World Health Organization uses different criteria for surveillance in countries where different exposures are likely and laboratory-based diagnostic criteria are less useful because of cost or unavailability.

[5]CD4 T cells are so named because the glycoprotein CD4 is found on their plasma membranes. CD4 is also found on B lymphocytes, monocytes, macrophages, stromal reticular cells of the bone marrow, and fibroblasts and related cells, such as glial cells in the brain. CD4 is the primary receptor for HIV attachment and entry into cells.

[6]Circulating viruses are the measurable part of an individual's viral burden. Much more virus—both actively replicating and latent—may be harbored in tissues. Indeed, viral load (i.e., the amount of HIV RNA) in mononuclear cells in lymph nodes may be 1 to 3 logs higher than in peripheral blood.

[7]Human immunodeficiency virus is a retrovirus, a type of virus that routes genetic information from RNA to DNA and then cleaves to an infected cell's chromosomal DNA and replicates synchronously with it.

[8]New drugs are continually being added to the available repertoire. The number of non–cross-resistant drugs is limited, however.

[9]*Pneumocystis carinii* pneumonia (PCP), toxoplasmic encephalitis, cryptosporidiosis, microsporidiosis, tuberculosis, disseminated *Mycobacterium avium* complex (MAC), *Streptococcus pneumoniae* and *Haemophilus influenzae* pneumonias, bartonellosis, candidiasis (oropharyngeal, esophageal, and vaginal), cryptococcosis, histoplasmosis, coccidioidomycosis, cytomegalovirus (CMV), herpes simplex virus (HSV), varicella-zoster virus (VZV), human papillomavirus infection (HPV), and bacterial enteric infections.

[10]The debate may be reopened as CD4-cell counts rise after falling viremia in response to more potent antiretroviral therapies. It is not yet clear to what extent immunity is actu-

ally replenished. Hence, whether and for how long to continue prophylaxes when counts have risen, or to what level they should rise before prophylaxes could be discontinued, must be empirically studied.

[11]Until recently, many articles directed at PWAs that promoted holistic approaches to health and well-being also included arguments that HIV did not cause AIDS—long after debate among scientists had ceased. These articles frequently argued that antiretrovirals were useless, even dangerous. AIDS activists' concern about drug costs, coupled with the drugs' limited sustained efficacy and frequent, sometimes severe adverse effects, seemed to lend plausibility to these arguments.

REFERENCES

Adinolfi, A. (1996). The role of the nurse in the care of patients with HIV infection. In Glaxo Wellcome Health Education Department (Ed.). *Care and management of patients with HIV infection.* (pp. 215–259). Durham NC: Glaxo Wellcome.

Barrett, E. A. M. (1983). An empirical investigation of Martha E. Rogers' principle of helicy: The relationship of human field motion and power. (Doctoral dissertation, New York University, New York, NY).

Barrett, E. A. M. (1990). *Visions of Rogers' science-based nursing.* New York: National League for Nursing.

Bennett, J. A. (1988). Helping people with AIDS live well at home. *Nursing Clinics of North America, 23,* 731–748.

Bennett, J. A. (1995). Acquired immunodeficiency syndrome and social disease. *Holistic Nursing Practice, 10*(1), 77–89.

Carwein, V. L., & Sabo, C. E. (1997). The use of alternative therapies for HIV infection: Implications for patient care. *AIDS Patient Care 11*(2), 79–85.

Casey, K. M. (1997). Malnutrition associated with HIV/AIDS: II. Assessment and interventions. *Journal of Association of Nurses in AIDS Care, 8,* 39–48.

Casey, K. M., Cohen, F. L., & Hughes, A. M. (1996). Preface. In K. M. Casey, F. Cohen, & A. M. Hughes (Eds.). *ANAC's core curriculum for HIV/AIDS nursing.* Philadelphia, PA: Nursecom for The Association of Nurses in AIDS Care, 24.

Catanzaro, M. (1990). Transitions in midlife adults with long-term illness. *Holistic Nursing Practice, 4*(3), 65–73.

Coffin, J. (1996, July). HIV viral dynamics. Paper presented at the 11th International Conference on AIDS and Sexually Transmitted Diseases. Vancouver.

Cooper, E. C., & Horn, T. (1997). *AIDS/HIV Treatment Directory.* New York: American Foundation for AIDS Research.

Fowke, K. R., D'Amico, R., Chernoff, D. N., Pottage, J. C., Benson, C. A., Sha, B. E., Kessler, H. A., Landay, A. L., & Shearer, G. M. (1997). Immunologic and virologic evaluation after influenza vaccination of HIV-1 infected patients. *AIDS, 11,* 1013–1021.

Heckman, T. G., Somlai, A. M., Sikkema, K. J., Kelly, J. A., Franzoi, S. L. (1997). Psychosocial predictors of life satisfaction among persons living with HIV infection and AIDS. *Journal of Association of Nurses in AIDS Care, 8,* 21–30.

Herek, G. M., & Glunt, E. K. (1988). An epidemic of stigma: Public reactions to AIDS. *American Psychologist, 43,* 886–891.

Kanki, P. (1997). Epidemiology and natural history of human immunodeficiency virus type 2. In V. T. DeVita, Jr., S. Hellman, & S. A. Rosenberg (Eds.). *AIDS: Etiology, diagnosis, treatment, and prevention* (4th ed., pp. 127–135). Philadelphia: Lippincott-Raven.

Kitahata, M. M., Koepsell, T. D., Deyo, R. A., Maxwell, C. I., Dodge, W. T., & Wagner, E. H. (1996). Physicians' experience with the acquired immunodeficiency syndrome as a factor in patients' survival. *New England Journal of Medicine, 334,* 701–706.

Lehman, R. H., Muurahainen, N., Guenter, P., & Cauterruci, M. (1996, July). "Cooking for life:" A nutrition education course for people with HIV/AIDS. *Proceedings of IXth International Conference on AIDS, 2,* 342. Vancouver.

Liss, M., Chan, R. S. K., McKinley, M., Ilaria, G., & Jacobs, J. (1996, July). Implementation of a cooking group to address the nutritional and home management needs of people with HIV. *Proceedings of IXth International Conference on AIDS, 2,* 102. Vancouver.

McEnany, G. W., Hughes, A. M., & Lee, K. A. (1996). Depression and HIV. *Nursing Clinics of North America, 31,* 57–79.

Miller, J. F. (1992). *Coping with chronic illness: Overcoming powerlessness* (2nd ed.). Philadelphia: FA Davis.

Morse, J. M. (1997). Responding to threats to integrity of self. *Advances in Nursing Science, 19*(4), 21–36.

Murphy, P., Sr., Bass, G., Donovan, C., & Selman, B. (1988). The patient with AIDS: Care and concerns. In I. B. Corless & M. Pittman-Lindeman (Eds.), *AIDS: Principles, practices, & politics* (pp. 151–166). Washington DC: Hemisphere Publishing.

Nelkin, D. & Gilman, S. L. (1988). Placing blame for devastating disease. *Social Research, 55,* 360–378.

Nokes, K., & Kendrew, J. (1996). Sleep quality in people with HIV disease. *Journal of the Association of Nurses in AIDS Care, 7,* 43–50.

Office of AIDS Research (OAR) Panel of Clinical Practices for Treatment of HIV Infection. (1997). *Preliminary guidelines for the use of antiretroviral agents in HIV-infected adults and adolescents.* Bethesda, MD: U.S. Department of Health and Human Services.

Pantaleo, G., Demarest, J. F., Schacker, T., Vaccarezza, M., Cohen, O. J., Daucher, M., Graziosi, C., Schnittman, S. S., Quinn, T. C., Shaw, G. M., Perrin, L., Tambussi, G., Lazzarin, A., Sekaly, R. P., Soudeyns, H., Corey, L., & Fauci, A. S. (1997). The qualitative nature of the primary immune response to HIV infection is a prognosticator of disease progression independent of the initial level of plasma viremia. *Proceedings of the National Academy of Sciences of the United States of America, 94(1):* 254–258.

Prochaska, J. O., & DiClemente, C. C. (1984). The transtheoretical approach: Crossing the traditional boundaries of therapy. Homewood, IL: Dow Jones-Irwin.

Prochaska, J. O., & Norcross, J. C. (1992). In search of how people change: Applications to addictive behaviors. *American Psychologist, 47,* 1102–1114.

Report of the Presidential Commission on AIDS. (1988). (p. xvii). Washington, DC:

Simpson, D. M., & Tagliati, M. (1997). Neuromuscular syndromes in human immunodeficiency virus disease. In J. R. Berger & R. M. Levy (Eds.), *AIDS and the nervous system* (2nd ed.). Philadelphia: Lippincott-Raven.

Sowell, R. L., Moneyham, L., Guillory, J., Seals, B., Cohen, L., & Demi, A. (1997). Self-care activities of women infected with human immunodeficiency virus. *Holistic Nursing Practice, 11*(2), 18–26.

Ungvarski, P. J., & Rottner, J. E. (1997). Errors in prescribing HIV-1 protease inhibitors. *Journal of Association of Nurses in AIDS Care, 8,* 55–61.

U.S. Centers for Disease Control. (1981a). Kaposi's sarcoma and *Pneumocystis* pneumonia in homosexual men: New York City and California. *MMWR, 30,* 305.

U.S. Centers for Disease Control. (1981b). *Pneumocystis* pneumonia: Los Angeles. *MMWR, 30,* 250.

U.S. Centers for Disease Control. (1985). Revision of the case definition of acquired immunodeficiency syndrome for national reporting: United States. *MMWR, 34,* 373.

U.S. Centers for Disease Control. (1986). Classification system for human T-lymphotropic virus type III/lymphadenopathy-associated virus infections. *MMWR, 35,* 334.

U.S. Centers for Disease Control. (1987). Revision of the CDC surveillance case definition for acquired immunodeficiency syndrome. *MMWR, 36*(Suppl. 1S):1S.

U.S. Centers for Disease Control and Prevention. (1992). 1993 revised classification system for HIV infection and expanded surveillance case definition for AIDS among adolescents and adults. *MMWR, 41*(RR-17), 1–9.

U.S. Centers for Disease Control and Prevention. (1994). Revised classification system for human immunodeficiency virus infection in children less than 13 years of age. *MMWR, 43*(RR-12).

USPHA/IDSA Prevention of Opportunistic Infections Working Group. (1995). USPHA/IDSA guidelines for the prevention of opportunistic infections in persons infected with human immunodeficiency virus: A summary. *MMWR, 44*(RR-8).

USPHA/IDSA Prevention of Opportunistic Infections Working Group. (1997). 1997 USPHA/IDSA guidelines for the prevention of opportunistic infections in persons infected with human immunodeficiency virus. *MMWR, 46*(RR-12), 1–47.

Williams, A. (1997). New Horizons: Antiretroviral therapy in 1997. *Journal of the Association of AIDS Care, 8,* 26–38.

Zerwekh, J. V. (1991). A family caregiving model for public health nursing. *Nursing Outlook, 39,* 213–217.

Appendix A: Empowering Persons Affected by AIDS

I. HIV/AIDS challenge
   A. The disease course
      1. Symptoms
         a. Diarrhea
            (1) Intervention
         b. HIV wasting
            (1) Intervention
         c. Fatigue
            (1) Intervention
         d. Encephalopathy and neuromuscular syndromes
         e. Sensory-perceptual alterations
         f. Pain, depression, and suicidal vulnerability
II. Empowered or overwhelmed?
   A. Implications for AIDS care
      1. Partnership
      2. Championing self-help
III. Assessment
   A. History
   B. Self-care resources, skills, and strategies
      1. Social support
         a. Information for self-care and illness management
         b. Planning and managing finances
   C. Stigma
   D. Supportive care
IV. Medical interventions
   A. Antiretroviral options
      1. Principles guiding antiretroviral therapy
   B. Preventing and treating opportunistic illness
      1. Client teaching
      2. Screening
      3. Secondary chemoprophylaxis
   C. Nonallopathic therapies
VI. Case study

Appendix B: National Hotline Numbers

These are useful sources of up-to-date information about HIV treatments and services that may be accessed locally as well as nationally.

AIDS Clinical Trials Information Service	800-874-2572*
	800-243-7012 TTY/TTD*
AIDS Treatment Data Network	800-734-7104*,†
American Foundation for AIDS Research (AmFAR)	
AIDS/HIV Treatment Directory	800-38A-mFAR†
Association for Drug Abuse Prevention & Treatment (ADAPT)	800-542-2347†
Body Positive (association for HIV-positive people)	800-566-6599†
Canadian HIV Trials Network	800-263-1638†
CDC National AIDS Clearinghouse	800-458-5231*
Gay Men's Health Crisis National Hotline	212-807-6655†
Good Samaritan Project (teen-to-teen hotline)	800-234-8336
	(4-8 PM CST)
National Association of People With AIDS (NAPWA)	202-898-0414†
National Patient Air Transport Hotline	800-296-1217
People with AIDS Coalition	800-828-3280*,†
Project Inform National Hotline (about treatment)	800-822-7422†
Sister Connect (for women)	800-747-1108
Women Alive (for women)	800-554-4876

*Spanish spoken.
†Newsletter(s) also available.

PART IV ➤

Selected Nursing Strategies

➤ Selected categories of nursing strategies are developed in this section. Innovative strategies to enhance quality of life of the chronically ill are presented by prescribing the use of literature (Chapter 15) and imagery (Chapter 16). Hobus presents selected literary passages and poems to be used as therapy. Storytelling, use of metaphors, and journal writing are included in Chapter 15. The theoretical bases and psychotherapeutic effects of imagery are described by Stephens in Chapter 16.

Ryan presents a framework for selecting strategies to facilitate behavior change in the chronically ill in Chapter 17. Theories that have been proposed to explain behavior change are reviewed, including self-efficacy, social support, social-cognitive theory, and macrosocial theory. Types of changes needed to improve and maintain health are described. Knowledge is the power resource that is developed in this chapter.

Detailed analyses of self-esteem and hope (two power resources) are included in Chapters 18 and 19. Newly developed models of nursing strategies to enhance self-esteem and inspire hope are presented. Clinical assessment and research instruments to measure these phenomena are reviewed.

15

Literature

A Dimension of Nursing Therapeutics*

➤ RUTH HOBUS

The use of literature is one of many innovative nursing interventions. Creative and selective use of readings, written journals, and storytelling is therapeutic in terms of enabling persons to cope with health alterations, to have hope and feel comforted, and to manage their life demands.

Literature, as a treatment modality, may empower the spirit, enable problem solving, provide fresh understanding of an event, or simply reassure (Gorelick, 1987; Hobus, Hansen, Evans, & Woodard, 1987; Mazza, 1988). Literature that focuses on the meaning of existence, transitions in health (Travelbee, 1971), or passages of time can "mirror well the life situation of clients" (Chavis, 1988, p. 232). Literature is a form of empowerment. Giving a voice and words to the client so that the experience, frustrations, and emotions can be shared enables the person to name the distress. "Naming" is an important aspect of psychological and spiritual care. Once clients can recognize and deal with their principal spiritual distress, other areas of care often fall into line. A clinical synopsis at the end of this chapter illustrates this point.

Varied terms referring to therapeutic use of literature include the following:

*Special recognition and thanks to A. Thomas Hansen, Humanist and Associate Professor of English, Northern State University, South Dakota, for his contributions, manuscript review, and support in development of this chapter. The author also thanks D. Evans, T. Hansen, L. Hasselstrom, and K. Norris for making their manuscripts from the Humanities in the Healing Arts Dialogue Series available.

1. *Bibliotherapy* (from the Greek words for book and healing): a bibliography that may be used, sometimes in a prescriptive fashion, to bring new thoughts to an individual or to determine the content of existing thought
2. *Transitional reading:* readings especially suited to those experiencing a change in their life cycle, such as the birth of a child; sudden incapacitation, illness, or injury; or a loss by death (Hobus, 1987)
3. *Interactive bibliotherapy:* a dialogue between a therapist and a client relative to the literary work to bring about a therapeutic interaction
4. *Reading bibliotherapy:* a newer concept consisting of assignment of self-help guided reading without discussion groups or a bibliotherapist (Cohen, 1989)

Bibliotherapy may restore the mind and spirit just as medical and other nursing interventions restore the body. Poetry therapy, journal writing, oral stories, teaching tales, and use of metaphors are some of the strategies used in bibliotherapy that are discussed.

All human interactions encompass a spiritual component (Tournier, 1965). The life a person lives in the body is evidenced in the mind and the spirit and reflects the client's belief systems (Nagai-Jacobsen & Burkhardt, 1989). It is not possible to be in a position of therapeutic helpfulness if one disregards the reality of the spirit (Nagai-Jacobsen & Burkhardt, 1989; Travelbee, 1971).

CHOICE OF THERAPEUTIC LITERATURE

Literature, in the context of therapy, may include anything that will be of probable value in helping the client and the caregiver to understand, to come to terms with, or to therapeutically redirect (reshape) a situation. Literary contributions can also bring humor to the situation (Schunior, 1989).

A common misconception is that nurses are not equipped to use literature as therapy because of inadequate knowledge of "good" or classical literature. Nurses, in fact, have a rich repertoire of personal interactions and previous experiences from which to draw either comforting, amusing, or teaching anecdotes. A point may be illustrated with a newspaper or magazine clipping or something from a journal. Literature used as therapy may include classics such as Tolstoy's *Ivan Ilych* or Robert Frost's "The Road Not Taken," depending on the client's needs, interests, and reading ability.

What is important in the selection of literature for a specific client is that it reflects his or her environment and understanding. Regional writers are especially useful in this realm (Hasselstrom, 1990). Regional writers discuss areas, topics, and values that are familiar and may be comforting or instructive. Poems, articles, and stories about the feelings of war veterans or the topics of growing old, abuse, women's issues, or the disabled are useful. Many anthologies are available by topic. *Despite This Flesh: The Disabled in Stories and Poems* is an example (Miller, 1985). Prescriptive readings by developmental life stages (Gold, 1988) can be found in Table 15.1.

"What you will look for in a poem," or writing of any type for therapy purposes, "is a statement of concentrated and psychic power, an inward-looking vision which expresses the dynamic conflicts and tensions of the inner life and one which will appear to fit many particular situations" (Jaskoski, 1987, p. 9). Such writing expresses universal truths: truths that endure and are valid for people of all ages. Literature that provokes reminiscences is generally a good choice, even if the memories are painful. Literature can assist recall and catharsis through the reminiscing process (Clements, 1986). Clements recommends this as an aid to families in distress whose children are hospitalized because of a serious illness or accident.

Short stories and short prose poems have the advantage of being compressed and getting a thought across in a few lines (Gorelick, 1987). Brevity can be an important factor for persons who are doing their own reading and may have a short attention span because of pain or medication. Others, with long hours to spend, such as in rehabilitation settings, may enjoy more lengthy writings.

Gorelick (1987) described how literature can be of help with family crises. The family tragedy may be abuse, addiction, chronic disease, or prolonged aftermath of an accident. The family at such an impasse "must discover a way to move their situation or they will ultimately succumb to defeat, despair or whatever else is fated by genes or the environment" (p. 42). A poem or good short piece may tell the story with sufficient power to give the reader a shock of recognition and offer new solutions to the client as reshaping takes place in the reader's mind (Gorelick, 1987).

Hasselstrom (1990) detailed this use of literature from a personal experience. A friend called one day with the intention of saying one last farewell, after having taken a large overdose of tranquilizers. The friend lived hundreds of miles from Hasselstrom, who was not sure that she could get help to the friend in time. However, the friend was rescued and taken to a hospital. As soon as Hasselstrom determined that her friend was out of danger, she sent the woman a copy of Victoria Tokareva's *Centre of Gravity*. This is a warm-hearted story of a Russian woman who tried several ways to commit suicide, unsuccessfully, because she always got sidetracked doing a good deed for someone. In the end she was offered a helping hand, from a stranger, to get back to the safety of her apartment. This helping hand reminded her

Table 15.1 ► A TENTATIVE FORMULATION OF DEVELOPMENTAL TASKS: GENERAL DEVELOPMENT TABLES			
Life Stage	**General Tasks and Skill Growth**	**Goals, Needs, and Activities**	**A Sample of Reading Prescriptions**
Infancy	Learning a sense of trust; object differentiation, phonic and visual coordination, etc.	Holding on/letting go, mother tongue, physical senses, and identity	Finger games, rhythm and rhyme, peek-a-boo-repetition, "this little pig," "ride a cock-horse," "rock-a-bye baby"
Early and middle childhood	A sense of initiative; family relations and roles; I/thou reality and rules, power, etc.; fears of desertion	The simplest adventure stories—projected danger and exploring—testing—feeling small stories Identity	Enid Blyton, Beatrix Potter, Babar, fairy tales, folk tales, animal sameness and differentiation, Disney, Just So Stories, Aesop's Fables, Toad and Ratty, Sendak
Preadolescence	Achieving a sense of industry, responsibility, social skills, body acceptance, competition	Living concepts, political and moral awareness, socialization, sexual awareness preparation, concepts of group structure and institutions; achieving personal independence, tastes and personal goal awareness, values adoption	Judy Blume, Nancy Drew, Hardy Boys, C. S. Lewis, L. M. Alcott, L. M. Montgomery, V. and B. Cleaver, Robert N. Peck, Farley Mowat
Adolescence	Sexual roles, economic independence, negotiation skills, achieving emotional stability, body awareness, clothing styles, skills and talents discoveries, deepening friendships, religious questioning	Acquiring information, developing power, sexual adjustment, modeling on chosen figures, developing language power, leaving home, career planning, future fantasies	S. E. Hinton, Betsy Byars, Mark Twain, Stephen King, Jane Austen, Charles Dickens, Lewis Wyndham

Early adulthood	Achieving intimacy, sharing, self-knowledge, mate selection, starting a family, education and training	Learning parenting and planning, investment, recreational skills and selection, social volunteer role selection, self-acceptance, and understanding	John Steinbeck, Philip Roth, Alice Munro, the Brontes, D. H. Lawrence, Margaret Atwood, Ernest Hemingway, Helen Keller
Middle adulthood	Rearing children, vocation and family planning, estate management, vocation stabilization, civic responsibility, social group formation, mediating, grandparenting, and family obligation	Coping with family stress, possible group work, values transmission, job anxiety, marriage enrichment or divorce, life review, physiological adjustment, reality acceptance	F. Scott Fitzgerald, Mordecai Richler, Nancy Thayer, Iris Murdoch, Mavis Gallant, George Eliot, Thomas Hardy, Erica Jong, James Carrol, Judith Guest, Virginia Woolf
Late adulthood	Grief for loss of friends, etc., retirement, reduced income, grandparenting, diminishing strength or health, loss of power, social or civil service interests, death planning	Normalizing loss and loneliness, aging and frustration; keeping mentally alert and interested, networking with peers, accepting failed plans and disappointments; coping with death, doubts, and fears; appropriate recreation	Margaret Laurence, Mavis Gallant, Charles Dickens, biographies of famous people, Bernard Malamud, Doris Lessing, Morley Torgov, May Sarton

Source: Gold, J. (1988). The value of fiction as a therapeutic recreation and developmental mediator: A theoretical framework. *Journal of Poetry Therapy, 1*(3), 135–147. Reprinted with permission of Plenum Publishing Corporation, New York, New York.

of the times she had stretched out her hands to others. In a few days Hasselstrom called her friend, who was then able to talk about her feelings and reevaluate her life. The story had intervened in a nonthreatening way.

Sometimes a poem may be written as part of a group therapy activity where each person furnishes input into the poem's construction. The result may not be a good poem from a literary viewpoint, but it often exquisitely meets the needs of the group (Hasselstrom, 1990). The self-catharsis takes place in a protective therapeutic manner.

Poems and short stories written by nurses, aides, and victims of abuse and chronic illness may often say very well what the client has not been able to articulate. This author has participated in workshops in which the participants have said, "How can I describe how I feel? I have no words for it." Literature of various kinds can help clients to focus and give voice to their innermost thoughts by furnishing the words.

Stories from literature often contain guidance as well as being a form of diversion and entertainment. Judeo-Christian stories, Christian and Zen parables, and the stories of Hans Christian Anderson are all examples of guidance embedded in stories. These forms are an indirect and nonthreatening means of instruction. "Direct teaching of behavioral laws and principles is often met with resistance" on the part of those being taught "because the message is too direct, too personal, too shocking . . . or too hard to understand" (Barker, 1985, p. vii).

There is a tradition of using literature as therapy within nursing. Travelbee (1971) advised nurses to use parables, metaphors, and personal experiences in a therapeutic use of self. The goal was to assist clients to cope with the illness and to accept their own humanness. Travelbee's basic assumption is that illness is a part of life, and finding meaning in illness or suffering can be a growth experience for both the client and the nurse (Travelbee, 1971). Meleis (1997) summarized two other noteworthy assumptions of Travelbee's theory:

1. Human beings are motivated to search for meaning and understanding in life's experiences.
2. Illness and suffering are not only physical encounters but are emotional and spiritual as well.

Paterson and Zederad's (1988) humanistic nursing model recognized the need for clients to know how other persons experience their own existence. They recognized literature as a realistic source of this information, stating that the commonalities of suffering and other dilemmas of the human condition described in poetry, drama, and fiction surpass textbooks in being concrete and realistic. Younger (1990) thought of literature as a way for nurses to learn compassion.

Moch (1989) expressed the need for the client to "get in touch with the message within illness" (p. 23) in an effort to find what remains of health within the illness. In Moch's plan, treatment would be decided by the client and would include bibliotherapy, journal keeping, meditation, and aesthetic art experiences.

LITERATURE USE WITH THE CHRONICALLY ILL

Reports on the functions of the right brain and left brain have provided some important links between metaphor, client's symptoms, and therapeutic interventions; the left brain is associated with analytic, orderly, and cognitive processing of information (Mills & Crowley, 1986). Barker (1985) stated, "the left brain processes literal, sequential, and logical aspects of language," whereas "metaphor is the language of the *right* cerebral hemisphere . . .. Therapy methods that address the right brain directly—such as the use of stories, . . . metaphor," and "embedded statements . . . seem to produce results more quickly" (p. 21). The right brain is also active in processing emotional information and physical symptomatology (Mills & Crowley, 1986). Right-hemispheric mediation of both client symptomatology and embedded suggestion through metaphors, or stories, allows this type of information to go "straight to the target area, the right-brain processes" (pp. 17–18). Flowers (1988) stated this concept aptly: "We could say that poetry calls the brain cells together, making the image-processing of the right brain collaborate with the word-processing of the left brain, and enticing the mind to dance with the heart and the body" (p. 27).

Metaphor has been variously defined as "a figure of speech that makes an implicit comparison between two unlike entities" (Lankton & Lankton, 1983, p. 78); "a story which means more than it appears to say, and says more than it appears to mean" (McAbee, 1987, p. 2); and "personal experiences or make-believe tales told to illustrate a particular viewpoint, make some concept clear by comparison, or lead someone's thinking toward a particular conclusion" (Laborde, 1984, p. 173).

The therapeutic benefits of storytelling and metaphor have been acknowledged because of the work of psychotherapist Milton Erickson, whose teaching tales and use of metaphors are now well known (Barker, 1985; Mills & Crowley, 1986; Rosen, 1982; Wallas, 1985). The uses of metaphors, imagery, and literature are also found in the family therapy of Minuchin, Satir, and Andolfi (Mazza, 1987).

Schrodes (1949) developed an early model for bibliotherapy as an interaction between the reader and literature in which the "readers see similarities between their own problems and those of characters in literary works" (Cohen, 1989, p. 79). "Schrodes listed the curative elements of bibliotherapy as identification, catharsis and insight" (p. 79) (Fig. 15.1). Yalom (1985) identified therapeutic factors in bibliotherapy similar to those found in group therapy. Cohen recognized a relationship

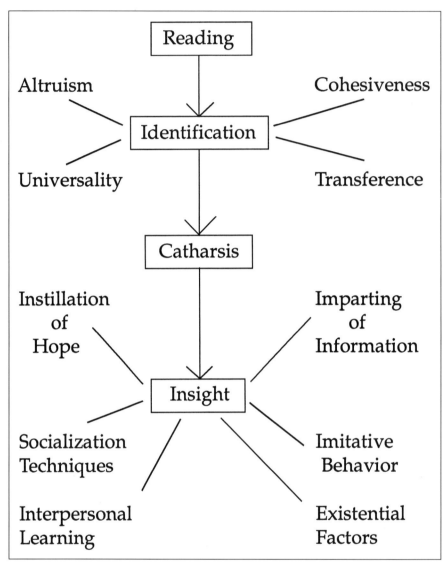

FIGURE 15.1 ➤ Proposed model for healthy pathway of bibliotherapy. (From Cohen, L. J. (1989). Reading as a group process phenomenon: A theoretical framework for bibliotherapy. *Journal of Poetry Therapy, 3*(2), 73–83. Reprinted with permission of Plenum Publishing Corporation, New York, New York.

between Schrodes's curative elements of bibliotherapy and Yalom's therapeutic components of group therapy and merged the two models, as seen in Figure 15.1. Yalom's elements of cure, altruism, universality, cohesiveness, and transference can take place in Schrodes's category called identification. Yalom's group tasks of socialization, instillation of hope, imparting of information, and so forth, fit in with Schrodes's view of the insight one gathers from reading (Cohen, 1989).

EXEMPLARS: LITERATURE IN CLINICAL USE

The author began to use literature as therapy in a variety of areas in 1985. The following poems and incidents illustrate some of the ways in which bibliotherapy can be used for clients and for health-team members.

A small, close-knit community that had never experienced any losses of small children to accident or violent death suddenly experienced the death of two children and a traumatic leg amputation of a third child. These accidents occurred over 3 months in a single summer. Staff members and the physician all grieved. Many of the health-team members were parents of children the same ages as those who died, some of whom had been friends. Throughout the summer, many emergency-room nurses voiced anxiety and verbalized feelings of not wanting to come to work. In nursing reports and in individual sessions the following poem helped several members of the health team.

Sad Summer*

We must have been eight or nine then,
because Jess was twelve, neighbor kid,
an authority on marbles, and other things.
We last saw him in the crowd on the 4th of July
at Bohson Park; he was laughing and excited,
and there was money in his pocket,
because he bought a boat ride and we only watched.

Remember when Dad came home and said
that Jess was dead!
We listened through the screen-door
while he talked to Mom.
Jess had gotten a rifle for his birthday,
climbed the hayloft in the barn to shoot pigeons . . ..
We had to guess the rest.

That night we got into the Model A
and drove over to their farm.
Mom went in and Dad went to the barn . . ..
In a sandy spot by the house, we could tell the place
where Jess always drew the circle,
set his marbles, and aimed his shooter.
Real slow and low you said, "Jess shoulda
stayed with marbles."

Our family sat in the second row,
Too close to the whiteness of the flowers,
and the cold coffin and the dreary sermon.

---

*Carlee Swann (1977), with permission.

That night we pooled our marbles in a shoe-box
and pushed it far back in the dark upstairs closet.
But all the rest of that summer
we saw the pigeons
that had always flown back and forth
from our barn to his.

The universality of experience found in this poem provided comfort to the health team. They were helped to see that they were not isolated. Members of the staff who had lost their enjoyment in coming to work could empathize with the children in the poem who put their marbles away. It was seen as a form of distancing. Health-care workers decided that, metaphorically, they "had been putting their marbles away." Once this was named, it afforded considerable relief. A final metaphor was found in the pigeons, likened to memories, which would continue to fly back and forth all summer between the farms (Hobus, 1987).

This poem changed the internal environment for the health-care workers as their understanding increased; it sensitized the health-team members to each other's anguish, and it encouraged verbalization of feelings.

The following poem exemplifies what an elderly or chronically ill client may be feeling. This is a desirable type of distancing (Lazarus, 1979) in which the client was able to help herself escape when the realities of critical care overpowered her.

Through the Window*

A colorless canopy
Covers the town tonight,
The arms of the elm
are lost in the lingering fog;
The bell in the clock tower
measures its might
By the answering bark
of the dog . . ..

I have passed my limit of
three-score years and ten,
And I hear the nurse as she walks
the sterile hall;
But she doesn't know that I'm sitting
across the street
Swinging my feet against
A wet brick wall.

"Through the Window" was written after its author had been discharged from a regional medical center. In addition to being a form of

---

*Carlee Swann (1978), with permission.

therapy for the client, it instructs and sensitizes the health-care team about the feelings of that client. It is universal.

The next poem, "Darkness," is useful in instructing one about the feelings of an elderly client, awake in the nursing home at night. All that is being asked is relief from loneliness. Imposed powerlessness is implicit. The author has used this poem in a number of workshops to sensitize family and health-care providers to needs of the elderly.

Darkness*

I lay securely positioned
curled up in an unfamiliar bed
in a dark unfamiliar room.
I feel empty, weak, old and alone.
I cannot sleep.
I see the call bell dangling on
the rails that surround my bed.
I push the bell and wait.
And wait.
The light goes on and a white figure
scolds, "What do you want?"
I want to be in my own home again,
surrounded by my own things
and the people I love.

I want to be young and alive again,
to feel and touch and move and create.
I want another day laughing with my friends
or scolding my children, or a walk in the wood,
or an evening by a bright fire.
What do I say?
Touch me. Hold me.
Reach out and reassure me that I am still alive.
Please, just a smile to warm me
so I don't feel so alone.
What do I say?—I say
"I feel cold."
I am covered. The room darkens.
Again I lay alone, imprisoned.

Barker (1985) reviewed clinical uses of anecdotes and stories. They can make or illustrate a point, suggest solutions to problems, help people recognize themselves, seed ideas, reframe or redefine a problem, model a way of communicating, embed directions in a pleasant manner, help to build egos, decrease resistance, allay fear, or remind people of their own resources. The following poem does several of these, depending on whose point of view is taken when reading it.

---

*L. S. Pike (1979), with permission.

What Have You Done to My Mother?*

How often these words are directed to me.
As they search for the "Mother" that used to be.
"Have you given her drugs or spoken unkindly?"
"I brought her some cookies, she stared at me. Blindly—"
"Not seeing the daughter who loves her dearly."
"She seems not to care that I've come all this way."
"What's wrong with this place, anyway?" . . .
"She strikes out in anger and curses my name."
"I know she can't mean it—it hurts just the same!" . . .
"But, if I leave now, will she be here tomorrow?"
Call it pain or grief—call it guilt or fear.
It sounds the same when it reaches my ear.
It's love, pure and simple, needs no explanation—
Will it be the same in the next generation?
"What have you done to my mother," they say.
"She's not the same person I left yesterday!"

The author, a nurse at the time this was written, gives voice to the universal phenomenon of parental decline and the pain that it brings to adult children. Many adult children have seen themselves in this poem.

Literature can help to name an experience so that one can consciously think about it and discuss it (Kissman, 1989). Naming the experience also implies the universality of the experience so that one no longer feels alone against overwhelming loss. Literature can be a way of knowing, informing, and finding oneself (Pies, 1988), as associations are made with the central story characters or with the voice of the poet.

"In time of loss, it is important to see what remains in our lives" (Woodard, 1987). Woodard (1990) illustrated the efficacy of literature in understanding overwhelming loss with a personal experience. A very close friend of his died suddenly without warning, leaving a wife and small child. Woodard was asked to go to his friend's city and arrange for the memorial service.

In the days that followed, alone with his deep grief, Woodard found that he was angry at people around him for no apparent reason. This vague, unsettling anger followed him everywhere he went. He was perplexed and unhappy with himself for feeling this way. Surely he had expected grief, but why this vague anger, always ready to surface?

Then, out of his literary background came the scene from *King Lear,* in which the old king holds his beautiful, dead youngest daughter in his arms. Woodard recalled these words from the king at that terrible moment: "Why should a dog, a horse, a rat, have life, and thou no breath at all? Thou'lt come no more. Never, never, never, never, never!" (Shakespeare, *King Lear*).

---

*L. G. Davey (1983), with permission.

Anger and frustration are often seen in the face of untimely death. When he remembered the scene from *King Lear,* Woodard stated that it comforted him. He realized that his grief reaction was universal. Remembering this scene from the play empowered him by giving permission for and understanding of the anger; it clarified his problem; it provided a rationale for understanding the anger; it gave him words with which to verbalize the pain.

A second example of the rage that one feels in the loss of a loved one is eloquently expressed in the words of Dylan Thomas (1957) at the death of his father*:

Do not go gentle into that good night,
Old age should burn and rave at close of day;
Rage, rage against the dying of the light.

Though wise men at their end know dark is right . . ..

And you, my father, there on the sad height,
Curse, bless me now with your fierce tears, I pray.
Do not go gentle into that good night.
Rage, rage against the dying of the light.

Death is the prototype of all injustices (May, 1975). Many clients and their families need permission or the words to voice rage, even if the death was of a parent whose timely end was to be expected. There is also rage in the permanent loss of abilities, as in chronic illness. To the extent that there is sufficient rapport between the client, or family, and the nurse, the poem may be comforting.

For those who enjoy classic literature, *King Lear* has other applicable themes for therapy. Some of them include pessimism, evil, failure as a king, feelings of failure as a father, and the "incompatibility between rational man and an absurd universe" (Trilling, 1967, p. 129). These qualities continue to make it a favorite.

Adolescents often face losses that forever change their world. Poetry therapy and interactive bibliotherapy for adolescents were reported by Cohen-Morales (1989), Mazza (1981), and Morris-Vann (1983). This therapy covers a wide range of conditions. Chronic disability, spinal cord injury, incest, and deaths of loved ones are several of the topics that have been discussed in the literature.

A therapeutic result of poetry writing is naming the pain when the client is ready, thus setting the stage for discovering meaning in the experience (Bardarah-McCandless, 1989). Control is in the hands of the writer. "Poetic imagery may perform a distancing function without denying the existence of the problem" (p. 148).

---

*by Dylan Thomas, from THE POEMS OF DYLAN THOMAS. Copyright © 1952 by Dylan Thomas. Reprinted by permission of New Directions Publishing Corp.

Finally, as the client moves into integration of the experience, there is an accepting of "previously forbidden feelings . . . such as rage, loneliness, . . . fear" and a reinterpretation of the earlier situation in the light of new understanding (Bardarah-McCandless, p. 149). The following poem expresses some of the rage and pain felt by a young man who lost his father to cancer.

A Farmer Dying*

What is there of justice, Father,
in the 57 years of droughts and blizzards
you have coughed up onto my bedroom floor?
What is left for me at 16
when you have told me
there is no room for God
in malignant tumors,
that a heart attack
would have been prettier
and much more quiet?
Can you see better than I
In this candle-lit darkness?
I ask you this, Father,
before I go
to my Hail Marys.

Norris (1987) wrote that younger children reveal the truth through their poetry and that you can discover events that are taking place in the children's lives, some of their longings and their fears. Norris described working as a poet-in-residence in a classroom. A poem, "My Very First Dad," by one of the young students described the father in glowing terms, "like God in my heart." In fact, the father had abandoned the child and the mother on the day the child was born. "The poem revealed, as perhaps nothing else could, that the child was carrying a load of pain" (Norris, 1990, p. 2). Norris states that this is typical of the "self-healing children engage in. It told the truth about the burden the child was carrying within and confronted the adults with a cry for help" (Norris, 1990, p. 2). Through poetry therapy, the child was able to name a pain that no one had suspected. Gorelick and Monser (1988), Kramer (1987), and Leedy (1985) are among those in support of poetry therapy as a therapeutic intervention for children.

Norris spoke of listening attentively to children and suggested that "listening sometimes requires a leap of the imagination. Sometimes the truth of what a child is saying is so unpleasant that our instinct is to deny it" (Norris, 1990, p. 3). The following prose poem illustrates Norris's own catharsis of a troubling event concerning a child.

---

*Kevin Woster (1978), with permission.

Saturday Afternoon at the Library*

I let him climb on my lap
Because he wanted to be held
by a woman;
he'd lost three already
by the age of five.
His mother in a wreck
when he was a baby
then his grandmother
who'd taken care of him;
and then
just last week
the stepmother, young,
with a baby of her own.
She was a sweet thing
who read self-help books;
Norman Vincent Peale,
How To Be Your Own Best Friend.
His dad beat her
and was drinking up
most of their money . . ..

What does the boy understand
of this? He knows
that she and the baby were gone
one day, when he and his dad came back from town.

He holds me tightly and says:
"I'm going to kill you.
"I'll shoot you
and cut you up in little pieces
and keep you in my refrigerator."
I look at him and say
"Don't put me there,
I'll be too cold."
He says: "I'll keep you
in my closet then."
I say: "Closets are too dark."
He giggles, slides down and away,
out the door.

And the boy just wanted
to be held close
to soft woman flesh
and loved. That was all he wanted.

Norris (1990) said of this incident, ". . . they were the words he
needed to say and someone needed to hear them" (p. 4). Norris spoke of

---

*Kathleen Norris (1988), with permission of the author.

sharing anecdotes and personal stories, as suggested by Travelbee. A child who grieved over being abandoned by the father was helped with an account of poet Diane Wakoski's similar experience and her subsequent choice of George Washington as her symbolic father. A child who grieved over a family suicide gained solace from hearing Norris share a similar family experience (Norris, 1990).

Smith (1989) compiled an excellent annotated bibliography of reading resources for children regarding death and grieving. Gold (1988) reported on the value of fiction as a mediator of the developmental life stages. The prescriptive reading suggestions for the various developmental states may be found in Table 15.1 (Gold, 1988).

Successful use of stories, anecdotes, and metaphors in clinical practice have been documented by Barker (1985), Larkin and Zahourek (1988), Mills and Crowley (1986), and Rosen (1982). Rosen (1982) identified advantages for using anecdotes and stories in client communication:

1. Anecdotes are interesting, hold attention, and "tag memory."
2. Anecdotes are nonthreatening and are told in the third person.
3. Stories and anecdotes bypass natural resistance to change because they are only a story.
4. Control over what is heard is in the ear of the client. One will hear only what the psyche will allow it to pick up.

METAPHORS AND STORYTELLING

Bornstein (1988) and Larkin and Zahourek (1988) pointed out that metaphors and stories are easily incorporated into many areas of nursing practice. The authors give a negative example of this in the horror stories clients hear from friends and relatives, including stories pregnant women hear. Positive stories, of course, are more therapeutic and can help to instill positive expectations of the treatment outcome (Larin & Zahourek, 1988). The authors pointed out that the phrase "I had a patient once . . ." is similar to "Once upon a time . . ." and sets the stage to illustrate how the healing process occurs or how someone will be encouraged.

Larkin and Zahourek (1988) also reported that indirect healing suggestions may be used in a number of acute care settings. "Waking suggestibility," according to the authors, is a time when the client is comfortable after medication for pain relief and is a prime time for the introduction of indirect metaphoric suggestion. Morgan (1988) suggested doing this in a very offhand way, almost as an afterthought. One lead-in is "I remember a patient who . . ." This is also the ideal time to intersperse needed information and embedded suggestions with the story.

Larkin and Zahourek (1988) related their use of therapeutic story-telling and of metaphors in pediatric clinical practice. A case study is presented of a 9-year-old boy with leukemia who was dying in a pediatric intensive-care unit. He was in much pain and afraid of approaching death. Larkin told him the story of "another boy who learned to go inside his mind and find a special big tree with a hidden opening . . . . So he went into the opening and found the warm, comforting home of a friendly chipmunk. It felt really peaceful there" (p. 50). Messages of "feeling comfort, feeling better and sitting by the fireside, talking to your friend" (p. 50) were interspersed throughout the story as embedded suggestion. The boy was encouraged to go within this sanctuary whenever the pain was too intense or he needed comfort. The child was able to die with little apparent distress (Larkin & Zahourek, 1988).

Mutual storytelling is also a strategy to keep the mind occupied when painful debridement and change of burn dressings must be done (Larkin & Zahourek, 1988). A story of a giraffe with purple spots was used to help a child explore the idea that her scars would make her somewhat different from other children when she was discharged from the hospital (Larkin & Zahourek, 1988).

"The most important requirement for an effective metaphor is that it meet the client at his model of the world . . . .. The metaphor preserves the structure of the client's problematic situation" (Gordon, 1978, p. 171). Metaphors can be derived from any acceptable source, including folklore, biblical tales, mythology, Mother Goose, or one's own personal experiences.

JOURNAL WRITING

Writing in a journal is another means of validating self, testing ideas, ventilating feelings, or expressing pain in privacy. "The journal becomes a therapy tool where a person's own emotions can be voiced without fear" (Hasselstrom, 1987).

Advantages in journal writing as a therapy form are:

1. A journal is liberating.
2. A journal can be a best friend and confidante.
3. A journal builds esteem as one later looks back and identifies solutions and power to cope with past problems (Hasselstrom, 1990).

There are people who have great difficulty expressing their deepest and most troublesome or even therapeutic thoughts in a group. If these clients have any interest in writing, prescriptive bibliography may include journal writing, which they may or may not discuss with a therapist. The client may never read it. The point of therapy is to gather thoughts and clarify and dispose of the painful emotions. Occasionally a prescriptive therapy may include assigning the client to read literature and to record his or her reactions in a journal (Aleksychik, 1989).

A clinical application of journal writing from the author's practice concerns a young male client who had just graduated from high school and was in a tragic motorcycle accident with a truck. He remembered nothing of the first weeks after the accident, but the young man's mother started a journal recounting his struggle to survive. After he was able to return to his home, with surgeries and rehabilitation still ahead of him, he began to keep the journal for himself.

Several years have passed, and the young man has enrolled in college, with some residual injuries. "When I have a bad week, I read the journal. The issues then were would I ever be continent? Would I walk? Reading the journal shows me how far I have come. It becomes a good attitude adjustment" (personal communication, 1990).

The young man had been a football player in high school and also had a close relationship with his family, especially his father. During the 2 years of convalescence and rehabilitation, the following poem by David Allan Evans helped to sustain him.

The Touchdown in Slow Motion*

. . . Here I go
    in the shape
of my father's hope
    on a 30 sweep right
ranging out cutting
    now turning it on
turning the corner
    to give up turf and
snatch what I need to be nifty
    with a last fake
in a farewell wave of my hand

Stretching out
    I find my light
and a way to move
    in the green world.

There was sustaining power in thinking about issues of rehabilitation as a different kind of football game. It implied to the client the need to give the strenuous rehabilitation routine as much dedication as had gone into football. This game was even more important. A final empowering image was the idea that he would walk again, "in the shape of his father's hope," a love that was there to sustain him just as it had been in his football victories.

---

*David Allan Evans (1974), with permission.

This anecdote illustrates that, as an outcome, the young man has grown spiritually and found meaning in his illness as Travelbee suggests. It also supports Hasselstrom's observation (1990) that confidence and empowerment are gained as the client looks back into the journal and can finally see the almost imperceptible gains.

The lines, "Here I go/in the shape/of my father's hope" are an applicable introduction of hope for victims of any number of conditions. Many clients who suffer chronic illness persevere in treatment largely because of their loved ones' enabling hope.

HEALING OF WAR VETERANS

Veterans often have special needs in therapeutic literature. In addition to the chronic illness or injury that is the focus of their medical treatment, the spiritual component may include a load of guilt and pain from service-related incidents, unresolved conflicts, and survivor guilt.

Most veterans no longer talk about their experiences because the general perception is that no one is interested. Nurses are poorly prepared to discuss these issues with clients who are veterans. A good strategy is to enroll in a course in war literature within a college humanities department. This will allow the caregiver to discover some of the issues in a relatively pain-free environment as Younger (1990) previously suggested.

In choosing literature for the veteran who is still dealing with service-connected spiritual and emotional conflicts, poems of Wilfred Owen and carefully chosen poems of Walt Whitman, such as "The Wound-Dresser," may be useful. Anthologies of war literature and poetry are available.

The veterans of the Vietnam era have special problems that have been addressed under posttraumatic stress disorder in *Military Medicine* and the nursing journals. Significant works of prose about the Vietnam experience include: *Going After Cacciato* (O'Brien), *In Country* (Mason), *Dispatches* (Herr), *Meditations in Green* (Wright), and *Short Timers (Full Metal Jacket)* (Hasford). "Each truthfully reveals important aspects of the Vietnam experience while maintaining its integrity as an achieved work of art" (Stewart, 1988, p. 123). Others of interest are: *American Experiences in Viet Nam: A Reader* (Sevy, 1989) and *Carrying the Darkness: American Indochina Poetry of the Vietnam War* (Erhardt, 1985).

Stewart (1989) suggested the potential of story making as a means of coming to terms with war experiences. The obvious therapeutic nursing intervention is to encourage the veteran to write his own story, even if it is never shared with others. Others who are willing to preserve their story for family and friends might find it a source of empowerment. Reminiscences may be recorded as an oral history.

ENHANCING SELF-ESTEEM AND ENABLING HOPE

Literature can aid survival by creating good feelings and enhancing self-esteem (Evans, 1990). Self-esteem is necessary for hopefulness and for empowerment. Evans believed that there is an example of enhancement of self-esteem in this poem by Emily Dickinson.

It Dropped So Low in My Regard*

It dropped so low-in my Regard—
I heard it hit the Ground—
And go to pieces on the Stones
At the bottom of my Mind—

Yet blamed the Fate that fractured—less
Than I reviled Myself
For entertaining Plated Wares
Upon my Silver Shelf—

There is a convincing imagery, a metaphoric example of someone else's values or opinions that are "silver-plated wares" compared with the "silver shelf" of the author's own insight and understanding (Evans, 1990). "The poem says, give yourself credit; trust yourself; what else can you do but trust yourself" (p. 2).

This poem can also serve as a warning to nurses who might think of this poem as paralleling the readiness of a client to adopt a new health style. To the extent that the client may not be convinced of the value of the new information, the health teaching may drop so low in the client's judgment that it does "go to pieces . . . at the bottom" of the hearer's mind.

Sometimes it is comforting to "know the problems can't be completely solved, you just have to do the best that you can" (Evans, 1987). There is a Zen parable about a man who drops over a cliff while trying to escape a tiger and clings tightly to a vine. But there is another tiger below him, snapping and snarling. "All he can do, then, is with his free hand pluck a strawberry on that same vine and eat it, and enjoy its sweetness! To be an adult is to realize that some problems and dilemmas simply cannot be 'worked out.' You might as well make the most of what you have left in life" (Evans, 1990, p. 3). This metaphorically restates Moch's concept; find any elements of health left within the illness.

Connectedness is important in establishing hope. Poetry and literature deal with connectedness of family and friends. "Bess," by William Stafford, may bring courage to family members grieving over the loss of

---

a mother. "Bess would have no meaning without her relationships with others. She is defined by those relationships" (Evans, 1990, p. 2).

Bess*

Ours are the streets where Bess first met her
cancer. She went to work every day past the
secure houses. At her job in the library,
she arranged better and better flowers, and when
students asked for books her hand went out for help.
In the last year of her life
she had to keep her friends from knowing
how happy they were. She listened while they
complained about food or work or the weather . . ..

Pain moved where she moved. She walked
ahead; it came. She hid; it found her . . ..
It was almost as if there was no room
left for her on earth. But she remembered
where joy used to live. She straightened its flowers;
she did not weep when she passed its houses . . ..

Another poem about connections is "A Flat One," by W. D. Snodgrass (1968) about an old man in a veterans' hospital who wasted away to nothing and then died. The voice is that of the male aide who attended the veteran. He "felt the old man's energy, learns from him, responds to him, even if he thinks there is no hope for his surviving" (Evans, 1990, p. 4).

A final and important source of empowerment and hope for many people is found in the words and music of hymns or readings from the bible; many reassuring portions can be read to satisfy varied needs such as love, hope, and self-worth.

Hansen (1990) stated, "Those who have suffered utterly devastating losses might find themselves tempted (or encouraged by others) to read the story of Job, whose life seems to be a case study in unrelenting disaster" (p. 1). Far from providing easy answers, the story of Job shows us how false and how "wrong" easy answers can be (Hansen, 1990). "Job lost his wealth, his life's work and his children. His wife told him to curse God and die. His friends suggested to him that he was being punished for his sins. He rejected that notion, but finally demanded an explanation from God" (Hansen, 1987, p. 2).

The story can teach compassion. Job suffered through no fault of his own, as many clients in today's world suffer. Job did eventually have his fortune and children restored to him—a happy ending that can be misleading. "This is the popular view of the story of Job—that it is inspiring

---

*"Bess" copyright 1970, 1998 by the Estate of William Stafford. Reprinted from *The Way It Is: New & Selected Poems* by William Stafford with the permission of Graywolf Press, Saint Paul, Minnesota.

because it gives hope to the hopeless. But we all know that goodness is rarely rewarded in the here and now. People suffer and don't know why, and unlike Job they are unlikely to get the kind of clear and unequivocal answer God gave to Job" (Hansen, 1990, p. 4).

The role of literature in the healing arts, as stated by Hansen (1990), is not to give comfort by falsifying, even if there is much to be said for positive thinking. "The role of literature in healing is to get the feelings out in the open, to articulate painful emotions we too often can't put into words. It admits that our sorrow is sometimes inconsolable, that our problems are sometimes unsolvable . . .. Even when it does this, it shows us that we are not alone—that others have been there before us and have found ways of living with what they could not change" (p. 4).

CLINICAL SYNOPSIS

Mr. B. was admitted to acute care after a 2-year battle with leukemia. He had been under the care of an oncologist and a surgeon. A splenectomy had been done 1 year previously, after which he had gone back to managing his business. He had several admissions to the hospital for complications of immunosuppression, pneumonia that would not clear, weakness, and fatigue. His white blood cell count was extremely low. With this admission he was placed in protective isolation.

For some time his primary physician had wanted him to transfer to a large university medical center for consultation and advanced care. Medical team members were convinced that he needed technologies available in a designated cancer treatment center. Mr. B. refused to go, telling the physician that he had unlimited faith in him. Mr. B. had not drawn up a will in the 2 years of illness and was currently talking of expanding his business. The team helplessly watched Mr. B.'s symptoms of lung involvement heighten and his blood studies deteriorate.

The author started a program of bibliotherapy and guided reading to suggest to Mr. B. that he really needed to set his affairs in order. Mr. B. was bored with the protective isolation and could not find enough to read or do. The author's first step, as primary nurse, was to spend as much time with him as possible, to build rapport with the client, who could receive few visitors in isolation. Mr. B.'s interests were assessed. He liked a certain cowboy humorist of national renown.

The author brought Mr. B. cassette tapes of those books. The next step was to bring humorous poems by the same author and regional poetry about the Midwest. The visits were continued whenever possible, allowing the client to vent his frustrations concerning his continued and worsening symptoms of pneumonia. He was not emotionally ready to hear the interspersed suggestions that we wished for him to go out for highly advanced care. He could not "hear" us. Over the next few days his reading was guided from purely recreational to regional literature, then to occasional stories or poems about men who had retired or had left their land, all from regional authors. On the fifth day, as the author stopped for the daily visit, the client looked up and said, "These stories are taking a strange twist. Are you trying to tell me something?" He had understood the stories intuitively, and with his psychological and spiritual battle behind him, that of denial, he was now ready to make arrangements for his physical care. He put his affairs in order that afternoon and sought care the next day.

CONCLUSION

As with any nursing intervention, the first step in using bibliotherapy or transitional reading is to establish rapport with the client and the family. Determine the reading interests and the reading skills of the client through a progression of short stories or poems. How receptive is the client to guided reading? A comment like, "I just happen to have a story about . . . at home," will give you valuable clues to this receptivity. Think of your own bookshelves as storerooms of untapped creative energy for your client (Cohen, 1988). Save, clip, and collect for future use. Some general guidelines about literature include (Cohen, 1988):

1. The readings should be enjoyable.
2. Short excerpts are effective. The whole book is not necessary.
3. Never force a book on a client.
4. Select literature that reflects as closely as possible the situation the client is facing. First-person accounts of similar experiences are helpful to some clients.
5. Know the literature you recommend. The client could be offended by alternative values.
6. Make friends with a research librarian and ask about book lists by topic, such as aging, life transitions, or loss.
7. Consult therapy resource lists such as "Poetic Resources" found in the *Journal of Poetry Therapy.*

A list of prescriptive readings is included at the end of this chapter for use with clients at varied ages and stages of health and illness.

REFERENCES

Aleksychik, A. (1989). Bibliotherapy: An effective principal and supplementary method of healing, correcting and administering relief. *Journal of Poetry Therapy, 3*(1), 19–21.

Bardarah-McCandless, J. (1989). Agony, a womb of poetry. *Journal of Poetry Therapy, 2*(3), 145–154.

Barker, P. (1985). *Using metaphors in psychotherapy.* New York: Brunner/Mazel.

Berger, A. (1988). Working through grief by poetry writing. *Journal of Poetry Therapy, 2*(1), 11–19.

Bornstein, E. (1988). Therapeutic storytelling. In R. Zahourek (Ed.), *Relaxation and Imagery: Tools for therapeutic communication and intervention* (pp. 101–118). Philadelphia: WB Saunders.

Chavis, G. G. (1988). Poetic resources. *Journal of Poetry Therapy, 1*(4), 232.

Clements, D. B. (1986). Reminiscence: A tool for aiding families under stress. *Maternal Child Nursing, 11,* 114–117.

Cohen, L. J. (1988). Bibliotherapy: The right book at the right time. *Journal of Psychosocial Nursing and Mental Health, 26*(8), 7–12.

Cohen, L. J. (1989). Reading as a group process phenomenon: A theoretical framework for bibliotherapy. *Journal of Poetry Therapy, 3*(2), 73–83.

Cohen-Morales, P. J. (1989). Poetry as a therapeutic tool within a group adolescent setting. *Journal of Poetry Therapy, 2*(3), 155–160.

Davey, L. G. (1983). What have you done to my mother? *Journal of Gerontological Nursing, 9*(2), 133.

Dickinson, E. (1983). It dropped so low in my regard. In T. H. Johnson (Ed.), *The poems of Emily Dickinson.* Cambridge, MA: The Belknap Press of Harvard University Press.

Erhardt, W. D. (1985). *Carrying the darkness: American Indochina poetry of the Vietnam War.* New York: Avon.

Evans, D. A. (1974). The touchdown in slow motion. *Train windows* (p. 35). Athens: Ohio University Press.

Evans, D. A. (1987, November). *The use of literature in healing.* Address presented at Humanities in the Healing Arts Dialogue #2, Sioux Falls, SD.

Evans, D. A. (1990). *Notes on nursing and literature.* Unpublished manuscript. Brookings: South Dakota State University.

Flowers, B. S. (1988). Poetry, healing and making whole. *Journal of Poetry Therapy, 2*(1), 25–31.

Fox, M. (1983). *Original blessing* (p. 85). Santa Fe, NM: Bear.

Gold, J. (1988). The value of fiction as a therapeutic recreation and developmental mediator: A theoretical framework. *Journal of Poetry Therapy, 1*(3), 135–147.

Gordon, D. (1978). *Therapeutic metaphors* (p. 19). Cupertino, CA: Meta Publications.

Gorelick, K. (1987). Greek tragedy and ancient healing: Poems as theater and Asclepian temple in miniature. *Journal of Poetry Therapy, 2*(1), 41–45.

Gorelick, K., & Monser, R. (1988). Consultation corner. *Journal of Poetry Therapy, 2*(1), 41–45.

Hansen, A. T. (1987, September). *Literature pertaining to parenting, home and family, and the story of Job.* Address presented at Humanities in the Healing Arts, Dialogue #1, Aberdeen, SD.

Hansen, A. T. (1990). *The story of Job and the use of literature in the healing arts.* Unpublished manuscript, Aberdeen, SD: Northern State University.

Hasselstrom, L. (1987, November). *Writing in a journal: How to turn blank pages into your private physician, personal psychiatrist and best friend.* Address presented at Humanities in the Healing Arts, Dialogue #3, Pierre, SD.

Hasselstrom, L. (1990). *Using journals as therapy.* Unpublished manuscript.

Hobus, R. M. (1987). *A professional framework for the application of literature in nursing.* Address presented at Humanities in the Healing Arts, Dialogue #1, Aberdeen, SD, and Dialogue #2, Sioux Falls, SD.

Hobus, R. M., Hansen, A. T., Evans, D. A., & Woodard, C. L. (1987). *Humanities in the healing arts.* A dialogue series. South Dakota Committee on the Humanities, Box 7050, University Station, Brookings, SD 57007.

Jaskoski, H. (1987). Artesan or genius: Two views of poetic process. *Journal of Poetry Therapy, 1*(1), 5–13.

Kissman, K. (1989). Poetry and feminist social work. *Journal of Poetry Therapy, 2*(4), 221–230.

Kramer, A. (1987). Poetry as a key to unlocking self. *Journal of Poetry Therapy, 1*(2), 77–87.

Laborde, G. L. (1984). *Influencing with integrity.* Palo Alto, CA: Science and Behavior Books.

Lankton, S. R., & Lankton, C. H. (1983). *The answer within.* New York: Brunner/ Mazel.

Larkin, D. M., & Zahourek, R. P. (1988). Therapeutic storytelling and metaphors. *Holistic Nursing Practice, 2,* 45–53.

Lazarus, R. S. (1979). Positive denial: The case for not facing reality. *Psychology Today, 13*(4), 44–45, 47–48, 51–52, 57, 60.

Leedy, J. J. (1985). *Poetry as healer: Mending the troubled mind.* New York: Vangard Press.

May, R. (1975). *The courage to create* (p. 29). New York: Bantam.

Mazza, N. (1981). The use of poetry in treating the troubled adolescent. *Adolescence, 62*(3), 403–407.

Mazza, N. (1987). Editor's note. *Journal of Poetry Therapy, 1*(2), 65.

Mazza, N. (1988). Poetry and technical proficiency in brief therapy: Bridging arts and science. *Journal of Poetry Therapy, 2*(1), 3–10.

McAbee, P. (Ed.). (1987, Fall). *Brochure on the magic of metaphor.* (Available from the Philadelphia Training Institute for Neuro-Linguistic Programming, 569 North Main St., Doylestown, PA 18901.)

Meleis, A. I. (1997). *Theoretical nursing: Development and progress* (3rd ed., pp. 254–263). Philadelphia: JB Lippincott.

Miller, V. (1985). *Despite this flesh: The disabled in stories and poems.* Austin: University of Texas Press.

Mills, J., & Crowley, R. (1986). *Therapeutic metaphors for children and the child within.* New York: Brunner/Mazel.

Moch, S. D. (1989). Health within illness: Conceptual evolution and practice possibilities. *Advances in Nursing Science, 11*(4), 23–31.

Morgan, L. B. (1988). Metaphoric communication and psychotherapeutic process. *Journal of Poetry Therapy, 1*(3), 169–181.

Morris-Vann, A. M. (1983). The efficacy of bibliotherapy on the mental health of elementary students who have experienced loss. *Dissertation Abstracts International,* 44, 676A. (University Microfilms No. 83-15616)

Nagai-Jacobsen, M. G., & Burkhardt, M. A. (1989). Spirituality: Cornerstone of nursing practice. *Holistic Nursing Practice, 3*(3), 18–26.

Norris, K. (1987, September). Poetry therapy in classroom and acute care settings. Address to Humanities in the Healing Arts, Dialogue #1, Aberdeen, SD.

Norris, K. (1988). Saturday afternoon at the library. *The Year of Common Things* (pp. 2–3). Denver: Wayland Press.

Norris, K. (1990). Healing in the classroom: A memoir. Unpublished manuscript.

Paterson, J., & Zederad, I. (1988). *Humanistic Nursing.* New York: John Wiley & Sons.

Pies, L. S. (1988). The poet and the therapist. *Journal of Poetry Therapy, 2*(2), 84–88.

Pike, L. S. (1979). Darkness. *Journal of Gerontological Nursing, 5*(2), 46.

Rosen, S. (1982). *My voice will go with you: The teaching tales of Milton H. Erickson.* New York: WW Norton.

Schrodes, C. (1949). Bibliotherapy: A theoretical and clinical experimental study. Unpublished doctoral dissertation. University of California, Berkeley.

Schunior, C. (1989). Nursing and the comic mask. *Holistic Nursing Practice, 3*(3), 7–17.

Sevy, G. (1989). *American experiences in Vietnam: A reader.* Norman: University of Oklahoma Press.

Shakespeare, W. (1605). *King Lear,* Act V, Scene 3, Lines 307–309.

Smith, A. C. (1989). Reading guidance: Death and grief. *Journal of Poetry Therapy, 3*(1), 23–28.

Snodgrass, W. D. (1968). The flat one. *After experience.* New York: Harper & Row.

Stafford, W. (1977). Bess. *The Way It Is: New & Selected Poems.* St. Paul: Graywolf Press.

Stewart, M. D. (1989). Making sense out of chaos: Prose writing, fictional kind and the reality of Vietnam. *Dissertation Abstracts International.* (University Microfilms No. DA 8908032)

Swann, C. (1977). Sad Summer. *Wanna go to Sally's?* Aberdeen, SD: North Plains Press.

Swann, C. (1978). Through the window. *Pasque Petals, 52.* Sioux Falls: South Dakota State Poetry Society.

Thomas, D. (1957). Do not go gentle into that good night. *The collected poems of Dylan Thomas* (p. 128). New York: New Directions.

Tournier, P. (1965). *The healing of persons* (pp. 6–61). San Francisco, Harper & Row.

Travelbee, J. (1971). *Interpersonal aspects of nursing* (2nd ed.). Philadelphia: F. A. Davis.

Trilling, P. (1967). *The experience of literature* (pp. 124–132). New York: Holt, Rinehart, & Winston.

Yalom, E. D. (1985). *The theory and practice of group therapy* (3rd ed.). New York: Basic Books.

Younger, J. B. (1990). Literary works as a mode of knowing. *IMAGE—Journal of Nursing Scholarship, 22*(1), 39–42.

Wallas, L. (1985). *Stories for the third ear.* New York: WW Norton.

Woodard, C. L. (1987). *The power of literature in healing.* Address presented at Humanities in the Healing Arts, Dialogue #1, Aberdeen, SD.

Woodard, C. L. (1990, March). *Spirituality in literature.* Address to the United Campus Ministries, Brookings, SD.

Woster, K. (1978). A farmer dying. *Oakwood, 4,* 17. Brookings: South Dakota State University.

Appendix: Prescriptive Reading Suggestions Edited by Ruth Hobus

1. *Death of a Loved One, Incapacitation, and Aging*

Chekov, Anton	"A Lament" (story on the loss of a son)
Dickinson, Emily	"Apparently, with No Surprise"
Dickey, James	"The Hospital Window" (about dying father)
Hughes, Langston	"Dreams" (Hold fast to dreams)
Ignatow, David	"Sunday at the State Hospital"
Masters, Edgar Lee	"Fiddler Jones"
	"The Hill"
Stafford, William	"Bess"
	"At the Grave of My Brother"
Swann, Carlee	"A Sad Summer"
Thomas, Dylan	"Do Not Go Gentle into That Good Night"
Williams, William Carlos	"The Last Words of My English Grandmother"
Woster, Kevin	"A Farmer Dying"

2. *The Need for Peace, Self-Contentment*

Berry, Wendell	"The Peace of Wild Things"
Frost, Robert	"The Pasture"
	"The Road Not Taken"
Jeffers, Robinson	"To the Stone Cutters"
Masters, Edgar Lee	"Albert Schirding" (go for the simple things)
	"Paul McNeeley" (about a nurse who gave peace to a dying man)
King James Bible	Psalm 23

3. *Birth of A Handicapped Child*
Miller, Vassar (Ed.)

Despite This Flesh (an anthology of the handicapped) Some of the selections include:

Williams, Miller
"The Ones That Are Thrown Out"

Tyler, Anne
"Average Waves in Unprotected Waters"

Jacobsen, Josephine
"The Glen"

4. *Child's Awareness of Death*
Conrad, Pam
My Daniel (a book about death of a brother)

Donnelly, Elfie
So Long Grandpa (death of a grandparent)

Woolverton, Linda
Running before the Wind (death of an abusive father)

Zindel, Bonnie
A Star for the Latecomer (mother died of cancer)

5. *Death of A Child*
Aiken, Conrad
"All Lovely Things"
Dickey, James
"The Lifeguard"
Field, Eugene
"Little Boy Blue" (widely anthologized)

Frost, Robert
"Home Burial" (widely anthologized)

6. *Midlife and Marital Discord*
Justice, Donald
"Men at Forty"
Ciardi, John
"Suburban Homecoming"
Lyell, Ruth
Middle Age, Old Age (short stories, poems, and plays on aging)

Mueller, Lisel
"A Voice in the Dark"
Plath, Sylvia
"Mirror" (aging)
Snodgrass, W. D.
"Heart's Needle" (divorce)
7. *Journals*
Thoreau, Henry David
Journal
Sarton, May
Journal of a Solitude
Simons, G. F.
Keeping Your Personal Journal

West, Celeste
Words in Our Pockets

8. *Selected Books*

Bly, Carol (1985). *Backbone*. Minneapolis: Milkweed Editions. (Short stories, one about a woman who ran away from a nursing home.)

Daniels, Kate (1984). *The White Wave*. Pittsburgh: University of Pittsburgh Press. (Poems about a children's ward and other family relationships.)

Dwyer, David (1976). *Ariana Olisvos: Her Last Works and Days*. Amherst: University of Massachusetts Press. (Many poems are about cancer.)

Gold, Joseph (1990). *Read for Your Life*. Ontario, Canada: Fitzhenry & Whiteside. (Sometimes humorous poems and readings through the developmental cycle.)

Hasselstrom, Linda (1987). *Roadkill*. Spoon River Poetry Press. Peoria, IL. (Poems about life. Concludes with "Hannah: Dying In a Hospital.")

Lloyd, Roseanne (1985). *Tapdancing for Big Mom*. Minneapolis: New Rivers Press. (Many poems about incest and how it haunts survivors.)

Norris, Kathleen (1981). *The Middle of the World*. Pittsburgh: University of Pittsburgh Press. (Miscellany of poems; includes "At Killian's Grave" about the death of a child.)

Norris, Kathleen (1988). *The Year of Common Things*. Wayland Press: Denver. (Memorable poems about family, love, abuse and answered prayers.)

Olds, Sharon (1983). *The Dead and the Living*. New York: Knopf. (Honest poems about child abuse and how it affects a family.)

Woodard, Charles (1989). *As Far As I Can See*. Windflower Press, Lincoln, NE. (Inspiring anthology of memories, home, legacy, and loss.)

Zweig, Paul (1985). *Eternity's Woods*. Middletown, CT: Wesleyan University Press. (Thoughtful volume; last poems of a poet with cancer.)

16

Imagery as a Means of Coping

➤ REBECCA STEPHENS

Imagery is a nursing strategy that facilitates client coping and positive responses to altered health states. The review of imagery contained in this chapter is relevant for the practitioner who believes that attitudes, beliefs, and reactions to life experiences influence whether persons get sick and how quickly they recover.

Imagery is a strategy that can enhance behavioral, cognitive, and decisional control. Different types of imagery can be used for different needs. *Guided imagery* helps the client appraise his or her situation. *End-result imagery* and *process imagery* help redefine the client's situation, allowing rehearsal of new behaviors and changing the perceived powerlessness caused by the threatening diagnosis.

This chapter explores the use of imagery as a cognitive tool to reduce pain and stress, alter the course of disease, and/or improve health-seeking behaviors. Imagery techniques are doubly effective because they can be taught while the client is dependent and can later help the client maintain control, reduce stress, and alleviate pain with minimal assistance at home. Imagery techniques involve the use of fantasy to achieve health-related goals. Imagery can be used to achieve altered states of awareness, change the client's perception of the situation, and facilitate control of the autonomic nervous system and other physiological mechanisms. In addition, it can be used for bypassing neurological mechanisms in order to give generalized instructions to the body. Imagery can also be used to enhance other medical and nursing therapies. For example, in clients with cancer, imagery can be combined with chemotherapy and radiation to improve the client's prognosis (Brigham, 1994). It is effective in helping to control the debilitating symptoms of nausea and vomiting that accompany these treatments (Frank, 1985). Imagery is predominantly an adjunctive therapy, rather than a primary therapy. Focused imagery combined with cognitive-behavioral group therapy resulted in significant improvement in overall cognitive states of nursing home residents (Abraham, Neudorfer, & Currie, 1992). Persons with chronic bronchitis and emphysema experienced significant improvement in perceived quality of life after 4 weeks of guided imagery training (Moody, Fraser, & Yarandi, 1993).

Although imagery has its roots deep in cultural and religious beliefs as an ancient healing technique (Samuels & Samuels, 1975), recently the anecdotal evidence in academic literature strongly supports the use of imagery in modern-day medicine and suggests that it has great potential as a therapeutic intervention in nursing. Formal nursing research studies on imagery are beginning to appear in the literature as well.

DEFINITION OF IMAGERY

Imagery is only one of several mental processes that can be used to develop cognitive control and promote stress reduction. Other processes include biofeedback, meditation, and relaxation. Biofeedback has also proved effective in stress reduction (Brown, 1984) and continues to be used today. Benson and Klipper's (1975) work documented physiological changes that are produced by relaxation.

Achterberg (1985) defined imagery as an ancient healing technique whereby mental images are used purposefully and therapeutically to achieve a specific desired goal. These thought processes invoke and use the senses: vision, audition, smell, taste, as well as movement, position, and touch. They are a communication mechanism among perception, emotion, and bodily change and act as a bridge between body and mind. Sometimes the subject is alert, concentrating intensely, participating with his or her whole being and visualizing the scene as if it were real. At other times imagery is done in a relaxed state.

Although frequently used together, imagery and relaxation are different. Brown (1974) stated, "the release of the body's tension during relaxation stimulates a dream-like trance in which many mental images are released" (p. 143). In relaxation, the thoughts are free flowing and intentionally undirected. This state of relaxation calms the body, promotes rest, and provides an escape from daily pressures. The individual using imagery channels the energy generated by the images by performing a goal-directed activity. In this instance, the initial part of the guided imagery uses a relaxation exercise followed by a combination of process imagery and/or end-result imagery. Process images are images of the actual or fantasized mechanism by which a desired effect can be achieved. End-result imagery has a concrete image of the desired result as having already taken place (Dossey, 1995).

The following is an example of process imagery. Place the client in a relaxed state using progressive relaxation as described by Snyder (1984). With the nurse as the guide, have the client with a recent skin graft visualize this image. The new skin and the graft site have hands reaching out to each other. Each day the hands move closer together until they can grasp each other in a firm handshake with complete closure at the suture line. Holden-Lund (1988) used process imagery with 24 cholecystectomy clients. She found significantly lower anxiety and lower cortisol levels 1 day postsurgery, and less surgical wound erythema in the treatment group than in the control group.

Many practitioners believe that physiological change is possible with mental imagery (Blandhard, McCoy, Wittrock, Musso, Gerardi, & Pangburn, 1988; Holden-Lund, 1988; Simonton, Matthews-Simonton, & Sparks, 1980). To individualize process imagery, the nurse must (1) have a fundamental knowledge of the physiology involved in disease, (2) know the interaction of all treatments, such as medications and surgery, (3) understand the client's belief system, and (4) have a complete assessment of the client's psychophysiological condition (Achterberg & Lawlis, 1980).

All persons use various forms of imagery in their lives. Memory, daydreams, dreams, and hallucinations are all forms of imagery. Some of these states are voluntary, like memory and daydreams. Others, including the alpha periods that occur just before sleep or upon awakening, are only partially under voluntary control. Alpha periods also occur naturally after intense periods of concentration (Samuels & Samuels, 1975). When persons are staring out of a window, they are probably in an alpha period. Other types of imagery such as dreams and hallucinations are totally beyond voluntary control.

Carl Jung (1963) was one of the first psychologists to address the idea of imagery as a form of therapy. Jung believed that new insights could be gained by actively using alpha times to bypass the censorship of the ego. Imagery directly connects the mind to bodily processes, thus making physiological change possible. Clients can be taught to organize and use alpha periods to enhance the image they are working on, such as weight loss.

Thus imagery, with or without relaxation, can help clients regain a sense of control over their lives, a renewed sense of purpose to face the limitations of their illness, and the strength to make the necessary lifestyle changes. Imagery can be used in a generalized form with no reference to the client's presenting symptoms, or it may be tailored to address specific problems. This technique is helpful to clients with a chronic illness as a means of maintaining or regaining psychological stamina.

Theoretical Rationale

Theoretical speculation about how imagery works has evolved in the fields of medicine and psychology. Although an exhaustive review is not feasible here, one early model by Horowitz (1978) is described. This framework may not be consistent for all the different views of imagery; however, it is useful for explaining how different people have varying success with imagery.

Horowitz's (1978) conceptual framework of imagery examines the three modalities in which thought represents meaning: the enactive, lexical, and imagic modes. *Enactive thought* represents motor response memories. Thinking about lifting a heavy book lying on the table stimulates enactive thought, and a mild tensing of the muscle groups in the shoulders and arms occurs. Control of an enactive mode of thought lies in the limbic system. The limbic system controls emotions that manifest themselves through the tensing of facial muscles. The enactive mode can be accessed by way of the imagic mode. Images may be connected with emotions, which trigger enactive thought followed by observable behavior. The *lexical mode* uses words and grammar to think about objects. Lexical thought makes it possible to communicate clearly. The left hemisphere of the brain controls this mode. Studies of right- and left-hemispheric function indicate that the right and left hemispheres of the brain process information differently. The left hemisphere analyzes, abstracts ideas, counts, marks time, and plans logically, thereby forming lexical thought. In the *imagic mode,* persons perceive and process perceptual information in the form of dreams, fantasies, and images. Primarily, right-hemispheric activity controls imagic thought. The right hemisphere of the brain shows us how things exist in space and how pieces fit together. This mode creates ideas and draws new conclusions. Paradigm shifts and leaps of understanding—an "Ah! Huh! Now I understand" type of learning—characterizes right-brain functioning.

Researchers believe that images held by the brain may be lost when we try to translate them into language (Samuels & Samuels, 1975). For example, when one awakens from a dream, the meaning and image of that dream are clear. However, the meaning becomes confused and lost when the individual tries to share the dream in words to another person. The translation of an image into lexical thought can distort or change the image. That does not indicate that the person did not have a clear understanding of the dream, but simply that putting it into words obscured the meaning. Western culture often disregards or belittles ideas that cannot be articulated well in words. Eastern culture values this form of thinking, believing it demonstrates great wisdom.

The mind, by way of the senses in the form of images, transforms all stimuli into the enactive, lexical, or imagic modes of thought. All are equally important to cognitive functioning. Persons call upon the various modes of thought for different purposes, but each individual has a predominant mode of thought. For example, an athlete may use enactive thought more frequently and an artist may have a more highly refined ability to use imagic mode of thought. Accountants and lawyers use predominantly lexical thought.

Consequently, individuals differ in their ability to elicit visual or auditory images. Some persons report that they are unable to experience visual or auditory images, even with detailed descriptions. Kunzendorf (1981) studied individual differences in imagery abilities and control of skin temperatures. Kunzendorf suggested that those who frequently use visual, auditory, and tactile-proprioceptive images facilitate imagery and may have more control over their autonomic nervous systems.

Finally, reframing is a theoretic framework that is helpful in explaining imagery. Reframing is a technique to help persons contact parts of their minds that are keeping them stuck. Reframing suspends a person's old belief system, allowing reorganization of a problem or experience. In this manner, the person can move toward a healthier state (Stanton, 1989).

Dossey (1995) described this process as a dramatic psychophysiological change that occurs in hypnosis and imagery resulting from gaining access to state-dependent memory, learning, and behavior systems and making their encoded information available for problem solving. When one gains access to state-dependent memory, it can then be reassociated, reorganized, or reframed in a manner that resolves or replaces the negative memory.

Although theories of how imagery functions appear in the literature, little agreement exists at this time among researchers. Nevertheless, practitioners continue to find imagery effective, despite this academic dilemma, and use it in their practice.

SELECTED LITERATURE

Imagery and Psychology

Many studies in the psychotherapy literature are in anecdotal form, unique to a specific client situation. Most of these studies look at imagery as a therapy for pathological conditions (Ashen, 1983; Singer, 1974) and to improve the client's health (Sheikh, 1984, 1990). Meichenbaum (1983) described the outcome of psychotherapy studies using imagery as follows: (1) a feeling of control gained from image rehearsal, (2) a change in the internal dialogue associated with maladaptive behavior, (3) mental rehearsal of adaptive responses, and (4) the consequent decrease of fear. Hymen and Warren (1978), combining imagery with rational emotive therapy, found text anxiety lowered in the experimental imagery group. Ayres and Hopf (1985), while studying speech anxiety, found imagery more effective when persons visualized themselves having a problem and working through it to a successful completion (process imagery) than when they pictured the task accomplished (end-result imagery).

Imagery and Healing

The connection between imagery and the immune system has been studied with increasing frequency. Simonton et al. (1980) first used imagery as a psychological intervention in the treatment of clients with advanced cancer. Comparing the survival rates of their study population to nationally established survival times for breast, bowel, and lung cancer, they found that clients using imagery combined with traditional medical treatment had a prolonged life expectancy. The study followed up 159 clients diagnosed with incurable cancer and a 1-year life expectancy. Sixty-three subjects remained alive after 2 years. In addition, 22.2 percent showed no evidence of cancer and 19.1 percent demonstrated tumor regression. The median survival for these clients was 8 to 19 months longer than the national average (Simonton et al., 1980).

Interest in using imagery for treating clients with terminal cancer grew. Studies found great discrepancies in the effectiveness of similar traditional cancer treatments. Yet, these differences did not seem connected to the location or the type of cancer under treatment. Life span also varied drastically (Simonton et al., 1980).

The client's hardiness and desire to live seemed to play a major role in the client's recovery or, at the very least, an increase in life span (Justice, 1987). Imagery therapy was designed by the institute (Simonton et al., 1980) to foster the client's sense of control over life and ability to enact change in this frightening situation. This program to foster well-being and teach imagery strategies has gained worldwide recognition.

In no way did Simonton et al. (1980) claim that imagery explained all the differences found in this study. However, they did believe that the program increased motivation, mobilized internal resources, and increased the expectation that the treatment results would be positive.

Studies by Frank (1985), Greer and Morris (1978), and Maguire (1981) found that personal coping strategies significantly influenced patient outcomes in breast cancer treatment. Bridge, Benson, Pietroni, and Priest (1988) and Frank (1985) reported that clients practicing "guided imagery/relaxation" felt less emotional distress and nausea or vomiting following chemotherapy infusion. Both studies used control groups.

Effects of imagery on physiological changes in the immune system are being determined. Halliburton (1986) studied changes in the T-cell activity of clients with cancer who practiced relaxation with guided imagery. The role of the B and T cells is to recognize the presence of an antigen and to initiate specific mechanisms of disposal, a process vital to fighting of cancer cells. After 1 year, the subjects' blood samples showed improved T-cell activity, increased killer cell activity, and changes in some B-cell measures. Similarly, Kiecolt-Glaser (1987) studied the impact of imagery on killer cells in a healthy elderly population and found improved T-cell function. In addition, the subjects had lower resting heart rates, slower respirations, and diminished perspiration. They reported feeling more in control of their lives.

Imagery and Discomfort

ANXIETY

Stephens (1990) studied the effectiveness of imagery on moderate levels of nonpathological anxiety. Using a quasi-experimental pretest-posttest design, Stephens randomly assigned 159 undergraduate nursing students to two treatment groups and a control group. One treatment group listened to an audiotape containing guided end-result imagery. The second group used an audiotape with the same imagery combined with relaxation. The third group was a control group. Findings showed both treatment groups had significantly lower levels of anxiety than the control group, using Speilberger, Gorsuch, and Lushene's (1983) State-Trait Anxiety Inventory. Surprisingly, imagery alone was as effective as the imagery combined with relaxation. This contradicts most of the findings in the literature that indicate that imagery combined with relaxation is more effective than imagery alone.

King (1988) tested Donovan's Relaxation with Guided Imagery Tool with 33 graduate nursing students and also found imagery to be effective in lowering anxiety. The effect was short-lived in that subjects had returned to preimaging levels within a 2-week interval. Guided imagery and relaxation also had a significant effect on lowering the anxiety of persons undergoing magnetic resonance imaging (Thompson & Coppens, 1994).

PAIN

Imagery helps in the control of pain, both acute and chronic, by augmenting relaxation, providing distractions, and inducing a state of autohypnosis (Shiekh, 1990). Stressors associated with illness include inability to tolerate ambiguity, delayed gratification, fatalistic ideation, feeling out of control, and viewing oneself as inadequate to fight the illness. Imagery effectively reduces these stressors.

Anecdotal reports indicate that imagery is very effective in reducing pain, but surprisingly few formal studies have been done. Donovan

(1980) used imagery to decrease anxiety and pain in cancer patients. Weinstein (1976) found imagery effective in lowering anticipatory pain in burn patients.

Most strategies employed pleasant imagery as a distraction. Maltzman (1988), however, found that viewing unpleasant slides increased pain tolerance more than viewing pleasant slides of landscapes. Perhaps the unpleasant slides were more distracting and mentally absorbing, therefore holding the subjects' attention for longer periods of time.

Imagery and Art

Achterberg and Lawlis (1980) outlined the beginning steps on the use of art to clarify images. They found that when the client pictures the white blood cells as stronger than the cancer cells, there is a high predictor of success in persons with cancer and other forms of chronic illness.

Using drawings is an effective way to evaluate clients' reactions to imagery. Following instructions to imagine their cancer cells, immune system, and medical intervention, the subject is asked to draw his or her thoughts. Central themes emerging from this qualitative data include vividness, activity, strength, concreteness versus symbolism, and effectiveness. The researchers believe that persons' experiences as seen through their drawings have major implications for treatment. Prognostic tools need to be developed.

Controversies

Although guided imagery holds promise as a therapeutic tool, researchers are critical of imagery studies because of inconsistent methodological protocols. Studies define imagery differently, combining imagery with other treatment modalities, such as rational emotive therapy. Length of client relaxation training and the number of imagery sessions vary among studies. Nonprobability sampling techniques and control groups were not used in early studies. These factors make interpretation of the data difficult and cloud the question, Is imagery a legitimate intervention strategy? Differences in conceptual labels such as guided imagery, relaxation with guided imagery, hypnosis, and pleasant imagery also lead to wide variations in the way guided imagery can be used in a study. These factors make it difficult to compare treatment effects from one study to another.

IMPLICATIONS FOR NURSING PRACTICE

Despite the methodological issues, data continue to accumulate to support the therapeutic effectiveness of guided imagery. Nurses will continue to study the potential of guided imagery as a therapeutic modality and will find imagery useful in varied situations. The outcome desired helps the nurse and client determine the imagery technique that is appropriate.

When nurses wish to help the client to modify physiological function, they use techniques involving deep relaxation and the symbolic representation of physiological control mechanisms. Such techniques expound on the placebo effect enhancing the healing process. Rossman (1988) pointed out ". . . placebo does not mean the response isn't real. It simply means the results stem from the belief of the patient in therapy, rather than from the therapy itself. The important thing about the placebo response is that it demonstrates beyond doubt that thoughts can trigger the body's own healing abilities" (p. 48).

The previous example of the skin graft shows how imagery uses symbolism. The placebo effect of the imagery enhances healing. However, imagery in this situation is only an adjunctive therapy combined with more traditional medical therapy such as sterile dressing changes, good nutrition, and antibiotic therapy.

If the goal of the imagery is to develop insight or increase personal resources to combat stress, symbolic representation of conflict and its resolution is used. End-result imagery can be used for conditions such as weight loss or smoking cessation.

The ability of the client to use imagery will vary, and the client will need assistance in development of the technique. Still, clients of all ages find imagery effective. Anyone who can think can imagine. Success will be determined by the willingness of the client to learn and practice the process. Nurses need to remember that imagery needs energy, and therefore a well-rested client increases the chance of success.

While using guided imagery, nurses are to pay close attention to detect any signs of client distress or agitation. If the client is hesitant about beginning, explore what the experience might be like first. Some casual suggestions about how to proceed may help the client to continue. Relaxation will make the imagery more effective. Clients should be told that they are in complete control of the imagery and can change it at any time or discontinue the treatment by opening their eyes.

Imagery techniques to improve the body's ability to fight off disease appear frequently in the literature. Clients who feel that they are at the mercy of a medication, the physician, or the agency can use imagery to bring back a much-needed sense of control. It is important to allow the client to create and individualize the images.

Imagery, as an adjunct to chemotherapy, can occasionally cause some clients to feel guilty if the imagery is not effective in attenuating tumor growth. Nurses must be alert for this reaction. Severe side effects from chemotherapy may tempt a client to end conventional treatment. Clients should understand that the use of imagery alone is inadvisable. Imagery should give the client a sense of power, not provide an additional stressor. Stop the imagery therapy if distress occurs.

USES AND TECHNIQUES

Pain

Imagery helps clarify the client's perception of the pain experienced. Pain can be labeled and described more vividly with the use of imagery. Clients become aware of how the pain can be manipulated and changed. Then the practitioner can use imagery to relieve discouragement and increase hopefulness, changing the expectation that the pain will continue forever, shifting the focus of the client's life away from the pain, and helping increase the client's energy level needed to deal with the pain.

Guided imagery can be used to create a place of safety from the pain. Visual and auditory images seem more effective than kinesthetic images (Sodergren, 1985). For example, find the sights and sounds that are pleasing to the client. Imagining a wave hitting the beach, the wind moving through the trees, or lying on a soft cloud under a clear blue sky may relax a client and provide a retreat from continual pain. McCaffery (1989) called this "taking a vacation from the pain." Cognitive-behavioral strategies incorporating imagery and visualization were effective in enhancing pain control in women with metastatic breast cancer (Arathuzik, 1994).

Do not talk to the client during the guided imagery process unless the client has a question that must be answered immediately. The client is guided to release feelings and images during this time. Talking as a logical process will interfere with the flow of the images.

Precede the script with a general relaxation script. Pick up cues, such as restlessness, from the client's behavior and add words like "pleasant," "warm," or "comfortable" to help promote relaxation. Tell the client that imagery is a fast way to connect the body, mind, and spirit by quieting the body and focusing on a particular event.

The following script illustrates a way to promote pain reduction:

> Let your imagination choose a place that is safe and comfortable . . . retreat to this place of comfort . . . experience the warmth of the sun as you float on your own special cloud under a splendid blue sky . . . this is a healthy technique that you can use at any time to escape from the pressures of daily life which cause or increase pain . . . allow yourself the privilege of coming to your special place frequently . . . at the beginning it may take you longer to create a state of pain-free enjoyment, but with practice you will reach this state with increased ease.

Rehabilitation

Korn's (1983) work with neurological patients demonstrated that after a cerebrovascular accident clients can use imagery to relearn how to swallow or regain sitting balance, speech, and memory. Korn suggested that helping the client reexperience the psychomotor task activates sensory and neuromuscular mechanisms. This stimulates the original task. Experiments with athletes produced the same results.

Relaxation

Effective relaxation improves with guided imagery. Subjects can reach a relaxed state faster, achieve deeper relaxation, and remain for longer periods. Imagery augments outcome behaviors such as a decrease in blood pressure, anxiety, and muscle tension. Participants exposed to pleasant guided imagery experience a sense of timelessness and transcending boundaries. Butcher and Parker (1988) believed that timelessness is an expansion and increased motion in the human energy field, thus enhancing patterning and harmony with the environment. They used Roger's Theory of Unitary Human Beings as a framework for their study.

Meichenbaum (1983) found combining relaxation and imagery more effective as a treatment for phobias. Through imagery techniques, the meaning of the phobic object is changed and the client can rehearse confrontation with the phobia. Collins and Rice (1997) combined relaxation and imagery in a study of 50 persons on a cardiac rehabilitation program. State anxiety scores did not change; however, interpersonal sensitivity and depression decreased in the relaxation imagery group.

Problem Solving

Imagery is helpful when adjusting to drastic bodily change. A client with a new amputation can be asked to visualize himself or herself going home for the first time. With the use of imagery, the client confronts previously ignored realities. A client with an amputation can resolve the problem of getting from the car to the house. Although identified new problems are difficult, the result is to help the client successfully prepare for discharge.

Similarly, rehearsal of a stressful conversation allows the client to act out various scenarios and try out new behaviors. The client and the nurse explore the situation, identify what is causing the anxiety, and modify the client's response to the situation or the meaning of the situation to the client. This allows the client to gain a feeling of control in a situation that has been frightening in the past. Imagery was effective in decreasing stress in 39 persons who stopped smoking (Wynd, 1992). Significantly less recidivism occurred with the imagery versus the control ($N = 37$) group.

SUMMARY

Imagery is a cost-effective, noninvasive strategy that has been documented to decrease stress and pain, enhance therapeutic effects of other interventions such as chemotherapy or smoking cessation, and increase feelings of control. It is an effective coping mechanism. Imagery serves as a connector among the mind, body, and spirit (Dossey, 1995) and deserves further study and use.

REFERENCES

Abraham, I. L., Neudorfer, M. M., & Currie, L. J. (1992). The effects of cognitive group intervention on cognitive functioning and depressive symptomatology among nursing home residents. *Nursing Research, 41,* 196–202.

Achterberg, J. (1985). *Imagery in healing: Shamanism and modern science.* Boston: New Science Library.

Achterberg, J., & Lawlis, G. F. (1980). *Bridges of the body-mind: Behavioral approaches to health care.* Champaign, IL: Institute for Personality & Ability Testing.

Achterberg, J., & Lawlis, F. (1982). Imagery and health interventions. *Topics of Clinical Nursing, 3*(4), 55–60.

Arathuzik, D. (1994). Effects of cognitive-behavioral strategies on pain in cancer patients. *Cancer Nursing, 17,* 207–214.

Ashen, A. (1983). Eidetic imagery. In A. A. Sheikh (Ed.), *Imagery: Current theory, research and application.* New York: John Wiley & Sons.

Averill, J. (1973). Personal control over aversion stimuli and its relationship to stress. *Psychological Bulletin, 88,* 286–303.

Ayres, J., & Hopf, T. S. (1985). Visualization: A means of reducing speech anxiety. *Communication Education, 34*(4), 318–323.

Blandhard, E., McCoy, G., Wittrock, D., Musso, A., Gerardi, R., & Pangburn, L. (1988). A controlled comparison of thermal biofeedback and relaxation training in the treatment of essential hypertension. II. Effects on cardiovascular reactivity. *Health Psychology, 7*(1), 19–33.

Benson, H., & Klipper, M. X. (1975). *The relaxation response.* New York: William Morrow.

Bridge, L. R., Benson, P., Pietroni, O. C., & Priest, R. G. (1988). Relaxation and imagery in the treatment of breast cancer. *British Medical Journal, 297*(5), 1169–1172.

Brigham, D. D. (1994). *Imagery for getting well: Clinical applications of behavioral medicine.* New York: WW Norton.

Brown, B. B. (1974). *New mind, new body.* New York: Harper & Row.

Brown, J. M. (1984). Imagery coping strategies in the treatment of migraine. *Pain, 18,* 157–167.

Butcher, H. K., & Parker, N. I. (1988). Guided imagery within Rogers' science of unitary human beings: An experimental study. *Nursing Science Quarterly, 1*(3), 103–110.

Collins, J. A., & Rice, V. U. (1997). Effects of relaxation intervention in phase II cardiac rehabilitation: Replication and extension. *Heart & Lung, 26,* 31–43.

Donovan, M. I. (1980). Relaxation with guided imagery: A useful technique. *Cancer Nursing, 3*(1), 27–32.

Dossey, B. M. (1995). Awaking the inner healer. In B. M. Dossey, L. Keegan, C. Guzzetta, L. Kolkmeier (Eds.), *Holistic nursing* (pp. 607–666). Denver: Aspen.

Frank, J. M. (1985). The effects of music therapy and guided visual imagery on chemotherapy induced nausea and vomiting. *Oncology Nursing Forum, 12*(5), 47–52.

Gordon, M. (1994). *Nursing diagnosis: Process and application* (3rd ed.). St. Louis: CV Mosby.

Greer, S., & Morris, T. (1978). The study of psychological factors in breast cancer: Problems of method. *Social Science Medicine, 12,* 129–134.

Halliburton, P. (1986). Impaired immunocompetence. In V. Carrieri, A. M. Lindsey, & C. W. West (Eds.), *Pathophysiological phenomena in nursing: Human responses to illness* (pp. 319–342). Philadelphia: WB Saunders.

Holden-Lund, C. (1988). Effects of relaxation with guided imagery on surgical stress and wound healing. *Research in Nursing and Health, 11,* 235–244.

Horowitz, M. J. (1978). *Image formation and cognition.* (2nd ed.). New York: Appleton-Century-Crofts.

Hymen, S. P., & Warren, R. (1978). Evaluation of rational-emotive imagery as a component of rational-emotive therapy in treatment of test anxiety. *Perceptual and Motor Skills, 46*(3), 847–853.

Jung, C. G. (1963). *Memories, dreams, reflections.* New York: Pantheon Books.

Justice, B. (1987). *Who gets sick: Thinking and health.* Houston: Peak Press.

Kiecolt-Glaser, R. (1987). Cited in Squires, A. Visions to boost immunity. *American Health, 6*(6), 54–61.

King, J. V. (1988). A holistic technique to lower anxiety: Relaxation with guided imagery. *Journal of Holistic Nursing, 6*(1), 16–20.

Korn, E. R. (1983). The use of altered states of consciousness and imagery in physical and pain rehabilitation. *Journal of Mental Imagery, 7,* 25–34.

Kunzendorf, R. G. (1981). Individual differences in imagery and autonomic control. *Journal of Mental Imagery, 5,* 47–60.

Maguire, P. (1981). Psychological and social consequences of cancer. In C. J. Williams & J. W. Whitehouse (Eds.), *Recent advances in clinical oncology* (pp. 236–254). London: Churchill Livingston Press.

Maltzman, S. (1988). Visual stimuli in distraction strategies for increasing pain tolerance: The confounding of affect with other stimulus characteristics. *Pavlovian Journal of Biological Science, 23*(2), 67–74.

McCaffery, M. (1989). *Nursing management of the patient in pain* (3rd ed.). Philadelphia: JB Lippincott.

Meichenbaum, D. (1983). Why does using imagery in psychotherapy lead to changes? In J. Singer & K. S. Pope (Eds.), *The power of the human imagination.* New York: Plenum Press.

Moody, L., Fraser, M., & Yarandi, H. (1993). Effects of guided imagery in patients with chronic bronchitis and emphysema. *Clinical Nursing Research, 2,* 478–486.

Rossman, M. L. (1988). The healing power of imagery. *New Age Journal, 5*(2), 47–54.

Samuels, M., & Samuels, N. (1975). *Seeing with the mind's eye: The history, techniques and uses of visualization.* New York: Random House.

Shiekh, A. (1984). *Imagery and human development series: Imagination and healing.* Farmingdale, NY: Baywood Publishing.

Shiekh, A. (1990). *Psychophysiology of mental imagery: Theory research and application.* Amityville, CA: Baywood.

Simonton, O. C., Matthews-Simonton, S., & Sparks, T. F. (1980). Psychological intervention in the treatment of cancer. *Psychosomatics, 21,* 226–235.

Singer, J. L. (1974). *Imagery and daydream methods in psychotherapy and behavior modification.* New York: Academic Press.

Snyder, M. (1984). Progressive relaxation as a nursing intervention: An analysis. *Advances in Nursing Science, 14,* 47–58.

Sodergren, K. M. (1985). Guided imagery. In M. Snyder (Ed.), *Independent nursing interventions* (pp. 103–124). New York: John Wiley & Sons.

Speilberger, C. D., Gorsuch, R. E., & Lushene, R. W. (1983). *STAI Manual.* Palo Alto, CA: Consulting Psychologists Press.

Stanton, H. (1989). Ego-enhancement: A five-step approach. *American Journal of Clinical Hypnosis, 31*(3), 192–198.

Stephens, R. (1993). Imagery: A strategic intervention to empower clients. Part I. Review and research literature. *Clinical Nurse Specialist, 7,* 170–175.

Stephens, R. L. (1990). *Imagery: A treatment for adult anxiety.* Manuscript submitted for publication.

Thompson, M. B., & Coppens, N. (1994). The effect of guided imagery on anxiety levels and movement of clients undergoing magnetic resonance imaging. *Holistic Nursing Practice, 8,* 9–69.

Weinstein, D. J. (1976). Imagery and relaxation with a burn patient. *Behavior Research and Therapy, 14,* 481.

Wynd, C. (1992). Relaxation imagery used for stress reduction in the prevention of smoking relapse. *Journal of Advanced Nursing, 17,* 294–302.

17

Facilitating Behavior Change in Chronically Ill Persons

➤ POLLY RYAN

Whether it begins dramatically with a myocardial infarction, or insidiously with osteoarthritis, living with a chronic illness changes one's life. The individual, with assistance from significant others and health professionals, must deal with the symptoms, monitor the illness trajectory, and implement treatment. In addition, he or she is advised to change behaviors that directly contribute to the illness or place one at increased risk for developing other illnesses. Therefore, in addition to living with chronic illness, redefining personal and social self-concepts, managing symptoms, carrying out treatments, and compensating for taxed resources, persons with chronic illness benefit from making a number of long-term behavior changes.

At the time when persons with chronic illness are most vulnerable, they are also most challenged to change lifelong behavior patterns. Failure to change behavior not only risks physiological consequences but may affect one's self-concept and social functioning. Repeated failure to lose weight, quit smoking, take medication, and/or exercise can erode the individual's self-concept and self-respect, resulting in social withdrawal. Repeated failures at maintaining behavior change can be degrading and threaten access to continuing care. The managing health professional might conclude, "There is really nothing more I can do for you until you are able to make these changes." Repeated failure and seeming rejection by health professionals further erode one's self-confidence.

Therefore, inability to change behavior can decrease one's sense of power. Feelings of powerlessness contribute to failed attempts at behavior change, and the problem becomes cyclical: Powerlessness leads to failure and failure leads to an increased sense of powerlessness. Successfully changing behavior can break the cyclical nature of failure and despair.

Individuals can learn to change their behavior. Behavior change does not happen because of need or desire: rather, behavior change results from special skills and adequate support. Persons with chronic illnesses must learn the skills that facilitate behavior change, and they need professional and social support during the process.

The purpose of this chapter is to identify how persons with chronic illness can be assisted in changing behavior. The following areas will be discussed: (1) definition and types of change, (2) selected theories, (3) chronic illness and behavior change, and (4) a framework for selecting strategies that facilitate change. All strategies presented have been tested; however, the framework for organizing the strategies is still being studied.

DEFINITION

Although behavior change can occur spontaneously and unconsciously, the type of behavior change discussed in this chapter occurs when a habitual pattern of behavior is deliberately altered. The behavior pattern is changed because it represents a risk to the individual's health. The ultimate responsibility for change lies with the individual; however, the health-care professional must identify a need for the change, identify desired outcomes, suggest strategies that facilitate change, and provide continued care during the change process. Depending on the setting and outcome, behavior change has been termed compliance, alliance, adherence; prevention or lifestyle modification; or recovery and/or cure (Ryan, 1990).

At the turn of the century little was known about behavior change. The major health problems were infectious diseases and injuries. Diagnostic tests, medications, and treatments were limited; as a result, people died of acute illness or injury. As antibiotics were discovered and technology advanced, many acute illnesses were curable and life expectancy increased. Currently, persons live longer, but they may accrue multiple chronic illnesses. Client management of these illnesses requires behavior change. In addition, epidemiologists have targeted behaviors that place persons at risk for development of disease. Consequently, behavior change is an integral component of the treatment and prevention of chronic health problems.

TYPES OF BEHAVIOR CHANGE

There are three types of behavior change: removal, replacement, and addition. *Removal* refers to behaviors that must be completely eliminated; for example, the use of any form of tobacco or street drugs or uncontrolled use of alcohol. *Replacement* refers to behaviors for which a substitute behavior is needed; for example, dietary habits, whether for caloric or nutrient substitutes. *Addition* refers to behaviors that supplement or expand usual behavior pattern and include taking medications, scheduling and keeping appointments, and exercising. Selecting strategies that effect behavior change partly depends upon the type of behavior being modified. Although there is overlap, some strategies are specifically appropriate for removing behavior, replacing behavior, or adding behavior. These strategies are discussed in more detail in the intervention section of this chapter.

THEORIES OF BEHAVIOR CHANGE

Within the past two decades numerous theories of change have been proposed. Extensive research has tested the ability of these theories to both explain and predict change. The theories of behavior change describe change from multiple perspectives, including causation and the process of change. An overview of select theories from these two perspectives will be discussed. Theories explaining behavior change include (1) sociodemographic model, (2) medical model, (3) health belief model, (4) social support, (5) social cognitive theory, (6) self-efficacy, and (7) macrosocial forces. The process of behavior change discussed includes work by Marlatt and Gordon (1985) and Prochaska and DiClemente (1983).

FACTORS INFLUENCING BEHAVIOR CHANGE
Sociodemographic Characteristics

One of the earliest explanations for compliance (adherence to recommended change) was based on sociodemographic characteristics (Haynes, Taylor, & Sackett, 1979; Marston, 1970). The relationship of age, gender, education, race, income, social status, psychological status, and religion to compliance was studied. These studies demonstrated that extremes of age and a diagnosis of paranoid schizophrenia correlated positively with noncompliance. Gender, education, race, ethnicity,

income, social status, or religious affiliation did not correlate with behavior change.

The Medical Model

The medical model (DiMatteo & DiNicola, 1982; Haynes, 1979;
Koltun & Stone, 1986) assumes that an individual would comply with
medical prescription if the disease was serious. To study this assumption, physicians ranked characteristics of the disease (i.e., type of illness, complexity of regimen, discomfort associated with the illness, duration of therapy) and gravity of illness (i.e., seriousness, duration,
associated disability). Actual compliance was then compared with these
rankings. The results demonstrated no significant correlation between
the physician's assessment of the characteristics or gravity of an illness
and compliance.

The Health Belief Model

The health belief model (HBM) (Becker, 1974; Becker et al., 1979;
Janz & Becker, 1984) was developed to determine what factors influenced preventive health behaviors. It was later used to study illness and
compliance. The HBM states that motivation to change behavior equals
perception of the reward minus the perceived cost and the perceived
barrier.

$$\text{Motivation} = \text{reward} - (\text{cost} + \text{barriers})$$

Essentially, behavior change depends on the attractiveness of the
goal, the estimation of one's likelihood of success, and occurrence of a
cue to change behavior. The HBM uniquely focuses on the client's perceptions rather than on the professional's. The major components of the
HBM are health and willingness to accept medical direction; subjective
estimates of susceptibility, vulnerability, and extent of bodily harm; interference with social roles; and perception of the efficacy and safety of
the proposed regimen. (Multiple studies document a significant positive
correlation between the HBM and compliance. However, the HBM does
not *predict* compliance with health-care recommendations.)

Social Support

Social networks and support are positively or negatively related to
behavior change (Berkman, 1984; Bruhn & Phillips, 1984; Cohen &
Syme, 1985; Cwikel, Dielman, Kirscht, & Israel, 1988; DiMatteo & Di-
Nicola, 1982; Gottlieb & Green, 1984; Jacobson, 1986). Specifically,
social support relates positively to behaviors that lead to a healthy
lifestyle (Aaronson, 1989; Boyd-Franklin, 1987; Coppotelli & Orleans,

1985; Hansen et al., 1987; Hubbard, Muhlenkamp, & Brown, 1986; Mermelstein, Cohen, Lichtenstein, Baer, & Kamarck, 1986; Muhlenkamp & Sayles, 1986) and sometimes to behavioral change associated with illness (Glasglow & Toobert, 1988; Morisky, DeMuth, & Field-Fass, 1985; Somer & Tucker, 1988; Stanton, 1987). The relationship between health beliefs and social influence is reported by the Ajzen and Fishbein Theory of Reasoned Action, which states that an individual's intention to act is a function of the person's beliefs and attitudes toward that behavior and his or her beliefs about others' expectations. Although this theory has had limited testing compared to the HBM, a number of studies have demonstrated a positive association between attitudes and subjective norms (Ajzen & Fishbein, 1972; Ajzen & Fishbein, 1980; Ajzen & Madden, 1986; Pender & Pender, 1986; Saltzer, 1980).

Social Cognitive Theory

The social cognitive theory (Bandura, 1986), based on the social learning theory (Bandura, 1977a), proposes a reciprocal relationship between cognition and other personal factors, environment, and behavior. Each factor is interdependent. Essential to this theory are the beliefs that people can use symbols, think about things before they happen, learn from personal and communal experiences, make decisions based on personal and communal standards, and reflect on their own past. To facilitate change, the professional influences cognition, environment, behavior, or all three. A component of this theory currently being tested widely is self-efficacy.

Self-Efficacy

To change behavior, the individual must know what to do, believe it is beneficial, and believe it is attainable. Self-efficacy is defined as belief in one's ability to perform a task. Bandura (1977b) defined self-efficacy as "the conviction that one can successfully execute the behavior required to produce the outcomes" (p. 193). A number of studies have tested self-efficacy and found that persons with high self-efficacy are likely to initiate and maintain a specific behavior change (Baer, Holt, & Lichtenstein, 1987; Bandura, 1982; Barrios & Niehaus, 1985; Coelho, 1984; Colletti, Supnick, & Payne, 1985; DiClemente, Prochaska, & Gibertini, 1985; Godding & Glasgow, 1985; Yates & Thain, 1983).

Macrosocial Factors

In addition to personal relationships, macrosocial forces effect behavior change (Hymowitz, 1987; Killen et al., 1989; Lefebvre & Flora, 1988; McLeroy, Bibeau, Steckler, & Glanz, 1988; Minkler, 1989; Syme &

Alcalay, 1982). Several macrosocial forces that affect behavior are workplace (Hallet, 1986; Peterson et al., 1988), laws (such as the Clean Indoor Air Act), public policy (Breslow, 1982), warnings from authorities (e.g., Surgeon General), and mass communication such as television, radio, and newspaper (Best, 1980; Cummings, Sciandra, & Markello, 1987).

PROCESS OF BEHAVIOR CHANGE

Prochaska and DiClemente

Prochaska and DiClemente (1983) proposed five stages of behavior change: precontemplation, contemplation, action, maintenance, and relapse. Persons in a precontemplation stage avoid thoughts or actions related to behavior change. They are defensive and hold firm to old beliefs and behaviors. Persons contemplating behavior change are interested in changing behavior and actively gather opinions by talking, listening, and reading. Persons in the action stage are actively engaged in changing behavior. Once the change has occurred, either it is maintained or relapse occurs; if relapse occurs, the individual returns to precontemplation or contemplation.

During each stage individuals engage in behaviors consistently. Prochaska and DiClemente concluded that particular strategies are most effective during particular stages of behavior change. Education and feedback are most effective during contemplation. As individuals are in transition from contemplation to change, self-reflection is effective. During the stage of action, persons change their environment, rely on social support, and use reinforcements for their behaviors. During maintenance, persons decrease their use of reinforcements but continue to use environmental control.

Marlatt and Gordon

Rather than five stages of behavior change, Marlatt and Gordon (1985) proposed three stages of change: commitment and motivation (preparation for the change), implementation, and long-term maintenance of the behavior change. Their unique and significant contribution has been the reframing of relapse as an opportunity to learn rather than a failure. They also suggest specific strategies during specific stages including the relapse stage.

Summary of Theories

There is no singular theory that consistently predicts behavior change. Many new and revised theories of behavior change combine concepts from multiple theories. Although there is no singular theory explaining and predicting behavior change, there are selected dimensions that predictably influence behavior change. The two major factors influencing behavior change are personal characteristics and social characteristics.

Personal characteristics include such factors as knowledge, beliefs, attitudes, meaning and purpose, motivation, and past experiences. Social factors influencing behavior change include environment; interpersonal social relationships such as social networks, social support, social influences; and macrosocial factors, such as work site, community, and communication media.

Behavior change is a process with identifiable stages. Although individual theorists differ in the actual name and number of stages, they generally agree that preparatory activity precedes change. Once change occurs, it must be maintained. Relapse frequently follows behavior change. Relapse can be viewed as failure, or it can be an invaluable learning opportunity when the individual can identify those aspects of change that they were not prepared to manage.

Behavior change may be viewed as a multidimensional, dynamic process. Personal and social characteristics influence initiation and maintenance of behavior but differ during various stages of change. The initiation and maintenance are associated with altered personal and social characteristics. Normally, the individual deliberately and consciously alters personal and social characteristics to change behavior. However, behavior change for persons with a chronic illness can differ.

CHRONIC ILLNESS AND THE CHANGE PROCESS

Behavior change is recommended or prescribed by a health-care professional as a component of treatment for the chronic illness. Failure of the client to change erodes the efficacy of the treatment plan and can cause a downward trajectory of the chronic illness. Frequently individuals are advised to make several changes simultaneously and to actively change their behavior soon after the diagnosis is made. The change is monitored by the health-care professional. Behavior change in chronic illness is characterized by external recommendation for change, health risk of unmodified behavior, continued external monitoring, multiple simultaneous changes, and lack of preparatory phase.

FRAMEWORK FOR SELECTING INTERVENTIONS

The framework to determine which strategies will most likely effect behavior change is based on the stage of behavior change, personal characteristics, and social characteristics. Once these factors have been identified, specific strategies can be chosen (Bandura, 1986; Barofsky, 1977; Comoss, 1988; DiMatteo & DiNicola, 1982; Dishman, 1988; Falvo, 1994; Frenn, Borgeson, Lee, & Simandl, 1989; Green, Kreuter, Deeds, &

Partridge, 1980; Haynes, Taylor, & Sackett, 1979; Health and Public Policy Committee, American College of Physicians, 1986; Leventhal & Cleary, 1980; Pender, 1996; Ryan, 1987; Trower, Casey, & Dryden, 1988).

Strategies need to match the stage of change, the personal characteristics, and social characteristics. If the personal characteristics are inadequate to initiate or maintain the desired change, individuals can be provided with strategies that strengthen or alter personal characteristics during that stage of change. If social characteristics are inadequate, strategies that strengthen or alter social characteristics are desirable. If both the personal and social characteristics are inadequate to initiate or maintain the desired change, the individual can be provided with strategies that strengthen or alter both.

The categories of strategies include universal strategies, strategies specific to stages of change, and strategies for persons choosing not to engage in the change process. The strategies specific to the stages of change are subdivided into those strategies specific to personal and social characteristics.

Universal Strategies

Some strategies are universal. The goals of the universal strategies include: to provide persons with the knowledge of what, why, and how changes should be made; to ensure the individual's familiarity with available resources; and to provide continued care. The respective strategies are teaching, identification of resources, and continued supervision.

All persons whose treatment for chronic illness requires behavior change(s) should be taught the rationale for change, consequences of not making the change, specific behaviors involved in the change, and intended outcomes (Bartlett, 1982; Devine & Cook, 1983; Lorig & Lourin, 1985; Marshall, Penckofer, & Llewellyn, 1986; Mazzuca, 1982; Powers & Wooldridge, 1982; Ruzicki, 1989). Information should be presented in a manner consistent with the individual's coping style and locus of control. Structured educational programs are more effective than unstructured programs, but individual and group learning are equally effective. When possible, information should be prepared in at least two methods (e.g., written and small group), as the combined methods facilitate cognitive, affective, and psychomotor learning (Cohen, 1981; Falvo, 1994; Redman, 1996; Simonds, 1983; Wilson-Barnett & Osborne, 1983). According to Ley (1976), information is most effective if it has six characteristics:

1. *Primacy:* The most important facts should be presented first.
2. *Brevity:* Information should be presented succinctly.
3. *Organization:* Material should be organized in topics or categories; as like information that is clustered will be remembered longer than information presented randomly.

4. *Specificity:* Directions should be clear.
5. *Repetition:* Important information should be repeated frequently and presented in a variety of ways.
6. *Level:* Information should be presented at the individual's level of comprehension.

Written material prepared for use by the general public should have a reading level between the third and sixth grades (Doak, Doak, & Root, 1985; Redman, 1996). The reading level can be determined by sentence length and number of polysyllabic words. Therefore, to prepare written material for a lower reading level, one should shorten the sentence and word length and use simple pictures and diagrams.

It is equally important to consider the comprehension level of groups and audiences. Again, it is helpful to keep sentences short and words simple. Pictures and diagrams can be used as an aid to concept explanation.

Teaching can also be done in a manner that takes into account the individual's coping style (Thornburg, 1982) and locus of control. For example, persons who cope with an illness by using minimization should be given only essential information. Extensive explanations and detailed descriptions are generally counterproductive. On the other hand, those individuals who cope through vigilant focusing benefit from explanations and detailed descriptions.

All persons changing behavior should be encouraged to know, find, and use the available resources. Lists of compiled resources are most helpful; for example, a listing of all local smoking cessation programs or listings of alternate modes of transportation to clinics. People need to be informed of services available through various associations (e.g., The American Heart Association, The American Lung Association, and American Cancer Society). They should be apprised of published information dealing with the management of chronic illness and related behavior changes.

And, finally, all persons should be seen regularly during the phase of active change, and periodically during maintenance. Everyone should have accurate information regarding follow-up care and access to a contact person for questions and emergencies.

Change Strategies Dependent on Stage and Personal and Social Characteristics

Some individuals successfully initiate and maintain change by knowing what to do and receiving regular care. However, most people require additional help and support. The following framework has been proposed as one method of selecting strategies that best match the individual's stage in the change process with their personal and social characteristics (Table 17.1).

Table 17.1 ➤ **STRATEGIES TO FACILITATE CHANGE**

Stage	Personal	Social
Preparation	Consciousness raising Discussion Value clarification Self-monitoring Problem solving Reframing	Reference groups Assertiveness
Actual change	Goal setting Tailoring regimens Self-monitoring Cognitive restructuring Time management Management of withdrawal Thought stopping	Planned social and environmental change
Maintenance	Relaxation Exercise Self-monitoring	Involvement with formal programs
Relapse	Reframing Relapse preparation	Increased support

The goal of strategies is to facilitate the change process by altering personal beliefs and social characteristics influencing behavior change during a specific stage. For the purposes of this discussion, four stages of change are used: preparation, actual change, maintenance, and relapse. Although this is an implied order of occurrence, it has not been tested. It is likely that change is fluid and dynamic, rather than a linear process, and that several stages occur simultaneously or in different sequences, depending on the behavior being changed and the individual.

PREPARATION

The common sequence in chronic illness is diagnosis followed by recommendation or prescription to change several behaviors. Ideally, these changes should occur immediately after diagnosis. When the sequencing of diagnosis and prescribed changes are immediate, individuals are expected to skip preparation. Possible consequences of skipping preparation are a higher rate of relapse, increased difficulty of change, increased distress in making change, increased use of resources to change, and higher rates of refusal to change.

However, for some, the physiological need for change outweighs the need for gradual preparation (e.g., the need for insulin, antiarrhythmic medication, or dialysis). Therefore, to facilitate behavior change in persons with a chronic illness, both the normal change process and therapeutic requirements of the illness need to be blended in a manner consistent with the physical and psychosocial needs and desires of the individual. Professional judgment is required when selecting behavioral change strategies.

Persons in the preparatory phase are contemplating behavior change. At this time they are most receptive to specific information about behavior. Personal characteristics needed to effect a change include a desire for more information, belief in the value of changing behavior, belief in ability to change behavior, belief that the behavior change will result in the desired outcomes, and willingness to bring habitual behaviors to a conscious level. Social characteristics needed to change include the involvement with social networks that will allow and support behavior change. Therefore, strategies are directed toward the achievement of these characteristics.

Examples of strategies that affect personal characteristics during preparation include consciousness raising (value clarification, discussion, self-monitoring), problem solving (identification of intended and unintended consequences), and reframing. Strategies that affect social characteristics and are effective during this stage include assertiveness skills and involvement in reference groups.

Consciousness-raising strategies bring aspects of behavior to awareness. Included among the techniques are discussions, value clarification techniques, and self-monitoring. In discussion, the principles of guidance and counseling are used to enable the individual to explore feelings and beliefs about the desired behavior change.

With value clarification, the individual is assisted to identify multiple alternative behaviors and to explore their values related to specific alternatives (Berger, Hopp, & Raettig, 1975; Steele, & Harmon, 1993; Uustal, 1977). One value clarification technique is the Pie of Life. Two circles or pies are drawn. The individual is instructed to cut the first pie into slices that represent those behaviors they believe are associated with their health. The individual is then instructed to cut the second pie into slices that represent those behaviors that they regularly perform. Once this is done, the individual can visualize the discrepancy between what they believe they should do and what they do. This enables the person to make a conscious choice to perform behaviors that are more consistent with values and beliefs. It also provides them with an opportunity to identify why they have engaged in behaviors that are inconsistent with their values and beliefs.

Self-monitoring (Carnahan & Nugent, 1975; Mahoney, 1974; Oldridge & Jones, 1983), when used in the preparation phase of behavior, enables the person to identify the patterns of a behavior. Self-monitoring employs a written record that enables the individual to identify cues and consequences of a particular behavior. Although behavior patterns can generally be identified in 3 to 5 days, it will be the individual's tolerance for self-monitoring that determines the extent of information logged. A self-monitoring log can be as limited as identification of the frequency and time of a behavior, or it can be as detailed as the place, persons, feelings, and activities associated with the behavior. These records are reviewed and patterns of behavior emerge, enabling the individual to become aware of the habitual, frequently unrecognized aspects of their behaviors. This insight prepares them for making specific plans for change.

Reframing is a technique in which one sees alternative perspectives of a behavior change. For example, instead of viewing smoking cessation or dieting as a loss, one can see them as a gift to oneself. When individuals reframe their thinking, they are freed to act differently.

If persons are surrounded with social influences that oppose or fail to support a behavior change, the individual will benefit by enlarging social support to include persons who foster the desired change. Reference groups, or persons with shared concerns, can provide essential support. Examples of reference groups include Weight Watchers, Alcoholics Anonymous, or Mended Hearts Club. In addition, people will benefit from using assertiveness skills to manage the negative messages and pressures from their support systems. People need to identify the inconsistent messages given by social groups. For example, their significant other may express a desire for them to lose weight, yet be displeased with the individual when he or she chooses not to share the dessert. Assertiveness skills enable one to manage the conflict without alienating the significant other.

Macrosocial messages, especially if consistent, can be very influential in preparing persons to change. For example, during the spring of 1990 there was a major television, radio, and written media campaign on saving the earth. Local governments provided people with specific information on how and what to recycle. The amount of material recycled increased significantly.

ACTUAL CHANGE

Habits, such as smoking, drinking, and overeating, occur automatically. These behaviors are so ingrained that they occur without thought. That is, people generally do not consciously decide to smoke every cigarette or eat every cookie. To change a behavior, individuals must become consciously aware of the behavior and make a deliberate choice to change it. This process requires time, energy, and focus. Failure to remain focused places the individual at risk for returning to habitual behaviors. Likewise, new behaviors are added by the individual consciously electing to perform the behavior.

Active change occurs by consciously attending to actions. The stage of active change can last from weeks to months. During this period, time and energy remain focused on behavior. In addition to being very preoccupied with behavior, the person must deal with side effects of changing behaviors. The withdrawal symptoms of some behaviors, like smoking and drinking, are clearly recognized. But all behavior change has associated effects. Dietary changes are associated with food cravings, hunger, and gastrointestinal symptoms. There are intended and unintended effects of the medication. Exercise programs are associated with various levels of fatigue and muscle soreness or injury. Constantly focusing on one's behavior is, in itself, tiring and disorganizing.

Examples of strategies affecting personal characteristics that are appropriate during the stage of active change include goal setting (Czar, 1987; Eiser & Gentle, 1988; Haller & Reynolds, 1982), tailoring, self-monitoring, cognitive restructuring, time management, preparation for and management of withdrawal, reminders, relaxation (Donovan, 1980; Scandrett & Uecker, 1992), and thought stopping. Examples of strategies that affect social characteristics and are effective during active change include planned social and environmental changes.

Behavior change must be tailored to the individual's lifestyle. That is, new behaviors should fit with routines and preferences. Self-monitoring was discussed under the preparatory phase of behavior change. During active change, self-monitoring is done in the same way, but its purpose changes. Rather than for identification of the cues and rewards for behavior, self-monitoring is now done to assist the individual to be aware of his or her behavior. If a written food diary is kept daily, the individual will remain aware of everything eaten. When a behavior is monitored, the individual is aware of actions, and the performance of the behavior becomes increasingly consistent with the desire to change the behavior.

Individuals should prepare for and manage withdrawal symptoms. The effect of sensory preparation on withdrawal symptoms is currently being tested. Sensory preparation is an intervention that apprises persons of potential noxious symptoms by informing them prior to the experience about the anticipated sensations. In addition, people need suggestions on coping with specific withdrawal symptoms. For example, taking a long, slow, deep breath is very helpful to persons experiencing an urge for a cigarette.

Behavior patterns can be changed by actually altering the behaviors associated with the pattern (as discussed in altering cues and using alternative rewards), or they can be changed by altering one's perspective of the behavior, its causes, the perceived loss and distress, and the perceived consequences. A number of cognitive coping skills (e.g., cognitive restructuring, framing, thought stopping) effectively alter one's perspective (Bandura, 1986; Davis, Eshelman, & McKay, 1995; Ellis, 1988).

Reminders are stimuli that cue a desired behavior (Gabriel, Gagnon, & Bryan, 1977). Reminders are effective for problems associated with forgetting. They are effective only for a few days; when used consistently and as reminders become routine, they lose their effectiveness. Postcards or telephone calls have been an effective method to decrease the number of missed appointments or increase the number of rescheduled follow-up visits. Self-sticking labels can also be affixed to grocery lists to remind persons of ingredients to be avoided.

Any individual planning to change behavior should also be assisted to develop realistic plans during the period of active change. Any new behavior takes time. A new diet requires additional time to plan menus, shop, substitute foods, and prepare meals. In addition, the occasional fast-food solution to a busy day needs to be reworked. Increased attention by health-care professionals is an effective strategy for facilitating behavior change.

During active change it is essential to alter environmental and social factors. Deciding what to alter is based on understanding the behavior pattern. Social and environmental cues are associated with behavior. In addition, every behavior has consequences that both reward and reinforce the behavior. Therefore, once the cues are identified, they can be altered in a fashion more consistent with the desired change. For example, a woman was advised to quit smoking because she has chronic obstructive pulmonary disease. She agreed to try and monitored her smoking behavior for a week. Based on the results of monitoring, it became apparent that she smoked only in the kitchen or outside, always smoked while on the telephone, always smoked after meals and with coffee, and considered the cigarette a reason to take a break from her work. She worked with the nurse to identify specific environmental factors that could be changed to make cessation easier. These changes consisted of limiting time in the kitchen by using television and telephone in the living room, brushing her teeth immediately after eating, temporarily substituting tea for coffee, and using preplanned breaks in her daily schedule.

The social factors associated with maintenance of the smoking habit also need to be identified and changed. For example, if one always smokes while bowling, perhaps one could ask to play with a team of nonsmokers or enlist the support of a team member who has successfully quit smoking.

Smoking cigarettes and eating are self-reinforcing behaviors. Once these behaviors are changed, one may experience a loss due to absence of the reinforcement. Frequently, the rewards of a new behavior are not evident. It can take months to feel good from exercise. Therefore, it can be helpful during the stage of active change to teach the individual to use artificial rewards (i.e., use rewards that are not normally associated with the behavior). Persons can identify a list of rewards before initiating change. Initially persons should use these rewards every time they perform the new behavior; later the rewards should be used intermittently. Intermittent rewards seem to be more effective in locking the behavior. The reward should be as small as possible, yet still be seen as rewarding. The reward should be immediate; that is, it should be paired with the behavior. Remote rewards are not effective for reinforcing new behaviors. Examples of rewards include calling a friend, trip to the hardware store, extra minutes in the bath or shower, or setting aside time to read.

Maintenance

During maintenance, behaviors that have been consciously changed must become habituated, or done automatically (Swan & Denk, 1987). The long-term goal of maintenance is to perform the desired behavior without always making a conscious choice. Maintenance is the stage of behavior change that has been studied least. Clinically it is the stage of change that has the fewest numbers of programs, resources, or information. Most third-party payers do not financially support continued supervision of the maintenance phase. However, relapse remains the most frequent outcome of behavior change. Therefore, it is an area in which extensive work needs to be done.

It has been suggested that there is a positive association between persons successfully maintaining the removal of a behavior (smoking, alcohol) and the use of relaxation and exercise. Self-monitoring is an effective means of maintaining weight loss. Persons who maintain connections with formal programs, such as volunteering, experience greater success with maintenance. Successful maintenance is facilitated by environments and social systems that support the change.

Relapse

Relapse is a stage of behavior that occurs when the individual returns to the prechange patterns of behavior (Saunders & Allsop, 1987; Wewers & Lenz, 1987). Relapse can be a slip or total reversal. For many specific behavior changes, the consequences of a slip are undetermined. However, Marlatt and Gordon (1985) postulated that if a slip is perceived as a failure and attributed to the individual's ability to change, it is highly probable that the slip will result in total relapse.

Examples of strategies that affect personal characteristics and are appropriate to the stage of relapse include prevention and reframing (Baer, Kamarck, Lichtenstein, & Ransom, 1989; Cummings, Jaen, & Giovino, 1985; Eiser, van der Pligt, Raw, & Sutton, 1985; Harackiewicz, Sansone, Blair, Epstein, & Manderlink, 1987; O'Connell & Martin, 1987; Shiffman, 1984; Supnick & Colletti, 1984). Increasing support is a strategy that affects the social characteristics and is effective during relapse (Mermelstein, Lichtenstein, & McIntyre, 1983). Preventing relapse is facilitated by self-monitoring. Persons need to be aware of risky persons and situations. It is most helpful to know this before attempting the change, but actual experience is frequently the most effective method of identifying persons and situations that need to be altered or avoided. Rather than viewing relapse as another failure, the individual can view the relapse as an invaluable learning opportunity. Persons can prepare for relapse by preplanning alternative ways of managing the lapse (Supnick & Colletti, 1984). If a lapse is stopped and personal and social characteristics altered, a total relapse can be prevented.

Continued support from significant others and health-care professionals is essential for persons who have relapsed. The availability of a person during highly tempting situations can prevent relapse. A therapeutic person can assist the individual to reframe the lapse, provide reinforcement for positive actions and outcomes, and generate alternative ways of continuing to manage situations. Continued supervision conveys the belief that change is important and the individual, with appropriate help, can make the desired change.

Management of Treatment for Nonchangers

For any number of reasons, there are individuals who choose not to make a change, not to change at this time, not to change in this professional relationship, or not to change in the manner recommended. Individuals have the right to choose not to change, particularly if their behavior does not directly harm others. Health-care professionals have the right to choose not to care for a person who chooses not to change, as long as other sources of care are available and the behavior is not life threatening. However, if the individual continues to request care and if the health-care professional is willing to care for a person who chooses not to make the recommended changes, a number of strategies can be effective. If the individual fails to participate in the change process, care is directed toward achievement of these goals: (1) the establishment and maintenance of a relationship, (2) simplification and prioritizing care, and (3) identification of alternative resources.

Continued relationships enable the professional to have a foot in the door. The foot-in-the-door strategy was originally developed for marketing and sales. The individual is requested to have minimal involvement with some aspect of change, such as agreeing to take printed information. Once the individual has agreed to this minimal participation they will be more likely to continue with increasing involvement. Gradually, positive outcomes will be attained and it becomes increasingly possible to change behavior. Maintaining an open door (continued access to care), repetitive and consistent messages, and a supportive relationship set the stage for future behavior change.

For those individuals who would experience significant physiological consequences, strategies such as negation, graduated regimen implementation, and contracting can be effective.

Graduated regimen is a strategy in which complex behavior patterns are gradually changed by successfully changing small sequential behaviors. Individuals successfully master one step at a time, mastery being required for progression to the next step. The American Heart Association Cookbook outlines step-by-step details of restricting cholesterol and saturated fats by using a graduated regimen.

Contracts have been demonstrated to be very effective in changing behavior (Herje, 1980; Lewis and Michnich, 1977; Mahoney and Thoresen, 1974; Steckel, 1980, 1982). A contract is a process in which the practitioner and the client select a behavior that is to be changed, specify the conditions of change, and identify a reward for successfully completing the contract. Contracts involve a negotiation process, as both the practitioner and the client agree on the goals and specific behaviors. Contracts are most effective when written and positively stated. The target behavior needs to be measurable (i.e., counted, recorded, graphed, or observable to both parties).

Again, continued care is necessary, as the strategies effectively change behavior when used, but when stopped, the behavior reverts back to prechange patterns.

SUMMARY

Behavior change is an active, powerful way of dealing with and managing a chronic illness. Successful change creates feelings of control and power, feelings that enable even greater success. Change produces hope. When someone is able to change, there is a realistic hope that the consequences of the illness can be minimized or at least contained.

Behavior change is a multidimensional process. Although there are common factors that influence behavior change, and common stages in the process of change, it is always unique for the individual, different at every moment and with every experience. Many strategies that facilitate change have been identified, yet what we know is limited by our world view, contained by our morality and ethics, and restricted by our science. With such limitations it is imperative that we proceed with caution, judge with great reluctance, and always look first to ourselves and our systems as we prescribe change.

REFERENCES

Aaronson, L. (1989). Perceived and received support: Effects on health behavior during pregnancy. *Nursing Research, 38,* 4–9.

Ajzen, I., & Fishbein, M. (1972). Attitudes and normative beliefs as factors influencing behavioral intentions. *Journal of Personality and Social Psychology, 21,* 1–9.

Ajzen, I., & Fishbein, M. (1980). *Understanding attitudes and predicting social behavior.* Englewood Cliffs, NJ: Prentice-Hall.

Ajzen, I., & Madden, T. (1986). Prediction of goal-directed behavior: Attitudes, intentions, and perceived behavioral control. *Journal of Experimental and Social Psychology, 22,* 453–474.

Baer, J. S., Holt, C. S., & Lichtenstein, E. (1986). Self-efficacy and smoking reexamined: Construct validity and clinical utility. *Journal of Consulting and Clinical Psychology, 54,* 846–852.

Baer, J. S., Kamarck, T., Lichtenstein, E., & Ransom, C. C. (1989). Prediction of smoking relapse: Analyses of temptations and transgressions after initial cessation. *Journal of Consulting and Clinical Psychology, 57,* 623–627.

Bandura, A. (1977a). *Social learning theory.* Englewood Cliffs, NJ: Prentice-Hall.

Bandura, A. (1977b). Self-efficacy: Toward a unifying theory of behavioral change. *Psychological Review, 84,* 191–215.

Bandura, A. (1982). Self-efficacy mechanism in human agency. *American Psychologist, 37,* 122–147.

Bandura, A. (1986). *Social foundations of thought and action: A social cognitive theory.* Englewood Cliffs, NJ: Prentice-Hall.

Barofsky, I. (Ed.). (1977). *Medication compliance: A behavioral management approach.* Thorofare, NJ: Slack.

Barrios, F. X., & Niehaus, J. C. (1985). The influence of smoker status, smoking history, sex, and situational variables on smokers' self-efficacy. *Addictive Behaviors, 10,* 425–429.

Bartlett, E. (1982). Behavioral diagnosis: A practical approach to patient education. *Patient Counseling and Health Education, 4,* 29–35.

Becker, M. H. (Ed.). (1974). *The Health Belief Model and personal health behavior.* Thorofare, NJ: Slack.

Becker, M. H., Maiman, L. A., Kirsch, J. P., Haefner, D. P., Drachman, R. H., & Taylor, D. W. (1979). Patient perceptions and compliance: Recent studies of the Health Belief Model. In R. B. Haynes, D. W. Taylor, & H. D. Sacket, (Eds.), *Compliance in health care* (pp. 78–109). Baltimore: Johns Hopkins University Press.

Berger, B., Hopp, J., & Raettig, V. (1975). Values clarification and the cardiac patient. *Health Education Monograph, 3,* 191–199.

Berkman, L. F. (1984). Assessing the physical health effects of social networks and social support. *American Review of Public Health, 5,* 413–432.

Best, J. A. (1980). Mass media, self-management, and smoking modification. In P. O. Davidson & S. M. Davidson (Eds.), *Behavioral medicine: Changing health lifestyles* (pp. 371–390). New York: Brunner/Mazel.

Boyd-Franklin, N. (1987). Group therapy for black women: A therapeutic support model. *American Orthopsychiatric Association, 57,* 397–401.

Breslow, L. (1982). Control of cigarette smoking from a public policy perspective. *Annual Review of Public Health, 3,* 129–151.

Bruhn, J., & Phillips, B. (1984). Measuring social support: A synthesis of current approaches. *Journal of Behavioral Medicine, 7,* 151–169.

Carnahan, J., & Nugent, C. (1975). The effects of self-monitoring by patients for the control of hypertension. *American Journal of Medical Science, 269,* 69–73.

Coelho, R. J. (1984). Self-efficacy and cessation of smoking. *Psychological Reports, 54,* 309–310.

Cohen, S. A. (1981). Patient education: A review of the literature. *Journal of Advanced Nursing, 6,* 11–18.

Cohen, S. A., & Syme, S. (Eds.). (1985). *Social support and health.* New York: Academic Press.

Colletti, G., Supnick, J. A., & Payne, T. J. (1985). The smoking self-efficacy questionnaire: Preliminary scale development and validation. *Behavioral Assessment, 7,* 249–260.

Coppotelli, H. C., & Orleans, C. T. (1985). Partner support and other determinants of smoking cessation and maintenance among women. *Journal of Consulting and Clinical Psychology, 53,* 455–460.

Cummings, K. M., Jaen, C., & Giovino, G. (1985). Circumstances surrounding relapse in a group of recent exsmokers. *Preventive Medicine, 14,* 195–202.

Cummings, K. M., Sciandra, R., & Markello, S. (1987). Impact of a newspaper mediated quit smoking program. *American Journal of Public Health, 77,* 1452–1453.

Cwikel, J. M. G., Dielman, T. E., Kirscht, J. P., & Israel, B. A. (1988). Mechanisms of psychosocial effects on health: The role of social integration, coping style and health behavior. *Health Education Quarterly, 15,* 151–173.

Czar, M. (1987). Two methods of goal setting in middle-aged adults facing critical life changes. *Clinical Nurse Specialist, 1,* 171–177.

Davis, M., Eshelman, E., & McKay, M. (1995). *The relaxation and stress reduction workbook* (4th ed.). Richmond, CA: Harbinger.

Devine, E. C., & Cook, T. D. (1983). A meta-analytic analysis of effects of psychoeducational interventions on length of postsurgical hospital stay. *Nursing Research, 32,* 267–274.

DiClemente, C. C., Prochaska, J. O., & Gibertini, M. (1985). Self-efficacy and the stages of self-change of smoking. *Cognitive Therapy and Research, 9,* 181–200.

DiMatteo, M. R., & DiNicola, D. D. (1982). *Achieving patient compliance: The psychology of the medical practitioner's role.* New York: Pergamon Press.

Dishman, R. K. (1988). *Exercise adherence: Its impact on public health.* Champaign, IL: Human Kinetics Books.

Doak, C., Doak, L., & Root, J. (1985). *Teaching patients with low literacy skills.* Philadelphia: JB Lippincott.

Donovan, M. (1980). Relaxation with guided imagery: A useful technique. *Cancer Nursing, 3,* 27–32.

Eiser, J. R., & Gentle, P. (1988). Health behavior as goal-directed action. *Journal of Behavioral Medicine, 11,* 523–535.

Eiser, J. R., van der Pligt, J., Raw, M., & Sutton, S. R. (1983). Trying to stop smoking: Effects of perceived addiction, attributions for failure, and expectancy of success. *Journal of Behavioral Medicine, 8,* 321–341.

Ellis, A. (1988). Psychotherapies that promote profound philosophical change foster behavioral change. *Journal of Integrative and Eclectic Psychotherapy, 7,* 397–402.

Falvo, D. R. (1994). *Effective patient education: A guide to increased compliance* (2nd ed.). Rockville, MD: Aspen.

Frenn, M. D., Borgeson, D. S., Lee, H. A., & Simandl, G. (1989). Life-style changes in a cardiac rehabilitation program: The client perspective. *Journal of Cardiovascular Nursing, 3,* 43–55.

Gabriel, M., Gagnon, J. P., & Bryan, C. (1977). Improved patient compliance through use of daily drug reminder chart. *American Journal of Public Health, 67,* 968–969.

Glasgow, R. E., & Toobert, D. J. (1988). Social environment and regimen adherence among Type II diabetic patients. *Diabetes Care, 11,* 377–386.

Godding, P. R., & Glasgow, R. E. (1985). Self-efficacy and outcome expectations as predictors of controlled smoking status. *Cognitive Therapy and Research, 9,* 583–590.

Gottlieb, N., & Green, L. (1984). Life events, social network, life-style, and health: An analysis of the 1979 national survey of personal health practices and consequences. *Health Education Quarterly, 11,* 91–105.

Green, L. W., Kreuter, M. W., Deeds, S. G., & Partridge, K. B. (1980). *Health education planning: A diagnostic approach.* Palo Alto, CA: Mayfield.

Haller, K. B., & Reynolds, M. A. (1982). *Mutual goal setting in patient care; CURN Project.* New York: Grune & Stratton.

Hallett, R. (1986). Smoking intervention in the workplace: Review and recommendations. *Preventive Medicine, 15,* 213–231.

Hansen, W. B., Graham, J. W., Sobel, J. L., Shelton, D. R., Flay, B. R., & Johnson, C. A. (1987). The consistency of peer and parent influences on tobacco and alcohol use among young adolescents. *Journal of Behavioral Medicine, 10,* 559–561.

Harackiewicz, J. M., Sansone, C., Blair, L. W., Epstein, J. A., & Manderlink, G. (1987). Attributional processes in behavior change and maintenance: Smoking cessation and continued abstinence. *Journal of Consulting and Clinical Psychology, 55,* 372–378.

Haynes, R. B. (1979). Determinants of compliance: The disease and the mechanics of treatment. In R. B. Haynes, D. W. Taylor, & H. D. Sacket (Eds.), *Compliance in health care* (pp. 49–62). Baltimore: Johns Hopkins University Press.

Haynes, R. B., Taylor, D. W., & Sackett, D. L. (Eds.) (1979). *Compliance in Health Care.* Baltimore: Johns Hopkins University Press.

Health and Public Policy Committee, American College of Physicians. (1986). Methods for stopping cigarette smoking. *Annals of Internal Medicine, 105,* 281–291.

Herje, P. (1980). Hows and whys of patient contracting. *Nurse Educator, 5,* 30–35.

Hubbard, P., Muhlenkamp, A. F., & Brown, N. (1984). The relationship between social support and self-care practices. *Nursing Research, 33,* 266–270.

Hymowitz, N. (1987). Community and clinical trials of disease prevention: Effects on cigarette smoking. *Public Health Review, 15,* 45–81.

Jacobson, D. (1986). Types and timing of social support. *Journal of Health and Social Behavior, 27,* 250–264.

Janz, N. K., & Becker, M. H. (1984). The Health Belief Model: A decade later. *Health Education Quarterly, 11,* 1–47.

Killen, J. D., Robinson, T. N., Telch, M. J., Saylor, K. E., Maron, D. J., Rich, T., & Bryson, S. (1989). The Stanford adolescent heart health program. *Health Education Quarterly, 16,* 263–283.

Koltun, A., & Stone, G. C. (1986). Past and current trends in patient noncompliance research: Focus on diseases, regimens-programs, and provider-disciplines. *Journal of Compliance in Health Care, 1,* 21–32.

Lefebvre, R. C., & Flora, J. A. (1988). Social marketing and public health intervention. *Health Education Quarterly, 15,* 299–315.

Leventhal, H., & Cleary, P. D. (1980). The smoking problem: A review of the research and theory in behavioral risk modification. *Psychological Bulletin, 88,* 370–405.

Lewis, C., & Michnich, M. (1977). Contract as a means of improving patient compliance. In I. Barofsky (Ed.), *Medication compliance: A behavioral management approach.* Thorofare, NJ: Slack.

Ley, P. (1976). Towards better doctor-patient communication. In A. E. Bennett (Ed.), *Communication between doctors and patients.* London: Oxford University Press.

Lorig, K., & Lourin, J. (1986). Some notions about assumptions underlying health education. *Health Education Quarterly, 12,* 31–38.

Mahoney, M. (1974). Self-reward and self-monitoring techniques for weight control. *Behavioral Therapy, 5,* 48–57.

Mahoney, M. J., & Thoresen, C. E. (1974). *Self-control: Power to the person.* Monterey, CA: Brooks-Cole.

Marlatt, G. A., & Gordon, J. R. (1985). *Relapse prevention.* New York: Guilford Press.

Marshall, J., Penckofer, S., & Llewellyn, J. (1986). Structured postoperative teaching and knowledge and compliance of patients who had coronary artery bypass surgery. *Heart & Lung, 15,* 82–86.

Marston, M. V. (1970). Compliance with medical regimens: A review of the literature. *Nursing Research, 19,* 312–323.

Mazzuca, S. A. (1982). Does patient education in chronic disease have therapeutic value? *Journal of Chronic Disease, 35,* 521–529.

McLeroy, K. R., Bibeau, D., Steckler, A., & Glanz, K. (1988). An ecological perspective on health promotion programs. *Health Education Quarterly, 15,* 351–377.

Mermelstein, R., Cohen, S., Lichtenstein, E., Baer, J. S., & Kamarck, T. (1986). Social support and smoking cessation and maintenance. *Journal of Consulting and Clinical Psychology, 54,* 447–453.

Mermelstein, R., Lichtenstein, E., & McIntyre, K. (1983). Partner support and relapse in smoking-cessation programs. *Journal of Consulting and Clinical Psychology, 51,* 465–466.

Minkler, M. (1989). Health education, health promotion and the open society: An historical perspective. *Health Education Quarterly, 16,* 17–30.

Morisky, D., DeMuth, N., & Field-Fass, M. (1985). Evaluation of family health education to build social support for long-term control of high blood pressure. *Health Education Quarterly, 12,* 35–50.

Muhlenkamp, A., & Sayles, J. (1986). Self-esteem, social support, and positive health practices. *Nursing Research, 35,* 334–338.

O'Connell, K. A., & Martin, E. (1987). Highly tempting situations associated with abstinence, temporary lapse, and relapse among participants in smoking cessation programs. *Journal of Consulting and Clinical Psychology, 55,* 367–371.

Oldridge, N., & Jones, N. L. (1983). Improving patient compliance in cardiac exercise rehabilitation: Effects of written agreement and self-monitoring. *Journal of Cardiac Rehabilitation, 3,* 257–262.

Pender, N. (1996). *Health promotion in nursing practice* (3rd ed.). Norwalk, CT: Appleton & Lange.

Pender, N., & Pender, A. (1986). Attitudes, subjective norms, and intentions to engage in health behaviors. *Nursing Research, 35,* 15–18.

Petersen, L., Helgerson, S. D., Gibbons, C. M., Calhoun, C., Ciacco, K. H., & Pitchford, K. C. (1988). Employee smoking behavior changes and attitudes following a restrictive policy on worksite smoking in a large company. *Public Health Reports, 103,* 115–120.

Powers, M., & Wooldridge, P. (1982). Factors influencing knowledge, attitudes, and compliance of hypertensive patients. *Research in Nursing and Health, 85,* 171–182.

Prochaska, J. O., & DiClemente, C. C. (1983). Stages and processes of self-change of smoking: Toward an integrative model of change. *Journal of Consulting and Clinical Psychology, 51,* 390–395.

Redman, B. (1996). *Practice of patient education* (8th ed.). St. Louis, MO: CV Mosby.

Ruzicki, D. A. (1989). Realistically meeting the educational needs of hospitalized acute and short-stay patients. *Nursing Clinics of North America, 24,* 629–637.

Ryan, P. (1987). Strategies for motivating life-style. *Journal of Cardiovascular Nursing, 1,* 54–66.

Ryan, P. (1990). *Behavior change: A concept analysis.* Unpublished manuscript. Milwaukee: University of Wisconsin-Milwaukee.

Saltzer, E. (1980). Social determinants of successful weight loss: An analysis of behavioral intentions and actual behavior. *Basic and Applied Social Psychology, 1,* 329–341.

Saunders, B., & Allsop, S. (1987). Relapse: a psychological perspective. *British Journal of Addiction, 82,* 417–429.

Scandrett, S., & Uecker, S. (1992). Relaxation training. In G. Bulechek & J. McCloskey (Eds.), *Nursing interventions: Essential nursing treatments* (2nd ed.). Philadelphia: WB Saunders.

Shiffman, S. (1982). Relapse following smoking cessation: A situational analysis. *Journal of Consulting and Clinical Psychology, 50,* 71–86.

Shiffman, S. (1984). Cognitive antecedents and sequelae of smoking relapse crisis. *Journal of Applied Social Psychology, 14,* 296–309.

Simonds, S. K. (1983). Individual health counselling and education: Emerging directions from current theory, research, and practice. *Patient Counseling and Health Education, 4,* 175–181.

Somer, E., & Tucker, C. M. (1988). Patient life engagement, spouse marital adjustment, and dietary compliance of hemodialysis patients. *Journal of Compliance in Health Care, 3,* 57–65.

Stanton, A. L. (1987). Determinants of adherence to medical regimens by hypertensive patients. *Journal of Behavioral Medicine, 10,* 377–394.

Steckel, S. (1980). Contracting with patient selected reinforcers. *American Journal of Nursing, 80,* 1596–1599.

Steckel, S. (1982). *Patient contracting.* New York: Appleton-Century-Crofts.

Steele, S. M., & Harmon, V. M. (1993). *Values clarification in nursing* (2nd ed.). East Norwalk, CT: Appleton & Lange.

Supnick, J. A., & Colletti, G. (1984). Relapse coping and problem solving training following treatment for smoking. *Addictive Behaviors, 9,* 401–404.

Swan, G. E., & Denk, C. E. (1987). Dynamic models for the maintenance of smoking cessation: Event history analysis of late relapse. *Journal of Behavioral Medicine, 10,* 527–554.

Syme, S. L., & Alcalay, R. (1982). Control of cigarette smoking from a social perspective. *Annual Review of Public Health, 3,* 179–199.

Thornburg, K. (1982). Coping: Implications for health practitioners. *Patient Counseling and Health Education, 4,* 3–9.

Trower, P., Casey, A., & Dryden, W. (1988). *Cognitive-behavioural counselling in action*. Beverly Hills: Sage.

Uustal, D. (1977). Searching for values. *Image, 9,* 15–17.

Wewers, M. E., & Lenz, E. R. (1987). Relapse among ex-smokers: An example of theory derivation. *Advances in Nursing Science, 9,* 44–53.

Wilson-Barnett, J., & Osborne, J. (1983). Studies evaluating patient teaching: Implications for practice. *International Journal of Nursing Studies, 20,* 33–44.

Yates, A. J., & Thain, J. (1985). Self-efficacy as a predictor of relapse following voluntary cessation of smoking. *Addictive Behaviors, 10,* 291–298.

18

·Enhancing
Self-Esteem

➤ JUDITH FITZGERALD MILLER

Self-esteem is the evaluative component of self-concept. It is a judgment about one's worth. Rosenberg (1989) stated that self-esteem is an attitude of approval or disapproval of self. Self-esteem involves three principal senses of self-regard: self-love, self-acceptance, and a sense of competence (Wells & Marwell, 1976). Self-esteem combines evaluative and affective components. Discrepancies between self-ideal (cognitions and expectations for self) and the actual attainment or fulfillment of the expectations affect self-esteem. Individuals with high self-esteem perceive themselves as worthwhile and significant; they feel confident in influencing desired outcomes. However, persons with low self-esteem feel worthless, of little importance, and unable to affect outcomes. Wells and Marwell (1976) reviewed other labels for self-esteem such as self-love, self-confidence, self-respect, self-acceptance, self-satisfaction, self-regard, self-evaluation, self-appraisal, self-worth, sense of adequacy of personal efficacy, sense of competence, self-ideal congruence, and ego or ego strength. Self-shame would be an opposing label (Morrison, 1989).

Coopersmith (1981) specified the theoretical bases for self-esteem to include:

1. *Significance:* Result of acceptance, attention, and affection from others with a sense of being valued and cared about as a worthwhile person
2. *Competence:* Perception of successful performance of important tasks
3. *Virtue:* Adherence to moral and ethical standards
4. *Power:* Ability to influence and control events, to control one's own life, and to influence others

The developmental influences of self-esteem in children are acceptance of children by their parents, enforcement of clearly defined limits, and respect for children's latitude within set limits (Coopersmith, 1981).

Persons who have high self-esteem appear to be adjusted, happy, competent, and free from undue anxiety (Gilberts, 1983); take risks; interact with others with confidence (Hirst & Metcalf, 1984); and report less pain in pain-induced studies (Feldman, 1986). Persons with low self-esteem use negative self-statements (Crouch & Straub, 1983), expect rejection and failure, and project past failure into the future (Wells & Marwell, 1976). They are also dependent on others, shy, nonexplorative, and guarded (Rosenberg, 1989). Cohen (1959) noted that persons with low self-esteem incorporate negative information into their concepts of self; they are more sensitive to negative feedback.

Although self-acceptance is fundamental to high self-esteem, illness challenges self-acceptance. Chronic illness presents lifelong demands for coping with a health alteration and imposed health regimen. The diagnosis of a chronic illness may be accompanied by a change in the individual's view of self (self-perception). If the individual's view of self is one of physical strength, endurance, and wholeness, there is a greater likelihood that the individual will have a higher self-esteem than if the self-perception is one of physical weakness, lack of energy, and altered body function. A change in self-perception occurs in chronically ill persons when previous aspirations need to be modified, roles changed, and other adjustments made because of altered physical reserve. When physical ability deteriorates, individuals may conclude that they are worthless, undeserving of self-respect, and generally inadequate. This lowered self-esteem is present in all clients during some phase of the health problem.

Norris and Kunes-Connell (1985, 1988) conceptualized three types of self-esteem. *Basic self-esteem* is the stable core sense of self-worth. *Functional* or *situational self-esteem* is that self-worth that varies with situations, rewards, and failures. *Defensive self-esteem* protects individuals from situational threats. It is also referred to as *pseudo self-esteem*. Although their work has focused on validating three distinct types of self-esteem as nursing diagnoses (Norris & Kunes-Connell, 1988, 1985), no attempt is made throughout this chapter to distinguish among these three types of self-esteem. A review of self-esteem as a power resource, assessment of self-esteem, and nursing strategies to enhance self-esteem are included in this chapter.

POWER RESOURCE

High self-esteem empowers the chronically ill individual in the following ways:

- It enables the person to be an active participant in care.
- It helps the person develop confidence in interpersonal communication.
- It provides the person with accurate internal feedback as opposed to the inaccurate, derogatory feedback that occurs in persons with low self-esteem.
- It enhances the potential for successful role performance.
- It is a resource for coping (Walsh & Walsh, 1989).

The level of self-esteem is significant in motivating clients to work on lifestyle modification or to follow through with rehabilitation programs (McGlashan, 1988).

Being an active participant in care decisions and assuming responsibility for care to hasten independence in self-management depend on many factors, one of which is self-esteem. Self-esteem enables the client to assume an active role in controlling care. Being a self-care agent requires the clients to have motivation, knowledge, and self-worth (Kearney & Fleisher, 1979). Clients with high self-esteem feel that they are worth the time and effort needed to maintain and improve health and eagerly take responsibility to meet self-care needs. Conversely, individuals with low self-esteem may be unable to make self-care decisions and assume responsibility for care outcomes. For example, an obese individual with low self-esteem may feel undeserving of better health and unworthy of close dietary monitoring, health-care personnel's time, and his or her own effort.

The confidence and competence individuals have in their interpersonal relationships are positively influenced by high self-esteem. Interactions with significant others (those from whom acceptance is sought) and with strangers provide feedback about self. If the individual feels worthwhile and demonstrates self-approval during interactions, others will respond with similar feelings of respect and approval. These clients feel confident that their own concerns are not petty or foolish and are deserving of professional consultation.

High self-esteem enables individuals to more accurately interpret feedback about self, whereas low self-esteem causes individuals to distort feedback. Persons with low self-esteem may consistently engage in an internal dialogue that results in a negative interpretation about self. Guilt and self-pity may be induced. For example, consider Mr. C., who has a colostomy. When his dressing is changed on a particular day, his nurse is less talkative than usual. Mr. C. interprets this as being due to her repugnance toward him. The client may carry on a silent dialogue to reaffirm his false interpretation. It seems as though the client seeks reinforcement for his own negative feeling of low self-worth. Instead of being open in interactions and validating the meaning of the feedback, the client may interpret the message in a way that is destructive to self.

High self-esteem breeds success in performing life roles. Self-esteem provides confidence in undertaking new roles (such as assuming the role of self-care agent) and a recognition of personal potential for accomplishing goals associated with familiar roles. The belief in one's own ability to be successful operates as a self-fulfilling prophecy. The client with high self-esteem confidently anticipates success, which in fact does materialize.

Coping mechanisms of persons with high and low self-esteem may be distinctly different. Cohen (1959) stated that preferred defenses (mental coping mechanisms) of persons with high self-esteem include denial and repression or ignoring conflicting impulses. Persons with low self-esteem used projective and expressive defenses. Therefore, persons who had low self-esteem before the onset of chronic illness may experience greater threats to self-esteem as a result of the illness than do persons with high premorbid self-esteem. This may be especially true if development of the illness is viewed as a personal shortcoming or a negative component of self.

Because self-esteem is a power resource, nursing efforts to enhance self-esteem help to increase the client's perceived power (alleviating powerlessness). Ascertaining the client's level of self-esteem is an important first step.

ASSESSMENT OF SELF-ESTEEM

To determine the nature of the client's self-esteem, information is gathered through observation, an interview, analysis of the client's role performance, and identification of changes in social interaction.

Observation of Self-Derogatory Comments

Nursing observations of patient behavior include noting the pattern of verbal comments by the patient over time. Self-derogatory verbal comments indicate low self-esteem. Examples are the following statements:

I feel I am no longer whole and therefore not a good productive person.
I can't do anything anymore. Now I am good for nothing, I'm useless.
I feel guilt and embarrassment when I have to ask for help.
I've lost my independence; that is mighty rough.
I've lost faith in myself.
Sometimes I feel my body has turned against me.
I don't like myself this way.
I simply don't like myself.

These comments indicate feelings of insignificance, uselessness, and worthlessness.

Other observations of client interaction may indicate low self-esteem. The client may be hesitant to bother the nurse or ask for help. The person with low self-esteem may avoid direct eye contact when communicating with others, especially when interacting with authority figures. The client's reluctance to participate in the medical plan may also indicate low self-esteem.

Interview

After a trusting nurse-client relationship has been established, specific questions can be raised to gather information about the client's self-esteem. Besides gathering data for self-esteem assessment, interview questions enable the client to review existing abilities and develop self-insight, thereby providing an opportunity to enhance self-esteem. The following questions are helpful in gathering self-esteem information:

How has having arthritis (or whatever the health problem is) changed the way you feel about yourself?

In evaluating your abilities, how would you describe yourself?

Would you say you had a positive or negative attitude toward yourself?

What do you like best about yourself?

What are your weak points?

What do you do to feel good about yourself?

Are you able to complete the care needed as a result of the illness?

What changes in your life will occur as a result of the illness? Are important losses involved?

Do you anticipate any differences in the way your family and friends will respond to you?

Tell me about your accomplishments and disappointments in life.

Information gathered by using client self-report (responses to the above or similar questions) can be validated with the client by asking the questions again or by confirming responses later. The self-report is compared with observations, social interaction, and role performance.

Role Performance

Role changes may be imposed by illness. Sometimes previous work roles are no longer possible. The more important the role is in determining the person's self-concept, the more devastating the role loss is to the person's self-esteem. For example, if a symphony pianist suffered a traumatic amputation of three fingers, the concept of self as a pianist would be threatened. The client's breadwinning capacity may be threatened temporarily until the client can accept a substitute role, for example, teaching piano or developing a related talent such as vocal music performance. Questions to be considered in assessing role performance include the following:

> How threatening is the health problem to the individual's definition of self or self-concept?
>
> Will the health problem interfere with established career goals or the present employment role?
>
> Does the health problem cause the client to feel less sexually attractive? (Joint deformities and decreased mobility of arthritis may limit activities the individual views as important for developing and maintaining sexual relationships.)
>
> Does the client perceive self to be less adequate in social relationships because of the health problem? (Clients with chronic diarrhea from Crohn's disease may hesitate to become involved in group activities to avoid the embarrassment of having to take frequent trips to the rest room.)

Changes in Social Interaction

Although information about self-esteem and social interaction relates closely to role performance, specific changes in social interaction can be noted. Have social activities been eliminated, leisure activities changed, or relationships with family and significant others altered? The client's family and friends may relate that the client's interaction themes focus on negative self-talk. Self-derogatory comments may dominate conversation. Friends may eventually withdraw. The resulting social isolation may contribute to further lowering of self-esteem.

Valued social activities may be eliminated. For example, the client with severe emphysema may avoid the weekly card party at the senior citizens' center to avoid exposure to crowds and respiratory infections. Although the decision may be a good one in terms of health maintenance, unless acceptable substitutes are found, positive feelings about self may diminish. The nurse can help the client find an alternative activity; for example, the client could select three friends to meet weekly at the client's home to play cards.

Low self-esteem indicators (verbalizations and behaviors) can be summarized in three categories: changes in role performance, changes in interpersonal relationships, and presence of negative self-talk (Table 18.1).

Assessment of self-esteem is important for designing appropriate individual strategies to enhance self-esteem. Individuals evaluate themselves highly in situations in which they achieve a sense of mastery. A sense of mastery is based on the person's behavior.

Table 18.1 ➤ **INDICATORS OF LOW SELF-ESTEEM**		
Interpersonal Relationships	**Negative Self-Talk**	**Role Performance**
Feels unworthy of nurses' time, care, attention	Verbalizations convey: Self-blame	Expresses having few accomplishments
Hesitant to ask for help	Guilt over disease	Expresses doubts about ability to fulfill roles
Pessimistic	Self-derogatory comments	Feels inferior; compares self to others
Feels undeserving of praise	Negative attitude toward self	Feels own actions will have little effect on an outcome (feels ineffective)
Resentful of others who are well	(physical self, personal self, and spiritual self)	
Lacks assertiveness		
Lacks self-confidence in one-to-one and/or group interactions	Feeling of uselessness	Feels insignificant
Self-conscious	Lack of self-respect	Unable to take pride in accomplishing goals
Expresses a sense of worthlessness		Unable to set goals
		Feels has failed in life's mission
		Lacks a sense of competence

Specific Tools for Self-Esteem Assessment

Paper-and-pencil tests to measure self-esteem include Rosenberg's Self-Esteem Scale (1989); Coopersmith's Self-Esteem Scale (1981, 1982) which has both a child and an adult version; and the Children's Self-Esteem Questionnaire by Busse, Mansfield, and Messinger (1974).

Taylor (1982) developed another self-esteem assessment guide based on the four theoretical bases of self-esteem (significance, competence, virtue, and power). Questions are posed to clients about the importance of each of the four theoretical bases and the extent to which they are present in their lives.

SELF-ESTEEM AND CHRONIC ILLNESS

Although the research findings about whether or not persons with chronic illness have lower self-esteem than healthy persons have been inconclusive (Weinberg-Asher, 1976; Wright, 1983), high self-esteem has been correlated with adjustment to disability and chronic illness (Burckhardt, 1985; Linkowski & Dunn, 1974). Self-esteem, low negative attitude, internal control over health, and perceived social support all contributed significantly to quality of life in 94 adults with arthritis (Burckhardt, 1985). A significant relationship between self-esteem and acceptance of disability in 55 disabled college students was reported by Linkowski and Dunn (1974). Self-esteem was also identified as a positive factor influencing medication compliance in adolescents with rheumatoid arthritis (Litt, Cuskey, & Rosenberg, 1982). Antonucci and Jackson (1983) found in their national survey of 2264 adults that not only was self-esteem lower in persons with a health problem, but there was also a linear relationship between severity of illness and low self-esteem. The linear relationship was stronger for men than women. Similar findings are reported for elderly persons in that those with poorer health, more daily pain, and greater disability had lower self-esteem (Hunter, Linn, & Harris, 1981–1982). Persons in their sample with low self-esteem had more anxiety, greater external control, and greater depression. Lisanti (1989) found that persons with continuous chronic back pain had lower self-esteem scores than those with intermittent chronic pain. On the other hand, although subjects reported significant differences in health status, self-esteem was not significantly different among groups of women with rheumatoid arthritis or systemic lupus erythematosus and those who were healthy (Cornwell & Schmitt, 1990). Body image was significantly lower in women with lupus. Hastings (see Chap. 12) found significant relationships between hope and social support, and between hope and adaptation in 30 persons with multiple sclerosis (MS). These findings were supported by Foote, Piazza, Holcombe, Paul, and Dattin (1990), who also found significant positive relationships between self-esteem and hope and self-esteem and social support in 40 persons with MS. Persons with MS who had severe limits in mobility (no walking) had significantly lower self-esteem than those depending on assistive devices or a wheelchair (Walsh & Walsh, 1989). Walsh and Walsh also reported that a positive affect was predictive of high self-esteem.

Crigger (1992) studied the influence of selected variables on adaptation of 90 women to MS including self-esteem, disease disability, social support, uncertainty, and spiritual well-being and mastery. The findings support the importance of self-esteem in achieving a sense of mastery. Social support positively affected self-esteem in this sample. Among all the variables, spiritual well-being was found to have the greatest total positive effect on mastery. Factors influencing perceptions of quality of life in 126 persons with chronic obstructive pulmonary disease were studied by Anderson (1995). Although dyspnea, functional status, and depression had a significant negative impact on quality of life, Anderson (1995) found that the individual's self-esteem had a positive influence on perceptions of quality of life. In another study on quality of life in 149 persons with coronary artery disease surviving a cardiac arrest, Motzer and Stewart (1996) found that when poor health vulnerability, perceived social support, and self-esteem were held constant, a sense of coherence improved quality of life.

Chronic illnesses that have an effect on sexuality also threaten self-esteem. LeMone (1996) studied the physical effects of diabetes on sexuality by interviewing 20 women with diabetes. Problems affecting sexuality and ultimately self-esteem included fatigue, changes in perimenstrual blood-glucose control, vaginitis, decreased libido, decreased vaginal lubrication, and increased time to reach orgasm.

Chronic Illness as Loss of Self

Charmaz (1983) studied the nature of suffering of 57 adults with various chronic health problems. Her work illustrates the impact of chronic illness as a threat to self-perception and provides a framework for nursing care directed at preserving self-esteem in chronically ill persons. Through in-depth interviews Charmaz identified that chronic illness meant suffering a loss of self because of:

1. Living a restricted lifestyle
2. Existing in social isolation
3. Experiencing discredited definitions of self
4. Becoming a burden

Living a restricted lifestyle means that the individual is unable to do the things once valued and enjoyed. In the most severe stage of illness progression, it may resemble an all-consuming retreat into illness. Recall the stages of illness progression from an earlier chapter: interrupted time, time intrusion, and encapsulation.

Social isolation occurs because of a restricted social network, little ability or energy to share leisure activities, and increasing amounts of time spent on illness management. Positive feedback about self is dependent in part upon social interaction. Persons with MS who belonged to a support group had higher self-esteem than those who did not (Walsh & Walsh, 1989). Orr, Reznikoff, and Smith (1989) found that of the 121 adolescents and young adults suffering burns, those who had more social support had higher self-esteem, more positive body image, and less depression.

Discrediting definitions of self occur because of feedback from others as well as from unmet expectations of the ill person. Ill persons may scrutinize encounters with others, finding hints of negative self-reflections, or, in some instances, the negative feedback may be blatant. Charmaz (1983) found that discrediting is more likely to occur when the ill person feels vulnerable or identifies with the individual providing the discrediting message.

Becoming a burden occurs when the individual becomes more dependent and immobilized. When one perceives one's self as a burden, self-worth is lowered. Physical, economic, and psychological dependency all play a role in perceiving self as a burden to others.

Constructing Positive Views of Self

Wright (1983) provided a framework for disabled persons to view themselves positively and avoid the devaluation that results from losses due to illness by focusing on (1) enlarging their scope of values, (2) subordinating physique, (3) containing disability effects, and (4) avoiding emphasis on comparative asset values.

Enlarging the scope of values refers to persons recognizing their own assets or abilities and that they can participate in desired activities in their own way despite limitations. It is moving beyond grieving over the losses due to illness. It may require accepting a new way of walking or receiving sexual gratification.

Subordinating physique means there is less psychic energy spent on worrying about the physical component of self in terms of appearance and physical prowess, and more energy is spent recognizing that an individual's definition of self extends beyond the physical self.

Containing disability means preventing the disability from consuming the entire identity of the person.

Avoiding comparison of asset values means spending less time ruminating and comparing present abilities to past abilities or to others' abilities and more time on valuing and accepting self and others.

Other works are helpful in designing a model of strategies to enhance self-esteem. Turk (1979) proposed the following to be essential components for adaptation to chronic illness: (1) knowledge about the nature of the illness (including therapy), (2) ability to use coping strategies, (3) presence of a social support system, (4) problem-solving attitude in facing the challenges of illness management, (5) sense of personal control, and (6) motivation to implement the required behaviors for illness management. Development of these personal resources contributes to self-worth.

Miller (1987) recommended the following categories of strategies to enhance self-esteem in adolescents: (1) establishing a trusting relationship, (2) promoting social interaction and involvement in groups, and (3) helping the adolescent discover his or her own assets. Although few studies on strategies to enhance self-esteem have been conducted, Thomas (1988) tested the effect of a meditation-relaxation training program on 11 black women and found that it had a significant impact on self-esteem and life satisfaction. A comparison didactic stress management information group ($N = 10$) had lower scores (Thomas, 1988). Goldberg and Fitzpatrick (1980) found that the 15 elderly persons who participated in movement therapy had higher self-esteem and morale than the 15 persons in the control group.

NURSING STRATEGIES TO ENHANCE SELF-ESTEEM

Another model for enhancing self-esteem based on literature and research findings as well as on study of the chronically ill is presented here. Specific areas for enhancing self-esteem may include developing the following: cognitive control, self-affirmation, positive perception of role performance competence, interpersonal relationships, social activities, and self-care competence. It should be noted that the proposed strategies have not been systematically studied to verify the outcomes suggested.

Cognitive Control

Helping persons become sensitized to thoughts and self-talk that are self-derogatory will reduce this self-initiated reinforcement of low self-worth. A direct reflective communication technique can be used to help the patient become aware of negative self-talk, to reappraise the statements and consequent feelings, and to find substitute positive statements. The goal is to change the person's internal dialogue as well as to change the negative thoughts and perceptions (McKay & Fanning, 1994; Meichenbaum, 1986). Examples of positive statements may have to be suggested to the person, such as, "Today I'm the best me possible. Because I am human, I am worthwhile. I am special. There is no one like me in the entire world." Helping the person become aware of distorted thinking such as catastrophizing, filtering out all positive details, and maximizing negative possibilities is helpful (McKay, Davis, & Fanning, 1981). The person is to be helped to have accurate perceptions of the situation and to avoid a totally devastating, demoralizing view.

The intended *outcome* of this strategy is positive self-talk and an accurate, not a distorted perception of the situation.

Self-Affirmation

Self-rejecting behaviors as indicated, as well as berating self, feeling embarrassed about disabilities, believing self to be unattractive, and giving credit deserved for self to others, all need to be eliminated before self-affirmation can occur. Self-affirmation includes giving self approval, talking gently to self, forgiving self, having fun without feeling guilty, rewarding self with a special treat (quiet time alone, listening to a favorite piece of music, or any appropriate reward), liking self and accepting affection from others (Bloomfield & Kory, 1988).

The *outcome* of self-affirmation is greater self-regard.

Role Performance Review and Role Modification

Despite disability, not all roles are abolished. Preventing negative spread of the view that the entire body is dysfunctional can be expanded beyond body image to social aspects of the individual as well. Roles that remain intact should be reviewed, and role supplementation strategies should be made for roles that must be modified. Together the nurse and client review intact roles making a verbal listing. Helping the client re-define roles may also be needed. Just because the client is no longer able to perform the physical task according to previous criteria does not mean that he or she no longer has the role. On the other hand, some roles will have to be surrendered, but this giving up of roles is necessary as well for healthy individuals at various times in their lives. An example of role modification may be the father of a 12-year-old whose father-ing role was defined, in part, by his active participation in his son's soccer plays. Because of an illness progression such as arthritis, the physical participation may become more limited; however, the nurse can review how the father can fulfill this role in other ways: watching the games, taking notes regarding specific plays, reviewing game strategies, critiquing drills, and so forth.

Role performance review is akin to reminiscing used with elderly persons, which has had positive results in terms of life satisfaction, adjustment, and ego integrity.

The *outcome* of role performance review is perceived self-competence.

Self-Care Competence

Achieving mastery in managing the health problem will enhance the client's perception of control. Perceived control has been correlated with high self-esteem in persons with cancer, for example (Lewis, 1982). Mastery includes the client's having knowledge about the specific pre-scribed health regimen and desired outcomes as well as having the skill to carry out the regimen. It also includes helping the client develop internal awareness of physiological and psychological cues that demand attention and, at times, medical intervention. Training in new skill development may need to begin with activities of daily living. Reinforcing independence with activities such as dressing and performing hygiene highlights progress and enhances self-esteem as the person becomes aware of new accomplishments.

The *outcome* of developing self-care competence is perceived control.

Interpersonal Relationships

The nature of the relationship between the nurse and client should be characterized by unconditional acceptance, positive regard, mutual respect, and an expectation for mutual growth because of the relationship. Eventually the nurse can share with the client how he or she benefited from knowing the client. Recognition of the client's knowledge or unique abilities and expressions of appreciation for insights gained from knowing the client enhance self-esteem. The nurse is to communicate sincere interest in the client as a whole person and not just an interest in the health problem.

Families need to be helped to understand the powerful role they play in the self-esteem of the client. They may need counseling to help them grieve over the losses experienced by their loved one as well as to help them see the richness of the personality of their loved one. They need to know that persons who are questioning their self-worth readily interpret messages from others as negative (Shrauger & Rosenberg, 1970), so any cues conveying a pseudorepugnance should be avoided.

It is through relationships with others that individuals receive affirmation of their worth. Preventing alienation and isolation from previously enjoyed activities is necessary. Helping the client conserve energy and make plans to continue whatever social activities previously contributed to positive self-esteem is worthwhile in preserving self-acceptance.

It should be noted that self-help groups do not have positive effects for all persons with disabilities. Dixon's (1981) study of 142 persons with disabilities revealed that group identification was strong among those with visible handicaps (persons with amputations, spinal cord injuries, and strokes), whereas persons with arthritis and emotional disorders preferred dissociation with others having the same diagnosis. Little research has been done on the specific effects of support groups for persons with physical handicaps. The results of one study of 34 women with rheumatoid arthritis concluded that group counseling had a significant effect on improving the self-concept and knowledge of the women (Kaplan & Kozin, 1981).

The *outcome* of experiencing healthy interpersonal relationships is positive feedback about self. Clients may realize that others accept and enjoy them despite the illness. Self-acceptance is the desired end result.

The model in Figure 18.1 summarizes the strategies to enhance self-esteem. Outcomes for each strategy are suggested. Although not discussed in this text, the impact of each opposing strategy and specified outcome are presented in the model. For example, the strategies and outcomes leading to decreased self-esteem (Fig. 18.2) include:

- Cognitive distortion resulting in negative self-talk
- Self-denial and self-doubt resulting in self-rejection
- Fixation on role incompetence resulting in reinforced self-incompetence
- Self-care incompetence resulting in powerlessness
- Social isolation resulting in lack of affirmation of worth

Self-esteem has been studied as it relates to other aspects of life. Barron (1987) discovered a relationship between learned helplessness and low self-esteem in 36 women who were divorced after their first marriage. When causal explanations for the divorce were found to be internal, stable, and global (dimensions of learned helplessness), then more emotional distress and lower self-esteem were present. Spouses

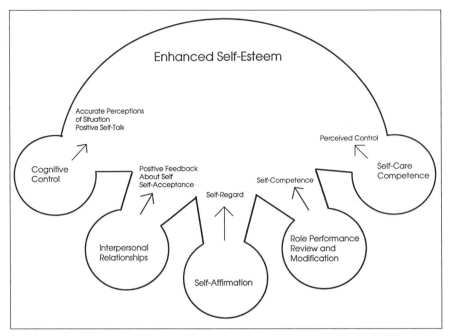

FIGURE 18.1 ➤ Strategies to enhance self-esteem.

have an impact on each other's self-esteem. The more positive a husband's appraisal of his wife, the higher the woman's self-esteem (Meisenhelder, 1986). Self-esteem has also been associated with positive health behaviors (Muhlenkamp & Sayles, 1986).

SUMMARY

A basic human need is to feel worthwhile to self and others. Personal worth is needed for all individuals, sick or well. Self-esteem has been identified as a central concern influencing the behavior of all persons. Helping persons find intrinsic worth, that is, not meeting some other-stipulated criteria for what is worthwhile, is the goal. In our Protestant work ethic ideology, we may be challenged to help persons to be more satisfied over being and less concerned about doing. Quality of life is not possible for persons with low self-esteem. High self-esteem could insulate individuals with a disability against the debilitating psychological problems of hopelessness and depression. Acceptance means viewing the loss due to chronic illness as nondevaluing (Dembo, Leviton, & Wright, 1975). Self-esteem levels in turn may reflect the levels of acceptance by the individual of the illness. The need for more research on self-esteem in the chronically ill is evident.

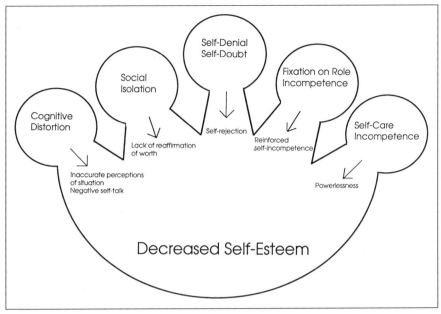

FIGURE 18.2 ➤ Mechanisms that decrease self-esteem.

REFERENCES

Anderson, L. (1995). The effect of chronic obstructive pulmonary disease on quality of life. *Research in Nursing and Health, 18,* 547–556.

Antonucci, T., & Jackson, J. (1983). Physical health and self-esteem. *Family and Community Health, 6,* 1–9.

Barron, C. (1987). Women's causal explanations of divorce: Relationships to self-esteem and emotional distress. *Research in Nursing and Health, 10,* 345–353.

Bloomfield, H., & Kory, R. (1988). *Inner joy: New strategies for adding more pleasure to your life.* New York: Berkley Publishing.

Burckhardt, C. (1985). The impact of arthritis on quality of life. *Nursing Research, 34,* 11–16.

Busse, T. V., Mansfield, R. S., & Messinger, L. J. (1974). *Activities in child and adolescent development.* New York: Harper & Row.

Charmaz, K. (1983). Loss of self: A fundamental for suffering in the chronically ill. *Sociology of Health and Illness, 5,* 168–195.

Cohen, A. (1959). Some implications of self-esteem for social influence. In C. Hovland & I. Janis (Eds.), *Personality and persuasibility.* New Haven, CT: Yale University Press.

Coopersmith, S. (1981). *Antecedents of self-esteem* (2nd ed.). San Francisco: Freeman.

Coopersmith, S. (1982). *Self-esteem inventories.* Palo Alto, CA: Consulting Psychologist Press.

Cornwell, C., & Schmitt, M. (1990). Perceived health status, self-esteem, and body image in women with rheumatoid arthritis or systemic lupus erythematosus. *Research in Nursing and Health, 13,* 99–107.

Crigger, N. J. (1992). *An adaptation model for women with multiple sclerosis*. Unpublished doctoral dissertation, Gainesville: University of Florida.

Crouch, M. A., & Straub, V. (1983). Enhancement of self-esteem in adults. *Family and Community Health, 6,* 65–78.

Dembo, T., Leviton, G. L., & Wright, B. A. (1975). Adjustment to misfortune: A problem of social-psychological rehabilitation. *Rehabilitation Psychology, 22,* 1–100.

Dixon, J. K. (1981). Group-self identification and physical handicap: Implications for patient support groups. *Research in Nursing and Health, 4,* 299–308.

Feldman, H. R. (1986). Self-esteem, types of attributional style, and sensation and distress pain ratings in males. *Journal of Advanced Nursing, 11,* 75–86.

Foote, A., Piazza, D., Holcombe, J., Paul P., & Daffin, P. (1990). Hope, self-esteem and social support in persons with multiple sclerosis. *Journal of Neuroscience Nursing, 22,* 155–159.

Gilberts, R. (1983). The evaluation of self-esteem. *Family and Community Health, 6,* 29–49.

Goldberg, W., & Fitzpatrick, J. (1980). Movement therapy with the aged. *Nursing Research, 29,* 339–346.

Hirst, S., & Metcalf, B. (1984). Promoting self-esteem. *Journal of Gerontological Nursing, 10,* 72–77.

Hunter, K. I., Linn, M. W., & Harris, R. (1981–1982). Characteristics of high and low self-esteem in the elderly. *International Journal of Aging and Human Development, 14,* 117–126.

Kaplan, S., & Kozin, F. (1981). A controlled study of group counseling in rheumatoid arthritis. *Journal of Rheumatology, 8,* 91–99.

Kearney, B., & Fleisher, B. (1979). Development of an instrument to measure exercise of self-care agency. *Research in Nursing and Health, 2,* 25–34.

LeMone, P. (1996). The physical effects of diabetes on sexuality in women. *The Diabetes Educator, 22,* 361–366.

Lewis, F. A. (1982). Experienced personal control and quality of life in late-stage cancer patients. *Nursing Research, 31,* 113–119.

Linkowski, D. C., & Dunn, M. (1974). Self-concept and acceptance of disability. *Rehabilitation Counseling Bulletin, 14,* 236–244.

Lisanti, P. (1989). Perceived body space and self-esteem in adult males with and without chronic low back pain. *Orthopaedic Nursing, 8,* 49–56.

Litt, T. F., Cuskey, W. R., & Rosenberg, A. (1982). Role of self-esteem and autonomy in determining medication compliance among adolescents with juvenile rheumatoid arthritis. *Pediatrics, 69,* 15–17.

McGlashan, R. (1988). Strategies for rebuilding self-esteem for the cardiac patient. *Dimensions of Critical Care, 7,* 28–38.

McKay, M., Davis, M., & Fanning. P. (1981). *Thoughts and feelings: The art of cognitive stress intervention.* Richmond, CA: New Harbinger Publications.

McKay, M., & Fanning. P. (1994). *Self-esteem.* New York: Fine Communications.

Meichenbaum, D. (1986). Toward a cognitive theory of self-control. In G. Schwartz & D. Shapiro (Eds.), *Consciousness and self-regulation: Advances in research* (Vol. 1.). New York: Plenum Press.

Meisenhelder, J. B. (1986). Self-esteem in women: The influence of employment and perception of husband's appraisals. *Image—Journal of Nursing Scholarship, 18,* 8–13.

Miller, S. (1987). Promoting self-esteem in the hospitalized adolescent: Clinical interventions. *Issues in Comprehensive Pediatric Nursing, 10,* 187–194.

Morrison, A. (1989). *Shame: The underside of narcissism.* Hillsdale, NJ: Analytic Press.

Motzer, S. U., & Stewart, B. (1996). Sense of coherence as a predictor of quality of life in persons with coronary heart disease surviving cardiac arrest. *Research in Nursing and Health, 19,* 287–298.

Muhlenkamp, A., & Sayles, J. (1986). Self-esteem, social support, and positive health practices. *Nursing Research, 35,* 334–338.

Norris, J., & Kunes-Connell, M. (1985). Self-esteem disturbance. *Nursing Clinics of North America, 20,* 745–761.

Norris, J., & Kunes-Connell, M. (1988). A multimodal approach to validation and refinement of an existing nursing diagnosis. *Archives of Psychiatric Nursing, 2,* 103–109.

Orr, D., Reznikoff, M., & Smith, G. (1989). Body image, self-esteem and depression in burn-injured adolescents and young adults. *Journal of Burn Care and Rehabilitation, 10,* 454–461.

Rosenberg, M. (1989). *Society and the adolescent self-image.* Hanover: University Press of New England.

Shrauger, J., & Rosenberg, M. (1970). Self-esteem and the effects of success and failure feedback on performance. *Journal of Personality, 33,* 404–406.

Taylor, M. (1982). The needs for self-esteem. In H. Yura & M. Walsh (Eds.), *Human Needs 2 and the Nursing Process* (pp. 117–153). Norwalk, CT: Appleton-Century-Crofts.

Thomas, B. (1988). Self-esteem and life satisfaction. *Journal of Gerontological Nursing, 14,* 25–30.

Turk, D. (1979). Factors influencing the adaptive process with chronic illness. In E. G. Sarason & C. D. Spielberger (Eds.), *Stress and anxiety* (Vol. 6). Washington, DC: Hemisphere Publishing.

Walsh, A., & Walsh, P. A. (1989). Love, self-esteem and multiple sclerosis. *Social Science and Medicine, 29,* 793–798.

Weinberg-Asher, N. (1976). The effects of physical disability on self-perception. *Rehabilitation Counseling Bulletin, 20,* 18–20.

Wells, L. E., & Marwell, G. (1976). *Self-esteem: Its conceptualization and measurement.* Beverly Hills, CA: Sage.

Wright, B. (1983). *Physical disability: A psychosocial approach* (2nd ed.). New York: Harper & Row.

19

Inspiring Hope

➤ Judith Fitzgerald Miller

One of a person's most valued, private, and powerful resources is hope. Hope is an intrinsic component of life that provides dynamism for the spirit (Adams & Proulx, 1975), saving individuals from apathetic inaction. It is the affect that accompanies faith (belief system). Although faith could not be sustained without hope, the basis of hope is faith. Hope means anticipating success, yet having some uncertainty. It is the negation of the worst possible outcome (Beck, Kovacs, & Weissman, 1975).

HOPE AS A POWER RESOURCE

Hope is a power resource in that it (1) enables transcendence (Bloch, 1970), as from earthly suffering; (2) is a buffer for stress (Korner, 1970); (3) creates a sense of well-being, combating a futile painful state of despair (Fromm, 1968); (4) enables healthy ego functioning (Heagle, 1975); (5) provides a sense of freedom during times of suffering (Lynch, 1987; Marcel, 1962); and (6) plays a role in psychotherapeutic and physical healing (Aardema, 1984; Diez-Manrique, 1984; Frank, 1968, 1975; Menninger, 1959; Pruyser, 1963).

HOPE DEFINED

Although Stotland (1984) defined hope as an expectation greater than zero of achieving a goal, hope is more than anticipating goal accomplishment.

Hope is a state of being, characterized by an anticipation of a continued good state, an improved state or a release from a perceived entrapment. The anticipation may or may not be founded on concrete, real world evidence. Hope is an anticipation of a future that is good and is

523

based upon: mutuality (relationships with others), a sense of personal competence, coping ability, psychological well-being, purpose and meaning in life, as well as a sense of "the possible." (Miller, 1986, p. 52)

Dufault (1981) described two spheres of hope: particularized and generalized. Particularized hope refers to the anticipation of achieving a specific desired goal. Generalized hope contributes to a feeling of well-being and provides a sense that life is worthwhile. It is an impetus to carry on with life's responsibilities and to transcend any dependence on particular objects of hope (Dufault & Martocchio, 1985). There are varied characteristics and dimensions of hope, including affective (sensations and emotions), cognitive (thoughts, insights, and imagination), affiliative (connectedness with others), temporal (time sense), and contextual (life circumstance) (Dufault & Martocchio, 1985). Hope cannot exist alone, but is dependent upon communion with another (Marcel, 1962). When significant others believe in the possibility of a positive outcome and convey a willingness to share the crisis, hope is enlivened. "Hope is an inner readiness, that of an intense but not yet spent activeness" (Fromm, 1968, pp. 11–12). Everything human beings do in life is based on some level of hope.

Owen (1989) proposed six hope attributes: goal setting, positive personal attributes (courage, optimism, positive attitude), future redefinition, meaning of life, peace, and energy. Stanley's (1978) definition of hope resulted from a qualitative study of 100 college students and concluded hope to be "a confident expectation that a future good, although accompanied by doubt and fear, is realistically possible through active endeavor, supportive interpersonal relationships and a religious faith" (p. 50). Stanley proposed seven common elements of hope: (1) expectation of a significant future outcome, (2) feeling of confidence in the outcome, (3) transcendence, (4) interpersonal relatedness, (5) a comfortable feeling, (6) an uncomfortable feeling, and (7) action to affect outcomes. For additional definitions, see the matrix of 16 hope definitions derived from research, clinical practice, conceptual, and conjectural orientations in Miller (1986, appendix A). Although there are varied definitions of hope, there is a consensus that hope is a multidimensional, complex construct.

Levels of Hope

Three levels of hope can be described, as shown in Figure 19.1. The first level is the most elementary, in which superficial wishes—as for basic material goods or a nice day—are included. Shallow optimism characterizes this level. When this level of hope is not actualized, little despair occurs and little psychic energy is expended.

The second level of hope includes hoping for relationships, self-improvement, and self-accomplishments. When hope at this level is

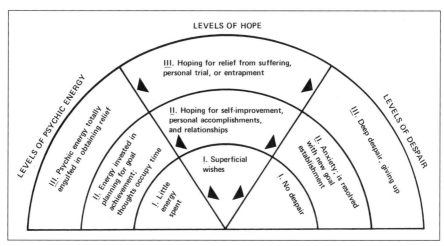

FIGURE 19.1 ➤ Levels of hope, despair, and psychic energy.

thwarted, the resultant level of despair is characterized by anxiety. The anxiety is relieved with new goal establishment. Psychic energy investment is greater than at the first level but less than at the next stage. Thoughts about goal achievement occupy considerable time and energy.

The third level of hope arises out of suffering, personal trial, or state of captivity. Marcel (1962) stated that it is in a situation tempted by despair that hope has its true meaning. Deep despair or giving up occurs when relief is not imminent by the evaluation of the individual. Total engulfment of psychic energy occurs at this point.

This chapter deals with the third level of hope—hope at its most intense and powerful level. Maintaining hope despite a downward physical course is a challenge (coping task) of the chronically ill. Included in this chapter is a discussion of the assessment of hope-hopelessness and nursing strategies to inspire hope.

Chronic illness, by virtue of its unpredictable nature and concomitant losses, precipitates powerlessness. When powerlessness is not contained, hopelessness can result. As shown in Figure 19.2, the cycle of powerlessness leads to depression and low self-esteem, causing hopelessness that, in turn, immobilizes the individual. The cycle continues until the giving up associated with prolonged hopelessness with no relief in sight leads to total despair and thought of self-harm may occur. The hastening of death may appear desirable. A clinical description of hopelessness leading to death is described in Chapter 8.

Losses of the Chronically Ill

Cumulative losses suffered by chronically ill patients can lead to hopelessness. Not only does the chronically ill individual suffer from

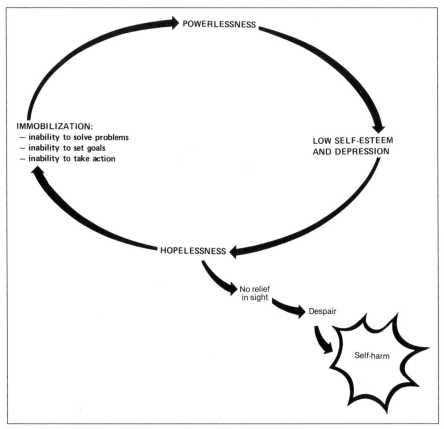

FIGURE 19.2 ➤ Powerlessness-hopelessness cycle.

loss of health status and body-function control—for example, coordination—but also the person may suffer loss of body parts, loss of roles, loss of self-esteem, loss of certainty, loss of sexual attractiveness, loss of social relationships, loss of independence, and loss of finances. Categories of losses recorded in 81 chronically ill adults are included in Table 19.1. Grieving over these losses is a crucial process for the chronically ill person. Grief resolution may be needed to prevent the accumulated losses from becoming overwhelming, thereby causing hopelessness. The client's degree of hopelessness can be understood by determining the client's perceived sense of powerlessness, duration of powerlessness, and severity of losses suffered.

Critical Elements of Hope

Based on an exploratory research study of hope in persons who are critically ill (Miller, 1989) and a comprehensive review of literature in-

Table 19.1 ➤ **CATEGORIES OF LOSSES OF THE CHRONICALLY ILL**

Health status losses—functions
  Energy
  Strength-vitality
  Ability to communicate verbally
  Muscle coordination
  Bowel and bladder control
Loss of body parts
  Organs
  Hair
  Weight
Loss of roles
  Loss of breadwinner role
  Loss of secure future
Loss of self-esteem, dignity
Loss of certainty, predictability from day to day
Loss of sexual performance abilities
  Loss of intimacy
Loss of relationships with others
Loss of independence—ability to care for self
Loss of finances

cluding the etymology of hope, theology, philosophy, sociology and anthropology, psychology, biology, nursing, and health perspectives, the following critical elements of hope were identified (Miller, 1986; Miller & Powers, 1988).

- *Mutuality and affiliation:* Interpersonal relationships that are characterized by caring, sharing, and a feeling of belonging, being needed (Lynch, 1987). Trust in another, having someone who shares the period of trial, and experiencing unconditional love are all descriptive of mutuality as an element of hope.
- *Sense of the possible:* Despairing effects of a futile attitude and a global impression that all of life is hopeless are avoided.
- *Avoidance of absolutizing:* Not imposing rigid all-or-nothing criteria on an aspect of life or hoped-for situation (Lynch, 1987).
- *Anticipation:* Looking forward to a future that is good, an expectation of a positive outcome coupled with acceptance of the necessity of patient waiting and trusting.
- *Establishing and achieving goals:* Objects of one dimension of hope.
- *Psychological well-being and coping:* Elements that enable individuals to have psychic energy needed to sustain hope. Hope has been described as an elementary strength of the human ego (Meissner, 1973).

- *Purpose and meaning in life:* Enables individuals to have something to live for, to devote energy to, and to feel a sense of life satisfaction.
- *Freedom:* Opposite of the sense of entrapment that accompanies hopelessness (Lynch, 1987; Marcel, 1962). With hope there is a way out of difficulty and a recognition that one's own freedom may be used to influence an outcome or create a positive attitude.
- *Reality surveillance:* Cognitive task in which individuals search for clues to confirm that maintaining hope is feasible. Activities may include comparing one's self to others, holding out for new therapeutic discoveries, reviewing strengths, and affirming self-competence (Wright & Shontz, 1968).
- *Optimism:* Prerequisite for hope (Gottschalk, 1974; Raleigh, 1980).
- *Mental and physical activation:* Energy that combats the apathy of despair.

Hope Antecedents, Concomitants, Sources, and Threats

Dufault (1981) studied 35 elderly persons with cancer over a 2-year period using a participant observation method to determine the critical indicators of hope: antecedents, concomitants, and sources of and threats to hope. Antecedents are the experiences and emotions that are present when hope arises and include the experience of captivity, loss, stress, major decision making, hardship, suffering, and challenges with uncertainty. Concomitants are the emotions and cognitions that are present when hope is alive and include faith, trust, love, courage, patience, uncertainty, peace, joy, humor, involvement, and well-being.

Dufault (1981) found that sources of hope were supportive behavior and sustaining relationships of significant others, pets, valued objects, spiritual factors, relief of symptoms, receiving a sense of personal worth, past positive life experiences, and having overcome adversity. Other sources of hope may include having faith in caregivers and in therapy; relying on an existential philosophy—viewing human beings as having limitless potential for growth; using select mental mechanisms such as a rationalizing chain or reality surveillance; and finding meaning in suffering.

Raleigh (1992) found that the most commonly reported sources of hopefulness in 45 persons with cancer and in 45 persons with other chronic illnesses included support from family, friends, and religious beliefs. Herth (1990a) interviewed 30 terminally ill adults to discover factors that fostered and hindered their hope. She found that hope was fostered by (1) interpersonal connectedness—presence of a meaningful shared relationship with another; (2) lightheartedness—feeling of delight, joy, or playfulness; (3) selected personal attributes such as determination, courage, and serenity; (4) attainable aims—efforts directed at some purpose; (5) spiritual base—presence of active spiritual beliefs and practices; (6) uplifting memories—recalling positive moments and times in life; and (7) affirmation of worth—having one's individuality accepted, honored and, acknowledged. Herth (1993) also found these categories to be relevant for inspiring hope in 60 older adults residing in either the community or a long-term care facility. Added categories included use of purposeful activities such as volunteering, reading to others, writing letters for others; cognitive strategies or thought processes to transform perceptions into a positive frame; redefining time by avoiding viewing the future in terms of seasonal events but rather as today, tomorrow, and/or eternity. Factors that interfered with maintaining hope in the terminally ill included a sense of physical and emotional abandonment, uncontrolled pain, and devaluation of the individual's personhood (Herth, 1990a). Persons with acquired immunodeficiency syndrome (AIDS) used four major ways to maintain hope. These included belief in miracles, use of religion, intense involvement in work or vocation, and dependence on support from family or friends (Hall, 1994).

Threats to hope in persons with cancer, in order of decreasing prevalence, included evidence of deteriorating health; behavior of the physician, nurses, and family (such as despairing behaviors and abruptness); negative aspects of therapies, diagnostic tests, and hospital environment; lack of information; ambiguity; a sense of being a burden and imposing on others; spiritual distress; and past negative life experiences (Dufault, 1981).

Hope Metaphors

Metaphoric expressions of hope were collected from books such as thesauri, dictionaries, novels, folk writings, and political speeches to provide another perspective in understanding hope (Averill, Catlin, & Chon, 1990). A total of 108 basic metaphors were categorized into eight groups depicting hope as (1) a vital principle, (2) a source of light and warmth, (3) an elevated space, (4) a form of support, (5) a physical object or thing, (6) a deception, (7) a pressure, and (8) miscellaneous metaphors. Each category has themes and subthemes. For example,

1. Hope as a vital principle has several themes, such as:
   a. Hope is the basis of life.
      (1) Where there's life there's hope.
      (2) Without hope the heart would break.
   b. Hope is a remedy for what ails a person.
      (1) Hope gives you strength.
      (2) The miserable have no other medicine but hope.

    c. Hope is itself a form of life.
      (1) Nourish hope.
      (2) Foster hope.
      (3) Keep hope alive (Averill, Catlin, & Chon, 1990, pp. 54–65).

These examples of the dynamics of hope provide increased understanding of hope and its complexities.

Can Hopelessness Be Induced by Others?

Jourard (1970) proposed that persons can be inspirited to live or dispirited to give up and die. A person dies in response to an invitation from others to stop living, such as when he or she is devalued, when his or her aims and purposes in life are diminished, and when the worth of another's existence is questioned. To dispirit another is to accelerate his or her rate of dying. To inspirit another is to augment another's worth and meaningful life. Jourard (1970) contended that by inspiriting another we can render the person more resistant to physical and mental problems, raising the spirit titer, so to speak.

ASSESSMENT OF HOPE AND HOPELESSNESS

Hope assessment modalities include observation of behaviors, being attentive to client verbalizations or conversation themes, and use of paper-and-pencil tests. Lange (1978) categorized behaviors as hopeful or despairing. For example, hopeful behaviors labeled *activation* included feeling energetic, alert, and interested in accomplishing goals. The opposite of activation is *hypoactivation,* for example, behaviors of feeling empty, drained, without energy, and being unable to take action because of feelings of heaviness. *Psychological comfort* is present with hope and includes a sense of well-being, feeling at peace, being free from conflict, able to release tension, and able to relax and be optimistic about the future. *Psychological discomfort* indicative of despair may include feelings of loss, deprivation, tension, and bearing a heavy burden. *Social engagement* is indicative of hope as noted by having a sense of being needed, benefiting from relationships with others, and expressing interest in others. *Social distancing* (withdrawing, keeping an emotional distance from others) is indicative of despair. *Sense of competence* is having self-assuredness, positive body image, and self-confidence. The opposite, *sense of incompetence,* is indicative of despair (Lange, 1978).

Behavioral indicators of hopelessness may include lack of participation in care activities when the client has the ability, withdrawal, despondency, lack of or change in interaction, less willingness to engage in conversation, expressions about wanting to be relieved of any more suffering, and requesting to have death hastened.

Engel (1968) has labeled the failure of coping mechanisms as the "giving-up–given-up complex." This complex includes (1) feelings of being at the end of one's rope, at an impasse, helpless and hopeless; (2) having a poor self-image and feeling incompetent and out of control; (3) having a loss of gratification from roles and relationships; (4) feeling a sense of disrupted continuity among past, present, and future; and (5) recalling memories of previous helpless states. Engel proposed that this psychological state creates a psychobiological condition that contributes to the emergence of disease. Engle (1971) also attributed deaths of subjects after experiencing sudden losses (e.g., death of a spouse) to the giving-up–given-up complex.

Isani (1963) described a nine-stage behavioral definition of progressive hopelessness (Table 19.2). Patient behaviors indicative of moving toward hope or moving toward despair are also identified in Table 19.2.

Table 19.2 ➤ **ANALYSIS OF CLIENT BEHAVIOR ACCORDING TO NINE-STAGE PROGRESSION OF HOPELESSNESS**

Client Behavior Indicates Moving Toward Hope	Definition of Hopelessness	Client Behavior Indicates Moving Toward Despair
Readily establishes personal goals and anticipated positive outcomes	1. The person has limited anticipation of an improved state of affairs related to achievement of goals	Unable to set goals
Continually modifies goals to allow perceived success	2. Repeatedly fails to achieve goals	Perceives unachieved outcomes as personal failure
Focuses on past successes as a sustaining force	3. Makes unfavorable comparisons of present situation of failure with past anticipations of success	Emphasizes failure in light of accomplishments while well
Modifies goals without self-punishment	4. Fails to modify goals or selected routes to goal achievement	Rigidly adheres to achieving goals possible only during healthy state
Plans for alternative action if one plan does not produce expected results	5. Reduces anticipations of finding clear-cut solutions	Makes no effort to consider alternatives
Promotes peace of mind through activity and motivation toward goal	6. Increasingly limits efforts to achieve goals	Becomes increasingly agitated over accomplishing nothing
Rationalizes why solution not found	7. Despairs of finding solutions	Verbalizes doubts in self, therapy, and life
Consensually validates with friends their belief in client	8. Loses faith in self and others	Verbalizes giving up as the only solution
Persists in motivating self, clings to positive signs and encouragement from respected others	9. Gives up trying, becomes hopeless	Gives up

Source: Adapted from Isani (1963).

Conversation themes indicative of hope include references about optimism over the future; receiving help, support, and sustenance from others or from self; being the recipient of good fortune, luck, or favor; achieving constructive outcomes; longevity; smooth interpersonal relationships (Gottschalk & Glesser, 1969). Conversation themes indicative of hopelessness include references about not being or wanting to be the recipient of God's favor or blessing; not getting help, support, sustenance; feeling hopeless, despairing; lacking ambition and interest; feeling pessimistic or discouraged (Gottschalk & Glesser, 1969).

Paper-and-pencil tests to measure hope do exist, and some of them are appropriate for nursing research and/or validation of a nursing diagnosis of decreased hope or hopelessness. These instruments include Herth Hope Scale (Herth, 1991), Herth Hope Index (1992), Hopefulness Scale for Adolescents (Hinds & Gattuso, 1991), The Miller Hope Scale (Miller, 1986; Miller & Powers, 1988), The Hope Scale (Erickson, Post, & Paige, 1975), the Stoner Hope Scale (Stoner, 1982), the Hope Index Scale (Obayuwana & Carter, 1981), the Herth Hope Scale (Herth, 1989), the Multidimensional Hope Scale (Raleigh & Boehm, 1994), and the Nowotny Hope Scale (Nowotny, 1989). The Miller Hope Scale does not limit the measure and definition of hope to an expectation for goal attainment as do those instruments based on Stotland's definition of hope (an anticipation of goal attainment). The intangible dimensions of generalized hope as described by Dufault (1981) are to be included in a comprehensive view of hope. The hope scales listed above have had varying degrees of psychometric evaluation and therefore need careful scrutiny before their use in clinical decision making.

RESEARCH SYNOPSES: SELECTED HOPE STUDIES

Hope has been credited with influencing survival against all odds, and when it is absent, recovery may be adversely affected and death may be hastened (Engle, 1968, 1971; Gottschalk, 1985; Jourard, 1970; Menninger, 1959; Richter, 1957; Seligman, 1995). The importance of hope to sustain persons through natural disasters (Henderson & Bostock, 1975, 1977), concentration camp experiences (Bettelheim, 1960; Frankl, 1962), and prisoner-of-war experiences (Nardini, 1952) has been well documented. Early studies noted that hope influences long-term survival in women with breast cancer (Greer, Morris, & Pettingale, 1979; Pettingale, 1984) as well as long-term survival on hemodialysis (Ziarnik, Freeman, Sherrard, & Calsyn, 1977). More recent qualitative and quantitative research has been completed.

Hope-inspiring strategies of 60 critically ill adults (ages 38 to 83 years) were discovered by use of a grounded theory method (Miller, 1989). A 20-item open-ended interview guide was used to solicit information about what sustained persons during a critical illness, a time when giving up was a possibility. Findings of this study provide ideas for nursing strategies to inspire hope. Transcriptions of verbatim interviews were analyzed, and the following were found to maintain hope (Miller, 1989):

- *Cognitive strategies:* Thought processes that individuals consciously used to change unfavorable perceptions to less threatening perceptions. These mental coping strategies included internal dialogues such as "I'd better get with it and get out of here." "I know I have to get through the tests, I am strong, I can do it."
- *Determinism:* Mental attitude reflecting a conviction that a positive outcome is possible. "There was no way I was going to give up." "You gotta aim high 'cause you might fall a little short and end up just where you belong." "The faintest glimmer of hope regarding recovery, even if it's recovery in a limited way, is worth going after."
- *Philosophy of life and world view:* View of life as having meaning and that growth takes place as a result of struggle and difficulty. Some clients had a deliberate day-to-day way of approaching recovery.
- *Spiritual strategies:* Beliefs and practices that enabled individuals to transcend suffering based on a relationship with God. "It's something you feel but find difficult to express. You know you're getting help from the Lord."
- *Relationship with caregivers:* Caregivers had a constructive view of the client and conveyed positive expectations for competent handling of stress. "They made you feel they wanted you to win." The relationships were described as having warmth and sincerity and being filled with strong encouragement.
- *Family bonds:* Sustaining relationships with loved ones who convey a sharing of the difficulty and provide reasons for living, goals to be accomplished, and directions for living. "My children are small, they need me."
- *Sense of being in control:* Perception that one's own knowledge and actions can affect an outcome. Being informed about progress and schedules and involved in care decisions enhanced control.
- *Goal accomplishment:* Desired activities to accomplish and valued outcomes to attain. Examples ranged from being able to perform a simple physical task ("go to the bathroom by myself") to being able to enjoy retirement (see pp. 25–26).

Other miscellaneous means of maintaining hope included use of humor, relaxation to improve a sense of well-being, and use of distraction to avoid thoughts of negative consequences.

The following threats to hope were identified by these critically ill clients: physical cues interpreted as setbacks, a feeling that no one cares (family does not visit or demonstrate support, family has fatalistic attitude), and negative hospital experiences such as receiving dehumanizing messages. A client described the experience ". . . like being put through one large-sized factory" (Miller, 1989, p. 27). Nurses can intervene in preventing these threats to hope.

Herth (1989) found a significant positive relationship between hope and level of coping in 120 persons with cancer receiving chemotherapy. Those persons categorized as having strong religious faith had significantly higher hope and coping than persons with weak, unsure, or lost faith. Persons whose disease did not interfere with performance of family role responsibilities had higher hope (Herth, 1989). Brandt's (1987) sample of 37 women on chemotherapy for breast cancer revealed that they had high levels of hope, received social support, and valued religious beliefs as helpful in coping with illness.

A significant positive relationship between hope and grief resolution was noted in 75 persons who had been widowed for 12 to 18 months (Herth, 1990b). Spouses of persons who died in hospice settings had significantly higher hope than spouses of those who died in hospitals or nursing homes. Significant negative correlations were found between hope and evasive, fatalistic, and emotive coping styles (Herth, 1990b).

Hope has been studied in adolescents. Hinds and Martin (1988) found that 59 adolescents with cancer relied on achieving a hopeful state as a process of comforting themselves. For these youths, hope was a component of a self-sustaining process leading to a sense of personal competence in resolving health threats. For adolescents, hope meant the degree to which the adolescent possessed a comforting, life-sustaining belief that a personal and positive future exists (Hinds, 1984, 1988).

A single core variable identified by 58 adolescents with cancer as directly promoting hopefulness was the nurses' use of humor (Hinds, Martin, & Vogel, 1987). Humor included being lighthearted, initiating or responding to teasing, and engaging in playful interactions. Using a grounded theory method, other nursing strategies identified as promoting hopefulness included the nurses' use of (1) truthful explanations, (2) participation in activities with the adolescent (cards, computer games, piano), (3) caring behaviors (hugging, demonstrating interest), (4) purposeful conversations diverted to neutral topics (use of cognitive clutter), (5) care competence, (6) sharing knowledge of survivors with a similar disease, (7) maintaining a future focus (Hinds, Martin, & Vogel, 1987).

Hope has been noted to be a prerequisite for effective coping and is considered by some to be a coping mechanism (Jalowiec & Powers, 1981; Korner, 1970; Stoner & Keampfer, 1985; Weisman, 1979). Maintaining hope is a coping task of the chronically ill (Greene, O'Mahony, & Rungasamy, 1982). Higher functional status and more years of education were significantly related to hope, as measured by the Miller Hope Scale, in 86 persons older than 65 years with cancer and in 88 elderly persons without cancer (McGill & Paul, 1993). Persons with a chronic illness perceived themselves in a "winning position" over their illness if they maintained hope (Forsyth, Delaney, & Gresham, 1984). Hope was noted to be a frequently used coping strategy by emergency-room clients (Jalowiec & Powers, 1981) and by hemodialysis clients (Baldree, Murphy, & Powers, 1982).

Hope has been identified as a primary need of family members of persons with cancer (Brockopp, Hayko, Davenport, & Winscott, 1989; Lewandowski & Jones, 1988; Weisman, 1979), of the critically ill (Coutu-Wakulczyk & Chartier, 1990; Leske, 1986; Norheim, 1989; Norris & Grove, 1986), and of brain-injured clients (Campbell, 1988). In 30 persons with multiple sclerosis and their 30 family member "carers," hope and psychological well-being were predictive of client adaptation (Miller & Hastings, submitted for publication). Similar findings were noted by Christman (1990) in 55 men receiving radiotherapy for cancer, in that lower hope and more uncertainty were associated with more adjustment problems.

NURSING STRATEGIES

Nursing strategies to inspire hope are countless in number and nature, limited only by lack of sensitivity to the uniqueness of each client and family response as well as lack of creativity. Figure 19.3 summarizes the categories of nursing strategies described in this chapter. These strategies have been gleaned from the literature, particularly from Miller (1985, 1991). The strategies are based upon an existential frame of reference in which human beings are viewed as having a never-ending possibility of improving their own being (Marcel, 1962). Nurses can inspire hope, focusing on living the moment as fully as possible. There may not be hope of returning to previous functioning or of being cured, but hope in maximizing the moment, benefiting optimally from relationships or aesthetic surroundings. Examples of maximizing experiences include:

- Savoring the richness of black coffee at breakfast
- Feeling the tartness of grapefruit waking up the taste buds

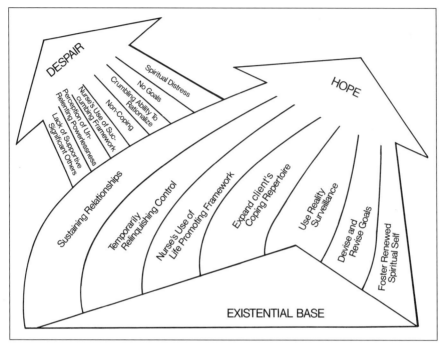

FIGURE 19.3 ➤ Hope-despair model.

- Noting the crystal-clear blue of the sky
- Feeling the warmth of a sunbeam
- Watching activities of animals in a tree outside the window
- Benefiting from each encounter with another human being
- Sharing experiences children are having
- Noting loving characteristics of spouse
- Appreciating expressions of caring concern
- Working out intricate plans, such as for rebuilding the summer cottage
- Planning to rearrange the living room furniture
- Building highlights into each day, such as meals, visits, Bible reading
- Writing messages to grandchildren, nieces, or nephews
- Planning volunteer work to help others
- Studying a favorite painting
- Listening to a symphony as a means of escape

It is recognized that not all patients benefit from isolated reconstructed experiences such as the melting of snowflakes on their cheeks. However, all patients benefit from renewed appreciation of making the most of the moment, not letting the moment pass by without appreciating its beauty. Using these experiences helps to achieve a sense of personal fulfillment.

Following are categories of strategies to inspire hope.

Affiliative Dimension: Use of Sustaining Relationships

The affiliative dimension of hope means that hope depends on a sense of connectedness with others and involvement beyond self, including intimacy and attachment, mutuality and sharing, and other-directed social interaction and relationships (Dufault, 1981). Specific strategies are (1) to use attachment ideation and (2) to develop significant others' awareness of their powerful role in influencing hope states of their ill loved ones. Attachment ideation is a preoccupation with a principal attachment figure, that is, with loved ones and significant others such as spouse, child, girlfriend, or boyfriend. With attachment ideation, the nurse helps the client review attributes, that is, unique, important, and loving characteristics of the attachment figure. Reviewing clients' peak life experiences and how their relationships are caring may be helpful. Even if clients are unconscious, attachment ideation may be used by repeating the loved one's name to the client, reviewing their special devotion and concern, relating experiences shared by the loved one as reminders of joy, and being needed throughout life as well as now. The nurse helps re-create mental images of the attached figure, enabling the client to fixate on someone for whom to live and maintain hope.

Significant others need to realize how powerful they are in sustaining the client. They may benefit from reviewing their role in maintaining hope that will have a reciprocal benefit for their loved one (client). Those persons who are the closest are the most meaningful in the client's life and have the most contagious influence in terms of hope and other mental states. Nurses may need to help family focus on goal-directed interactions that emphasize unfinished work waiting for the client, life goals to be accomplished, and how they are vitally needed in the lives of their family. The nurse may model this type of communication and also model use of touch and closeness so that the family member is not hesitant to use these modalities. Lack of supportive significant others leads to despair.

Enhance Control and Support the Temporary Relinquishing of Control

Enhancing control by providing clients with the skills to manage self-care and monitor self, or in times of acute need assuring them that relinquishing control is temporary, may affect hope states. The perception of unrelenting powerlessness leads to hopelessness.

Use of a Life-Promoting Interpersonal Framework

A deliberate interaction style that focuses on surviving adversity and growing as a result is a constructive life-promoting framework (Wright, 1980). Clients are regarded as potentially powerful, unique persons having coping resources that can be uncovered. Client resources can be reviewed and their use reinforced. Confrontation with problems is interpreted as being part of life, and the client's ability to resolve and/or adapt is emphasized. Getting on with living without unduly dwelling solely on problems is the goal. The interaction that focuses on survival with discovery of new meaning in life will have an impact on hope.

The opposite approach is a succumbing framework in which the nurse concentrates on the devastation of the crisis; what the client can no longer do, spreading a theme of disability throughout all aspects of the person's life (negative spread). A disabling theme is evident in the interaction. The problem is not that the disability is recognized but that constructive forces in the person's life are neglected (Wright, 1980).

Expand Client and Family Coping Repertoire

Persons receive a sense of strength knowing there are ways to respond (cope) to control negative affects and anxiety. Weisman (1979) defined coping as what one does about a problem to bring about relief, quiescence, and equilibrium. Noncoping leads to powerlessness, depression, and eventually despair. Coping mechanisms as described in Chapter 2 can be taught, such as use of self-instructional internal language, imagery, stress inoculation, rational inquiry, and mutuality. All these mechanisms support the belief that there is a way out of difficulty and may enable anticipation of a future. Noncoping leads to despair.

Reality Surveillance

Reality surveillance is a cognitive task in which the individual searches for clues to confirm that maintaining hope is feasible (Wright & Shontz, 1968). Also called reality or phenomenal grounding, this mental mechanism provides some tangible evidence from the real world as a basis for hope. Korner (1970) referred to constructing hope from examining bits of reality held together by logic and reasoning, using a rationalizing chain. Table 19.3 contains selected categories of reality surveillance with exemplar client behavior and the related nursing role. The opposite phenomenon is a crumbling ability to rationalize, leading to despair.

Devise and Revise Goals

Hope is energized by the belief in the ability to accomplish something (Lynch, 1987; Stotland, 1984). Clients may need help in devising goals and recognizing their accomplishments. These goals may include (1) physical strides, (2) work to be accomplished, (3) responsibility to discharge, and (4) love relationships to renew and/or sustain. Specific feedback about progress in healing, returning to previous or new levels of functioning, and so forth, needs to be consistently provided. Setting physical goals that are realistic must be considered, for example, walking distance and other amounts of exercise to be tolerated. Work can be accomplished through others. Clients may be helped to see that providing guidance without needing to personally carry out all work plans provides a sense of accomplishment. Having someone and something to live for inspires hope. Renewing and being able to sustain love relationships maintain hope. In hopelessness, the future is tolerable if the client feels there is unconditional love from someone and that there is someone with whom to share the future.

Foster Renewed Spiritual Self

Spiritual life is a major source of hope for some persons. This includes maintaining a relationship with God or deity and having a sense of purpose and meaning in life. Providing opportunity for prayer, reading hope-filled scripture, and creating an environment in which the client feels comfortable expressing hope in God are examples of nursing strategies. If appropriate, nurses can remind clients of the boundless, infinite love God has for each person. Marcel (1962) stated, "Hope is the radical refusal to set limits." When all in life looks grim, that is, when what is happening is beyond the individual's influence, hopelessness is prevented by turning to God. Spiritual distress is the opposite phenomenon, which contributes to despair.

Hope may also be inspired by use of humanities resources such as literature, poetry, art, and music. See Chapter 15 for poignant poems and suggested literature sources for use in comforting clients. Careful use of humor is another strategy to help put stress in perspective, alleviate excess tensions, and maintain some sense of life as having moments of lightheartedness. Helping clients find meaning in suffering, in their existence in life, in their current challenges may also be an effective strategy to mobilize hope.

Farran, Herth, and Popovich (1995) conceptualized hope as consisting of experiential, spiritual and transcendental, relational, and ratio-

Table 19.3 ➤ ANALYSIS OF REALITY SURVEILLANCE		
Selected Categories of Reality Surveillance*	**Examples of Client Behavior Indicative of the Category**	**Nursing Role**
Reviewing changing environmental conditions	"I must be improving; the nurses are not monitoring me as closely; they come less often."	If client's interpretations are accurate, confirm them; that is, the VNA will visit less frequently because of these signs of improvement. Review indicators of improvement.
Reviewing assets	"I have a good health history; I have never been hospitalized before." "I still have one good leg." "I have always exercised to keep physically fit." "Now that I have an ileostomy, at least I won't get cancer of the bowel."	Help client review assets, which include physical, interpersonal, and role-function abilities.
Comparing self with other individuals or groups	"It took my neighbor longer to recover from his heart attack." "I didn't realize I would be able to wear my same clothes after my colostomy surgery." "The patient representative from the ostomy association was so helpful."	Information on self-help groups can be provided. Listen to client's need to compare own better progress to other clients with slower progress.
Planning for assuming self-care responsibilities	"I realize now, the diabetes will not be going away. I'd better start learning to take care of myself."	Provide assistance through teaching and support so client gradually assumes responsibility for care and realizes that self-care is not an impossible, overwhelming task.

Avoiding confrontation with negative outcomes	"The chemotherapy has got to be effective after all this suffering with side effects. It's got to be killing something."	Listen with empathy; help client with internal dialogue to increase client's insight.
Plans are contingent upon if-then events	"If I remain in remission until Christmas, I will plan the trip."	Foster positive expectations for remaining physically stable. Teach importance of optimistic mind-set, influencing body response. Inform client of mind-body pathways and holistic response to health.
Holding out for future discoveries	"Who knows, maybe they will find a cure for multiple sclerosis."	Share knowledge of advances in caring for clients with debilitating diseases. Acknowledge discoveries in medicine that were unheard of years ago.
Using statements of uncontestable truisms	"God will help me through this." "All that is needed is for me to do my best and to follow the medical orders."	Recognize that this verbalization is comforting to the client and the client is watching the nurse's response.
Making testimonials	"I've read of miraculous cures of arthritis."	Demonstrate interest without scientific interrogation or "putting the client down," repudiating the client for the claims.

Source: Adapted from Wright and Shontz (1968).

nal thought processes. They proposed strategies related to each process. The *experiential process* refers to hope being born and tested in suffering and loss. Interventions related to the experiential process include creating a climate that fosters self-expression and ventilation of fears, questions, and expectations. Denial may be necessary and should be respected if it sustains the person's integrity and assists the person during a waiting period until hope begins to surface. The *spiritual and transcendental process* refers to finding purpose and meaning in life. Focusing on aesthetics, cherishing small joys in life, keeping a journal on feelings and experiences, and encouraging creative expressions of hope may all be relevant strategies. The *relational process* refers to open, caring relationships needed to mobilize and support hope. Nurses can maintain a sense of connectedness by being present, using active listening, fostering family support systems, involving the family in the plan of care and ultimately as a source of hope, and finding someone or something for the client to care about (pets, plants, friends, hobbies). The *rational thought process* refers to goals to be accomplished. Reviewing these goals, reinforcing their accomplishment, and referring to the future with positive outlook are possible strategies (Farran et al., 1995).

Tollett and Thomas (1995) used a specific intervention with homeless veterans to attempt to change their levels of hopelessness, self-esteem, self-efficacy, and depression. Twelve 60-minute small group sessions were held during which veterans were helped to find reasons for hope, identify their strengths, form a vision of a future, define goals, and engage in success mapping (Tollett & Thomas, 1995). Significant improvements in hope, self-esteem, and depression were found in the 40 veterans in the experimental group, and significant differences were found between the 40 experimental subjects and 19 veterans in the control group.

SUMMARY

"To hope" is different from "to hope that." To hope is an existential orientation to achieve a generalized state of being. "To hope that" means there is a specific object of hope, and the individual is subjected to the vulnerable insecurity of not having his or her particular object of hope realized. A focus of nursing strategies to inspire hope needs to include generalized hope and not be exclusively devoted to hope for goal accomplishment. In general, by increasing clients' levels of hope, we are empowering them to be in control of their lives, to anticipate a future that is good, and to have a restored sense of well-being.

REFERENCES

Aardema, B. (1984). *The therapeutic use of hope.* Unpublished doctoral dissertation. Western Michigan University, Kalamazoo, MI.

Adams, C., & Proulx, J. (1975). The role of the nurse in the maintenance and restoration of hope. In B. Scheonberg et al. (Eds.), *Bereavement: Its psychosocial aspects* (pp. 256–263). New York: Columbia University Press.

Averill, J. R., Catlin, G., & Chon, K. K. (1990). *Rules of hope.* New York: Springer-Verlag.

Baldree, K. S., Murphy, S., & Powers, M. J. (1982). Stress identification and coping patterns in patients on hemodialysis. *Nursing Research, 31,* 107–112.

Beck, A., Kovacs, M., & Weissman, A. (1975). Hopelessness and suicidal behavior: An overview. *Journal of the American Medical Association, 234,* 1146–1149.

Bettelheim, B. (1960). *The informed heart: Autonomy in a mass age.* Glencoe, IL: Free Press.

Bloch, E. (1970). *Man on his own.* New York: Herder & Herder.

Brandt, B. (1987). The relationship between hopelessness and select variables in women receiving chemotherapy for breast cancer. *Oncology Nursing Forum, 14,* 35–39.

Brockopp, D. Y., Hayko, D., Davenport, W., & Winscott, C. (1989). Personal control and the needs for hope and information among adults diagnosed with cancer. *Cancer Nursing, 12,* 112–116.

Campbell, C. H. (1988). Needs of relatives and helpfulness of support groups in severe head injury. *Rehabilitation Nursing, 13,* 320–325.

Christman, N. (1990). Uncertainty and adjustment during radiotherapy. *Nursing Research, 39,* 17–20.

Coutu-Wakulczyk, G., & Chartier, L. (1990). French validation of the Critical Care Family Needs Inventory. *Heart and Lung, 19,* 192–196.

Diez-Manrique, J. F. (1984). Hope as a means of therapy in the work of Karen Horney. *American Journal of Psychoanalysis, 44,* 301–310.

Dufault, K. (1981). *Hope of elderly persons with cancer.* Unpublished doctoral dissertation. Case Western Reserve University, Cleveland, OH.

Dufault, K., & Martocchio, B. (1985). Hope: Its spheres and dimensions. *Nursing Clinics of North America, 20,* 370–391.

Engel, G. (1968). A life setting conducive to illness: The giving-up–given-up complex. *Annals of Internal Medicine, 69,* 293–300.

Engle, G. (1971). Sudden and rapid death during psychological stress: Folklore or folk wisdom? *Annals of Internal Medicine, 74,* 771–782.

Erickson, R., Post, R., & Paige, A. (1975). Hope as a psychiatric variable. *Journal of Clinical Psychology, 31,* 324–330.

Farran, C., Herth, K., & Popovich, J. (1995). *Hope and hopelessness: Critical clinical constructs.* Thousand Oaks, CA: Sage.

Forsyth, G., Delaney, K., & Gresham, M. (1984). Vying for a winning position: Management style of the chronically ill. *Research in Nursing and Health, 7,* 181–188.

Frank, J. (1968). The role of hope in psychotherapy. *International Journal of Psychiatry, 5,* 383–385.

Frank, J. (1975). Mind-body relationships in illness and healing. *International Academy of Preventive Medicine, 2,* 46–59.

Frankl, V. (1962). *Man's search for meaning.* New York: Simon Delta.

Fromm, E. (1968). *The revolution of hope.* New York: Harper & Row.

Gottschalk, L. (1974). A hope scale applicable to verbal samples. *Archives of General Psychiatry, 30,* 770–785.

Gottschalk, L. (1985). Hope and other deterrents to illness. *American Journal of Psychotherapy, 39,* 515–524.

Gottschalk, L., & Glesser, G. (1969). *The measurement of psychological states through the content analysis of verbal behavior.* Berkeley: University of California Press.

Greene, S., O'Mahony, P., & Rungasamy, P. (1982). Levels of measured hopelessness in physically ill patients. *Journal of Psychosomatic Research, 26,* 591–593.

Greer, S., Morris, T., & Pettingale, K. (1979). Psychological responses to breast cancer: Effect on outcome. *Lancet, 2,* 768–787.

Hall, B. (1994). Ways of maintaining hope in HIV disease. *Research in Nursing and Health, 17,* 283–293.

Heagle, J. (1975). *Contemporary meditation on hope.* Chicago: Thomas More Press.

Henderson, S., & Bostock, R. (1975). Coping behaviour: Correlates of survival on a raft. *Australian and New Zealand Journal of Psychiatry, 9,* 221–223.

Henderson, S., & Bostock, R. (1977). Coping behavior after shipwreck. *British Journal of Psychiatry, 131,* 15–20.

Herth, K. (1989). The relationship between level of hope and level of coping response and other variables in patients with cancer. *Oncology Nursing Forum, 16,* 67–72.

Herth, K. (1990a). Fostering hope in terminally ill people. *Journal of Advanced Nursing, 15,* 1250–1259.

Herth, K. (1990b). Relationship of hope, coping style, concurrent losses and setting to grief resolution in the elderly widow(er). *Research in Nursing and Health, 13,* 109–117.

Herth, K. (1991). Development and refinement of an instrument to measure hope. *Scholarly Inquiry for Nursing Practice, 5,* 39–51.

Herth, K. (1992). An abbreviated instrument to measure hope: Development and psychometric evaluation. *Journal of Advanced Nursing, 17,* 1251–1259.

Herth, K. (1993). Hope in older adults in community and institutional settings. *Issues in Mental Health Nursing, 14,* 139–156.

Hinds, P. (1984). Inducing a definition of hope through the use of grounded theory methodology. *Journal of Advanced Nursing, 9,* 357–362.

Hinds, P. (1988). Adolescent hopefulness in illness and health. *Advances in Nursing Science, 10,* 79–88.

Hinds, P., & Gatusso, J. (1991). Measuring hopefulness in adolescents. *Journal of Pediatric Oncology Nursing, 8,* 92–94.

Hinds, P., & Martin, J. (1988). Hopefulness and the self-sustaining process in adolescents with cancer. *Nursing Research, 37,* 336–340.

Hinds, P., Martin, J., & Vogel, R. (1987). Nursing strategies to influence adolescent hopefulness during oncologic illness. *Journal of the Association of Pediatric Oncology Nurses, 5,* 14–22.

Isani, R. (1963). From hopelessness to hope. *Perspectives in Psychiatric Care, 1,* 15–20.

Jalowiec, A., & Powers, M. (1981). Stress and coping in hypertensive and emergency room patients. *Nursing Research, 30,* 10–15.

Jourard, S. (1970). Living and dying: Suicide an invitation to die. *American Journal of Nursing, 70,* 269–275.

Korner, I. (1970). Hope as a method of coping. *Journal of Consulting and Clinical Psychology, 34,* 134–139.

Lange, S. P. (1978). Hope. In C. E. Carlson & B. Blackwell (Eds.), *Behavioral concepts and nursing intervention* (pp. 171–190). Philadelphia: JB Lippincott.

Leske, J. (1986). Needs of relatives of chronically ill patients: A follow-up. *Heart and Lung, 15,* 189–193.

Lewandowski, W., & Jones, S. L. (1988). The family with cancer: Nursing interventions throughout the course of living with cancer. *Cancer Nursing, 11,* 313–321.

Lynch, W. F. (1987). *Images of hope: Imagination as the healer of the hopeless.* Notre Dame, IN: University of Notre Dame Press.

Marcel, G. (1962). *Homo viator: Introduction to a metaphysic of hope.* Translated by E. Craufurd. New York: Harper & Row.

McGill, J., & Paul, P. (1993). Functional status and hope in elderly people with and without cancer. *Oncology Nursing Forum, 20,* 1207–1213.

Meissner, W. W. (1973). Notes on the psychology of hope. Part I. *Journal of Religion and Health, 12,* 7–29.

Menninger, C. (1959). Hope. *American Journal of Psychiatry, 146,* 481–491.

Miller, J. F. (1985). Nursing strategies to inspire hope. *American Journal of Nursing, 85,* 22–25.

Miller, J. F. (1986). *Development of an instrument to measure hope.* Unpublished doctoral dissertation. University of Illinois, Chicago.

Miller, J. F. (1989). Hope inspiring strategies of the critically ill. *Applied Nursing Research, 2,* 23–29.

Miller, J. F. (1991). Developing and maintaining hope in families of the critically ill. *Clinical Issues in Critical Care Nursing.*

Miller, J. F., & Hastings, D. (Submitted for publication.) Family member response and patient adaptation to multiple sclerosis: The influence of hope.

Miller, J. F., & Powers, M. J. (1988). Development of an instrument to measure hope. *Nursing Research, 37,* 6–10.

Nardini, J. E. (1952). Survival factors in American prisoners of war of the Japanese. *American Journal of Psychiatry, 109,* 241–248.

Norheim, C. (1989). Family needs of patients having coronary artery bypass graft surgery during the intraoperative period. *Heart and Lung, 18,* 622–626.

Norris, L., & Grove, S. (1986). Investigation of selected psychosocial needs of family members of critically ill adult patients. *Heart and Lung, 15,* 194–199.

Nowotny, M. (1989). Assessment of hope in patients with cancer: Development of an instrument. *Oncology Nursing Forum, 16,* 57–61.

Obayuwana, A., & Carter, A. (1981). *Hope Index Scale.* Silver Spring, MD: Institute of Hope.

Owen, D. (1989). Nurses' perspectives on the meaning of hope in patients with cancer: A qualitative study. *Oncology Nursing Forum, 16,* 75–79.

Pettingale, K. W. (1984). Coping and cancer prognosis. *Journal of Psychosomatic Research, 28,* 363–364.

Pruyser, P. (1963). Phenomenology and dynamics of hoping. *Journal of Science and the Study of Religion, 3,* 86–96.

Raleigh, E. (1980). *An investigation of hope as manifested in the physically ill adult.* Unpublished doctoral dissertation. Wayne State University, Detroit, MI.

Raleigh, E. (1992). Sources of hope in chronic illness. *Oncology Nursing Forum, 19,* 443–448.

Raleigh, E., & Boehm, S. (1994). Development of the Multidimensional Hope Scale. *Journal of Nursing Measurement, 2,* 155–167.

Richter, C. P. (1957). On the phenomenon of sudden death in animals and man. *Psychosomatic Medicine, 19,* 190–198.

Seligman, M. (1995). *Helplessness: On depression, development and death.* San Francisco: WH Freeman.

Stanley, A. T. (1978). *The lived experience of hope: The isolation of discrete descriptive elements common to the experience of hope in healthy young adults.* Unpublished doctoral dissertation. Catholic University, Washington, DC.

Stoner, J. (1982). *Hope and cancer patients.* Unpublished doctoral dissertation. University of Colorado, Denver.

Stoner, J., & Keampfer, S. (1985). Recalled life expectancy information, phase of illness and hope in cancer patients. *Research in Nursing and Health, 8,* 269–274.

Stotland, E. (1984). *The psychology of hope.* San Francisco: Jossey-Bass.

Tollett J., & Thomas, S. (1995). A theory-based nursing intervention to instill hope in homeless veterans. *Advances in Nursing Science, 18,* 76–90.

Weisman, A. (1979). *Coping with cancer.* New York: McGraw-Hill.

Wright, B. (1980). Person and situation: Adjusting the rehabilitation focus. *Archives of Physical Medicine and Rehabilitation, 61,* 59–64.

Wright, B., & Shontz, F. (1968). Process and tasks in hoping. *Rehabilitation Literature, 29,* 322–331.

Ziarnik, J. P., Freeman, C. W., Sherrard, D. T., & Calsyn, D. A. (1977). Psychological correlates of survival on renal dialysis. *Journal of Nervous and Mental Disease, 164,* 210–213.

An "f" following a page number indicates a figure; a "t" indicates a table.